MALIGNANT LYMPHOMAS
Etiology, Immunology, Pathology, Treatment

BRISTOL-MYERS CANCER SYMPOSIA

Series Editor
MAXWELL GORDON
Science and Technology Division
Bristol-Myers Company

MALIGNANT LYMPHOMAS

Etiology, Immunology, Pathology, Treatment

Edited by

SAUL A. ROSENBERG
Divisions of Oncology and Radiation Therapy
Stanford University School of Medicine
Stanford, California

HENRY S. KAPLAN
Cancer Biology Research Laboratory
Department of Radiology
Stanford University School of Medicine
Stanford, California

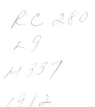

1982

ACADEMIC PRESS

A Subsidiary of Harcourt Brace Jovanovich, Publishers

New York   London
Paris   San Diego   San Francisco   São Paulo   Sydney   Tokyo   Toronto

ACADEMIC PRESS, INC.
111 Fifth Avenue, New York, New York 10003

United Kingdom Edition published by
ACADEMIC PRESS, INC. (LONDON) LTD.
24/28 Oval Road, London NW1 7DX

Library of Congress Cataloging in Publication Data
Main entry under title:

Malignant lymphomas.

(Bristol-Myers cancer symposia series ; v. 3)
Papers presented at a symposium held at Stanford
University, Nov. 20-21, 1980.
Includes bibliographical references and index.
1. Lymphoma--Congresses. I. Kaplan, Henry S.,
Date. II. Rosenberg, Saul A. III. Series.
[DNLM: 1. Lymphoma--Congresses. W3 BR429 v. 3 1980 /
WH 525 M249 1980]
RC280.L9M337   616.99'446   81-22822
ISBN 0-12-597120-6   AACR2

Contents

1

In Vitro Cultivation and Characterization of the Giant Neoplastic Cells of Hodgkin's Disease: Some Unresolved Problems

HENRY S. KAPLAN, LENNART OLSSON, JEROME S. BURKE, ELLIOTT F. OSSERMAN, WERNER HENLE, and GERTRUDE HENLE

2

Phenotypic Characterization and Induced Differentiation of Established Human Non-Hodgkin's Lymphoma Cell Lines

KENNETH NILSSON

3

Marker Profiles of 55 Human Leukemia–Lymphoma Cell Lines

JUN MINOWADA, KIMITAKA SAGAWA, IAN S. TROWBRIDGE, PATRICK D. KUNG, GIDEON GOLDSTEIN

8 Tumor Antigen–Antibody Interactions in Murine Lymphomas: Possible Implications for Human Lymphomas

I. WEISSMAN, E. PILLEMER, D. KOOISTRA, A. TSUKAMOTO,
L. JERABEK, D. HUMPHREY, R. COFFMAN, M. McGRATH, S. NORD,
and R. ELLIS

9 The Role of Epstein–Barr Virus in the Etiology of Burkitt's Lymphoma and Nasopharyngeal Carcinoma

GEORGE KLEIN

10 Feline Lymphomas and Leukemias as Models for Human Neoplasia

M. ESSEX

11 Expression of C-Type RNA Viral Proteins by a Human Lymphoma Cell Line

ROBERT S. GOODENOW, SAI-LING LIU, KIRK E. FRY, RONALD LEVY,
and HENRY S. KAPLAN

21

A Working Formulation of Non-Hodgkin's Lymphomas: Background, Recommendations, Histological Criteria, and Relationship to Other Classifications

RONALD F. DORFMAN, JEROME S. BURKE, and COSTAN W. BERARD

22

Radiation Therapy in the Management of Stage IIIA Hodgkin's Disease

RICHARD T. HOPPE, RICHARD S. COX, HENRY S. KAPLAN, and SAUL A. ROSENBERG

23

The Curative Potential of Chemotherapy in the Treatment of Hodgkin's Disease and the Non-Hodgkin's Lymphomas

VINCENT T. DEVITA, JR. and SUSAN MOLLOY HUBBARD

24

Primary Chemotherapy for Hodgkin's Disease and Non-Hodgkin's Lymphoma

JOHN M. GOLDMAN

25
Chemotherapy of Malignant Lymphomas of Unfavorable Histology
STEPHEN E. JONES and THOMAS P. MILLER

26
The Role of Radiation Therapy in the Treatment of Stage I and II Hodgkin's Disease
PETER MAUCH, ALAN LEWIN, and SAMUEL HELLMAN

27
A Working Formulation of Non-Hodgkin's Lymphomas for Clinical Usage: Clinicopathological and Prognostic Correlations
RICHARD T. HOPPE

28
The Place of Radiation Therapy in the Management of Patients with Localized Non-Hodgkin's Lymphoma
R. S. BUSH and M. GOSPODAROWICZ

33 *In Vivo* Effects of Murine Hybridoma Monoclonal Antibody in Human T-Cell Neoplasms
RICHARD A. MILLER and RONALD LEVY

34 A Survey of Pediatric Hodgkin's Disease at Stanford University: Results of Therapy and Quality of Survival
SARAH S. DONALDSON and HENRY S. KAPLAN

35 Pediatric Non-Hodgkin's Lymphomas: The Children's Cancer Study Group Experience—An Interim Report
R. D. T. JENKIN, J. R. ANDERSON, R. CHILCOTE, P. COCCIA, P. EXELBY, J. KUSHNER, A. MEADOWS, S. SIEGEL, J. WILSON, S. LEIKIN, D. HAMMOND, and J. KERSEY

36 LSA₂-L₂ in Childhood Non-Hodgkin's Lymphoma
NORMA WOLLNER

Contributors

Numbers in parentheses indicate the pages on which the authors' contributions begin.

R. H. ADAMSON (239), Laboratory of Chemical Pharmacology, National Cancer Institute, National Institutes of Health, Bethesda, Maryland 20205

J. R. ANDERSON (591), Children's Cancer Study Group, Los Angeles, California 90031

LEIF C. ANDERSSON (75), Transplantation Laboratory and Department of Pathology, University of Helsinki, SF 00290 Helsinki 29, Finland

E. BAJETTA (537), Istituto Nazionale Tumori, Milan 20133, Italy

A. BANFI (537), Istituto Nazionale Tumori, Milan 20133, Italy

COSTAN W. BERARD (351), Division of Pathology and Clinical Laboratories, St. Jude Children's Research Hospital, Memphis, Tennessee 38101

CHARLES P. BIEBER (219), Department of Cardiovascular Surgery, Stanford University Medical Center, Stanford, California 94305

MARCIA M. BIEBER (285), Cancer Biology Research Laboratory, Department of Radiology, Stanford University School of Medicine, Stanford, California 94305

G. BONADONNA (537), Istituto Nazionzale Tumori, Milan 20133, Italy

MICHAEL R. BRISTOW (627), Division of Cardiology, Stanford University School of Medicine, Stanford, California 94305

SHERRI BROWN (95), Howard Hughes Medical Institute, and Division of Oncology, Department of Medicine, Stanford University, Stanford, California 94305

JEROME S. BURKE (1, 259, 351), Department of Pathology, Stanford University School of Medicine, Stanford, California 94305

R. S. BUSH (485), The Princess Margaret Hospital, Toronto, Ontario, Canada

R. BUZZONI (537), Istituto Nazionale Tumori, Milan 20133, Italy

R. CANETTA (537), Istituto Nazionale Tumori, Milan 20133, Italy

R. CHILCOTE (591), Children's Cancer Study Group, Los Angeles, California 90031

P. COCCIA (591), Children's Cancer Study Group, Los Angeles, California 90031

R. COFFMAN (131), Laboratory of Experimental Oncology, Department of Pathology, Stanford University School of Medicine, Stanford, California 94305

C. NORMAN COLEMAN (259), Division of Radiation Therapy, Department of Radiology, and Division of Medical Oncology, Department of Medicine, Stanford University Medical Center, Stanford, California 94305

CHARLES A. COLTMAN, JR. (523), Department of Medicine, University of Texas Health Sciences Center, San Antonio, Texas 78284

RICHARD S. COX (369), Division of Radiation Therapy, Department of Radiology, Stanford University, Stanford, California 94305

EDWARD J. DE PERSIO (523), Department of Radiology, University of Texas Medical Branch, Galveston, Texas 77550

VINCENT T. DEVITA, JR. (379), National Cancer Institute, Bethesda, Maryland 20205

JEANETTE DILLEY (95), Howard Hughes Medical Institute, and Division of Oncology, Department of Medicine, Stanford University, Stanford, California 94305

DENNIS O. DIXON (523), Southwest Oncology Group, Statistical Center, Houston, Texas 77030

SARAH S. DONALDSON (571), Division of Radiation Therapy, Department of Radiology, Stanford University School of Medicine, Stanford, California 94305

RONALD F. DORFMAN (351), Department of Pathology, Stanford University Medical Center, Stanford, California 94305

R. ELLIS (131), Laboratory of Experimental Oncology, Department of Pathology, Stanford University School of Medicine, Stanford, California 94305

EDGAR G. ENGLEMAN (295), Department of Pathology, Stanford University School of Medicine, Stanford, California 94305

M. ESSEX (175), Department of Microbiology, Harvard University School of Public Health, Boston, Massachusetts 02115

P. EXELBY (591), Children's Cancer Study Group, Los Angeles, California 90031

KIRK E. FRY (185), Cancer Biology Research Laboratory, Department of Radiology, Stanford University School of Medicine, Stanford, California 94305

LILLIAN A. FULLER (523), Department of Radiotherapy, M. D. Anderson Hospital, Houston, Texas 77030

CARL G. GAHMBERG[1] (75), Department of Bacteriology and Immunology, University of Helsinki, 00290 Helsinki 29, Finland

ROBERT C. GALLO (201), Laboratory of Tumor Cell Biology, National Cancer Institute, National Institutes of Health, Bethesda, Maryland 20205

ELI GLATSTEIN (503), Radiation Oncology Branch, Clinical Oncology Program, Division of Cancer Treatment, National Cancer Institute, Bethesda, Maryland 20205

ARVIN S. GLICKSMAN (639), Department of Radiation Oncology, Rhode Island Hospital, and Section on Radiation Medicine, Brown University, Providence, Rhode Island 02902

JOHN M. GOLDMAN (419), MRC Leukaemia Unit, Royal Postgraduate Medical School, London W12 0HS, England

GIDEON GOLDSTEIN (53), Immunobiology Division, Ortho Pharmaceutical Corporation, Raritan, New Jersey 08869

ROBERT S. GOODENOW (185), Division of Biology, California Institute of Technology, Pasadena, California 94305

M. GOSPODAROWICZ (485), The Princess Margaret Hospital, Toronto, Ontario, Canada

PETRE N. GROZEA (523), Oklahoma Medical Research Foundation, Department of Medicine, University of Oklahoma College of Medicine, Oklahoma City, Oklahoma 73190

D. HAMMOND (591), Children's Cancer Study Group, Los Angeles, California 90031

RUSSELL HARDY (107), Division of Tumor Immunology, Sidney Farber Cancer Institute, Harvard Medical School, Boston, Massachusetts 02115

ADA HATZUBAI (95), Howard Hughes Medical Institute, and Division of Oncology, Department of Medicine, Stanford University, Stanford, California 94305

SAMUEL HELLMAN (453), Joint Center for Radiation Therapy, Department of Radiation Therapy, Harvard Medical School, Boston, Massachusetts 02115

WERNER HENLE (1), Division of Virology, Children's Hospital, Philadelphia, Pennsylvania 19104

GERTRUDE HENLE (1), Division of Virology, Children's Hospital, Philadelphia, Pennsylvania 19104

RICHARD T. HOPPE (369, 469, 513), Division of Radiation Therapy, Department of Radiology, Stanford University School of Medicine, Stanford, California 94305

SANDRA HORNING (513), Division of Oncology, Department of Medicine, Stanford University School of Medicine, Stanford, California 94305

[1]Present address: Department of Biochemistry, University of Helsinki, Helsinki, Finland 00170.

SUSAN MOLLOY HUBBARD (379), Scientific Information Branch, Division of Cancer Treatment, National Cancer Institute, Bethesda, Maryland 20205

D. HUMPHREY (131), Department of Pathology, University of Texas Health Sciences Center, San Antonio, Texas 78284

R. D. T. JENKIN[2] (591), Children's Cancer Study Group, Los Angeles, California 90031

L. JERABEK (131), Laboratory of Experimental Oncology, Department of Pathology, Stanford University School of Medicine, Stanford, California 94305

STEPHEN E. JONES (439), Department of Medicine and Section of Hematology/Oncology, Department of Internal Medicine, University of Arizona Health Sciences Center, Tucson, Arizona 85724

HENRY S. KAPLAN (1, 185, 259, 285, 369, 513, 571), Cancer Biology Research Laboratory, Stanford University School of Medicine, Stanford, California 94305

J. KERSEY (591), Children's Cancer Study Group, Los Angeles, California 90031

GEORGE KLEIN (155), Department of Tumor Biology, Karolinska Institutet, S 104 01 Stockholm 60, Sweden

D. KOOISTRA (131), Laboratory of Experimental Oncology, Department of Pathology, Stanford University School of Medicine, Stanford, California 94305

PATRICK D. KUNG[3] (53), Division of Immunosciences, Ortho Pharmaceutical Corporation, Raritan, New Jersey 08869

PAULA KUSHLAN (513), Division of Oncology, Department of Medicine, Stanford University Medical Center, Stanford, California 94305

J. KUSHNER (591), Children's Cancer Study Group, Los Angeles, California 90031

A. LATTUADA (537), Istituto Nazionale Tumori, Milan 20133, Italy

S. LEIKIN (591), Children's Cancer Study Group, Los Angeles, California 90031

RONALD LEVY (95, 185, 553), Howard Hughes Medical Institute, and Division of Oncology, Department of Medicine, Stanford University, Stanford, California 94305

ALAN LEWIN (453), Joint Center for Radiation Therapy, Department of Radiation Therapy, Harvard Medical School, Boston, Massachusetts 02115

SAI-LING LIU (185), Cancer Biology Research Laboratory, Department of Radiology, Stanford University School of Medicine, Stanford, California 94305

Present address:

[2]Ontario Cancer Foundation, Toronto-Bayview Clinic, Toronto, Ontario M4N 3M5, Canada.

[3]Present address: Human Immunology Centocor, Inc., Malvern, Pennsylvania 19355.

ROBERT J. LUKES (309), Department of Pathology, Hematopathology Section, and the Cancer Center of the University of Southern California School of Medicine, Los Angeles, California 90033

M. McGRATH (131), Laboratory of Experimental Oncology, Department of Pathology, Stanford University School of Medicine, Stanford, California 94305

DAVID MALONEY (95), Howard Hughes Medical Institute, and Division of Oncology, Department of Medicine, Stanford University, Stanford, California 94305

PETER MAUCH (453), Joint Center for Radiation Therapy, Department of Radiation Therapy, Harvard Medical School, Boston, Massachusetts 02115

A. MEADOWS (591), Children's Cancer Study Group, Los Angeles, California 90031

THOMAS P. MILLER (439), Department of Medicine and Section of Hematology/Oncology, Department of Internal Medicine, University of Arizona Health Sciences Center, Tucson, Arizona 85724

RICHARD A. MILLER (553), The Howard Hughes Medical Institute, Division of Oncology, and Department of Medicine, Stanford University Medical Center, Stanford, California 94305

JUN MINOWADA (53), Department of Immunology, Roswell Park Memorial Institute, New York State Department of Health, Buffalo, New York 14263

S. MONFARDINI (537), Istituto Nazionale Tumori, Milan 20133, Italy

ELEANOR MONTAGUE (523), University of Texas System Cancer Center, M. D. Anderson Hospital, and Department of Radiotherapy, Tumor Institution at Houston, Houston, Texas 77030

JOSEPH W. MYERS (523), Department of Medicine, University of Texas Health Sciences Center, San Antonio, Texas 78284

LEE M. NADLER (107), Division of Tumor Immunology, Sidney Farber Cancer Institute, Harvard Medical School, Boston, Massachusetts 02115

KENNETH NILSSON (35), The Wallenberg Laboratory, Uppsala University, Uppsala, Sweden

S. NORD (131), Laboratory of Experimental Oncology, Department of Pathology, Stanford University School of Medicine, Stanford, California 94305

LENNART OLSSON[4] (1, 121), Cancer Biology Research Laboratory, Department of Radiology, Stanford University Medical Center, Stanford, California 94305

THOMAS F. PAJAK (639), Cancer and Leukemia Group B, Scarsdale, New York 10583

JOHN W. PARKER (309), Department of Pathology, Hematopathology Sec-

---

[4]Present address: Medical Department A, State University Hospital, Copenhagen, Denmark 2100.

tion, and the Cancer Center of the University of Southern California School of Medicine, Los Angeles, California 90033

JOHN L. PENNOCK (219), Department of Cardiovascular Surgery, Stanford University Medical Center, Stanford, California 94305

E. PILLEMER (131), Laboratory of Experimental Oncology, Department of Pathology, Stanford University School of Medicine, Stanford, California 94305

BRACHA RAMOT (277), Department of Hematology, Chaim Sheba Medical Center, Sackler Medical School, Tel Aviv University, Tel Aviv, Israel

ELLIS L. REINHERZ (107), Division of Tumor Immunology, Sidney Farber Cancer Institute, Harvard Medical School, Boston, Massachusetts 02115

BRUCE A. REITZ (219), Department of Cardiovascular Surgery, Stanford University Medical Center, Stanford, California 94305

JEROME RITZ (107), Division of Tumor Immunology, Sidney Farber Cancer Institute, Harvard Medical School, Boston, Massachusetts 02115

SAUL A. ROSENBERG (259, 369, 513), Divisions of Oncology, Medicine, and Radiation Therapy, Stanford University School of Medicine, Stanford, California 94305

KIMITAKA SAGAWA (53), Department of Immunology, Roswell Park Memorial Institute, New York State Department of Health, Buffalo, New York 14263

STUART F. SCHLOSSMAN (107), Division of Tumor Immunology, Sidney Farber Cancer Institute, Harvard Medical School, Boston, Massachusetts 02115

S. M. SIEBER (239), Laboratory of Chemical Pharmacology, National Cancer Institute, National Institutes of Health, Bethesda, Maryland 20205

S. SIEGEL (591), Children's Cancer Study Group, Los Angeles, California 90031

JOSEPH V. SIMONE (663), Hematology–Oncology Department, St. Jude Children's Research Hospital, Memphis, Tennessee 38101

PHILIP STASHENKO (107), Department of Immunology and Forsyth Dental Center, Harvard School of Dental Medicine, Boston, Massachusetts 02115

SAMUEL STROBER (285), Division of Immunology, Department of Medicine, Stanford University School of Medicine, Stanford, California 94305

CLIVE R. TAYLOR (309), Department of Pathology, Immunopathology Section, and the Cancer Center of the University of Southern California School of Medicine, Los Angeles, California 90033

IAN S. TROWBRIDGE (53), Department of Cancer Biology, The Salk Institute for Biological Studies, San Diego, California 92138

A. TSUKAMOTO (131), Laboratory of Experimental Oncology, Department of Pathology, Stanford University School of Medicine, Stanford, California 94305

P. VALAGUSSA (537), Istituto Nazionale Tumori, Milan 20133, Italy

ANNA VARGHESE (259), Division of Radiation Therapy, Stanford University Medical Center, Stanford, California 94305

ROGER A. WARNKE (231), Department of Pathology, Stanford University School of Medicine, Stanford, California 94305

I. WEISSMAN (131), Laboratory of Experimental Oncology, Department of Pathology, Stanford University School of Medicine, Stanford, California 94305

J. WILSON (591), Children's Cancer Study Group, Los Angeles, California 90031

NORMA WOLLNER (603), Department of Pediatrics, Memorial Sloan-Kettering Cancer Center, New York, New York 10021

Editor's Foreword

The first and second Bristol-Myers cancer symposia dealt with cancer research primarily at the preclinical level. The first symposium was held at the Baylor College of Medicine and described the effects of drugs on the cell nucleus. The second symposium at Yale University was on the topic of molecular actions and targets for cancer chemotherapeutic agents.

In this, the third symposium volume, we shift to a clinical topic in cancer research. The Stanford symposium, held on November 20–21, 1980, dealt with advances in the treatment of malignant lymphomas. In that symposium, which was attended by speakers and participants of international note, striking progress was described in the treatment of lymphomas which occur in both children and adults.

Hodgkin's disease is one type of lymphoma which is among the most curable of cancers, with a 5-year survival rate of 90% among patients receiving modern radiotherapy and chemotherapy treatments. Survival rates of lymphomas are now so good that we need to be alerted to the possibility of the emergence of new tumors in long-term survivors who have been treated by radiation and chemotherapy. This incidence of new tumors was about 3% out of 1096 adult Hodgkin's disease patients treated at Stanford since 1968 with chemotherapy and radiation. Thus, the follow-up of patients should include not only monitoring of the recurrence of the original tumor but also the occurrence of new tumors.

This volume discusses the current knowledge of immunologic markers, including the use of hybridomas to produce monoclonal antibodies to tumor antigens. Also, the results of an international comparison of the major pathologic classification systems for lymphomas are detailed.

The fourth Bristol-Myers Symposium on Cancer Research was held at Johns Hopkins University in December 1981 and discussed the heterogeneity of cancer cells. The proceedings of this conference will be the subject of the fourth volume of this series.

Maxwell Gordon
Series Editor

Foreword

When Bristol-Myers initiated its program of unrestricted cancer research grants in 1977, we took particular pride in the series of academic symposia to be sponsored by the recipient institutions.

The third annual Bristol-Myers Symposium on Cancer Research reflected the unique contribution made by the Stanford University School of Medicine to the understanding of malignant lymphomas.

From the standpoint of both basic science and clinical research, Stanford has long been a world leader in lymphoma research. While lymphomas are much less common than either lung or breast cancer, they have proven to be much more responsive to treatment. The advances in therapy achieved during the past two decades against Hodgkin's disease, for example, have been so dramatic as to result in cure for the great majority of patients.

Much of this research has been conducted by Henry S. Kaplan and Saul A. Rosenberg. Under their distinguished co-chairmanship, the Stanford symposium was a significant contribution to the exchange of current understanding of lymphatic cancers.

These proceedings join the published volumes of the first and second Bristol-Myers symposia. The first, "Effects of Drugs on the Cell Nucleus," was held at Baylor School of Medicine in 1978; the second, "Molecular Actions and Targets for Cancer Chemotherapeutic Agents," was organized by Yale University School of Medicine in 1979.

The Johns Hopkins Oncology Center organized the fourth symposium, "Tumor Cell Heterogeneity: Origins and Implications" in December 1981, and the proceedings should be published later this year. Future symposia will be organized by the other grant recipient institutions: The University of Chicago, the Institute for Cancer Research at the Royal Marsden Hospital in London; the

Istituto Nazionale per lo Studio e la Cura dei Tumori in Milan; the Georgetown University School of Medicine, and the Memorial Sloan-Kettering Cancer Center.

At the same time, we have increased our commitment to the unrestricted research grant program initiated in 1977. These grants now total $3.86 million at seven United States and two foreign institutions.

When we began this program, we recognized that our efforts could be only a modest increment to the massive support for cancer research the federal government provides. We considered it important, however, to demonstrate the fact that private enterprise also contributes to cancer research and to identify our company as one of those contributors.

We do this because we share your concern for finding the answer to the many questions about cancer that still remain unanswered. This is why—while the marketing of anti-cancer drugs affects only three of our twelve divisions—it is, on balance, our most important endeavor—and it regularly receives our highest priorities in terms of both resources and hopes.

Richard L. Gelb
Chairman of the Board
Bristol-Myers Company

Preface

The Symposium on Malignant Lymphomas, held at Stanford University on November 20–21, 1980, was the third in a series of such symposia generously supported by the Bristol-Myers Company.

The advances in understanding and treatment of the malignant lymphomas have been significant during the last decade. Invited participants to the symposium included many of the world leaders in their fields. The symposium was divided into four areas: etiology, immunology, pathology, and treatment.

As organizers of the symposium and guest editors of the proceedings, we are gratified by the results. The symposium was stimulating and current, and the proceedings provide valuable documentation of the progress and research opportunities in this dynamic field.

Saul A. Rosenberg
Henry S. Kaplan

Abbreviations

ABVD, adriamycin-bleomycin-vinblastine-dacarbazine
ACIF, anticomplement immunofluorescence
ADCC, antibody-dependent cellular cytotoxicity
AFP, alpha fetoprotein
ALL, acute lymphoblastic leukemia
AML, acute myeloid leukemia
AMoL, acute monocytic leukemia
ANAE, acid-naphthylacetate esterase
ANLL, acute non-lymphatic leukemia
ASV, avian sarcoma virus
ATG, antithymocyte globulin
ATL, adult T-cell leukemia

B-MOPP, bleomycin + N-mustard+vincristine+procarbazine+prednisone
BACOP, bleomycin + adriamycin + cyclophosphamide + vincristine + pro-
carbazine
BL, Burkitt's lymphoma
BNLI, British National Lymphoma Investigation
BX, testicular biopsy

CALGB, cancer acute leukemia group B
cALL, common acute lymphoblastic leukemia
CAT, cytosine arabinoside-adriamycin-thioguanine
CCNU, 1-(2-chloroethyl)-3-cyclohexyl-1-nitrosourea
CCSG, Children's Cancer Study Group
CEA, carcinoembryonic antigen
CHOP, cyclophosphamide-adriamycin-vincristine-prednisone

CLL, chronic lymphocytic leukemia
CML-BP, chronic myelogenous leukemia in the blastic phase
CMV, cytomegalovirus
COMLA, cyclophosphamide-vincristine-methotrexate with leucovorin-ara C
COMP, cytoxan-vincristine-methotrexate-prednisone
CPRC, California Primate Research Center
CS, clinically staged
CT, computed tomographic scanning
CVB, CCNU-vinblastine-bleomycin
CVP, cytoxan-vincristine-prednisone
CyIg, cytoplasmic immunoglobulin
CX, chemotherapy

DARR, direct antiglobulin rosetting reaction
DHL, diffuse histiocytic lymphoma
DL, diffuse large cell malignant lymphoma
DLID, diffuse lymphocytic intermediately differentiated lymphoma
DLPD, diffuse lymphocytic poorly differentiated lymphoma
DLWD, diffuse lymphocytic well-differentiated lymphoma
DM, diffuse mixed malignant lymphoma
DSC, diffuse small cleaved cell

EA, early antigen
EAC, erythrocyte–antibody–complement
EBNA, Epstein–Barr virus associated nuclear antigen
EBV, Epstein–Barr virus
ELISA, enzyme-linked immunoabsorbent assay
E-RFC, E-rosette-forming cells

FACS, fluorescence-activated cell sorter
FCC, follicular center cell lymphoma
FCS, fetal calf serum
FFP, freedom from progression
FM, follicular mixed malignant lymphoma
FOCMA, feline oncornavirus—associated cell membrane-antigen
FeLV, feline leukemia virus

G-6PD, glucose 6-phosphate dehydrogenase

HA, *Helix pomatia* antigen
HCL, hairy cell leukemia

HD, Hodgkin's disease
HL, histiocytic lymphoma
HLA, human leukocyte antigen
HP, binding protein
HZV, *Herpes zoster* varicella

IF, involved field irradiation
Ia-like, immune associated antigen
IgM-EAC$_{3d}$, erythrocyte-IgM antibody-C$_{3d}$ component of complement

LCL, lymphoblastoid cell lines
LD, lymphocytic depletion
LL, lymphocytic lymphoma
LOAP, chlorambucil-vincristine-cytosine arabinoside-prednisone
LOPP, chlorambucil-vincristine-procarbazine-prednisone
LP, lymphocytic predominance
LS, lymphosarcoma
LSA$_2$-L$_2$, cytoxan-vincristine-methotrexate-prednisone-daunomycin-Ara-C-
 6-thioguanine-L-asparaginase-methotrexate-BCNU

M-BACOD, methotrexate + BACOD
MC, mixed cell lymphoma
MC, mixed cellularity
MGP, methyl green-Pyronine
ML, malignant lymphoma
MLC, mixed lymphocyte culture
MLR, mixed leukocyte reactions
MM, multiple myeloma
MNU, 1-methylnitrosourea
MOPP, nitrogen mustard-vincristine-procarbazine-prednisone
MPMV, Mason–Pfizer mammary virus
MSV, murine sarcoma virus
MVPP, nitrogen mustard-vinblastine-procarbazine-prednisone

NASDAE, naphthol AS-D esterase
NHL, nodular histiocytic lymphoma
NLPD, nodular lymphocytic poorly differentiated lymphoma
NML, nodular mixed lymphoma
NPDL, nodular poorly differentiated lymphoma
NS, nodular sclerosis
NSE, nonspecific esterase

PAS, periodic acid-Schiff
PAVe, procarbazine-alkeran-vinblastine
PBL, peripheral blood lymphocytes
PBML, peripheral blood mononuclear leukocyte
PBS, phosphate buffered saline
PEPA, protected environment + prophylactic antibiotics
PHA, phytohemagglutinin
PMH, Princess Margaret Hospital
PS, pathological stage
PVC, polyvinyl chloride
PWM, pokeweed nitrogen

RER, rough endoplasmic reticulum
RT, radiotherapy

SCAB, streptozotocin-CCNU-adriamycin-bleomycin
SDS, sodium dodecyl sulfate
SL, small lymphocytic malignant lymphoma
SLE, systemic lupus erythrymatosus
SRBC, sheep red blood cells
SWOG, Southwest Oncology Group
SmIg, surface membrane immunoglobulin

TCGF, T-cell growth factor
THF, thymic humoral factor
TLI, total lymphoid irradiation
TNI, total nodal irradiation
TPA, 12-tetradecanoyl-phorbol 13-acetate

VN, virus negative

1

In Vitro Cultivation and Characterization of the Giant Neoplastic Cells of Hodgkin's Disease: Some Unresolved Problems

HENRY S. KAPLAN, LENNART OLSSON, JEROME S. BURKE,
ELLIOTT F. OSSERMAN, WERNER HENLE, AND GERTRUDE HENLE

I. Introduction

The neoplastic nature of Hodgkin's disease is now widely accepted, but the identity and origin of its tumor cell population remain controversial. To make an unambiguous histopathological diagnosis of Hodgkin's disease, a pathologist must observe one or more characteristic Reed–Sternberg cells against an appropriate pleomorphic stromal background. In formalin-fixed tissue sections stained with hematoxylin and eosin, these cells typically are binucleate, are multinucleate, or have hyperlobated nuclei with densely staining nuclear membranes, vacuolated or clear nucleoplasm, large to enormous nucleoli, and abundant, slightly amphophilic or pale-blue cytoplasm (1). Mononuclear cells of identical nuclear morphology are also seen in such tissue sections; these cells, though referred to as "Hodgkin's cells," are not regarded as diagnostic of the disease, since they may be encountered in other clinical situations. Indeed, although Reed–Sternberg cells were once regarded as pathognomonic of Hodgkin's disease, morphologically indistinguishable cells have now been demonstrated in tissue sections from patients with infectious mononucleosis (2), certain diffuse large-cell ("histiocytic") lymphomas, and occasionally even nonlymphomatous neoplasms (3).

The large size, distinctive morphology, and ominous appearance of Reed–Sternberg cells have long suggested that they constitute the tumor cell population of Hodgkin's disease. However, this view has been difficult to reconcile with the remarkably sparse numbers of these cells in most tissue specimens. In striking contrast to the monotonous abundance of tumor cells in all other malignant lymphomas, Reed–Sternberg cells seldom constitute more than 1%, and often less than 0.01% of the cells in an involved lymph node or spleen. The abundant stromal cell population is made up of varying proportions of apparently normal small and medium-sized lymphocytes, eosinophils, plasma cells, fibroblasts, and benign, pale-staining histiocytes.

Cytogenetic studies have revealed two populations of mitotic cells in fresh biopsy material and in short-term cultures treated with colchicine or vinblastine. One of these populations has a diploid complement of 46 chromosomes and is believed to represent the normal stromal cell population, whereas the second class of mitotic cells, usually seen in small numbers and occasionally lacking, is clearly aneuploid and often hypotetraploid. Structurally abnormal marker chromosomes are often present, sometimes in multiple cells of the same case, thus providing unambiguous evidence for their origin from the same aneuploid clone (4). An extensive review of the evidence for the clonal derivation of aneuploid cell populations in Hodgkin's disease has been presented elsewhere (5).

Doubt concerning the identity of the tumor cell population was also raised by early studies suggesting that the Reed–Sternberg cells lacked the capacity to divide, whereas the mononuclear Hodgkin's cells were mitotically active and capable of DNA synthesis, as reflected in the incorporation of tritiated thymidine (^{3}H-TdR) (6,7). Thus, the concept has been proposed that Hodgkin's cells comprise the true neoplastic cell population and that Reed–Sternberg cells are merely end-stage degenerative forms which, though important for diagnosis, have little or no replicative potential. However, more recent studies on fresh biopsy material, as well as cell culture studies to be described below, have revealed definitive evidence of the incorporation of ^{3}H-TdR into the DNA of binucleate and multinucleate giant cells, as well as the occasional presence of binucleate or multinucleate mitotic figures (8–12).

Debate has also focused on the cell of origin of Hodgkin's and Reed–Sternberg cells. On the basis of their size and morphology, they were once thought to be derived from the reticulum cell or histiocyte (1,13). However, nonspecific esterase, an enzyme characteristically observed in histiocytes, could not be detected in these giant cells by cytochemical techniques (14). With increasing awareness of the remarkable changes in morphology and mitotic activity which occur during blastogenic transformation of lymphocytes, the suggestion has emerged that the giant cells of Hodgkin's disease may be derived from lymphocytes which have undergone blastogenic transformation *in vivo* (15,16). More specifically, some investigators have regarded them as derived from T lymphocytes (15,17), and others from B lymphocytes (18–21). The latter interpretation derives primarily from the observation in these cells of positive immunofluorescence or immunohistochemical staining reactions for surface (SIg) or intracytoplasmic (CIg) immunoglobulin. However, additional studies have shown that such cells may contain both lambda and kappa light chains (22–25), whereas a normal B lymphocyte may contain either lambda or kappa, but not both (26). Incubation with radiolabeled IgG has revealed that the IgG sometimes detected in these cells is internalized from the extracellular environment, perhaps through an Fc receptor, rather than endogenously synthesized (25). Moreover, Reed–Sternberg cells consistently yielded negative immunoperoxidase reactions for the J chain of immunoglobulin, a marker characteristically observed in B-cell malignancies (27).

Ultrastructural studies have also failed to yield definitive evidence concerning the cell of origin of Reed–Sternberg cells. Some investigators have been impressed by structural features suggesting origin from the lymphocyte (28), whereas others have called attention to the presence of lysosomes and cytoplasmic processes suggestive of a macrophage lineage (11).

Various techniques of cultivation *in vitro* or in diffusion chambers *in vivo* have been used in efforts to learn more about the nature of the giant cells of Hodgkin's disease. The literature concerning earlier cell culture studies has been reviewed elsewhere (5). Some of the multinucleated cells described in the early reports appear to have been foreign body giant cells rather than Hodgkin's cells.

Many, and perhaps all, of the earlier serially passaged cultures were almost certainly banal lymphoblastoid cell lines (LCLs) derived from B lymphocytes naturally infected with the Epstein–Barr virus (EBV). Overgrowth by LCLs has been a frequent pitfall in attempts to culture human malignant lymphomas (29).

It is only in the past few years that significant successes have been reported in the cultivation of cells which, on the basis of their morphological, biological, functional, and marker properties, seem reasonably likely to have been authentic Reed–Sternberg or Hodgkin's cells. In some of these instances, although varying degrees of active proliferation could be maintained for some months, the cultures ultimately died out (30,31). However, several groups of investigators have now reported the successful establishment of permanent cell lines of giant cells purportedly derived from Reed–Sternberg and Hodgkin's cells (32–35). The validity of these interpretations is considered further in Section IV, in light of our own observations which extend the earlier studies of Kaplan and Gartner (31).

II. Materials and Methods

A. Sources of Tissues and Cells

Involved spleens obtained at staging laparotomy from patients with biopsy-proven, previously untreated Hodgkin's disease comprised about 95% of the initial material. Involved lymph nodes were occasionally obtained from treated patients undergoing excisional biopsy for confirmation of suspected relapse. In rare instances, cultures were initiated from cell populations pelleted from pleural, pericardial, or peritoneal effusion fluids which had been examined cytologically and found to contain cells morphologically compatible with Hodgkin's or Reed–Sternberg cells. Control cultures of normal spleen macrophages were prepared as described previously (36).

B. Cell Culture Procedures and Conditions

The methods used for the preparation of cell suspensions, for monitoring of cell viability, and for the cultivation of cell suspensions or explant fragments in liquid medium were those previously described by Kaplan and Gartner (31). After difficulty was repeatedly encountered in attempts to trypsinize the large, round adherent cell population for subpassage, we tried other methods of cell harvest, including scraping with a rubber policeman, treatment with lidocaine (37), and incubation in cold Ca^{2+}- and Mg^{2+}-free Hanks' balanced salt solution (38). We also explored the use of other substrates to which cells would be expected to adhere less firmly, if at all. These attempts included the cultivation of cells at the interface between liquid medium and a layer of solid 0.5% Noble agar, 3% agarose, or semisolid 0.8–1.25% methylcellulose (31); in liquid medium in flasks or dishes coated with Teflon; and in liquid medium in which the Hodgkin's cells were overlaid on feeder layers of pediatric fibroblasts or normal spleen macrophages.

The culture medium most commonly employed was RPMI-1640 containing 15–20% fetal calf serum (FCS), 5–15% pooled normal human serum (HS), and antibiotics and vitamins as previously described (31). In individual experiments, supplements such as mouse L-cell-conditioned medium, phytohemagglutinin, lipopolysaccharide, 2-mercaptoethanol, and L-cysteine were added.

C. Morphological Studies

1. Light Microscopy

Cell samples removed from the cultures for morphological examination by light microscopy were deposited on glass slides by cytocentrifugation, air-dried, fixed in absolute methanol for 2 minutes, and stained in Wright–Giemsa as previously described (31). Cells were tested for nonspecific esterase activity by the α-naphthyl acetate procedure of Yam, Li, and Crosby (39).

2. Electron Microscopy

Cells from trypsinized monolayers were plated in 10×35 mm plastic tissue culture dishes (Falcon Plastics, Oxnard, California) or eight-chamber glass slides (Miles Laboratory, Westmount, Illinois). The cultures were maintained in medium at 37°C for 2 days to 1 week until approximately 50% confluence of an adherent cell population was obtained. The monolayers were then washed three times in phosphate-buffered saline (PBS), pH 7.2, fixed *in situ* in a mixture of 2% glutaraldehyde and 1% sucrose in 0.067 M sodium cacodylate buffer, pH 7.4, for 1 hour, washed in 0.067 M sodium cacodylate, pH 7.4, and 4% sucrose for 10 minutes, and postfixed in 2% osmium tetroxide for 30 minutes at 4°C. After fixation the monolayers were washed twice in sodium maleate buffer, pH 5.2, counterstained with uranyl acetate for 30 minutes at 4°C, and the sodium maleate buffer wash repeated. Following dehydration in graded alcohols, the monolayers were infiltrated with a 1:1 mixture of 100% alcohol and Epon overnight, and the residual 1:1 mixture was subsequently pipetted. Epon was then added to the plastic tissue culture dishes and allowed to polymerize at 60°C overnight; inverted Epon-filled capsules were added to the surface of the eight-chamber glass slides, and following polymerization these were snapped off.

In case 93, cell suspensions were also examined. Cells were removed from the culture surface by trypsinization during the same passage, and 6×10^6 cells centrifuged for 8 minutes at 1000 rpm. Following decantation of the culture medium, the cell pellet was fixed in an identical glutaraldehyde–sucrose–

cacodylate mixture and a subsequent cacodylate–sucrose wash. The cell pellet was then processed for electron microscopy by conventional procedures.

D. Surface Marker Studies

The method of Rabellino *et al.* (40) using goat anti-human IgM was used to test cells for SIg. Sheep erythrocytes supplied fresh weekly in Alsever's solution were used to test cells for their capacity to form spontaneous (E) rosettes as described by Bentwich *et al.* (41). Tests for IgG-EA, IgM-EA, IgM-EAC$_{3b}$, and IgM-EAC$_{3d}$ rosette formation were carried out by previously described methods (42–44).

E. Phagocytic Activity Tests

Tests for the capacity of cultured cells to phagocytize carbon particles (sterile India ink), heat-killed *Candida,* or antibody-coated sheep erythrocytes were performed as previously described by Kaplan and Gartner (31).

F. Lysozyme Assays

The supernatant fluids of long-term cultures were assayed, sometimes at serial intervals, for the presence of increased concentrations of lysozyme by the lysoplate method of Osserman and Lawlor (45). Serum samples from untreated patients with Hodgkin's disease were also assayed by this procedure. During the last 2 years, these assays have been performed by a more sensitive radioimmunoassay procedure developed in the same laboratory (V. P. Butler, D. T. Eng, and E. F. Osserman, unpublished). Human lysozyme isolated from the urine of patients with myelomonocytic leukemia was used as the reference standard in all assays.

G. Epstein–Barr Studies

The sera of patients were titrated for antibodies to EBV-related antigens. Indirect immunofluorescence (IF) tests (46,47) were used to measure antibodies to the Epstein–Barr viral capsid antigens (VCAs) and to the diffuse (D) and restricted (R) components of the EBV-induced early antigen (EA) complex. An anticomplement immunofluorescence (ACIF) procedure was used to measure antibodies to the EBV-associated nuclear antigen (EBNA) (48). For detection of the corresponding EBV-related antigens in cultured cells, cultures were transferred to medium devoid of human serum for 24 hours, at which time the cells were harvested. Smears or cytocentrifuge preparations on coverslips or glass slides were air-dried, fixed for 3 minutes at $-20°C$ in acetone or acetone and methanol, and tested by the above-cited procedures for VCA, D and R, and EBNA. In selected instances, attempts were made to infect viable cells with EBV by the procedure of Rocchi *et al.* (49).

H. Heterotransplantation

Tests of the capacity of the Hodgkin's cell cultures to "take" and grow progressively after heterotransplantation were performed by intracerebral inoculation of suspensions of cultured cells into congenitally athymic, nude mice, as previously described by Epstein *et al.* (50).

I. Autoradiography and Chromosome Studies

Cells from selected cultures were incubated for varying intervals, ranging from 2 to 24 hours with ^{3}H-TdR, usually at 1 μCi/ml. They were then processed for autoradiography as described by Kaplan and Gartner (31). Cultures of giant cells were examined for mitotic activity following incubation with colchicine. Chromosome numbers were determined by treatment of mitotic cells with hypotonic potassium chloride and acetic acid–ethyl alcohol and staining with Wright–Giemsa as previously described (31).

III. Results

A. Giant Cell Identification in Involved Tissues

Involved tissues or effusion fluids from more than 100 cases of Hodgkin's disease have been placed in culture to date. In five instances, the tissue source was an involved lymph node; seven were cytologically positive or probably positive pleural or pericardial effusion fluids; and the remainder were involved spleens. Touch imprints of areas of involvement in the spleens and lymph nodes were made to verify the presence in them of binucleate or multinucleate giant cells with morphological features consistent with those of Reed–Sternberg cells (Fig. 1). Cell suspensions prepared from involved spleens were routinely depleted of erythrocytes and granulocytes by Ficoll–Hypaque gradient centrifugation (51), following which samples of the residual cell suspension were cytocentrifuged, stained, and checked for the presence of giant cells of similar morphology. It was usually possible to identify such cells with reasonable confidence, and in a few instances the presence of characteristic lymphocyte rosettes (52) added to the certainty of their identification (Fig. 2). The viability of cells harvested from the Ficoll–Hypaque gradients was also verified by dye exclusion. Thus, it was possible to ensure that the cell suspensions placed in culture actually contained viable giant cells.

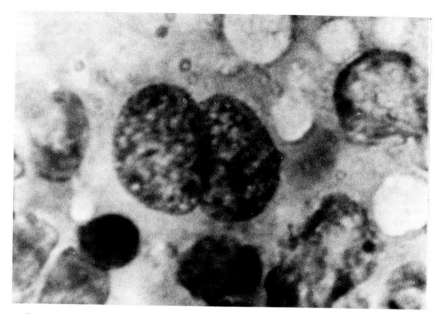

Fig. 1. A binucleate Reed–Sternberg cell is clearly identifiable in this Wright–Giemsa-stained touch imprint of an involved area in the spleen of a patient with Hodgkin's disease.

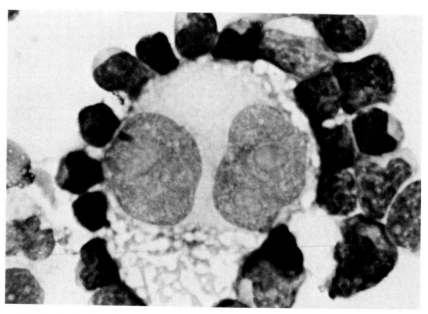

Fig. 2. Typical lymphocyte rosette around a classic binucleate Reed–Sternberg cell in a cell suspension prepared from an involved lymph node of a patient with relapsing Hodgkin's disease.

B. Culture Morphology and Fate

Two major subpopulations of cells could readily be distinguished when the cell suspension or tissue fragment cultures were examined with an inverted microscope within the first few days after culture initiation. The first was a nonadherent population of small cells with the typical dimensions of lymphocytes; these usually died off rapidly, though small numbers of lymphocytes persisted for as long as 3–4 weeks in some cultures. The other subpopulation was an adherent population of much larger cells, most of which were round or oval in shape and some of which could be seen to contain two or more nuclei. This population was assumed, on the basis of cell size alone, to include neoplastic giant cells. In addition, however, it also included large numbers of macrophages when the tissue source was the spleen, and variable numbers of fibroblasts from either spleen or lymph nodes. When cultures were started from pleural or pericardial effusion fluids, the large, round adherent cell population also included normal mesothelial cells. The largest macrophages could easily be distinguished because they acquired enormous dimensions, became extensively spread on the surface of the tissue culture plate or flask, and failed to divide. The remainder of the large, round cell population frequently showed a distinct increase in cell number during the first few weeks in culture, and in several instances continued to increase in number through several subpassages. When active proliferation of the large, round adherent cell population was observed, it led typically to the formation of grapelike clusters (Fig. 3) or nearly confluent sheets of cells.

These large, round adherent cells were often so tightly adherent that they could not readily be trypsinized for subpassage. However, they could be harvested with good yields and high viability by incubation in an ice-cold Ca^{2+}-, Mg^{2+}-free balanced salts solution (38). When aliquots of cells removed from the cultures were cytocentrifuged, stained, and examined by light microscopy, many had the typical morphological features of macrophages or normal mesothelial cells, but giant binucleate or multinucleate cells with morphological features consistent with those of Reed–Sternberg cells were not difficult to identify (Fig. 4). In a few cultures, particularly those initiated from lymph nodes, these cells were mixed with fibroblast-like cells which were readily trypsinizable and could easily be distinguished morphologically from the Hodgkin's giant cell population.

The least successful cultures persisted for only 3–4 weeks and contained very few if any Hodgkin's giant cells at the end of that interval. In other instances, however, the cultures exhibited active proliferation and could be carried through variable numbers of subpassages for as long as 8 months. Ultimately, however, the proliferative capacity of the large, round adherent cells appeared to diminish and the cultures were lost through gradual attrition. Attempts to clone the cells in semisolid 0.3% agarose were unsuccessful, with the exception of a single clone (Fig. 5) from the culture of case 83, which could not be subpassaged. As noted by Kaplan and Gartner (31), liquid cultures on solid agar substrates grew well for

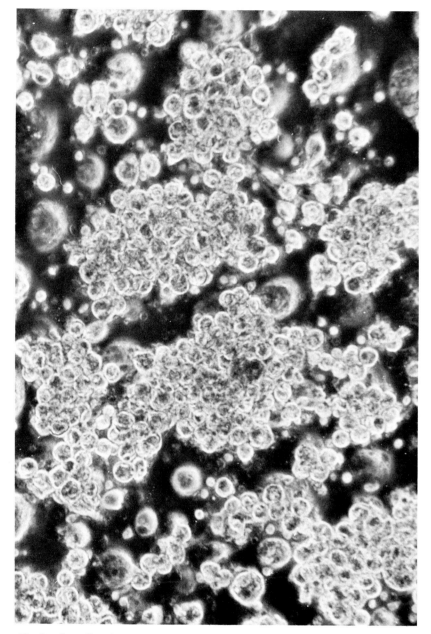

Fig. 3. Grapelike clusters of large, round adherent cells in a 3-week-old flask culture of cells from an extensively involved spleen (case 83). The size of these cells may be appreciated by comparison with that of the sparse lymphocytes still persisting in the culture. The even larger, solitary cells in the background are macrophages.

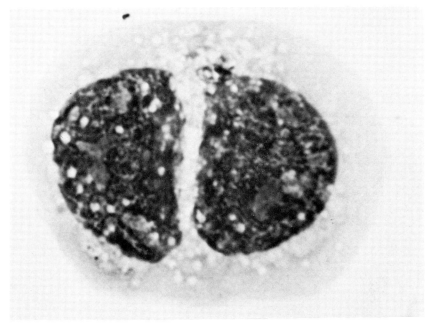

Fig. 4. Binucleate giant cell in a cytocentrifuge preparation of cells harvested from an involved spleen culture similar to that in Fig. 3. Wright–Giemsa stain.

3–4 weeks but then deteriorated rapidly, apparently as a result of phagocytosis of the agar, which accumulated in the cytoplasm of the giant cells as metachromatically staining amorphous material.

We have not succeeded to date in achieving the permanent establishment in culture of a cell line comprised of unambiguously identifiable Hodgkin's and Reed–Sternberg cells. However, three cultures deserve special comment.

One culture initiated in March 1976 from an extensively involved spleen (case 25) grew progressively and generated large numbers of obviously bizarre binucleate, trinucleate, and multinucleate giant cells. Slightly more than 2 months after initiation of the culture, when the giant cells were still growing slowly but actively, the culture was suddenly overrun by the outgrowth of a typical B-lymphoblastoid cell line, apparently originating from the few viable B lymphocytes still persisting in the culture at that time. It proved impossible to rid the giant cell population of the lymphoblastoid cells. Meanwhile, at an earlier stage, cells from this culture had been inoculated intracerebrally into nude mice. Successful heterotransplants were obtained from which the human cells were reinitiated in secondary culture. Giant cells of similar morphology once again began to grow actively and might well have yielded a permanent cell line but for the unfortunate development of a fungal infection which destroyed the culture.

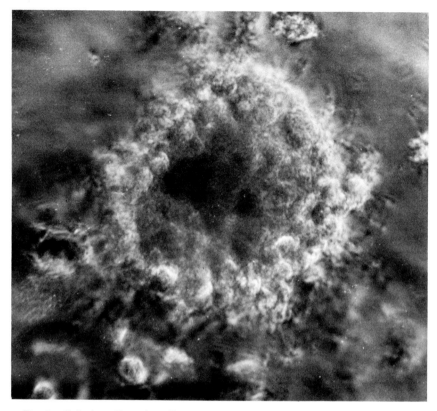

Fig. 5. Cells from the culture illustrated in Fig. 3 growing as a solitary clone in 0.3% agarose supplemented with conditioned medium at 24 days after transfer and 52 days after initiation of the primary culture.

A second culture (case 56) which was initiated in August 1977 from a cytologically positive pleural effusion (Fig. 6) in a patient with relapsing stage IVB Hodgkin's disease grew actively in primary culture and could be subpassaged for approximately 3.5 months, after which the proliferative activity of the giant cells diminished and the culture died out. Once again, a successful intracerebral heterotransplant yielded a source of giant cells for secondary culture. These cells, after a lag period of 2–3 weeks, began to grow actively, once again forming typical clusters of giant cells (Fig. 7). When aliquots of these cultures were examined by indirect immunofluorescence, the presence in them of variable proportions of cells staining positively with antihuman antibody could be verified. In addition, however, other cells of very similar size and morphology were present which, by their immunofluorescent staining reactions, appeared to be of murine origin. Chromosome preparations were then made which verified the presence of mitotic figures containing mouse chromosomes. Thus, normal brain cells of the nude mouse host had apparently undergone spontaneous transformation *in vitro* during cocultivation with the Hodgkin's giant cells. Several attempts to rid these cultures completely of the contaminating murine cell population by the use of anti-mouse brain antibody plus complement failed, though appreciable enrichment of the human cell population could be detected by indirect immunofluorescence. Aliquots of these cultures, after enrichment of the human cell population, were frozen and stored in liquid nitrogen awaiting the availability of a fluorescence-activated cell sorter (53) with which a greater degree of purification of the human cell population might be achieved. These studies are now pending, and it is hoped that a permanent line composed exclusively of human giant cells can still be established from this case.

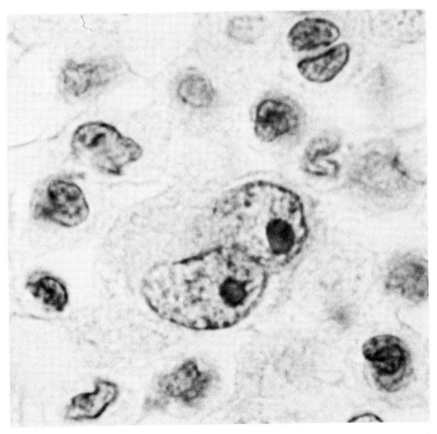

Fig. 6. Classic binucleate Reed–Sternberg cell in the sectioned pleural effusion pellet of case 56.

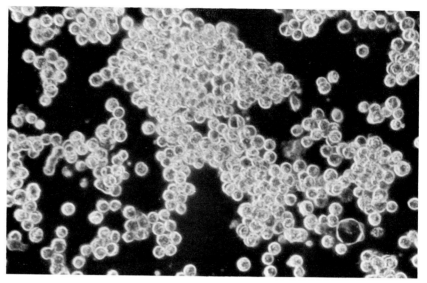

Fig. 7. Clusters of large, round cells from case 56 growing in liquid medium above a substrate layer of 3% agarose. These cells were placed in secondary culture after successful heterotransplantation of the primary culture into the nude mouse brain. This culture became an established line but contained a mixture of human and murine cells of similar size and morphology, the latter apparently derived by spontaneous *in vitro* transformation of normal mouse brain cells.

The final culture deserving comment did indeed result in the establishment of a permanent cell line, but in this instance the cells which have grown out have certain features, discernible by electron microscopy, which appear to be incompatible with those of the Hodgkin's and Reed–Sternberg giant cells of Hodgkin's disease. This culture was also initiated from a cytologically positive pleural effusion (Fig. 8) of a patient (case 93) with documented relapsing Hodgkin's disease who died at another hospital soon thereafter. No autopsy was performed, and it is thus impossible to exclude the possibility that this patient had a second malignant neoplasm, presumably of epithelial cell origin.

The tumor cells were unusually large and began to grow actively as adherent monolayers (Fig. 9) almost immediately after being placed in culture. The culture was cloned by the limiting dilution technique, and three single-cell clones (Fig. 10) were successfully derived from the parental culture. As early as day 4, aliquots of the actively growing culture yielded near-triploid mitotic figures containing approximately 70 chromosomes and a distinctive giant marker chromosome (54). Cytocentrifuge preparations revealed that the cells were binucleate or multinucleate, with morphological features on light microscopy which were compatible with those of Reed–Sternberg cells, and cytochemical

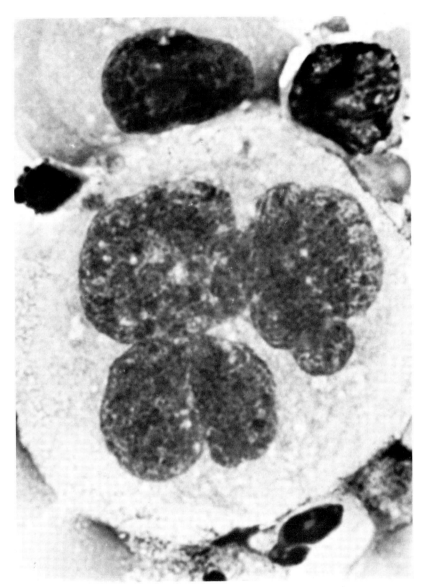

Fig. 8. Giant multinucleate cell, initially presumed to be a Reed–Sternberg cell, in the pleural effusion fluid of a patient with relapsing Hodgkin's disease (case 93). This patient died at another hospital, and no autopsy was performed. As indicated in the text, the permanent cell line established from these cells was subsequently found to have ultrastructural features suggesting its origin from a malignant epithelial neoplasm.

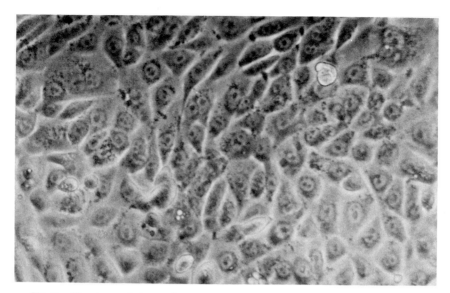

Fig. 9. Monolayer of giant cells, some binucleate, established as a permanent cell line from the malignant cells of the pleural effusion illustrated in Fig. 8. Note the presence of prominent and occasionally huge nucleoli.

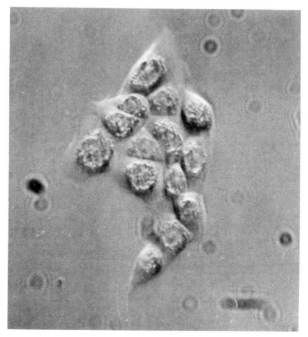

Fig. 10. Early clone of 14 cells derived from the culture of Fig. 9 after single-cell plating by the limiting dilution procedure.

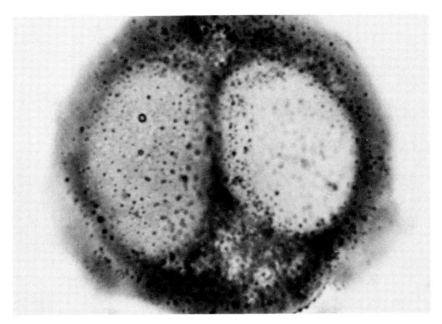

Fig. 11. Intensely positive nonspecific esterase reaction in a binucleate giant cell from the culture of Fig. 9 (case 93).

studies revealed the presence of strongly positive reactions for nonspecific esterase (Fig. 11). Some of the cells displayed weakly positive phagocytic activity for heat-killed *Candida* and definite phagocytic activity for India ink. Lysozyme studies, as indicated below, were weakly positive for the parental culture, negative for one clone, and definitely positive for the other two clones. Thus, many features of these cells were consistent with those previously observed for other Hodgkin's cell cultures, and it was provisionally concluded that we had at long last succeeded in establishing a permanent line of Hodgkin's giant cells. However, electron micrographs, to be described below, clearly revealed the existence of desmosomes and other features suggestive of an epithelial origin when the monolayers were examined in the plane of the culture vessel.

C. Cell Morphology

1. *Light Microscopy*

The majority of cells in the Wright–Giemsa cytocentrifuge preparations of case 93 were mononuclear, but many were binucleated or multinucleated forms. The nuclei tended to be eccentric and confined to one pole of the cell. The nuclear chromatin generally was condensed and aggregated, and in occasional

cells the chromatin was finely reticulated. Although small, nucleoli were prominent and blue-staining; in these preparations perinucleolar clear zones were not
observed. The cytoplasm was abundant and stained intensely basophilic; the
basophilia frequently was confined to a bandlike configuration at the cell border.
The cytoplasm also was usually finely vacuolated, but in many of the larger
binucleated and multinucleated cells the vacuoles were large, clear, well-
defined, and often appeared to compress the nuclei; occasional large vacuoles
often appeared to contain basophilic inclusions. In most respects, these
morphological characteristics were consistent with those of the large, round
adherent cell population of the long-term cultures described by Kaplan and
Gartner (31).

2. *Electron Microscopy*

Ultrastructure of the suspensions obtained from case 93 revealed cells with
irregularly indented nuclei and small surface cytoplasmic extensions (Fig. 12).
Nucleoli were large and frequently displayed exceedingly prominent nucleo-
lonema; occasional cells appeared binucleated (Fig. 13). There were numerous mitochondria, abundant free ribosomes, and occasional scattered short cisternae of endoplasmic reticulum. Examination of the *in situ* monolayer from the
same case revealed similar nuclear and cytoplasmic features; however, in this
preparation autophagosomes were apparent and numerous cells contained intracytoplasmic lumina (Fig. 14). The surface cytoplasmic extensions noted in the
cell suspensions appeared more prominent, forming acinar-like arrangements
between adjacent cells (Fig. 15). Moreover, where cells were closely apposed,
desmosomes were prominent (Fig. 15, inset).

Electron microscopy of monolayers obtained from three other cases (105, 107,
and 108) showed features similar to each other; these were in contrast to those of
the monolayers from case 93. The majority of cells were large and spindle-
shaped, with oval nuclei, small nucleoli, and chromatin condensation confined to
the region of the nuclear envelope. Cell surface contact was infrequent, and
desmosomes, intracellular lumina, or microvilli were not observed. Cytoplasmic
features were variable; in some areas there was a paucity of organelles, while
other regions of the same cell were more heterogeneous, with clusters of ribosomes, short cisternae of rough endoplasmic reticulum, scattered mitochondria,
and occasional dense bodies. Particularly striking was a subplasmalemmal net-
work of microfilaments. Examination of an early monolayer cultivated on glass
in one of these cases (105) revealed more irregular nuclear profiles and more
prominent nucleoli (Fig. 16). Although cytoplasmic organelles were essentially
similar to those seen in later cultures, there appeared to be more rough endoplasmic reticulum and numerous lucent degenerative vacuoles. Occasional cells
showed attachment points, but desmosomes were not observed (Fig. 16, inset).

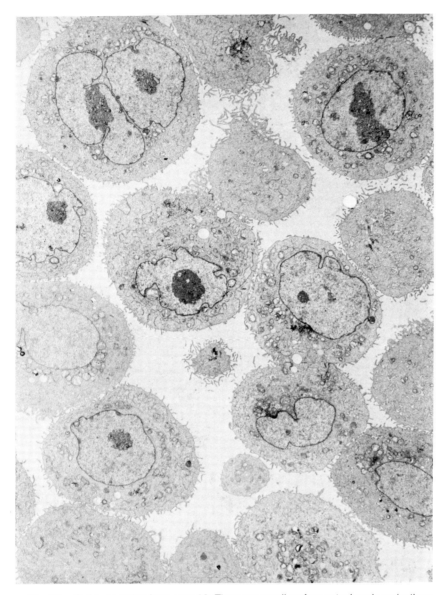

Fig. 12.   Cell suspension from case 93. There are small surface cytoplasmic projections, and many cells have prominent nucleoli. ×2400.

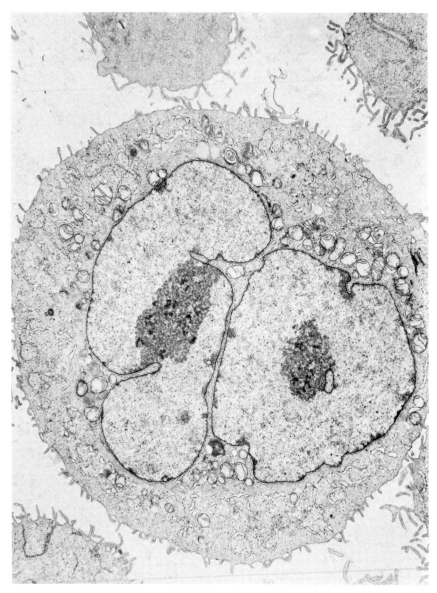

Fig. 13. Detail of binucleate cell resembling a Reed–Sternberg cell seen in Fig. 12. ×5400.

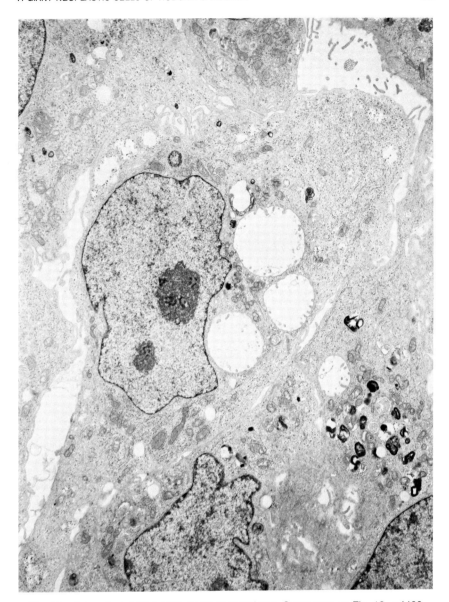

Fig. 14. Intracytoplasmic lumina found in monolayer. Same case as Fig. 12. ×4400.

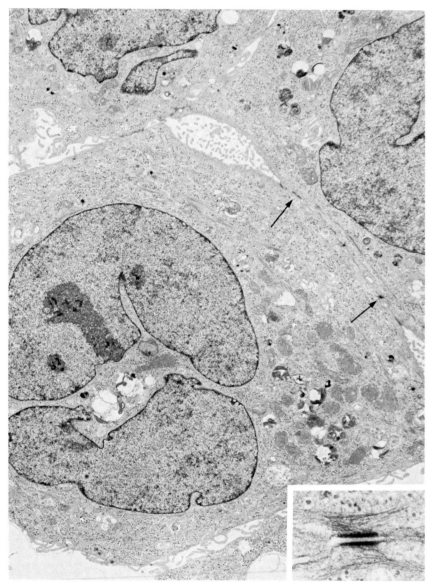

Fig. 15. Surface microvilli forming acinar-type configurations and numerous desmosomes (arrows) between apposing cells. Case 93. ×4600. Inset: Detail of desmosome. ×45,000.

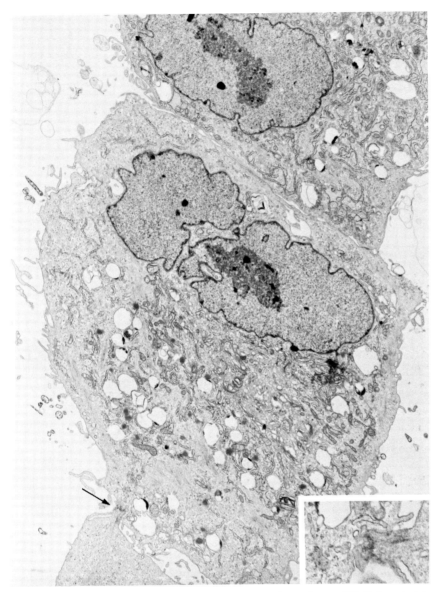

Fig. 16. Irregular nuclei and large nucleoli of early culture of case 105. Cell contact is focal (arrow). ×5000. Inset: Detail of cellular attachment point ×12,500.

D. DNA Synthesis and Mitotic Activity

As previously observed by Kadin and Asbury (30) and by Kaplan and Gartner (31), autoradiographs of cultures incubated with ³H-TdR readily revealed simultaneous labeling of both nuclei of binucleate giant cells (Fig. 17). In case 15, binucleate and multinucleate labeled cells comprised 0.2% (18/809) of all labeled cells. However, there was great variability from one preparation to another; in one preparation, 20.7% of all binucleate and multinucleate cells were labeled (31). When labeled cells were cocultivated overnight with unlabeled cells from the same culture and reexamined by autoradiography, all binucleate cells were either unlabeled or were labeled in both nuclei, indicating that the binucleate cells had developed by endocellular reduplication rather than by cell fusion (31). In contrast to the cultures containing giant cells from involved tissues of patients with Hodgkin's disease, cultures of normal spleen macrophages revealed no incorporation of ³H-TdR into cellular DNA.

Mitotic figures were readily demonstrable in colchicine-treated Hodgkin's cultures. In some instances such mitotic figures were binucleate, indicating that the binucleate cells were indeed capable of nuclear division as well as DNA

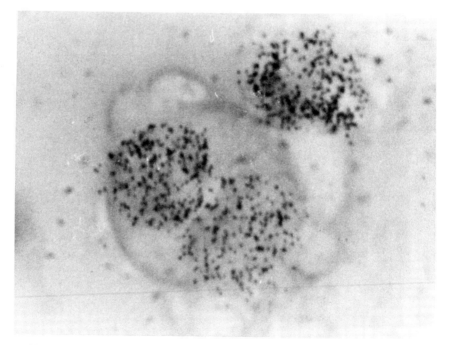

Fig. 17. Autoradiograph of large, round adherent cells from a long-term culture of involved spleen tissue. DNA synthesis, indicated by the incorporation of tritiated thymidine, is evident in a binucleate as well as a large mononuclear cell.

synthesis. Cultures of normal spleen macrophages revealed no mitotic figures (36). It thus appears that the capacity for DNA synthesis and for mitosis are two criteria whereby the Hodgkin's disease giant cell population can be distinguished with reasonable confidence from normal spleen macrophages.

E. Tests for Neoplastic Attributes of the Cultured Cells

1. Cytogenetic Studies

Aneuploidy demonstrable in the early passages of a cell culture is generally accepted as a fundamental attribute of neoplasia (55). Chromosome preparations of the colchicine-treated cells in case 15, examined after 3 weeks in culture, revealed 70 countable mitotic figures, all of which were aneuploid. They included 63 hyperdiploid cells, with a modal chromosome number of 53; 6 hypotetraploid cells, with 77–91 chromosomes; and 1 hyperoctoploid cell, with approximately 190 chromosomes (31). Chromosome studies from several other cultures have also revealed aneuploid cells, usually with hypotetraploid chromosome numbers. However, the total numbers of mitotic figures available for analysis have been relatively small. The permanent cell line established from the cytologically positive pleural effusion of case 93, as mentioned above, revealed mitotic figures with a near-triploid chromosome number and a distinctive long marker chromosome. More detailed analysis of the karyotype of this cell line will be presented elsewhere (55a).

2. Heterotransplantability

Kaplan and Gartner (31) observed successful intracerebral heterotransplants of giant cells from six of eight cases of Hodgkin's disease carried in long-term culture. Since that earlier report, we have observed several additional successful heterotransplants in the nude mouse brain. Histological sections have revealed infiltrates composed of mono-, bi-, and occasionally multinucleate cells extensively invading the brain and sometimes also the meninges. Frozen sections stained by indirect immunofluorescence, using rabbit anti-human spleen serum preabsorbed with mouse spleen and liver, confirmed the human origin of these infiltrating cells. In several instances, including cases 15 and 56, cells recovered from the brains of nude mice were again successfully grown in secondary culture. As indicated above, the secondary culture of case 15 was aborted by a fungal infection, and the secondary culture of case 56 was partially overgrown by spontaneously transformed mouse brain cells which could not readily be distinguished, with respect to size or morphology, from the human cells in these cultures. When cultures of normal human spleen macrophages were similarly inoculated intracerebrally into nude mice, no takes were observed during an observation period of more than 200 days (31).

F. Surface Marker Studies

As previously observed by Kaplan and Gartner (31), the large, round adherent cells in these Hodgkin's disease cultures displayed the capacity to ingest India ink particles. Uptake was delayed, relative to that in normal macrophages, but after 48 hours a high proportion of the presumptive Hodgkin's and Reed–Sternberg cells became labeled with India ink. After excess India ink was washed from the cultures and incubation resumed for several additional days, the cultures were observed to contain a mixture of ink-bearing and ink-free large, round adherent cells; in such cultures, the number of ink-free cells increased slowly but progressively in relation to the number of ink-labeled cells, providing further evidence for the proliferative capacity of the Hodgkin's giant cell population. Kaplan and Gartner (31) observed that nearly all the large, round adherent cells possessed Fc receptors, as indicated by their capacity to form IgG-EA rosettes. Controls showed no capacity to form IgM-EA rosettes. The large, round adherent cell population also displayed the capacity to form IgM-EAC$_{3b}$ rosettes, indicative of the presence of complement receptors. In one culture also tested for the capacity to form IgM-EAC$_{3d}$ rosettes, negative results were obtained. The capacity to form lymphocyte "rosettes" (Fig. 2), a distinctive feature of Reed–Sternberg cells in short-term culture (52), was also observed in some of our long-term cultures. In indirect immunofluorescence tests using antisera directed against human immunoglobulins, none of the cultured Hodgkin's cells revealed the presence of SIg. Tests for the capacity of the cultured cells to form spontaneous E rosettes with sheep erythrocytes were also entirely negative (31). Thus, the cultured giant cells lacked the classic surface marker attributes of either B or T lymphocytes. Nearly all the cultures tested revealed positive staining reactions for nonspecific esterase, an enzyme activity characteristically observed in cells of the monocyte–macrophage lineage.

G. Lysozyme Studies

Supernatant culture fluids assayed by either the lysoplate or radioimmunoassay procedure revealed significantly elevated concentrations of lysozyme in 11 of 19 long-term cultures from involved tissues of patients with Hodgkin's disease, and borderline positive values were obtained in 4 additional instances (58 and 79%, respectively). In contrast, significantly elevated lysozyme concentrations were not observed in any of 18 long-term cultures of non-Hodgkin's lymphomas; and only 5 of 18 (28%) had borderline positive levels. Supernatant culture fluids from eight uninvolved spleens (four Hodgkin's disease, four non-Hodgkin's lymphomas) also revealed none with significantly elevated levels, and four with borderline values. Of the six secondary cultures established from nude mouse brain heterotransplants, two revealed significantly increased lysozyme levels, and three others revealed borderline values. Antigenic analyses indicated, however, that the lysozyme in these instances was primarily of murine origin.

Serum lysozyme levels were measured in 68 patients with Hodgkin's disease, using the lyso-plate assay procedure of Osserman and Lawlor (45). Of these, a total of 31 (45%) revealed lysozyme levels of 11 μg/ml or greater, as compared to the established normal level of 5-10 μg/ml. Elevated serum lysozyme levels were encountered somewhat more often in patients with advanced (stage III or IV) disease (16 of 29, or 55%) than in patients with limited (stage I or II) disease (15 of 39, or 39%).

H. Epstein-Barr Virus Studies

Long-term cultures from 15 cases of Hodgkin's disease were transferred for 24 hours to medium lacking human serum and harvested, and cytocentrifuge preparations were made. These were then examined for the presence of EBNA by the anticomplement fluorescence test (48). In every instance, the giant cells in these cultures were consistently EBNA-negative. This was true even in instances in which the sera of the same patients revealed significantly elevated serum antibody titers to the major EBV antigens, VCA, EA, and/or EBNA. Earlier studies have established that patients with Hodgkin's disease often exhibit significantly elevated serum antibody titers to these EBV antigens (56-59). The fact that the giant cells in our cultures were EBNA-negative is consistent with the report (60) that EBV DNA could not be detected by molecular hybridization in the involved spleens of several patients with Hodgkin's disease.

IV. Discussion

Cell culture techniques offer the attractive possibility of elucidating many of the long-standing enigmas surrounding the biology of Hodgkin's disease. If the identity and the lineage of the neoplastic cell population could be unequivocally established, the functional properties of these cells and their responses to a number of stimuli could be ascertained. This information in turn might explain the progressive lymphocyte depletion observed in patients with advancing disease, their characteristic impairment of cell-mediated immunity, and the frequent occurrence of such atypical manifestations as fever, night sweats, itching, and alcohol-induced pain. However, it is essential that the cell cultures on which such studies are performed satisfy three essential criteria: (1) that they be permanently established cell lines from which one or more single cell clones have been successfully derived, thus eliminating the possibility that mixtures of cells of diverse types might persist in the cultures; (2) that they possess the essential attributes of neoplastic cells in culture, such as aneuploidy and heterotransplantability in nude mice in early passage generations; and (3) that they be unambiguously identifiable as having derived directly from authentic Reed–Sternberg and/or Hodgkin's cells *in vivo*.

Permanent cell lines established from the cultured cells of patients with a diagnosis of Hodgkin's disease have now been reported by several groups of investigators (32–35), and an additional permanent line has been established from the malignant pleural effusion of case 93. However, each of these cell lines is open to serious challenge. Errors or uncertainties in histopathological diagnosis may have been involved in some instances. A particularly instructive example is case 93, in which the presence of a coexistent malignant epithelial neoplasm is strongly suggested by the fact that the cultured cells exhibit the presence of desmosomes in monolayers examined by electron microscopy. Had this culture been examined solely by the usual technique of preparing trypsinized cell suspensions for electron micrographic study, the presence of desmosomes would not have been discovered, and this cell line might well have been accepted as an authentic example of a permanently established Hodgkin's cell line. The two long-term diffusion chamber cultures described by Boecker *et al.* (21) were derived from cytologically positive pleural effusions of patients in whom a diagnosis of Hodgkin's disease had been made. These cells were reported to exhibit positive immunofluorescence staining reactions for SIg, indicative of their origin from B lymphocytes. A later report from the same group (61) indicates that, on subsequent histopathological review, the diagnosis was revised in at least one of these cases to diffuse large-cell (histiocytic) lymphoma rather than Hodgkin's disease. Such an interpretation would be far more consistent with our own cell culture observations, in which diffuse histocytic lymphomas have often revealed B-lymphocyte charactistics (62), whereas the large, round adherent cells of Hodgkin's cultures, as described here, have been consistently SIg-negative. In a recent report by Ben-Bassat *et al.* (63), a permanent cell line with surface marker attributes indicating an origin from T lymphocytes was established in culture. However, although this patient is stated to have had a diagnosis of Hodgkin's disease, many of the clinical features of this case, such as the presence of superior vena caval obstruction syndrome, the rapid recurrence of the mediastinal mass and superior vena caval obstruction following one cycle of mechlorethamine–vincristine–procarbazine–prednisone (MOPP) combination chemotherapy, and the extremely rapid progression to death are far more suggestive of a T-lymphoblastic lymphoma than of Hodgkin's disease.

Still another pitfall is the erroneous identification of a banal B-lymphoblastoid cell line as having been derived from the neoplastic cell population. It is clear that many of the earlier long-term cultures (64–68) were examples of LCL overgrowth of Hodgkin's cultures. A recently described cell line (34) is probably an additional such instance, since it was reportedly EBNA-positive. The presence of binucleate cells is not at all uncommon in B-lymphoblastoid cell lines; such binucleate cells could readily be mistaken for Reed–Sternberg cells.

Another problem is the contamination of cell cultures by extraneous cell lines. Of four permanent cell lines purportedly derived from patients with Hodgkin's disease described by Long *et al.* (32), three have been shown by cytogenetic and other rigorous criteria to have been derived from an owl monkey kidney cell line (69). The fourth of these cell lines, though cytogenetically confirmed as human in origin, apparently came from a spleen which was both grossly and microscopically uninvolved at the time of laparotomy. In this instance, and perhaps also in recent reports of established cell lines, the characteristics of which seem atypical (33,34), the possibility must be entertained of spontaneous transformation of initially normal, nonneoplastic cells during the course of cultivation. Although spontaneous transformation of human cells is rare, relative to its frequency in murine cultures, it might conceivably be more common in the microenvironment provided by cocultivation with Hodgkin's and Reed–Sternberg cells. This possibility is also suggested by our observation of the apparently spontaneous transformation of nude mouse brain cells during cocultivation with the Reed–Sternberg and Hodgkin's cells of case 56.

Thus, it must be concluded that no permanent cloned cell line unambiguously derived from the neoplastic giant cell population of a patient with a verifiable diagnosis of Hodgkin's disease has been established to the present time. This in turn suggests that new culture techniques are needed, and perhaps that a search for specific growth factors required by these neoplastic cells may be helpful in achieving this long-elusive goal.

It is clearly essential that cultured cells be shown to possess the biological attributes of neoplasia. At this time, perhaps the single most reliable criterion is the presence of an aneuploid chromosome constitution in early passages of a culture. It is well established that the B-lymphoblastoid cell lines which not infrequently arise in and overgrow Hodgkin's cultures are initially diploid, though they may become aneuploid during subsequent continuous cultivation (29). In several of our cultures, the colchicine-treated large, round adherent cells were shown to be aneuploid. Hyperdiploid chromosome numbers were observed frequently, and hypotetraploid chromosome numbers, presumably derived from binucleate cells, were also observed with significant frequency. In rare instances, giant hyperoctoploid mitotic figures were seen. Heterotransplantability in immunosuppressed rodents or in the congenitally athymic nude mouse was formerly deemed an equally rigorous criterion of neoplasia and was accepted as such in our earlier studies on permanent cell lines established from a variety of non-Hodgkin's lymphomas (50). However, two groups (70,71) have recently shown that EBV genome-positive, diploid, B-lymphoblastoid cell lines are also capable of successful heterotransplantation into the brains of nude mice. Thus, although heterotransplantability still distinguishes neoplastic cells from normal cells, it is not capable of distinguishing neoplasia from the virus-induced proliferative response of LCLs, which appear to occupy a state intermediate between normalcy and true neoplasia.

EBV is now widely accepted as the major causative agent of infectious mononucleosis (72). Moreover, it appears to have a biologically significant association with at least two human neoplasms, endemic Burkitt's lymphoma and nasopharyngeal carcinoma, as indicated by epidemiological evidence and by the consistent presence of multiple copies of the EBV genome, detectable by molecular hybridization and by the EBNA test, in the DNA of the tumor cells (cf. Ref. 73 for review). Interest in the possibility that EBV might also contribute to the genesis of Hodgkin's disease was stimulated by the observation of cases in which infectious mononucleosis appeared to precede the onset of lymphadenopathy due to Hodgkin's disease (cf. Ref. 5 for review) and by the high titers of serum antibodies to the EBV antigens VCA, EA, and/or EBNA which are frequently observed in patients with Hodgkin's disease (56–59). Several recent epidemiological studies have revealed the occurrence of significantly increased numbers of cases of Hodgkin's disease in populations previously known to have had infectious mononucleosis (74–77). However, our studies have revealed that the large, round adherent cells of long-term cultures were consistently EBNA-negative, as were the cells of two permanently established lines (33,35), clearly indicating that these cells are devoid of EBV genomes. If the cultured cells are indeed the progeny of Reed–Sternberg and Hodgkin's cells, this would constitute evidence that EBV is not directly involved in the etiology of Hodgkin's disease, though prior EBV-induced infectious mononucleosis may well augment susceptibility to the as yet unknown causative agent.

Functional and surface marker studies have made it clear that the large, round adherent cell population of our cultures is not derived from either B or T lymphocytes; instead, these cells appear to have many of the attributes of cells of the mononuclear phagocyte–macrophage lineage. They lack SIg and the capacity to form E rosettes but appear to bear Fc and C' receptors, as indicated by their capacity to form IgG-EA and IgM-EAC$_{3b}$ rosettes, respectively (31,78). They are sluggishly but definitely phagocytic for India ink and are capable of ingesting sheep red blood cells after IgG-EA or IgM-EAC rosette formation. Moreover, their supernatant culture fluids frequently contained significantly elevated levels of lysozyme, an enzyme characteristically secreted into the extracellular environment by the macrophage (79). However, two notes of caution are in order. The first is that these were not cloned cultures derived from permanent cell lines and thus may well have contained variable admixtures of persisting nonproliferative normal cellular elements, such as splenic macrophages, pleural mesothelial cells, and other stromal elements. The second is that the recently developed radioimmunoassay may have made it possible to detect low levels of lysozyme secretion by cell types other than the macrophage; this possibility would perhaps explain the low but apparently significant lysozyme concentrations observed in the supernatant culture fluids of the permanent cell line established from case 93 and in the culture fluids from two of the three clones derived from this cell line, which was shown to form desmosomes and thus is presumably not of macrophage origin.

The variable ultrastructural appearance of the monolayers dramatically illustrates the caution that must be taken in the interpretation of Hodgkin's disease in culture. Initial examination of cell suspensions obtained in case 93 clearly showed nuclear and cytoplasmic features which approximated the ultrastructure of Reed–Sternberg and mononuclear Hodgkin's cells obtained from fresh tissues (11,28). Electron microscopy of monolayers from the same case, obtained at the same passage as the suspensions, however, revealed intracytoplasmic lumina, intercellular acinar-like formation, and unequivocal desmosomes. Although desmosome-like junctions have been described in epithelioid macrophages found in granulomas (80), the morphological features of the monolayers are diagnostic of epithelial cells such as those found in adenocarcinoma (81). It is of interest that in another study cells in monolayers thought to represent Hodgkin's disease were noted to contain surface microvilli and spaces within the cytoplasm recorded as "pseudoacinar spaces" (82). Subsequent ultrastructural examination of the same cell lines obtained from subcutaneous heterotransplants in nude mice has revealed more definite epithelial characteristics including intercellular junctions (69). Our current cultures do not show any features suggesting that they are derived from epithelial cells. Studies are ongoing to examine suspensions from these monolayers and tumors obtained after injection into nude mice, in addition to further study of the monolayers, in order to determine whether more than one structural population exists.

It is clear that no single morphological, surface marker, or functional attribute, or any presently definable combination of attributes, is sufficiently rigorous to permit the unambiguous identification of a giant cell in culture as having derived from a Reed–Sternberg or Hodgkin's cell. The recent successful development by two of us (83) of a technique for the establishment of human–human hybridomas producing monoclonal antibodies with predefined antigenic specificity may make it possible to generate human monoclonal antibodies against distinctive cell membrane antigens of the neoplastic giant cells of Hodgkin's disease. With the aid of such monospecific antibodies, it may be possible to demonstrate that these distinctive cell membrane antigens are shared by the large, round adherent cells of the cultures described in this report. If clonable permanent cell lines thus identifiable as authentic progeny of Reed–Sternberg and Hodgkin's cells can be obtained, they will undoubtedly contribute significantly to our understanding of the biology and immunology of this curious neoplastic disease and perhaps also to its therapeutic conquest.

Added in Proof: As this article was being completed, a paper appeared (84) concerning two cell lines (one of which died out after 7 months) from the malignant pleural effusions of two patients with Hodgkin's disease. Both were aneuploid and hyperdiploid, heterotransplantable, bore Ia-like antigens, formed rosettes with T lymphocytes, and were positive for α-naphthyl acetate esterase and acid

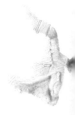

phosphatase. They lacked cytoplasmic or surface membrane light or heavy chains, lysozyme, immunophagocytic activity, and the capacity to form E, IgG-EA, or IgM-EAC rosettes. Further studies on the remaining cell line, L428, will be awaited with interest.

Acknowledgments

Suzanne Gartner, Nancy Pleibel, and Jean Lee provided invaluable assistance with the cell cultures and heterotransplantation studies. Darlene Whitney and Betty Talton provided expert technical assistance with the electron micrographic preparations. Marcia Bieber and Roger Warnke very kindly performed certain of the surface marker and indirect immunofluorescence studies, and Vincent P. Butler, Doris Tse Eng, and Joanna Shyong carried out the lysozyme assays. Ronald F. Dorfman and his staff reviewed all the surgical pathology and effusion cytology material.

These studies were supported by research contracts NO1-CP-43228, NO1-CP-91044, and NO1-CP-33272 and by grants CA-05838, CA-10372, and CA-21112 from the National Cancer Institute, National Institutes of Health, and by gifts from the Joseph Luetje and Jerry M. Tenney Memorial Funds for Lymphoma Research. Lennart Olsson was supported by a Danish Medical Research Council Postdoctoral Fellowship and by a grant from the Elizabeth Naumann Research Scholar Fund.

References

1. H. Rappaport, "Atlas of Tumor Pathology," Sect. III, Fasc. 8. Armed Forces Institute of Pathology, Washington, D.C., 1966.
2. R. J. Lukes, B. H. Tindle, and J. W. Parker, *Lancet* **2**, 1003 (1969).
3. S. B. Strum, J. K. Park, and H. Rappaport, *Cancer* **26**, 176 (1970).
4. G. S. F. Seif and A. I. Spriggs, *J. Natl. Cancer Inst.* **39**, 557 (1967).
5. H. S. Kaplan, "Hodgkin's Disease," 2nd ed. Harvard Univ. Press, Cambridge, Massachusetts, 1980.
6. A. M. Marmont and E. E. Damasio, *Blood* **29**, 1 (1967).
7. M. J. Peckham and E. H. Cooper, *Cancer* **24**, 135 (1969).
8. M. J. Peckham, *Br. J. Cancer* **28**, 332 (1973).
9. L. M. Schiffer, *Natl. Cancer Inst. Monogr.* **36**, 191 (1973).
10. M. Marinello, G. Tkachenko, J. Gavilondo, and B. Baeza, *Neoplasma* **22**, 185 (1975).
11. I. Carr, *J. Pathol.* **115**, 45 (1975).
12. M. Friedman, U. Kim, K. Shimaoka, A. Panahon, T. Han, and L. Stutzman, *Cancer* **45**, 1653 (1980).
13. G. A. Ackerman, R. A. Knouff, and H. A. Hoster, *J. Natl. Cancer Inst.* **12**, 465 (1951).
14. R. F. Dorfman, *Nature (London)* **190**, 915 (1961).
15. S. E. Order and S. Hellman, *Lancet* **1**, 573 (1972).
16. R. J. Lukes and R. D. Collins, *Cancer* **34**, 1488 (1974).
17. M. Biniaminov and B. Ramot, *Lancet* **1**, 368 (1974).
18. J. Leech, *Lancet* **1**, 265 (1973).
19. A. J. Garvin, S. S. Spicer, R. T. Parmley, and A. M. Munster, *J. Exp. Med.* **139**, 1077 (1974).
20. M. E. Kadin, S. R. Newcom, S. B. Gold, and D. P. Stites, *Lancet* **2**, 167 (1974).
21. W. R. Boecker, D. K. Hossfield, W. M. Gallmeier, and C. G. Schmidt, *Nature (London)* **258**, 235 (1975).
22. C. R. Taylor, *Eur. J. Cancer* **12**, 61 (1976).
23. T. O. Landaas, T. Godal, and T. B. Halvorsen, *Int. J. Cancer* **20**, 717 (1977).

24. S. Poppema, J. D. Elema, and M. R. Halie, *Cancer* **42**, 1793 (1978).
25. M. E. Kadin, D. P. Stites, R. Levy, and R. Warnke, *N. Engl. J. Med.* **299**, 1208 (1978).
26. P. J. Gearhart, N. H. Sigal, and N. R. Klinman, *Proc. Natl. Acad. Sci. U.S.A.* **72**, 1707 (1975).
27. P. Isaacson, *J. Clin. Pathol.* **32**, 802 (1979).
28. R. F. Dorfman, D. F. Rice, A. D. Mitchell, R. L. Kempson, and G. Levine, *Natl. Cancer Inst. Monogr.* **36**, 221 (1973).
29. K. Nilsson and J. Pontén, *Int. J. Cancer* **15**, 321 (1975).
30. M. E. Kadin and A. K. Asbury, *Lab. Invest.* **28**, 181 (1973).
31. H. S. Kaplan and S. Gartner, *Int. J. Cancer* **19**, 511 (1977).
32. J. C. Long, P. C. Zamecnik, A. C. Aisenberg, and L. Atkins, *J. Exp. Med.* **145**, 1484 (1977).
33. A. N. Roberts, K. L. Smith, B. L. Dowell, and A. K. Hubbard, *Cancer Res.* **38**, 3033 (1978).
34. C. Friend, W. Marovitz, G. Henle, W. Henle, D. Tsuel, K. Hirschhorn, J. G. Holland, and J. Cuttner, *Cancer Res.* **38**, 2581 (1978).
35. M. Schaadt, C. Fonatsch, H. Kirchner, and V. Diehl, *Blut* **38**, 185 (1979).
36. A. J. Treves, M. Feldman, and H. S. Kaplan, *J. Immunol. Methods* **13**, 279 (1976).
37. M. Rabinovitch and M. De Stefano, *J. Cell. Physiol.* **85**, 189 (1975).
38. R. M. Blaese, J. J. Oppenheim, R. C. Seeger, and T. A. Waldmann, *Cell. Immunol.* **4**, 228 (1972).
39. L. T. Yam, C. Y. Li, and W. H. Crosby, *Am. J. Clin. Pathol.* **55**, 283 (1971).
40. E. Rabellino, S. Colon, H. M. Grey, and E. R. Unanue, *J. Exp. Med.* **133**, 156 (1971).
41. Z. Bentwich, S. D. Douglas, F. P. Siegal, and H. G. Kunkel, *Clin. Immunol. Immunopathol.* **1**, 511 (1973).
42. H. Huber, M. J. Polky, W. D. Linscott, H. H. Fudenberg, and H. J. Müller-Eberhard, *Science* **162**, 1281 (1968).
43. E. S. Jaffe, E. M. Shevach, M. M. Frank, C. W. Berard, and I. Green, *N. Engl. J. Med.* **290**, 813 (1974).
44. F. M. Griffin, Jr., C. Bianco, and S. C. Silverstein, *J. Exp. Med.* **141**, 1269 (1975).
45. E. F. Osserman and D. P. Lawlor, *J. Exp. Med.* **124**, 921 (1966).
46. G. Henle and W. Henle, *Cancer Res.* **27**, 2442 (1967).
47. G. Henle, W. Henle, and G. Klein, *Int. J. Cancer* **8**, 272 (1971).
48. B. Reedman and G. Klein, *Int. J. Cancer* **11**, 99 (1973).
49. G. Rocchi, J. Hewetson, and W. Henle, *Int. J. Cancer* **11**, 637 (1973).
50. A. L. Epstein, M. M. Herman, H. Kim, R. F. Dorfman, and H. S. Kaplan, *Cancer* **37**, 2158 (1976).
51. A. Böyum, *Scand. J. Clin. Lab. Invest.* **21**, Suppl. 97, 77 (1968).
52. A. E. Stuart, A. R. W. Williams, and J. A. Habeshaw, *J. Pathol.* **122**, 81 (1977).
53. H. R. Hulett, W. A. Bonner, J. Barrett, and L. A. Herzenberg, *Science* **166**, 747 (1969).
54. H. S. Kaplan, *Cancer* **45**, 2439 (1980).
55. A. L. Epstein and H. S. Kaplan, *Cancer* **34**, 1851 (1974).
55a. B. Kaiser-McCaw, F. Hecht, J. Lee, and H. S. Kaplan, in preparation.
56. B. Johansson, G. Klein, W. Henle, and G. Henle, *Int. J. Cancer* **6**, 450 (1970).
57. P. H. Levine, D. V. Ablashi, C. W. Berard, P. P. Carbone, D. E. Waggoner, and L. Malan, *Cancer* **27**, 416 (1971).
58. W. Henle and G. Henle, *Natl. Cancer Inst. Monogr.* **36**, 79 (1973).
59. G. Rocchi, G. Tosato, G. Papa, and G. Ragona, *Int. J. Cancer* **16**, 323 (1975).
60. M. Nonoyama, Y. Kawai, C. H. Huang, J. S. Pagano, Y. Hirshaut, and P. H. Levine, *Cancer Res.* **34**, 1228 (1974).
61. W. M. Gallmeier, W. R. Boecker, U. Bruntsch, D. K. Hossfeld, and C. G. Schmidt, *Haematol. Blood Transfus.* **20**, 277 (1977).
62. A. L. Epstein, R. Levy, H. Kim, W. Henle, G. Henle, and H. S. Kaplan, *Cancer* **42**, 2379 (1978).

63. H. Ben-Bassat, S. Mitrani-Rosenbaum, H. Gamliel, E. Naparstek, R. Leizerowitz, A. Korkesh, M. Sagi, R. Voss, G. Kohn, and A. Polliack, *Int. J. Cancer* **25**, 583 (1980).
64. J. A. Sykes, L. Dmochowski, C. C. Shullenberger, and C. D. Howe, *Cancer Res.* **22**, 21 (1962).
65. J. Pontén, *Int. J. Cancer* **2**, 311 (1967).
66. Y. Ito, O. Shiratori, S. Kurita, T. Takahashi, Y. Kurita, and K. Ota, *J. Natl. Cancer Inst.* **41**, 1367 (1968).
67. T. Tsubota, *Acta Haematol. Jpn.* **35**, 156 (1972).
68. R. A. Adams, G. E. Foley, S. Farber, E. E. Hellerstein, and L. Pothier, *Birth Defects, Orig. Artic. Ser.* **9**, 200 (1973).
69. N. L. Harris, D. L. Gang, S. C. Quay, S. Poppema, W. A. Nelson-Rees, and S. J. O'Brien, *Nature (London)* **289**, 228 (1981).
70. B. Giovanella, K. Nilsson, L. Zech, D. Yim, G. Klein, and J. S. Stehlin, *Int. J. Cancer* **24**, 103 (1979).
71. M. Schaadt, H. Kirchner, C. Fonatsch, and V. Diehl, *Int. J. Cancer* **23**, 751 (1979).
72. G. Henle, W. Henle, and V. Diehl, *Proc. Natl. Acad. Sci. U.S.A.* **59**, 94 (1968).
73. M. A. Epstein and B. G. Achong, eds., "The Epstein-Barr Virus." Springer-Verlag, Berlin and New York, 1979.
74. R. R. Connelly and B. W. Christine, *Cancer Res.* **34**, 1172 (1974).
75. N. Rosdahl, S. O. Larsen, and J. Clemmesen, *Br. Med. J.* **2**, 253 (1974).
76. N. Muñoz, R. J. Davidson, B. Witthoff, J. E. Ericsson, and G. de Thé, *Int. J. Cancer* **22**, 10 (1978).
77. G. Kvale, E. A. Hoiby, and E. Pedersen, *Int. J. Cancer* **23**, 593 (1979).
78. S. V. Payne, D. G. Newell, D. B. Jones, and D. H. Wright, *Am. J. Pathol.* **100**, 7 (1980).
79. Z. A. Cohn and B. Benson, *J. Exp. Med.* **121**, 153 (1965).
80. B. MacKay, *Ultrastruct. Pathol.* **1**, 67 (1980).
81. F. Gyorkey, K. W. Min, I. Krisko, and P. Gyorkey, *Hum. Pathol* **6**, 421 (1975).
82. D. L. Gang, J. C. Long, P. C. Zamecnik, S. Y. Chi, and A. M. Dvorak, *Cancer* **44**, 543 (1979).
83. L. Olsson and H. S. Kaplan, *Proc. Natl. Acad. Sci. U.S.A.* **77**, 5429 (1980).
84. M. Schaadt, V. Diehl, H. Stein, C. Fonatsch, and H. H. Kirchner, *Int. J. Cancer* **26**, 723 (1980).

2

Phenotypic Characterization and Induced Differentiation of Established Human Non-Hodgkin Lymphoma Cell Lines

KENNETH NILSSON

I. Introduction

During the last decade numerous attempts have been made to establish continuous cell lines from explanted human malignant lymphoma biopsies. As a rule, however, these attempts have met with little success, the exception being Burkitt's lymphoma (BL) (1). To date only a limited number of cell lines, which will be described in the following discussion, are available for the analysis of phenotypic properties.

MALIGNANT LYMPHOMAS

35

The reasons for the lack of success with human lymphoma *in vitro* cultivation seem to be twofold. First, the standard tissue culture conditions do not supply the demands of the lymphoma cells for special nutrient factors and/or specific hormonal growth factors. This is best exemplified by the individually distinct nutritional requirements of the SU-DHL lines demonstrated by Epstein and Kaplan (2) and by the T-cell growth factor (TCGF) dependency of mycosis fungoides biopsies observed by Gallo and co-workers (3). It is probably significant in this context that most non-BL cell lines were derived from pleural effusions of unusually malignant cases of lymphoma, as the pleural effusion may be regarded as an *in vivo* tissue culture in which lymphoma cells have adapted and/or selected to grow. BL cells, in contrast, are less strict in their medium requirements and can be established with comparative ease (Table I), both in simple media such as Eagles' minimal essential medium (MEM) and richer media, e.g., RPMI-1640.

The second difficulty encountered in attempts to establish human lymphoma cell lines is the overgrowth of Epstein–Barr virus (EBV)-carrying lymphoblastoid cell lines (LCL) of nonneoplastic origin. Such lines, which grow out at a particularly high frequency from biopsies of Hodgkin's lymphoma (Table I), usually have a selective growth advantage and eventually overgrow the lymphoma cells and become predominant in the cultures (7). There seems to be some EBV-associated property of LCL cells which makes them particularly well adapted to the conventional tissue culture medium, as EBV-carrying BL lines easily become established *in vitro,* and particularly since EBV conversion of EBV genome-negative lymphoma lines *in vitro* makes them require less medium and serum supplementation (8).

This article will deal only with the phenotypic characteristics of non-Hodgkin lymphoma cell lines, as the properties of Hodgkin lymphoma cell lines are

TABLE I

Frequency of Establishment of Human Lymphoma Cell Lines

| | | Established cell lines | | | | |
| | | Lymphoblastoid lines | | Tumor cell lines | | |
Type of biopsy	Number of biopsies	No.	Percent	No.	Percent	Reference
Burkitt's lymphoma	46	2	4	24	52	1
Burkitt's lymphoma	47	0	0	34	72	4
Lymphocytic lymphoma	26	9	35	2	8	1
Histiocytic lymphoma	19	1	5	1	5	1
Histiocytic lymphoma	10	0	0	10	100	5,6
Hodgkin's disease	41	35	85	0	0	1

described elsewhere in this volume (9). It will particularly emphasize (1) the phenotypic heterogeneity encountered within cell lines originating from each histopathological entity [Rappaport's classification (10)], and (2) that human lymphoma cells do not always seem to be irreversibly arrested at a particular stage of differentiation, as exemplified by the inducible differentiation in the U-937 histiocytic cell line.

II. Phenotypic Properties of Nonneoplastic Epstein–Barr Virus-Carrying Lymphoblastoid Cell Lines

Lymphoblastoid cell lines become established from both normal blood and lymphoid tissue from various types of hematopoietic malignancies. With a special grid organ culture, the Spongostan grid technique (11), the frequency of established LCLs from malignant lymphomas varies from 85% in Hodgkin's disease to 4% in BL (Table I). These cell lines have polyclonal derivation, a normal karyotype, and characteristic morphological, functional, and surface membrane properties. The defining features of an LCL are summarized in Table II.

Lymphoblastoid cell lines are derived from EBV-carrying precursor B cells present among the tumor cells in explants from EBV-seropositive individuals. It is possible that polyclonal LCLs are derived not only by the direct outgrowth of B cells, latently infected by EBV *in vivo,* but also from B cells infected *in vitro* by EBV liberated from *in vivo* infected B cells which undergo a lytic EBV producer cycle *in vitro* as demonstrated by Epstein and co-workers (17).

TABLE II

Characteristics of Lymphoblastoid Cell Lines

Defining features of newly established lines[a]	Reference
Presence of the EBV genome	7
Typical morphology	7
Polyclonal derivation	12
Diploid karyotype	13,14
Typical surface glycoprotein profile	15
Lack of tumorigenic potential subcutaneously in nude mice	16

[a] It is urgent that characterization of cell lines derived from biopsies of EBV-seropositive donors be done shortly after their establishment, since LCL-type cell lines will become monoclonal, aneuploid, or even tumorigenic subcutaneously in nude mice after prolonged *in vitro* culture (usually >6 months). The only stable markers are the presence of the EBV genome and the basic surface glycoprotein profile (15).

The mere fact that EBV may be released into the culture medium when lymphoma biopsies are explanted *in vitro* from EBV cell-positive patients may also be a prerequisite for the establishment of EBV-carrying truly neoplastic non-BL lymphoma lines from EBV genome-negative lymphoma biopsies (Section III,B).

III. Phenotypic Heterogeneity of Human Lymphoma Cell Lines

A. Burkitt's Lymphoma Cell Lines

More than 100 BL cell lines have been established during the last 15 years. The vast majority of these lines are EBV-positive, but a minority of the African and non-African BLs (five biopsies) have yielded EBV-negative lymphoid cell lines.

With few exceptions (LCL) Table I), BL-derived cell lines originate from the monoclonal tumor cell population as shown by comparative studies on tumor biopsy cells and derived cell lines using glucose-6-phosphate dehydrogenase (G-6-PD) isoenzymes and pattern of immunoglobulin production as markers (12,18). The neoplastic nature of the BL lines is also demonstrated by their cytogenetic characteristics (Table III) and biological behavior *in vitro* and *in vivo*. The majority of BL cell lines, as well as BL biopsy cells, have a very characteristic and probably reciprocal translocation of a fragment of one chromosome 8 to the long arm of one chromosome 14 (Table III) (13,19,20). Some BL lines have been shown to have alternative cytogenetic markers [t(2;8) and t(8;22)] (21). Burkitt's lymphoma lines usually form colonies in agarose and will grow as progressively growing tumors when explanted subcutaneously into nude mice (16).

TABLE III

Cytogenetic Markers in Human Lymphoma Cell Lines

Cell line[a]	Model chromosome number	Common marker chromosome
Burkitt's lymphoma (EBV+)	46–53	t(8;14), t(8;22), t(2;8)
Burkitt's lymphoma (EBV−)	45–46	t(8;14), t(8;22)
Lymphocytic lymphoma	46–52	t(8;14)
		14q+, +7, +8
Histiocytic lymphoma	43–79	14q+, +8, 6q−

[a] The lines have been designated according to the histopathological diagnosis (Rappaport's classification) of the tumor biopsy from which they originated.

1. Epstein–Barr Virus Genome-Carrying Burkitt Lymphoma Cell Lines

These cell lines have individually characteristic phenotypes but share some basic properties (for a detailed review, see Ref. 1). The cells are round and have a villous surface. The ultrastructural features are similar to those of resting lymphocytes. Studies on their dynamic morphology by time-lapse cinematography have revealed a very restricted capacity of these BL cells for translocation. In accordance with this BL cells stain comparatively faintly for actin by immunofluorescence and attach poorly to feeder cells (22). They usually grow as small, loose clumps in suspension, but rare lines adhere strongly to plastic or feeder cells, and some BL lines grow as single-cell suspensions.

With respect to surface characteristics heterogeneity was found in the expression of C3, Fc, and EBV receptors, common acute lymphoblastic leukemia (cALL) antigen, β_2-microglobulin, and human leukocyte antigen (HLA). All lines examined, however, have been highly agglutinable with concanavalin A (Con A) and have had a characteristic surface glycoprotein pattern as studied by galactose oxidase–tritiated NaB^3H_4 labeling, with two pairs of glycoproteins with apparent molecular weights of 69K and 71K, and 87K and 85K, respectively, as markers (gp69/71 and gp87/85). With very few exceptions BL lines express surface IgM but never IgD. Functionally BL cell lines have also displayed some heterogeneity. Analyses with respect to immunoglobulin production have shown that the majority of these lines, like small, resting B lymphocytes, produce surface immunoglobulins but fail to express cytoplasmic or secretory immunoglobulins. However, a few BL lines seem to represent more (e.g., Seraphina) or less (e.g., Raji) advanced stages of B-lymphoid differentiation.

2. Epstein–Barr Virus Genome-Negative Burkitt's Lymphoma Lines

The number of such cell lines is still so small that the results from phenotypic studies do not allow any general conclusions about the possible biological differences between them and EBV genome-positive BL lines. However, the same heterogeneity in growth properties, surface markers, functional characteristics, and tumorigenicity as that found for EBV genome-positive BL lines have been encountered in the few lines examined (Table IV).

It is notable that two of the lines (BJAB and JBL), although both aneuploid, lack the chromosome 14 marker (14q+). Compared to common BL cell lines EBV genome-negative BL lines have been difficult to establish, and the two tested lines (BJAB and Ramos) grow poorly at low concentrations of serum.

B. Lymphocytic Lymphoma Cell Lines

To date a few laboratories have reported the successful long-term cultivation of authentic tumor lines from patients with lymphocytic lymphoma (LL) (29–

TABLE IV

Characteristics of Epstein-Barr Virus Genome-Negative Burkitt's Lymphoma Lines

Characteristic	Cell line[a]				
	BJAB (16,23,24)	Ramos (13,16,25)	SU-AmB-1 (20,26)	JBL (27)	DG-75 (15,28)
Establishment	Slow, 8 weeks	Like BL (EBV+)	Feeder cells used	Slow, 8 weeks	Slow, 6 weeks
Growth in low serum concentration	Poor	Poor	Poor	NT	NT
Lymphocyte surface markers					
SmIg	IgM κ	IgM λ	IgM λ	IgM λ	IgM κ
Fc receptor (EA)	(+)	NT	–	+	NT
Fc receptor (aggr. Ig)	NT	(+)	(+)	NT	NT
C3 receptor (EAC)	+	+	–	+	–
SRBC receptor	–	–	–	–	–
EBV receptor	+	+	–	NT	–
Tumorigenicity (in nude mice)	+	+	+	+[b]	–
Chromosome 14q marker	–	+	+	–	+
BL (EBV+) surface glycoprotein pattern	–	+	NT	NT	+

[a] NT, not tested.
[b] Tumorigenic in hamsters.

36). In almost all cases the LL cell lines were established from pleural effusions of patients with advanced and therapy-resistant disease.

All tested lines have been aneuploid, with the chromosome 14q+ marker present in most cases (13,31–34) (Table III). However, the origin of the 14q+ marker in LL seems not to be identical to that in EBV-positive BL lines. The neoplastic nature of the lines is also proven by their monoclonal immunoglobulin production and by their capacity to form colonies in agar *in vitro* and tumors subcutaneously in nude mice.

With few exceptions LL lines have been found to be EBV genome-negative. The initial latent period before the explanted cells assumed logarithmic growth was variable. Some of the lines (e.g., K-LL-3) (33) became established without a lag phase, while in most cases 6–10 weeks elapsed before tumor cell proliferation was noted. In some cases feeder cells were required for sustained growth during a variable period after establishment. The growth rate was highly variable, and the population doubling time was usually longer than for BL lines (36–72 hours).

The morphology is always different from that of the prototype nonneoplastic LCL type of cell line and is basically similar to that described above for BL lines (uniform, mostly round, fairly immobile cells with ultrastructural features reminiscent of resting B lymphocytes). However, the morphology of each line represents a variation on this theme and is individually distinct. Also, with respect to surface characteristics a marked variability is found among the different LL lines. With one exception [K-LL-3 (33)] the lines express surface immunoglobulins. Most lines produce IgM, but IgG (30,32,35), IgD (29), and IgA (29,35) synthesis is also found. Thus LL lines seem to represent a stage of B-lymphocyte differentiation roughly corresponding to that of unstimulated B lymphocytes. Most, but not all, lines have C3 receptors, but only a few (e.g., U-715) have Fc receptors. All lines have HLA-DR. The two lines examined for surface glycoprotein pattern (U-698 and U-715) had the characteristic marker glycoproteins of BL (gp69/71 and gp85/87) (15). The expression of cALL antigen was variable (37).

A few EBV-carrying cell lines with phenotypic properties suggestive of a true malignant derivation have been established from patients with LL (30,34,35). These cell lines, when critically examined in early *in vitro* passages for the defining (Table II) and other common LCL features, were found to be unique and different from prototype LCLs. Many (34) had the 14q+ chromosome marker, only exceptionally present in secondarily chromosomally altered LCLs (38). In some cases even the presence of the same marker chromosome as in the *in vivo* tumor cells was demonstrated (34). However, the tumor biopsy cells were EBNA-negative. There seem to be a few possible explanations for this unexpected finding, as cross-contamination *in vitro* could be ruled out:

1. The lines are after all secondarily altered LCLs. Particularly because of the chromosomal findings, discussed above, this is a far-fetched explanation.

2. A very small minority of the lymphoma cells may have been EBV-carrying *in vivo* and escaped detection in the EBNA test. This is also unlikely since the tumors, as expected, seemed to be monoclonal as judged from karyotypic analyses and immunoglobulin phenotypes. In monoclonal BL *all* cells contain EBV genomes, and there is no reason to suspect a different situation in monoclonal LL.

3. The *in vivo* tumor cells may have carried EBV receptors and become infected *in vitro* by EBV liberated from contaminating EBV-carrying nonneo-plastic B cells. This cannot be critically excluded, since the conversion of EBV genome-negative lymphoma cells to an EBV carrier state *in vitro,* which was followed by improved growth, has been amply demonstrated (8). Although not proven, it is thus possible that some EBV-positive lines derived from LLs may be authentic tumor cells which picked up EBV *in vitro.*

C. Histiocytic Lymphoma Cell Lines

With the use of special and time-consuming tissue culture techniques which define the nutrient requirements for each individual tumor it has been possible to establish a panel of 12 lymphoma cell lines (SU-DHL-1–12) at a frequency approaching 100% from histiocytic lymphomas (HLs) (20). In addition to this two other HL lines have been reported (39,40). As the frequency of establishment of SU-DHL lines was so high, they may be regarded as representative of diffuse HL in general, and the phenotypic variation within this group of lines thus provides a good illustration of the biological heterogeneity of large-cell lym-phomas.

The features of the HL lines have recently been detailed (2,5,6,20,39–45). All HL lines are EBV genome-negative, aneuploid (Table III), and tumorigenic intracerebrally in nude mice, all features being consistent with a malignant deri-vation. On the basis of studies on morphology, growth properties, and functional (Table V) and surface characteristics (Tables V and VI and Fig. 1) three major categories of HL cell lines can be defined:

1. True histiocytic HL cell lines represented thus far only by the U-937 cell line (39). This cell line is of unequivocal monocytic origin as evidenced by its morphology, expression of myelomonocytic lysosomal enzyme profile, surface marker characteristics, surface glycoprotein pattern, and functional prop-erties [capacity for phagocytosis and lysozyme secretion, and activity as an effector cell in antibody-dependent cellular cytotoxicity (ADCC) (Tables V and VI and Fig. 1)]. (See also Section IV.)

2. Histiocytic lymphoma cell lines with lymphoid phenotypes (20). Most of these lines express surface immunoglobulins (SU-DHL-3–7 and -10–12) and must thus be classified as B-lymphoid cells. In accordance with this, SU-DHL-4, -5, and -7 express HLA-DR and *Helix pomatia* A (HP)-binding surface glycopro-

TABLE V

Some Phenotypic Characteristics of Epstein–Barr Virus Genome-Negative Human Histiocytic Lymphoma Cell Lines

Designation of cell line	Surface markers (% positive cells)				Phagocytosis, *Candida*	Lysozyme secretion	Cytochemical phenotype	Activity in ADCC assay	Reference
	SmIg	CR	FcR	SRBC					
U-937	0	29	31	0	(+)	+	Monocyte-like	+	(39,46,47)
SKW-4	>90	72	4	0	(+)	−	Nonspecific	−	(40)
SU-DHL-2	0	10	13	0	+	−	Monocyte-like	−	(25,15,20)
SU-DHL-4	>90	2	0	0	−	−	Nonspecific	−	(6,20)
SU-DHL-5	>90	1	2	0	−	−	Nonspecific	−	(6,20)
SU-DHL-7	>90	0	80	0	−	−	Nonspecific	−	(6,20)
SU-DHL-9	0	0	0	0	−	−	Nonspecific	−	(6,20)

TABLE VI

Expression of HP-Binding Surface Glycoproteins and HLA-DR and Common Acute Lymphocytic Leukemia Antigens in Human Histiocytic Lymphoma Cell Lines[a]

Designation of cell line	Major HP-binding surface glycoprotein			HLA-DR		cALL antigen
	210K	150K	75K	Immunofluorescence	Immunoprecipitation	
U-937	−	−	−	+	+	−
SKW-4	−	−	+	+	+	−
SU-DHL-2	(+)	−	+	−	−	−
SU-DHL-4	+	(+)	−	+	+	−
SU-DHL-5	+	−	−	+	+	−
SU-DHL-7	+	−	−	+	+	−
SU-DHL-9	−	+	−	+	+	+

[a] Adapted from ref. (45).

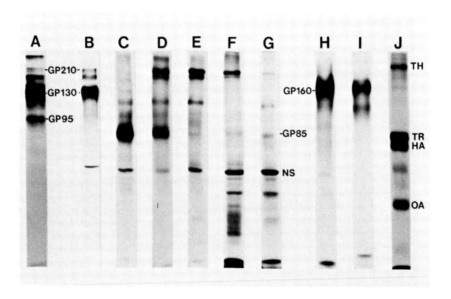

Fig. 1. Fluorography patterns of labeled surface glycoproteins of human blood monocytes (A), HL line U-937 (B), HL line SKW-4 (C), HL line SU-DHL-2 (D), HL line SU-DHL-4 (E), HL line SU-DHL-7 (F), LH line SU-DHL-9 (G), myeloid leukemia line HL-60 (H), normal blood granulocytes (I), and ^{14}C-labeled standard marker proteins: TH, Thyroglobulin (MW 210K); TR, transferrin (MW 85K); HA, human albumin (MW 68K); OA, ovalbumin (MW 43K) (J) (see ref. 43).

teins (gp210) (Table VI) similar to that of B-lymphoblastoid cells (45). Two
"lymphoid" HL cell lines (SU-DHL-8 and -9) have a non-T non-B surface
marker phenotype (Table V and Fig. 1) and, interestingly, SU-DHL-9 expresses
HLA-DR and the cAAL antigen of Greaves (45) (Table VI). The finding of an
HP-binding glycoprotein of 150K molecular weight in SU-DHL-9 (Table VI) was
unique among HL cell lines. An HP-binding glycoprotein of the same apparent
molecular weight has so far been detected only in T lymphocytes and chronic
lymphocytic leukemia (CLL) cells (48).

3. Essentially undefined HL cell lines (SU-DHL-1 and -2) with some features
(phagocytic and nonspecific esterase activity) suggestive of monocytic origin.
Important monocytic markers such as lysozyme production, effector cell activity
in ADCC (Table V), and the expression of characteristic surface glycoproteins
(Fig. 1) and HLA-DR are lacking in SU-DHL-2. (SU-DHL-1 has not been
examined.)

IV. Inducible Differentiation in a True Histiocytic Lymphoma Cell Line (U-937)

Like lymphoma cells *in vivo*, cell lines in general appear to be arrested at a
particular stage of differentiation (49). Attempts to induce differentiation with
mitogens have been essentially unsuccessful. However, recently inducible differentiation *in vitro* has been demonstrated for the U-937 HL cell line using
12-tetradecanoyl-phorbol 13-acetate (TPA) or the supernatant from mixed lymphocyte cultures (MLCs) (44,50) as an inducer.

TABLE VII

Phenotypic Changes in U-937 Cells after Exposure to TPA or Mixed Lymphocyte Culture Supernatant[a]

Characteristic
Morphological maturation
Increased content of nonspecific esterase (NASDAE, ANAE); decrease in peroxidase
Increased expression of Fc receptors
Increased expression of HLA-DR, β_2-microglobulin, and HLA
Specific changes in the surface glycoprotein pattern (altered glucosylation?)
Decreased sensitivity to NK cells
Increased activity as effector cell in ADCC
Increased phagocytic activity
Increased secretion of lysozyme
Concomitant inhibition of growth and DNA synthesis

[a] Adapted from ref. (44).

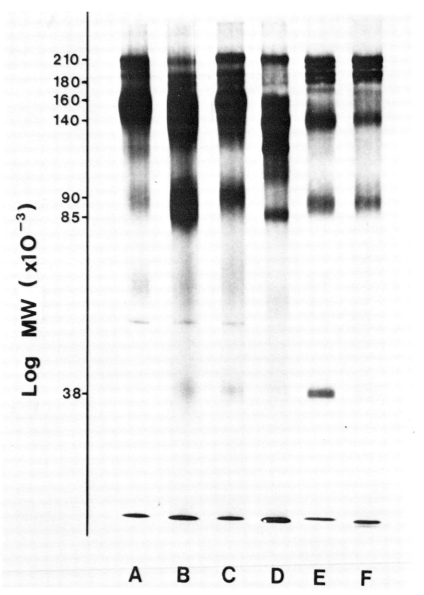

Fig. 2. Fluorography patterns of labeled surface glycoprotein obtained by SDS slab gel electrophoresis. Gel concentration 7.5%. (A) Untreated U-937 cells, (B) TPA-treated U-937 cells, (C) MLC supernatant-treated U-937, (D) untreated blood monocytes, (E) TPA-treated blood monocytes, (F) MLC supernatant-treated blood monocytes. Molecular weights calculated on the basis of the following markers: myosin (200K), phosphorylase a (100K), albumin (66K), and ovalbumin (43K) (see ref. 45).

As discussed above, the phenotypic features of U-937 suggest that they represent immature monocytoid cells frozen at a differentiation stage close to that of myelomonocytic stem cells, as the cells contain peroxidase. When exposed to TPA (10^{-12}–10^{-7} M) or an MLC supernatant (20–30%) for 3–4 days, U-937 cells will undergo a stepwise morphological and functional maturation process similar to that described for normal monocyte–macrophage differentiation (Table VII). The cells become larger, and 60–80% attach to the surface of plastic petri dishes or aggregate if the surface is covered by agarose.

Light and electron microscope studies have characterized the induced cells as macrophage-like cells. The cytochemical profile underwent changes. The frequency of peroxidase-positive cells decreased to 3–4%, and a simultaneous increase in the intensity of staining for the nonspecific esterases naphthol AS-D esterase (NASDAE) and acid α-naphthylacetate esterase (ANAE) was found.

The cell surface membrane undergoes drastic changes after TPA or mixed lymphocyte culture (MLC) treatment. Apart from increased adhesiveness, a number of surface alterations have been demonstrated (44). The frequency of Fc receptors for positive cells increased, and the amount of HLA-DR, A,-B, -C and β_2-microglobulin increased in a variable fraction of the cells (15–30%) as studied by single-cell photometry (44). Both TPA- and MLC supernatant-induced surface changes were also shown by the decrease in sensitivity to natural killer (NK) cells regularly found (46). The most direct demonstration of induced surface membrane alterations are, however, studies on the surface glycoprotein composition using galactose oxidase–tritrated NaB^3H_4 labeling (44). As shown in Fig. 2, the following major changes were noted: a 200K-molecular-weight band disappeared, and the 145K–160K and the 90K bands were more strongly labeled. Three "new" bands appeared with apparent molecular weights of 180K, 140K, and 85K, respectively. It is interesting that no changes occurred in the surface protein profile when lactoperoxidase-catalyzed surface labeling was used. This may suggest that differentiation-associated surface glycoprotein changes are due to changes in the carbohydrate portions (51).

Treatment with TPA has also induced several functional changes consonant with induced macrophage differentiation. The capacity for phagocytosis and lysozyme production increased, and the cells became more potent as effector cells in ADCC (46). Taken together it seems clear that at least a sizable fraction (20–30%) of U-937 cells undergo the phenotypic changes expected for maturing monocytic cells.

V. Conclusions

With BL cells as an exception, human lymphoma cells are difficult to establish *in vitro* as continuous cell lines. However, using special techniques diffuse

TABLE VIII

Non-Hodgkin Lymphoma Cell Lines: Tentative Morphological and Functional Differentiation and Relationship to the Normal B-Cell Lineage

Non-Hodgkin lymphoma cell line

Undifferentiated lymphoma	Poorly differentiated lymphocytic lymphoma	Well-differentiated lymphocytic lymphoma	Poorly differentiated lymphocytic lymphoma
K-LL-3	U-698		U-715 BALM-5
Histiocytic lymphoma SU-DHL-9			Histiocytic lymphoma SU-DHL-4,5,7 SKW-4

Burkitt's lymphoma
Raji Daudi Seraphina

Normal B-cell lineage

Morphology:

Multipotent stem cell	Lymphoid stem cell	Immature pre-B cell	B Lymphocyte	B Blast	Lympho-plasmacyte	Plasma cell

Functional differentiation:

	Multipotent stem cell	Lymphoid stem cell	Immature pre-B cell	B Lymphocyte	B Blast	Lympho-plasmacyte	Plasma cell
Surface Ig	−	−	−?	+++	++	+	(+)
Intracellular Ig	−	−	+	−	+	++	+++
Secreted Ig	−	−	−	−	+	++	+++
Fc Receptor	−	−	?	++	+	?	−
C3 Receptor	−	−	?	++	+	?	−
EBV Receptor	−	−	?	++	−	?	−
cALL Antigen	−	+	+	−	−	−	−
HLA-DR	−	+	+	+	+	+	±

large-cell (histiocytic) lymphoma cells have also been established at a rate close to 100%.

The *in vitro* studies on human lymphoma cell lines have defined the following neoplastic features of lymphoma cells: monoclonality suggesting monoclonal derivation *in vivo*, aneuploidy with some characteristic markers [t(8;14), t(8;22), t(2;8), +7, +8, 6q−], and a capacity for growth in agarose *in vitro* and intracerebrally in nude mice.

Human lymphoma cell lines derived from a given histopathological entity are phenotypically heterogeneous. This underlines the individuality of human lymphomas and may explain the variability in biological behavior encountered in lymphoma-bearing patients.

Although human lymphoma cell lines represent "frozen" stages of differentiation (Table VIII), it is possible that they are not irreversibly arrested at a particular differentiation stage as exemplified by the macrophage differentiation observed *in vitro* for the HL cell line U-937. It is tempting to speculate that differentiation-inducing substances may be clinically useful in the treatment of lymphomas, as induced terminal differentiation usually is associated with inhibition of proliferation.

Acknowledgments

The studies reported in this article have in part been supported by grants from the Swedish Cancer Society. The excellent secretarial assistance of Mrs. Eva Harryson and Mrs. Anna-Greta Lundquist is gratefully acknowledged.

References

1. K. Nilsson, *in* "The Epstein-Barr Virus" (M. A. Epstein and B. G. Achong, eds.), p. 225. Springer-Verlag, Berlin and New York, 1979.
2. A. L. Epstein and H. S. Kaplan, *Cancer Res.* **39**, 1748 (1979).
3. B. J. Poiesz, F. W. Ruscetti, J. W. Mier, A. M. Woods, and E. C. Gallo, *Proc. Natl. Acad. Sci. U.S.A.* **77**, 6815 (1980).
4. J. S. Nadkarni, J. J. Nadkarni, P. Clifford, G. Manolov, E. M. Fenyö, and E. Klein, *Cancer (Philadelphia)* **23**, 64 (1969).
5. A. L. Epstein and H. S. Kaplan, *Cancer (Philadelphia)* **34**, 1851 (1974).
6. A. L. Epstein, R. Levy, H. Kim, W. Henle, G. Henle, and H. S. Kaplan, *Cancer (Philadelphia)* **42**, 2379 (1978).
7. K. Nilsson and J. Pontén, *Int. J. Cancer* **15**, 321 (1975).
8. M. Steinitz and G. Klein, *Proc. Natl. Acad. Sci. U.S.A.* **72**, 3518 (1975).
9. H. S. Kaplan, *et al.*, this volume, Chapter 1.
10. H. Rappaport, "Atlas of Tumor Pathology," Sect. III, Fasc. 8. U.S. Armed Forces Inst. Pathol., Washington, D.C., 1966.
11. K. Nilsson, *Int. J. Cancer* **8**, 432 (1971).
12. J. M. Béchet, P. Fialkow, K. Nilsson, and G. Klein, *Exp. Cell Res.* **89**, 275 (1974).

13. L. Zech, U. Haglund, K. Nilsson, and G. Klein, *Int. J. Cancer* **17**, 47 (1976).
14. J. E. Jarvis, G. Ball, A. B. Rickinson, and M. A. Epstein, *Int. J. Cancer* **14**, 716 (1974).
15. K. Nilsson, L. C. Andersson, C. G. Gahmberg, and H. Wigzell, *Int. J. Cancer* **20**, 708 (1977).
16. K. Nilsson, B. C. Giovanella, J. S. Stehlin, and G. Klein, *Int. J. Cancer* **19**, 337 (1977).
17. A. B. Rickinson, J. E. Jarvis, D. H. Crawford, and M. A. Epstein, *Int. J. Cancer* **14**, 704 (1974).
18. R. van Furth, H. Gorter, J. S. Nadkarni, E. Klein, and P. Clifford, *Immunology* **22**, 847 (1972).
19. Y. Manolova, G. Manolov, J. Kieler, A. Levan, and G. Klein, *Hereditas* **90**, 5 (1979).
20. H. S. Kaplan, R. S. Goodenow, S. Gartner, and M. M. Bieber, *Cancer (Philadelphia)* **43**, 1 (1979).
21. A. Bernheim, R. Berger, and G. Lenoir, *C.R. Hebd. Seances Acad. Sci.* **291**, 237 (1980).
22. A. Fagraeus, K. Nilsson, K. Lidman, and R. Norberg, *JNCI, J. Natl. Cancer Inst.* **55**, 783 (1975).
23. J. Ménézes, W. Leibold, G. Klein, and G. Clements, *Biomedicine* **22**, 276 (1975).
24. G. Klein, J. Zeuthen, P. Terasaki, R. Billing, R. Honig, M. Jondal, A. Westman, and G. Clements, *Int. J. Cancer* **18**, 639 (1976).
25. G. Klein, B. Giovanella, A. Westman, J. Stehlin, and D. Mumford, *Intervirology* **5**, 319 (1975).
26. A. L. Epstein, W. Henle, G. Henle, J. F. Hewetson, and H. S. Kaplan, *Proc. Natl. Acad. Sci. U.S.A.* **73**, 228 (1976).
27. I. Miyoshi, S. Hiraki, I. Kubonishi, Y. Matsuda, H. Kishimoto, T. Nakayama, T. Tanaka, H. Masuji, and I. Kimura, *Cancer (Philadelphia)* **40**, 2999 (1977).
28. H. Ben-Bassat, N. Goldblum, S. Mitrani, T. Goldblum, J. M. Yoffey, M. M. Cohen, Z. Bentwich, B. Ramot, and E. Klein, *Int. J. Cancer* **19**, 27 (1977).
29. K. Nilsson and C. Sundström, *Int. J. Cancer* **13**, 808 (1974).
30. K. Nilsson, V. Ghetie, and J. Sjöquist, *Eur. J. Immunol.* **5**, 518 (1975).
31. W. M. Gallmeier, W. R. Boecker, U. Bruntsch, D. K. Hossfeld, and C. G. Schmidt, *Haematol. Blood Transfus.* **20**, 277 (1977).
32. M.-S. Lok, H. Kishiba, T. Han, S. Abe, J. Minowada, and A. A. Sandberg, *Int. J. Cancer* **24**, 572 (1979).
33. S. D. Smith and D. Rosen, *Int. J. Cancer* **23**, 494 (1979).
34. I. T. Magrath, P. A. Pizzo, J. Whang-Peng, E. C. Douglass, O. Alabaster, P. Gerber, C. B. Freeman, and L. Novikovs, *JNCI, J. Natl. Cancer Inst.* **64**, 465 (1980).
35. I. T. Magrath, C. B. Freeman, P. Pizzo, J. Gadek, E. Jaffe, M. Santaella, C. Hammer, M. Frank, G. Reaman, and L. Novikovs, *JNCI, J. Natl. Cancer Inst.* **64**, 477 (1980).
36. U. Bruntsch, W. M. Gallmeier, D. K. Hossfeld, W. R. Boecker, C. Hertenstein, J. Gasch, and C. G. Smidt. In preparation.
37. G. Janossy, M. F. Greaves, D. Capellaro, J. Minowada, and C. Rosenfeld, *Protides Biol. Fluids* **25**, 591 (1978).
38. G. Manolov, Y. Manolova, G. Klein, A. Levan, and J. Kieler, *Cancer Gen. Cytogen.* (in press).
39. C. Sundström and K. Nilsson, *Int. J. Cancer* **17**, 565 (1976).
40. K. Nilsson, L. Klareskog, P. Ralph, C. Sundström, and L. Zech. In preparation.
41. K. Nilsson, L. C. Andersson, C. G. Gahmberg, and K. Forsbeck, *in* "International Symposium on New Trends in Human Immunology and Cancer Immunotherapy" (B. Serrou and C. Rosenfeld, eds.), Doin Editeurs, Paris, p. 271, 1980.
42. A. L. Epstein, M. M. Herman, H. Kim, R. Dorfman, and H. S. Kaplan, *Cancer (Philadelphia)* **37**, 2158 (1976).
43. K. Nilsson, L. C. Andersson, and C. G. Gahmberg, *Leuk. Res.* **4**, 279 (1980).
44. K. Nilsson, K. Forsbeck, M. Gidlund, C. Sundström, T. Tötterman, J. Sällström, and P. Wenge, *in* "Modern Trends in Human Leukemia," Vol. 26, p. 215, Springer-Verlag, Berlin, Heidelberg, 1981.

45. K. Nilsson, A. Kimura, L. Klareskog, L. C. Andersson, C. G. Gahmberg, S. Hammarström, and H. Wigzell, *Leuk. Res.* **5**, 185 (1981).
46. M. Gidlund, A. Örn, P. Pattengale, M. Jansson, H. Wigzell, and K. Nilsson, *Nature* **292**, 848 (1981).
47. C. Huber, C. C. Sundström, K. Nilsson, and H. Wigzell, *Clin. Exp. Immunol.* **25**, 367 (1976).
48. S. Hammarström, U. Hellström, P. Perlmann, and M.-L. Dillner, *J. Exp. Med.* **138**, 1270 (1979).
49. K. Nilsson, *INSERM Symp.* **8**, 307 (1978).
50. H. S. Koren, S. J. Anderson, and J. W. Larrick, *Nature (London)* **279**, 328 (1979).
51. K. Forsbeck, personal communication.

3

Marker Profiles of 55 Human Leukemia–Lymphoma Cell Lines

JUN MINOWADA, KIMITAKA SAGAWA, IAN S. TROWBRIDGE,
PATRICK D. KUNG, AND GIDEON GOLDSTEIN

I. Introduction

Pulvertaft in 1964 (1), for the first time, succeeded in establishing an African Burkitt's tumor into continuously growing lymphoid cell lines. During the past decade an increasing number of permanent hematopoietic cell lines have been established from various human specimens of leukemia–lymphoma origin and

MALIGNANT LYMPHOMAS

even of normal origin (2,3). Until we established and characterized a set of sheep erythrocyte (E)-rosette-forming acute lymphoblastic leukemia (ALL) cell lines (MOLT 1-4) (4), immunological studies on human leukemia–lymphoma cells were rather unremarkable. The observations that E-rosette formation was a definitive T-cell marker and that surface membrane immunoglobulins were definitive B-cell markers (5) made it possible to identify various immunological subtypes of lymphoid malignancies (6). The role of permanent leukemia–lymphoma cell lines in this progress has increasingly been recognized, and in fact the leukemia–lymphoma cell lines thus far established represent all three subtypes of ALL (namely, common ALL, T-cell ALL, and B-cell ALL), acute myeloid leukemia (AML), chronic myelogenous leukemia in the blastic phase (CML-BP), chronic lymphocytic leukemia (CLL) of both the B- and T-cell types, hairy cell leukemia (HCL), acute monocytic leukemia (AMoL), and various lymphomas.

One of the recent advances in immunobiological research has been the development of murine monoclonal hybridoma technology by Köhler and Milstein (7). The monoclonal hybridoma antibody not only permits various antibody reagents to be prepared with uniformity and precision and in unlimited supply but also makes feasible their usage in clinical applications. However, vigorous and continued efforts must be made in characterizing and understanding the various aspects of this new technological development before its promised goals can be accomplished.

This article is therefore intended to characterize further a collection of 55 human leukemia–lymphoma cell lines with certain murine monoclonal antibodies. The results are presented in comparison with the previously known characteristics of these cell lines. A particular attempt has been made to improve and incorporate our findings into the hypothetical scheme of normal hematopoietic cell differentiation proposed earlier (8,9).

II. Materials and Methods

A. Leukemia–Lymphoma Cell Lines

Establishment, characterization, and maintenance of each cell line have been reported in detail (1-4,10-13). Numerous colleagues, who have established various unique leukemia–lymphoma cell lines have generously provided us with their cell lines. These cell lines have been similarily characterized and maintained in our laboratory. Medium RPMI-1640 supplemented with 5–10% (v/v) heat-inactivated fetal calf serum was used for all cultures. Mycoplasma and other microbial infections of the cell cultures were routinely monitored. All studies were thus undertaken with cell cultures free of infection at the time of the experiments. A list of the 55 leukemia–lymphoma cell lines used in the present

TABLE I

Human Leukemia-Lymphoma Cell Lines

	T-Cell			B-Cell			Non-T-non-B-cell	
No.	Cell line	Origin[a]	No.	Cell line	Origin[a]	No.	Cell line	Origin[a]
1	CCRF-CEM	ALL	1	NALM-1[b]	CML	1	K-562	CML
2	CCRF-HSB-2	ALL	2	BALL-1	ALL	2	HL-60	APL
3	MOLT 1-4	ALL	3	BALM 1-2	ALL	3	ML 1-3	AML
4	RPMI 8402	ALL	4	NALM 6-15[b]	ALL	4	KG-1	AML
5	HPB-ALL	ALL	5	NALM 17-18[b]	ALL	5	REH	ALL
6	JM	ALL	6	KOPN 1-8[b]	ALL	6	KM-3	ALL
7	MOLT-10	ALL	7	HPB-null[b]	ALL	7	NALL-1	ALL
8	MOLT-11	ALL	8	LAZ-221[b]	ALL	8	NALM-16	ALL
9	PEER	ALL	9	U-698-M	LS	9	U-937	LY
10	P12/Ichikawa	ALL	10	BALM 3-5	LB	10	SU-DHL-1	LY
11	DND-41	ALL	11	EB-3	BL			
12	HPB-MLT	ATL	12	RAJI	BL			
13	TALL-1	ATL	13	HR1K	BL			
14	HD-Mar 2	HD(?)	14	OGUN	BL			
15	SKW-3	CLL	15	B35M	BL			
			16	AL-1	BL			
			17	SL-1	BL			
			18	NK-9	BL			
			19	Daudi	BL			
			20	B46M	BL			
			21	Namalva	BL			
			22	Ramos	BL			
			23	BJAB	BL			
			24	DG-75	BL			
			25	Chevallier	BL			
			26	DND-39	BL			
			27	SU-DHL-4	LY			
			28	RPMI 8226	MM			
			29	U-266	MM			
			30	ARH-77	MM			

[a] ALL, Acute lymphoblastic leukemia; ATL, adult T-cell leukemia; HD, Hodgkin's disease; LS, lymphosarcoma; BL, Burkitt's lymphoma; CML, chronic myelocytic leukemia; LY, lymphoma, histiocytic; AML, acute myeloblastic leukemia; CLL, T-cell lymphocytic leukemia; LB, B-cell lymphoma; MM, multiple myeloma; APL, acute promyelocytic leukemia.
[b] Pre-B-cell leukemia.

study is shown in Table I in which the cell lines are divided for convenience into three groups, namely, T-cell, B-cell and non-T–non-B-cell groups, respectively.

B. Surface Marker Assays

Rosette formation with sheep erythrocytes was used as a positive T-cell surface marker. Rosette formation with a bovine erythrocyte–IgG antibody complex (EA) and a bovine erythrocyte–IgM antibody–complement complex (EAC) were also used, respectively. The expression of receptors for EA and EAC rosettes was rather unrestricted among cells in the lymphoid, myeloid, erythroid, and monocytoid lineages. The receptors for EA and EAC, nevertheless, were useful additional markers for delineating further within each cell line when other markers were used in combination. Surface membrane immunoglobulin (SmIg) as a positive B-cell marker was detected by direct membrane immunofluorescence using fluorescein-conjugated goat anti-human immunoglobulin chain-specific reagents (κ-, λ-, α-, δ-, γ-, or μ-chain specific). To identify a pre-B-cell phenotype lacking detectable SmIg, methanol-fixed cell smears were stained for μ chain in the cytoplasmic region by direct immunofluorescence (CyIg). Details of the test procedure have been described in previous reports (4,6,11,13).

Four xenoantigens, namely, common ALL-associated antigen (cALL) (14,15), immune-associated (Ia)-like gp28,30 antigen (Ia-like) (16,17), T-cell-specific antigen (T-Ag) (18), and myelomonocyte-specific antigen (MAg-I) (19) were detected by indirect membrane immunofluorescence using specific rabbit antibody preparations as the primary reagent and a fluorescein isothiocyanate (FITC)-conjugated goat anti-rabbit IgG reagent as the secondary reagent. Details of the preparation and specificity of these rabbit antisera have been reported previously (15,17–19). Briefly, the cALL antigen is expressed on cells from the common form of non-T–non-B-cell ALL, pre-B-cell ALL, a certain proportion of T- and B-cell leukemia–lymphomas, approximately 30% of CML-BP as a lymphoid blast crisis, and a few percent of normal bone marrow cells. The Ia-like antigens are expressed on cells from normal blood B lymphocytes, normal immature myeloid cells in the bone marrow, B-cell leukemia–lymphoma cells, common ALL, null cell ALL, the majority of AML and CML-BP, and a certain proportion of histiocytic lymphomas. The T-Ag is expressed on cells from normal blood T cells as well as thymocytes, and T-cell leukemia–lymphoma cells. The MAg-I antigens are expressed on cells from normal granulocytes, monocytes as well as immature meyloid cells in the bone marrow, the majority of AMLs and CMLs, and a certain proportion of histiocytic lymphomas.

Another series of xenoantigens detectable by murine monoclonal hybridoma antibodies in either an ascites preparation or a tissue culture fluid preparation were detected by indirect membrane immunofluorescence using monoclonal antibodies as a primary reagent and a FITC-conjugated goat anti-mouse IgG prepa-

TABLE II

Antibodies Used in Immunofluorescence

Reagent	Immunogen	Specificity	Reference
FITC goat polyclonal antibody			
Antiimmunoglobulin chain	Respective immuno-globulin chain	κ, λ, α, δ, γ, or μ chain	(11,12)
(κ, λ, α, δ, γ, or μ)			
Rabbit polyclonal antibody[a]			
Anti-cALL	NALM-1	cALL (gp 100)	(15)
Anti-Ia	Daudi's gp 28/30	Ia (gp 28/30)	(17)
Anti-T cells	MOLT-4	T Cells	(18)
Anti-MAg-I	HL-60	Myelomonocytes	(19)
Murine monoclonal antibody[a]			
B3/25	K-562	Erythroblasts plus ? (gp200)	(20)
B7/21	NALM-6	Ia (gp28,30)	(P.C.)[b]
I25/14	Daudi	B Cells plus ?	(P.C.)
T50/12	JM	T Cells plus ?	(P.C.)
T56/20	JM	Pan-leukocytes?	(P.C.)
OKT-1	Peripheral blood leukocytes	Pan-T Cells	(21)
OKT-9	Thymocytes	Replicating T Cells	(22)
OKI-1	Leukocytes	Ia (gp28/30)	(23)
OKM-1	Leukocytes	Myelomonocytes	(24)

[a] As the second reagent, FITC-labeled goat anti-rabbit or mouse IgG reagent was used.
[b] (P.C.) Personal communication, I. S. Trowbridge.

ration as a secondary reagent. Details of the preparation and specificity of each antibody have been reported previously for five of the nine preparations used. Four preparations of monoclonal antibodies are still under characterization for their specificity.

All antibody preparations used in this study are listed in Table II with the immunogens used, antibody specificity, and original references. Briefly, the B3/25 antibody (20) detects an unusual surface antigen which is expressed on cells from all human cell lines thus far tested, normal erythroblasts and unidentified blastic cells in the bone marrow, erythroleukemia, and a substantial portion of T-cell leukemia–lymphomas. The B7/21 antibody detects an antigenic determinant of the Ia-like gp28,30 molecule which appears to be a common structure of the molecule, and its distribution among various cell types is the same as that of the Ia-like antigen detectable by the rabbit anti-Ia-like antibody. The specificities of the I25/14, T50/12, and T56/20 antibodies are still under characterization and are so far known as described in Table II. The OKT-1 antibody detects an antigen shared by all human T cells (21) and T-cell-type CLL cells. The OKT-9 antibody detects antigens reported to be "prothymocytes" (22), but it reacts with cells from all human cell lines and a majority of T-cell leukemias (unpublished data). While the majority of normal thymocytes, however, do not react with OKT-9, normal erythroblasts in the bone marrow are reactive with this antibody. The OKI-1 antibody detects an Ia-like gp28/30 antigen similar to the reactivities of B7/21 antibody (23). The OKM-1 antibody detects an antigen on the peripheral blood monocytes (24) and cells of the majority of AMLs and AMoLs.

C. Assay for Terminal Deoxynucleotidyl Transferase

The method for the assay of terminal deoxynucleotidyl transferase (TdT) has been described in detail previously (25). In addition to the assay for enzyme activity, immunofluorescence with rabbit anti-TdT antibody on fixed cell smears has been employed for some experiments (Dr. Srivastava, unpublished data).

D. Detection of Epstein–Barr Virus Infection

The presence of Epstein–Barr virus (EBV) genome in the cells was determined by the anticomplement immunofluorescence test known as the EBNA test (26).

E. Cytogenetic Analysis

The chromosomal composition of each cell line was assessed by the banding procedure as described earlier in detail (27).

F. Assay for Stimulating Capacity in the Mixed Leukeocyte Culture

A stimulating capacity of normal allogeneic T lymphocytes in a "one-way" mixed leukocyte culture (MLC) system is known as a functional marker of non-T cells (28). This capacity in the MLC system was used for further characterization of each cell line.

III. Results

A. Marker Profiles of 55 Leukemia–Lymphoma Cell Lines

As listed in Table I, the 55 leukemia–lymphoma cell lines were, for convenience, subgrouped into a T-cell group having a definitive T-cell marker (T-Ag), a B-cell group having a definitive B-cell marker (SmIg and/or CyIg), and a group having neither a T- or a B-cell marker.

By means of a multiple marker assay which has been employed in our laboratory for characterizing various leukemia–lymphomas, all 55 cell lines were characterized. As shown in Table III, the 15 T-cell leukemia–lymphoma cell lines have two sets of common markers, i.e., positive for T-Ag and chromosomal abnormality, which are independent of each other, and negative for EA, Ia, SmIg, CyIg, MAg-I, EBV, and MLC-S. An exception to this finding is the MOLT-10 line derived from an ALL. A fraction of the cell population ranging from 10 to 40% in a given time period expressed Ia antigens but the remaining cells consistently had a T-cell phenotype. No satisfactory explanations can be offered at the present time for this observation with MOLT-10.

By taking detectable immunoglobulins such as SmIg and/or CyIg as definitive B-cell markers, the next 30 cell lines were categorized as B-cell leukemia–lymphoma cell lines. As shown in the previous study (12), each B-cell line demonstrated a monoclonal nature having a distinct immunoglobulin isotype (data are not shown in Table III). Among all B-cell lines, the presence of Ig, Ia, chromosomal abnormalities and MLC-S activity is a common denominator, but other markers are variable.

Ten cell lines of leukemia–lymphoma origin were grouped on the basis of the absence of either a T- or a B-cell marker into the non-T–non-B-cell type. Nonetheless, this group consisted of rather heterogeneous cell lines; three myeloid leukemia lines (HL-60, ML 1-3, and KG-1) had a common antigenic characteristic, MAg-I antigen expression. One of two histiocytic lymphoma lines, however, expressed MAg-I antigen. Both chromosomal abnormality and MLC-S activity were common characteristics of all cell lines in this group. Four

TABLE III

Origins and Markers of 55 Cell Lines[a]

No.	Cell line	Origin	E	EA	EAC	SmIg	CyIg	T-Ag	Ia-like	cALL	MAg-I	TdT	EBV	Chr	MLC-S
									Markers						
T-Cell leukemia–lymphoma cell lines															
1	CCRF-CEM	ALL	–	–	–	–	–	+	–	+	–	H	–	A	–
2	CCRF-HSB-2	ALL	–	–	–	–	–	+	–	+	–	L	–	A	–
3	MOLT 1-4	ALL	+	–	+	–	–	+	–	–	–	H	–	A	–
4	RPMI 8402	ALL	–	–	+	–	–	+	–	+	–	H	–	A	–
5	HPB-ALL	ALL	+	–	+	–	–	+	–	+	–	H	–	A	–
6	JM	ALL	+	–	+	–	–	+	–	–	–	H	–	A	–
7	MOLT-10	ALL	+	–	–	–	–	+	–/+	–/+	–	H	–	A	+
8	MOLT-11	ALL	+	–	+	–	–	+	–/+	–/+	–	H	–	A	–
9	PEER	ALL	+	–	–	–	–	+	–	–	–	L	–	A	–
10	P12/Ichikawa	ALL	+	–	+	–	–	+	–	–	–	H	–	A	–
11	DND-41	ALL	+	–	+	–	–	+	–	+	–	H	–	A	–
12	HPB-MLT	ATL	+	–	+	–	–	+	–	+	–	H	–	A	–
13	TALL-1	ATL	+	–	–	–	–	+	–	–	–	H	–	A	–
14	HD-Mar-2	HD?	+	–	+	–	–	+	–	+	–	H	–	A	–
15	SKW-3	CLL	+	–	–	–	–	+	–	–	–	L	–	A	–
B-Cell leukemia–lymphoma cell lines															
1	NALM-1	CML-BC	–	–	–	–	+	–	+	+	–	H	–	A/Ph[i]	+
2	BALL-1	ALL	–	+	+	–	+	–	+	–	–	L	–	A	+
3	BALM 1-2	ALL	–	–	+	+	+	–	+	–	–	L	+	A	+
4	NALM 6-15	ALL	–	–	–	–	+	–	+	+	–	H	–	A	+
5	NALM 17,18	ALL	–	–	–	–	+	–	+	+	–	H	–	A	+
6	KOPN 1-8	ALL	–	–	–	–	+	–	+	+	–	L	–	A	+
7	HPB-null	ALL	–	–	–	–	+	–	+	+	–	L	–	A	+
8	LAZ-221	ALL	–	–	–	–	+	–	+	+	–	H	–	A	+
9	U-698-M	LS	–	–/+	–	+	+	–	+	+	–	L	–	A	+
10	BALM 3-5	LB	–	–	–	+	+	–	+	–	–	L	+	A	+
11	EB-3	BL	–	–	–	+	+	–	+	+	–	L	+	A	+

Non-T-Non-B leukemia-lymphoma cell lines

No.	Cell line	Type										TdT	EBV	Chr	MLC-S
12	Raji	BL	−	−	+	+	−	+	−	−	+	L	−	A	+
13	HR1K	BL	−	+	+	+	−	+	−	−	+	L	+	A	+
14	OGUN	BL	−	−	+	+	−	+	−	−	+	L	−	A	+
15	B35M	BL	−	−	+	+	+	+	+	−	+	L	+	A	+
16	AL-1	BL	−	−	+	+	−	+	−	−	+	L	+	A	+
17	SL-1	BL	−	−	+	+	−	+	−	−	+	L	+	A	+
18	NK-9	BL	−	−	+	+	−	+	−	−	+	L	+	A	+
19	Daudi	BL	+	+	−	+	+	+	−	−	+	L	+	A	+
20	B46M	BL	−	+	−	+	−	+	−	−	+	L	+	A	+
21	Namalva	BL	+	+	−	+	−	+	−	−	+	L	−	A	+
22	Ramos	BL	−	−	+	+	−	+	−	−	+	L	−	A	+
23	BJAB	BL	−	+	+	+	−	+	−	−	+	L	−	A	+
24	DG-75	BL	−	−	+	+	−	+	−	−	+	L	−	A	+
25	Chevallier	BL	−	−	+	+	−	+	−	−	+	L	−	A	+
26	DND-39	BL	−	−	+	+	−	+	−	−	+	L	+	A	+
27	SU-DHL-4	LY	−	−	+	+	−	+	−	−	+	L	−	A	+
28	RPMI 8226	MM	−	−	−	−	+	+	−	−	−	L	−	A	+
29	U-266	MM	−	−	−	−	+	−	−	−	−	L	+	A	+
30	ARH-77	MM	+	−	+	+	+	+	+	−	+	L	−	A	+
1	K-562	CML-BC	−	+	−	−	−	−	−	−	−	L	−	A/Ph[I]	+
2	HL-60	APL	+	−	−	−	−	−	−	+	−	L	−	A	+
3	ML 1-3	AML	+	−	−	−	−	−	−	+	−	L	−	A	+
4	KG-1	AML	+	−	−	−	−	−	+	+	−	L	−	A	+
5	REH	ALL	−	−	−	−	−	+	+	+	+	H	−	A	+
6	KM-3	ALL	−	−	−	−	−	+	+	+	+	H	−	A	+
7	NALL-1	ALL	−	−	−	−	−	+	+	+	+	H	−	A	+
8	NALM-16	ALL	−	−	−	−	−	+	+	+	+	H	−	A	+
9	U-937	LY	+	+	−	−	−	−	−	+	+	L	+	A	+
10	SU-DHL-1	LY	−	−	−	−	−	+	−	−	−	L	−	A	+

a E, Sheep erythrocyte rosette; EA, rosette formed by bovine erythrocyte–IgG antibody complex; EAC, rosette formed by bovine erythrocyte–IgM antibody–complement complex; SmIg, surface membrane immunoglobulin; CyIg, cytoplasmic immunoglobulin; T-Ag, T-cell antigen; Ia-like, Ia-like B-cell-associated antigen; cALL, antigen specific to non-T–non-B ALL; MAg-I, antigen specific to myelomonocytes; TdT, terminal deoxynucleotidyl transferase (H, high activity 10–100/mg DNA; L, low activity ≤2/mg DNA); EBV, Epstein–Barr virus infection; Chr, chromosome constitution (A, abnormal; N, normal); MLC-S, stimulating activity in one-way MLC assay; NT, not tested.

common ALL lines expressed both Ia and cALL antigens but were negative for three definitive markers, namely, T-Ag, Ig, and MAg-I antigens.

As seen in Table III, in T-, B-, and non-T–non-B-cell-type leukemia–lymphoma cell lines, there exist rather heterogeneous marker profiles. Nevertheless, certain definitive markers, such as T-Ag, Ig, and MAg-I were found to be useful for defining respective lineage in hematopoietic cell differentiation.

Table IV lists the 29 cell lines with known derivation from a lymphoma or the

TABLE IV

Membrane Markers of Lymphoma Lines as Determined by Polyclonal and Monoclonal Antibodies[a]

						Markers (% positive)			
No.	Cell line	E	EA	EAC	SmIg	cALL	Ia	T-Ag	MAg-I
T-Lymphoma line									
1	MOLT-10	—	—	—	—	40	40	60	—
2	HPB-MLT	30	—	30	—	100	—	100	—
3	HD-Mar 2	30	—	20	—	100	—	100	—
B-Lymphoma line									
4	U-698-M	—	—	—	K-DM	100	100	—	—
5	BALM-3	—	—	—	K-G	—	100	—	—
6	BALM-4	—	—	—	K-G	—	100	—	—
7	BALM-5	—	20	—	K-G	—	70	—	—
8–12	EB-3[b]	—	—	—	λ-M	100	100	—	—
13	Raji	—	60	50	M	100	100	—	—
14	HR1K	—	80	—	M	100	100	—	—
15	B35M	—	—	50	K-M	100	100	—	—
16–17	AL-1[b]	—	—	50	M	—	100	—	—
18	NK-9	—	—	—	λ-M	—	100	—	—
19	Daudi	—	80	—	K-DM	100	100	—	—
20	B46M	—	80	—	K-DM	100	100	—	—
21	Ramos	—	—	—	λ-DM	100	100	—	—
22	Namalva	—	20	—	λ-M	100	100	—	—
23	OGUN	—	—	30	M	—	100	—	—
24	SU-DHL-4	—	—	—	K-G	100	100	—	—
B-Myeloma line									
25	RPMI 8226	—	—	—	λ	—	100	—	—
26	U-266	—	—	—	λ-E	—	100	—	—
27	ARH-77	—	—	70	κ-G	—	100	—	—
Non-T–Non-B lymphoma line									
28	U-937	—	90	—	—	—	—	—	100
29	SU-DHL-1	—	—	—	—	—	—	—	—

[a] Abbreviations used are shown in the footnotes to Table III.
[b] Cell lines 9, 10, 11, 23 (DG-75, Chevallier, DND-39, BJAB) exhibit the same profile as cell line 8 (EB-3). Cell line 17 (SL-1) exhibits the same profile as cell line 16 (AL-1).

leukemic phase of a lymphoma. Nine mouse monoclonal antibodies listed in Table II were used to further characterize these cell lines. All cell lines were reactive with both B3/25 and OKT-9 antibodies. The reactivity of B7/21 and OKI-1, which both have anti-Ia specificity, was generally the same as that of the rabbit anti-Ia antibody. While BALM-3, -4, and -5, which had been derived from a single specimen of a B-cell lymphoma in the leukemic phase, reacted with both rabbit anti-Ia antibody and B7/21 monoclonal anti-Ia antibody, OKI-1, another

B3/25	B7/21	I25/14	T50/12	T56/20	OKT-1	OKT-9	OKI-1	OKM-1
50	40	—	60	100	70	100	10	—
100	—	40	100	100	100	100	—	—
30	—	100	100	100	100	30	—	—
100	100	100	—	—	—	100	100	—
100	100	100	—	—	—	100	10	—
100	100	100	—	—	—	100	—	—
100	70	100	—	—	—	100	100	—
100	100	100	100	—	—	100	100	—
100	100	100	100	—	—	100	100	80
100	100	100	100	—	—	100	100	—
100	100	70	0	60	—	100	100	—
100	100	10	100	100	—	100	100	—
100	100	100	100	100	—	100	100	—
100	100	100	—	100	—	100	100	—
100	100	100	100	100	—	100	100	—
100	100	100	—	—	—	100	100	—
100	100	100	—	—	—	100	100	—
100	100	100	100	80	—	100	100	—
100	100	30	0	100	—	100	50	—
100	100	100	0	100	—	100	100	—
100	100	10	100	100	—	100	100	—
100	—	—	100	100	—	80	—	—
100	—	100	—	100	100	100	—	—

monoclonal anti-Ia, did not react with BALM-4 cells. These BALM-3, -4, and -5 lines were established in three separate flasks but originated from the same pleural effusion of a monoclonal B-cell lymphoma. It was shown that the differences in Ia antigens and other characteristics of these three cell lines were most likely due to different stages of B-cell differentiation within the same lymphoma clone (29). Sixteen cell lines derived from Burkitt's lymphoma (nos. 8–23) exhibited further heterogeneity in reactivity with these monoclonal antibodies (T50/12, T56/20, and OKM-1). Three myeloma-derived cell lines (nos. 25–27) exhibited a minimal difference with a T50/12 antibody. The SU-DHL-4 line was derived from a histiocytic lymphoma but was found to be a B-cell lymphoma. Two histiocytic lymphoma cell lines (U-937 and SU-DHL-1) differed from each other in reactivity with I25/14, T50/12, and OKT-1 antibodies.

B. Stability of Markers in Cell Lines

With regard to the possible alteration of marker expression in culture, it was found that such an antigen was detected with B3/25 and OKT-9 antibodies (Table IV). Next, five selected cell lines for which cryopreserved cells were available were tested with a set of Ortho monoclonal antibodies. Cells of four T-cell leukemia lines and a Burkitt's lymphoma cell line that had been frozen 6–8 years ago were compared with cells from each cell line that had been kept in actively growing culture for the same amount of time. The results are shown in Table V where only minimal alterations are seen in their reactivity with a few antibodies (OKT-4 and OKT-11). The observed changes may well have been due to the sensitivity limitations of the assay method rather than qualitative changes, but they suggested that a loss of antigen after prolonged *in vitro* cultivation seemed to occur. On the other hand, many of the surface markers were found to be unchanged after such prolonged culture.

C. Heterogeneity of T-Cell Leukemia as Determined by Monoclonal Antibodies

As already described in Section III,A (Table III), further detailed analysis was carried out with the monoclonal antibodies. Ten patients with T-cell ALL were also tested for marker profiles of their leukemic T blasts. For comparison, normal thymocytes from 10 patients who had no hematological malignancies were similarly tested. The results are shown in Table VI. It is evident that the heterogeneous profiles of the OKT-defined antigen expressions among 14 T-cell leukemia-lymphoma cell lines may well reflect similar heterogeneity in the antigen expression profile seen in the leukemic T blasts of the 10 patients. Because of the generally accepted notion that T-cell ALL might arise from a clone in the thymus, normal thymocytes from 10 patients were tested. All T-cell leukemia

TABLE V

Stability of Markers in Leukemia–Lymphoma Cell Lines as Determined by Ortho Monoclonal Antibodies[a]

Date tested		Markers (% positive)									
		OKT-1	OKT-3	OKT-4	OKT-5	OKT-6	OKT-8	OKT-9	OKT-10	OKT-11	OKI-1
CCRF-CEM	(cALL)										
3/8/74	70	100	100	100	0	20	0	100	100	50	0
8/80	100	100	50	100	0	20	0	100	100	0	0
CCRF-HSB-2											
5/12/74		50	0	0	0	0	0	100	30	0	0
8/80		10	0	0	0	0	0	100	100	0	0
MOLT-3	(E)										
3/19/73	90	100	0	100	0	100	100	100	100	100	0
8/80	90	100	0	100	0	100	100	100	100	100	0
RPMI 8402	(cALL)										
2/26/74	100	100	0	30	0	0	0	100	100	100	0
8/80	100	100	0	0	0	0	0	100	100	100	0
HR1K	(cALL)										
12/6/71	100	0	100	0	0	0	0	100	100	0	100
9/80	100	0	100	0	0	0	0	100	100	0	100

[a] Ortho monoclonal antibodies used have been previously reported (21-24).

TABLE VI

Reactivity of Ortho Monoclonal Antibodies with T-Cell Leukemia Cell Lines and Fresh, Uncultured ALL Cells"

No.	Specimen[b]	E	cALL	OKT-1	OKT-3	OKT-4	OKT-5	OKT-6	OKT-8	OKT-9	OKT-10	OKT-11	OKI-1
									Markers				
	T-Cell leukemia–lymphoma lines												
1	HPB-MLT	+	+	+	+	+	+	+	+	+	+	+	−
2	JM	+	−	+	+	+	+	+	+	+	+	+	−
3	HPB-ALL	+	+	+	+	+	−	−	+	+	+	+	−
4	HD-Mar 2	+	+	+	+	+	−	+	+	+	+	+	−
5	MOLT-3	+	−	+	−	+	−	+	+	+	+	+	−
6	MOLT-4	+	−	+	−	+	−	+	−	+	+	+	−
7	CCRF-CEM	−	+	+	+	+	−	+	+	+	+	+	−
8	TALL-1	+	−	+	+	+	−	−	−	+	+	−	−
9	DND-41	+	+	+	+	+	−	+	+	+	+	+	−
10	PEER	−	−	+	+	+	−	−	−	+	+	−	−
11	SKW-3	+	−	+	−	+	−	−	+	+	+	+	−
12	RPMI 8402	−	+	+	−	+	−	−	−	+	+	+	−

13 CCRF-HSB-2	−	−	+	−	−	+	+	+	+	+	−
14 MOLT-10[c]	+	+	+	+	+	+	+	+	+	+	+
Fresh, uncultured ALL cells											
1 New, 11 ♂	+	−	+	+	+	−	+	+	+	+	+
2 New, 3 ♂	+	−	+	+	+	−	+	+	−	+	+
3 New, 17 ♂	+	−	+	+	+	+	+	+	+	+	+
4 New, 6 ♀	+	+	+	+	+	+	+	+	+	−	−
5 Rel., 19 ♂	+	+	+	−	+	−	−	+	−	+	−
6 Rel., 10 ♂	+	−	+	−	+	−	+	+	+	+	+
7 Rel., 13 ♂	+	+	+	−	+	−	−	−	+	+	−
8 New, 17 ♂	+	+	−	+	+	+	N.T.	+	+	−	−
9 New, 14 ♀	−	+	−	−	−	−	−	−	−	−	−
10 New, 19 ♂	+	−	+	+	−	−	+	−	+	−	−
Normal thymus (10)	+	+	+	+	+	+	+	+	+	+	−
N = 10	+	+	+	+	+	+	+	+	+	+	+

[a] Positive reactions (+) vary in both intensity and percentage of reactive cells (20–100%). Negative reactions (−) include 0–5% positive reactions in the thymuses which represent a total of 10 patients with no hematological malignancies.

[b] New, Untreated T-ALL; Rel., relapsed T-ALL.

[c] Reactivity of MOLT-10 with all OKT antibodies except OKT-9 and OKT-10 varies 10–40%.

lines and 8/10 of fresh T-ALL lines were positive for an OKT-9 antigen but, in sharp contrast, only a minor population of the thymocytes (0–5%) reacted with OKT-9 antibody. It should be also noted that 5/13 T-ALL lines, excluding SKW-3 as a T-CLL line, and 2/9 of fresh T-ALL lines lacked antigens detectable by OKT-6 which is known to be a antithymus antibody (21–24). Although general findings in the present study confirmed what was previously reported by Reinherz *et al.* (22), who used some of the same OKT antibodies for T-ALL analysis, our results combined with those for other markers such as cALL and TdT were not readily interpretable to fit to the differentiation scheme we proposed (9).

IV. Hypothesis and Discussion

According to previous studies dealing with observed heterogeneity in leukemia membrane phenotype profiles, several investigators suggested a hypothetical scheme of human hematopoietic cell differentiation (8,9,22,30–34). Their view is based on the fact that, in spite of historical claims, all markers thus far identified as leukemia-specific antigens have turned out to be normal gene products present in either a small number in the peripheral blood or an extremely small number in normal bone marrow (6,8,16,35–37). Series of studies from this laboratory, which involved parallel studies with an ever-increasing number of leukemia–lymphoma cell lines and a large series of fresh leukemias (8,9,29,30–32), have proposed the hypothesis that respective marker profiles of leukemia–lymphoma cell lines can be viewed as reflecting normal hematopoietic cell differentiation. One of the puzzling facts exhibited in both leukemia–lymphoma cell lines and individual leukemia–lymphoma cases is a monoclonality of each case with remarkably fixed expression of a certain marker profile representing a specific point during hematopoietic cell differentiation.

Figure 1 shows our latest hypothetical scheme of human hematopoietic cell differentiation based on studies on the marker profiles of 55 leukemia–lymphoma cell lines as well as a large series of fresh leukemia–lymphoma cases. A possible relation of the megakaryocyte lineage is not included in the scheme, since no cell lines with these particular lineage characteristics are available to us. It is not known what marker profile may represent pluripotential stem cell compartment. Nevertheless, it is assumed that lymphoid, myeloid, erythroid, and monocytoid cell differentiation emerge from such a cell compartment. Figure 2 illustrates which combinations of multiple markers may be distributed and be expressed simultaneously in relation to the dynamics of cellular proliferation and differentiation. Based on the reasons already discussed, these 55 leukemia–lymphoma cell lines can each be assigned to a particular compartment on the basis of marker profiles (Fig. 3). The fact that, unlike the difficulties encountered

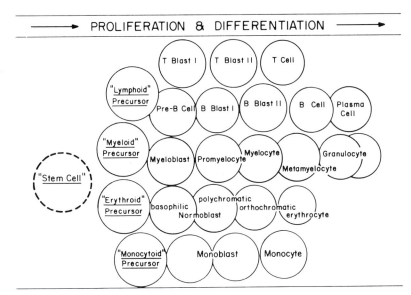

Fig. 1. A scheme of human hematopoietic cell differentiation. Each compartment has a particular marker expression, as shown in Fig. 2. This scheme excludes the megakaryocyte lineage, since there are no cell lines available in this lineage.

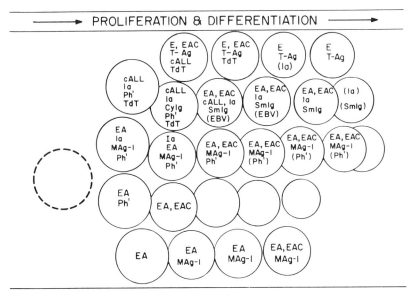

Fig. 2. Marker expression during hematopoietic cell differentiation. Various markers (abbreviations are shown in the footnotes to Table I) are expressed in combination in each compartment. A particular marker combination with a definitive marker, such as T-Ag, Sm-CyIg, or MAg-I, or an absence of these three antigens, identifies the particular lineage (T, B, myeloid–monocytoid, or erythroid) and degree of differentiation of the cells in question.

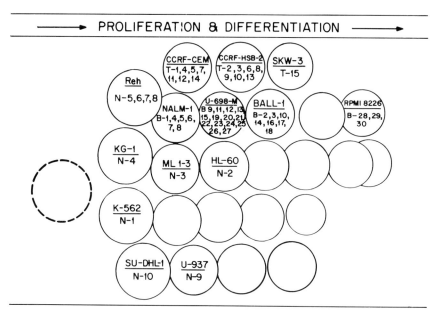

Fig. 3. Assigned compartments for 55 human leukemia–lymphoma cell lines. On the basis of marker profile, each cell line shown in Table III is assigned to a particular compartment. One cell line representative of each compartment is shown in the figure, and more than one cell line (shown as T-, B-, or N-followed by a number from Table III) is present in many compartments.

with lymphoid lines, several myeloid leukemia cell lines (such as HL-60, KG-1, ML 1–3, and K-562) have been shown to be inducible toward further maturation stages with various agents makes it possible to delineate changes in the marker profiles responsible for such cellular differentiation and maturation (38–41). It should be also noted that two leukemia cell lines, K-562 (40,42) and NALM-1 (13), each representing Philadelphia chromosome-positive CML blasts, are apparently erythroid stem cells and pre-B-cells, respectively. This finding is in agreement with the concepts previously advanced by a number of studies indicating that CML is a clonal stem cell disease (43–45).

Our attempt to hypothesize the marker profiles of leukemia–lymphomas into a scheme of normal hematopoietic cell differentiation may not be all correct, but it certainly provides not only a reasonable approach to a better understanding of hematopoietic malignancies but also insight into normal hematopoietic cell differentiation. Perhaps the scheme becomes more significant when one recognizes the tremendous heterogeneity in patients with leukemia–lymphoma in terms of their response to therapy, in addition to morphological, biochemical, and immunological marker profiles. Vigorous and continued efforts in studying every aspect associated with hematopoietic malignancy would certainly imporove potential deficiencies and defcct in the present scheme. It must be remembered that study of the cell lines has its limitations and should not be expected to substantiate all conceivable phenomena and characteristics observed in patients with this disease. For this reason, a parallel study involving the cell lines and fresh leukemia–lymphoma has to be an essential part of the progress. On the basis of our marker profile study, the fresh leukemia–lymphoma cases can be distributed as shown in Fig. 4.

Recent advances in the study of murine monoclonal antibodies (7) have provided much precise knowledge of the dynamic relationship between cell surface markers and their functional attributes (21,34,46–48). Application to the study of leukemia–lymphoma has already achieved much progress in which many conventional polyclonal xenoantibodies are to be replaced (23,24,35). It is also expected that many restricted antigens specific to or associated with leukemia–lymphoma cells will be found (49). Reinherz et al. (22) and Janossy et al. (50) have reported a possible relationship between a discrete membrane phenotype of ALL and its differentiative stage within thymus or bone marrow.

Our finding in the present study involving several monoclonal antibodies demonstrated that further heterogeneity in the marker profiles of 55 leukemia–lymphoma cell lines was evident. While the respective phenotypes of each cell

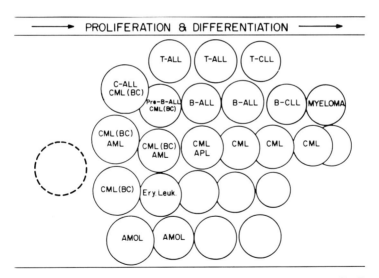

Fig. 4. Distribution of fresh leukemia–lymphomas on the basis of marker profile. Possible assignment of ALL, APL, AML, AMoL, CLL, CML, CML-BP, multiple myeloma, and histiocytic lymphoma is made on the basis of marker profile. Continuity among the various leukemias is apparent in terms of the hematopoietic cell differentiation pattern.

line are generally stable for years in *in vitro* cultivation, some alteration in the marker profiles does occur under culture conditions (Table V). The antigens defined by B3/21 and OKT-9 were found to be expressed on all cell lines examined (Table IV), though they were present only on fresh cells of certain restricted cell types. As tabulated in Table IV, it was found that the heterogeneity of marker profiles among lymphoma cell lines was similar to that found in leukemia cell lines.

Concerning the marker profiles of T-cell leukemia–lymphoma lines and T-cell ALL, our data confirm in principle those of Reinherz *et al.* (22). Nevertheless, we are unable at the present time to correlate their heterogeneity of antigen expression with our view of hematopoietic cell differentiation, notably placing a total of 14 T-cell lines into a coherent scheme relative to the previous scheme based on the study with conventional antisera (8,9). It seems possible that all monoclonal antibodies may not always define antigens linked to cellular differentiation. Although potential usage of monoclonal antibody is well proved, further characterization of the antibody is needed for a satisfactory interpretation.

In any event, human leukemia–lymphoma cell lines could be of great value for further biomedical research, notably leukemia–lymphoma research, provided that one recognizes their limitations and possible alterations in *in vitro* cultivation, as shown clearly in the present study.

V. Summary

A total of 55 human leukemia–lymphoma cell lines, which included 15 T-cell, 30 B-cell, and 10 non-T–non-B-cell types, were further characterized for their marker profiles. With the use of a multiple marker analysis consisting of rosette, immunofluorescence, enzyme, and cytogenetic assays, the identity of each leukemia–lymphoma cell line was established to represent a monoclonal cell population of leukemia or lymphoma origin. Although the majority of marker expression in the cell lines during prolonged cultivation was unchanged from that found in the original tumor cells *in vivo,* certain alterations did occur. Analysis with several murine monoclonal antibodies demonstrated that cells from all permanent hematopoietic cell lines expressed an antigen detectable in only a few cell types in normal bone marrow, all erythroleukemias, and the majority of T-cell leukemias. All the individual markers except a cytogenetic abnormality were determined to be for normal gene products and were generally stable for a prolonged period of *in vitro* cultivation.

Rather than being a tumor-specific feature, the observed heterogeneity in the marker profiles among these leukemia–lymphoma cell lines could be best interpreted as reflecting the heterogeneity of the hematopoietic target cell clone at a particular stage of cellular differentiation. Based on the present observations, the hypothetical scheme of hematopoietic cell differentiation proposed previously was further modified.

Acknowledgments

The authors gratefully acknowledge numerous colleagues who provided many of the unique leukemia–lymphoma cell lines, and T. Han, A. A. Sandberg, and B. I. S. Srivastava for MLC, cytogenetic, and enzyme analyses. We are also grateful to the staff of the Cell Culture Laboratory for their able technical and clerical assistance. Our colleagues in the departments of Pediatrics and Medical Oncology who provided various clinical materials are also greatly acknowledged. This study was supported in part by grants CA-14413, CA-17609, CA-20272, and AI-08899 from the National Institutes of Health, USPHS.

References

1. R. J. Pulvertaft, *Lancet* **1**, 238 (1964).
2. S. Iwakata and J. T. Grace, Jr., *N.Y. State J. Med.* **64**, 2279 (1964).
3. G. E. Moore, *J. Surg. Oncol.* **4**, 320 (1972).
4. J. Minowada, T. Ohuman, and G. E. Moore, *JNCI, J. Natl. Cancer Inst.* **49**, 891 (1972).
5. S. S. Frøland and J. B. Natvig, *Transplant. Rev.* **16**, 114 (1973).
6. M. F. Greaves, G. Janossy, G. Francis, and J. Minowada, *Cold Spring Harbor Conf. Cell Proliferation* **5**, 823 (1978).
7. G. Köhler and C. Milstein, *Nature (London)* **256**, 495 (1975).
8. J. Minowada, *in* "Human Lymphocyte Differentiation: Its Application to Cancer" (B. Serrou and C. Rosenfeld, eds.), p. 337. Elsevier/North-Holland Biomedical Press, Amsterdam and New York, 1978.
9. J. Minowada, K. Sagawa, M. S. Lok, I. Kubonishi, S. Nakazawa, E. Tatsumi, T. Ohnuma, and N. Goldblum, *in* "New Trends in Human Immunology and Cancer Immunotherapy" (B. Serrou and C. Rosenfeld, eds.), p. 188, Doin, Paris, 1980.
10. J. Minowada, G. Klein, P. Clifford, E. Klein, and G. E. Moore, *Cancer (Philadelphia)* **20**, 1430 (1967).
11. J. Minowada, T. Tsubota, M. F. Greaves, and T. R. Walters, *JNCI, J. Natl. Cancer Inst.* **59**, 83 (1977).
12. J. Minowada, M. Oshimura, T. Tsubota, D. J. Higby, and A. A. Sandberg, *Cancer Res.* **37**, 3096 (1977).
13. J. Minowada, H. Koshiba, G. Janossy, M. F. Greaves, and F. J. Bollum, *Leuk. Res.* **3**, 261 (1979).
14. M. F. Greaves, G. Brown, N. T. Rapson, and T. A. Lister, *Clin. Immunol. Immunopathol.* **4**, 67 (1975).
15. H. Koshiba, J. Minowada, and D. Pressman, *JNCI, J. Natl. Cancer Inst.* **61**, 987 (1978).
16. S. F. Schlossman, L. Chess, R. E. Humphreys, and J. L. Strominger, *Proc. Natl. Acad. Sci. U.S.A.* **73**, 1288 (1976).
17. K. Koyama, K. Nakamuro, N. Tanigaki, and D. Pressman, *Immunology* **33**, 217 (1977).
18. T. Tsubota, J. Minowada, and D. Pressman, *JNCI, J. Natl. Cancer Inst.* **59**, 399 (1977).
19. K. Sagawa, H. Koshiba, M. S. Lok, and J. Minowada, *Proc. Int. Leukocyte Culture Conf.* **13**, 109 (1979).

20. M. B. Omary, I. S. Trowbridge, and J. Minowada, *Nature (London)* **286,** 888 (1980).

21. P. O. Kung, G. Goldstein, E. L. Reinherz, and S. F. Schlossman, *Science* **206,** 347 (1979).

22. E. L. Reinherz, P. C. Kung, G. Goldstein, R. H. Levey, and S. F. Schlossman, *Proc. Natl. Acad. Sci. U.S.A.* **77,** 1588 (1980).

23. E. L. Reinherz, P. C. Kung, J. M. Pesando, J. Ritz, G. Goldstein, and S. F. Schlossman, *J. Exp. Med.* **150,** 1472 (1979).

24. J. Breard, E. L. Reinherz, P. C. Kung, G. Goldstein, and S. F. Schlossman, *J. Immunol.* **124,** 1943 (1980).

25. B. I. S. Srivastava and J. Minowada, *Biochem. Biophys. Res. Commun.* **51,** 529, 1973.

26. M. Reedman and G. Klein, *Int. J. Cancer* **2,** 499 (1973).

27. I. Hayata, M. Oshimura, J. Minowada, and A. A. Sandberg, *In Vitro* **11,** 361 (1975).

28. T. Han and J. Minowada, *Immunology* **35,** 33 (1978).

29. M. S. Lok, H. Koshiba, T. Han, S. Abe, J. Minowada, and A. A. Sandberg, *Int. J. Cancer* **24,** 572 (1979).

30. M. F. Greaves, *in* "Human Lymphocyte Differentiation: Its Application to Cancer" (B. Serrou and C. Rosenfeld, eds.), p. 253. Elsevier/North-Holland Biomedical Press, Amsterdam and New York, 1978.

31. K. Nilsson, *in* "Human Lymphocyte Differentiation: Its Application to Cancer" (B. Serrou and C. Rosenfeld, eds.), p. 307. Elsevier/North-Holland Biomedical Press, Amsterdam and New York, 1978.

32. M. Seligmann, J. L. Preud'Homme, and J. C. Brouet, *in* "Human Lymphocyte Differentiation: Its Application to Cancer" (B. Serrou and C. Rosenfeld, eds.), p. 133. Elsevier/North-Holland Biomedical Press, Amsterdam and New York, 1978.

33. S. Thierfelder, H. Rodt, E. Thiel, G. Hoffmann-Fezer, B. Betzel, R. J. Haas, G. F. Wundisch, and C. Bender-Gotze, *Recent Results Cancer Res.* **69,** 41 (1979).

34. E. L. Reinherz and S. F. Schlossman, *Cell* **19,** 821 (1980).

35. J. Ritz, J. M. Pesando, J. Notis-McConarty, H. Lazarus, and S. F. Schlossman, *Nature (London)* **283,** 583 (1980).

36. R. Billing, B. Rafizadeh, I. Drew, G. Hartman, R. Gale, and P. Terasaki, *J. Exp. Med.* **144,** 167 (1976).

37. R. S. Metzgar and T. Mohanakumar, *Semin. Hematol.* **15,** 139 (1978).

38. S. J. Collins, F. W. Ruscetti, R. E. Gallagher, and R. C. Gallo, *Proc. Natl. Acad Sci. U.S.A.* **75,** 2458 (1978).

39. H. P. Koeffler and D. W. Golde, *Science* **200,** 1153 (1978).

40. L. C. Anderson, M. Jokienen, and C. G. Gahmberg, *Nature (London)* **278,** 364 (1979).

41. M. A. Boss, D. Delia, J. B. Robinson, and M. F. Greaves, *Blood* **56,** 910 (1980).

42. B. B. Lozzio and C. B. Lozzio, *Leuk. Res.* **3,** 363 (1980).

43. P. J. Fialkow, S. M. Gartler, and A. Yoshida, *Proc. Natl. Acad. Sci. U.S.A.* **58,** 1468 (1967).

44. D. R. Boggs, *Blood* **44,** 449 (1974).

45. G. Janossy, M. Roberts, and M. F. Greaves, *Lancet* **2,** 1058 (1976).

46. E. L. Reinherz, P. C. Kung, G. Goldstein, and S. F. Schlossman, *Proc. Natl. Acad. Sci. U.S.A.* **76,** 4061 (1979).

47. C. Y. Wang, R. A. Good, P. Ammirati, G. Dymbort, and R. L. Evans, *J. Exp. Med.* **151,** 1539 (1980).

48. M. B. Omary, I. S. Trowbridge, and H. A. Battifora, *J. Exp. Med.* **152,** 842 (1980).

49. L. M. Nadler, P. Stashenko, R. Hardy, and S. F. Schlossman, *J. Immunol.* **125,** 570 (1980).

50. G. Janossy, J. F. Bollum, K. F. Bradstock, and J. Ashley, *Blood* **56,** 430 (1980).

4

Differentiation and Surface Membrane Glycoproteins in Hematopoietic Malignancies

LEIF C. ANDERSSON AND CARL G. GAHMBERG

Hematopoietic tissue undergoes continuous renewal throughout life. The functionally specialized cells of blood and lymphoid tissues originate from pluripotent stem cells and differentiate along discrete pathways. The maturation within the different lineages is strictly controlled by still incompletely understood mechanisms. In addition to the characteristic morphological changes occurring during normal hematopoiesis the differentiating cells express various histochemically detectable enzyme markers and surface membrane structures which often are defined as receptors and/or antigens.

Malignant transformation in the hematopoietic system induces a clonal cell proliferation which escapes normal homeostatic control. This leads to lymphoma or leukemia with an accumulation of cells arrested at a certain stage of differentiation.

I. Analysis of Membrane Markers in the Classification of Hematopoietic Malignancies

Despite an intense search, no tumor-specific antigens of general occurrence have been found in human hematopoietic malignancies. The reason for this might be that, if tumor-specific antigens really exist, they may carry specificities unique for each individual malignancy and are therefore not of wider clinical importance. But malignant hematopoietic cells express membrane structures also found in specific lineages and stages of differentiation of normal hematopoietic cells. Such differentiation antigens provide valuable information for the current classification of leukemias and lymphomas. Some of the differentiation antigens are specific for a certain cell lineage [e.g., glycophorin A for the erythroid lineage (1)], others are typical of early differentiation stages of lymphoid or myeloid cells [e.g., common acute lymphoblastic leukemia (ALL) antigen (2) and HLA-DR and Ia-like antigens (3)]. Polymorphism-expressing surface structures such as immunoglobulins permit a distinction between polyclonal and monoclonal B-cell proliferation. Finally, analysis for receptors, used in the identification of functional subpopulations of immunocompetent cells, is employed in the classification of hematopoietic malignancies.

The development of the monoclonal antibody technique by Köhler and Milstein (4) has revolutionized the analysis of cell surface antigens. Discrete structures specific for certain differentiation stages or even certain malignancies can now be detected with standardized reagents. It should, however, be kept in mind that monoclonal antibodies primarily react with epitopes and not with molecules, which in case of malignancy might provide false information about the biological derivation of a cell.

II. Analysis of the Surface Membrane Glycoprotein Pattern in Identification of the Normal and Malignant Hematopoietic Cell

Most if not all proteins exposed on the mammalian cell surface are glycoproteins (5). They consist of a hydrophobic segment(s) embedded in the lipid bilayer and a hydrophilic carbohydrate-containing portion on the external surface of the plasma membrane. Glycoproteins comprise most of the surface structures recognized as antigens and receptors.

We have been involved in developing two methods for selective radioactive labeling of the carbohydrate portions of cell surface exposed glycoproteins (and glycolipids). In the first method surface sialic acid residues are oxidized by treatment of intact cells with 1–2 mM sodium periodate on ice followed by reduction with sodium borotritiate. This introduces ^{3}H label in sialic acid residues. We earlier demonstrated that this reaction was specific for the outer surface when carried out at 0°C (6). In the other method, galactose and N-acetylgalactosamine residues are labeled after treatment of intact cells with galactose oxidase for 30 minutes at 37°C. The enzyme reaction is surface-specific. Because of its high molecular weight (70,000), galactose oxidase does not penetrate the intact cell membrane. To increase the labeling efficiency cells

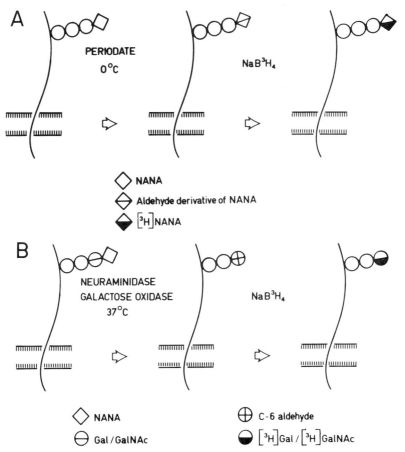

Fig. 1. (A) Schematic drawing of the periodate–sodium borotritiate surface-labeling method. (B) Schematic drawing of the neuraminidase–galactose oxidase–sodium borotritiate surface-labeling method.

are pretreated with neuraminidase which removes sialic acids and exposes more galactose residues. The enzymatic oxidation is followed by reduction with sodium borotritiate, and the original sugar is reformed and labeled with tritium (7). The principles of these procedures are shown in Fig. 1. The labeled glycoproteins are solubilized in detergent and analyzed by sodium dodecyl sulfate (SDS) polyacrylamide slab gel electrophoresis under reducing conditions. The radioactive proteins are visualized by modified autoradiography (fluorography) (8).

A. Surface Glycoproteins of Normal Hematopoietic Cells

Figure 2 shows the surface glycoprotein profiles of the major populations of blood leukocytes. The different cell types can easily be distinguished by their specific glycoprotein patterns (9). The functional involvements of most of the surface glycoproteins are still unknown. Some of these, such as the transplantation (HLA-ABC) (gp42) antigens and HLA-DR (Ia-like) gp31 and -24 molecules can be identified. As shown in Fig. 6A–C, the surface glycoprotein profiles of the main lineages of mature lymphocytes, T cells, B cells, and null lymphocytes also have different features. By using rabbit antisera specific for human T cells and thymocytes, combined with immune precipitation techniques from surface-labeled cells, surface molecules carrying T-cell-specific antigens have been identified (10). The T-lymphocyte-specific bands gp180, -170, -165,

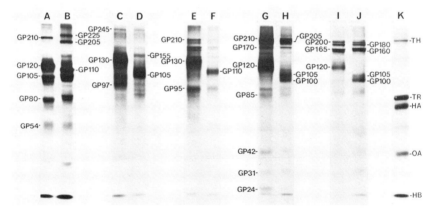

Fig. 2. Fluorography patterns of surface glycoproteins (GP) labeled with sodium borotritiate after neuraminidase (NE) and galactose oxidase (GO) or periodate (PI) treatment of purified populations of blood leukocytes. (A) Platelets with NE + GO; (B) platelets with PI; (C) granulocytes with NE + GO; (D) granulocytes with PI; (E) monocytes with NE + GO; (F) monocytes with PI; (G) non-T lymphocytes with NE + GO; (H) non-T lymphocytes with PI; (I) T lymphocytes with NE + GO; (J) T lymphocytes with PI; (K) ^{14}C-labeled standard proteins: TH, thyroglobulin; TR, transferrin; HA, human serum albumin; OA, ovalbumin; HB, hemoglobin. GP210 indicates a glycoprotein with an apparent molecular weight of 210,000, etc. [From Andersson and Gahmberg (9).]

and -160 reacted with these antisera. In addition, a molecule with an apparent molecular weight of 25,000, which may correspond to the rat and mouse Thy 1 (theta) antigen, was precipitated (Fig. 3).

The expression of T-cell-specific antigens in relation to differentiation was studied in isolated populations of human cortical and medullary thymocytes and peripheral T cells. As shown in Fig. 4, cortical and medullary thymocytes show different surface glycoprotein profiles. The bands of higher molecular weight, gp200 and -180, are present on medullary thymocytes and seem to appear concomitantly with the acquisition of immunological competence (10).

Another selective change in the surface glycoprotein was observed in both mouse (11) and human (12) T lymphocytes after *in vitro* and *in vivo* induced functional differentiation. When T cells were stimulated with allogeneic cells in

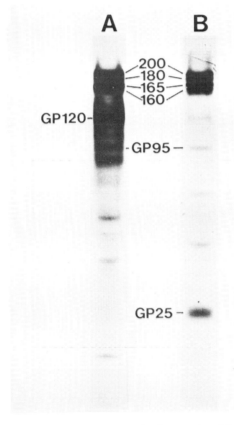

Fig. 3. Fluorography patterns of glycoproteins from surface-labeled (NE + GO) T lymphocytes (A) and immune precipitate obtained with rabbit anti-T-lymphocyte antibodies (B). [From Andersson and Gahmberg, *Mol. Cell. Biochem.* **27**, 117 (1979).]

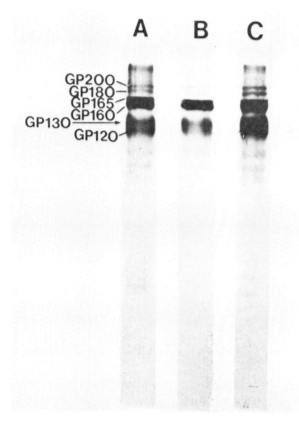

Fig. 4. Fluorography patterns of glycoproteins from surface-labeled (NE + GO) thymocytes. (A) Surface glycoproteins from unfractionated thymocytes; (B) surface glycoproteins from immature (cortical) thymocytes; (C) surface glycoproteins from mature medullary thymocytes.

mixed lymphocyte culture to differentiate into killer T cells, a glycoprotein with a mobility corresponding to a molecular weight of 130,000 (gp130) appeared. This protein was not strongly expressed on mitogen-activated T cells (Fig. 5). This phenomenon has further been analyzed in the mouse system by Kimura *et al.*, who found that the corresponding protein, called T 145, constitutes a selective marker for the cytotoxic T cell carrying the relevant Lyt phenotype (13). The occurrence of this differentiation determinant is not due to *in vitro* culturing, since apparently the same protein is observed on cytotoxic T lymphoblasts isolated from the blood of patients with acute infectious mononucleosis (14).

B. Surface Glycoproteins of Malignant Hematopoietic Cells

1. *Established Cell Lines*

To obtain basic information about the surface glycoprotein profiles of malignant human hematopoietic cells, we have analyzed a large panel of various established human leukemia and lymphoma cell lines. The results, which have previously been described in detail (15, 16), can be summarized as follows. The surface glycoprotein profiles of lymphoid cell lines of B-cell origin had basic similarities to those of blood B lymphocytes and *in vitro* activated B blasts. The

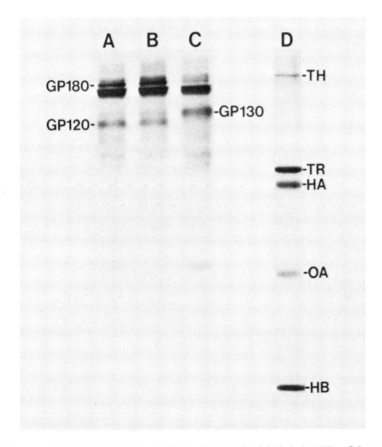

Fig. 5. Fluorography patterns of surface glycoproteins labeled after NE + GO treatment of T lymphoblasts cultured for 6 days. (A) Phytohemagglutinin (PHA)-stimulated blasts; (B) concanavalin A (Con-A)-stimulated blasts; (C) blasts stimulated with allogeneic cells in mixed lymphocyte culture; (D) standard proteins as in Fig. 2.

glycoprotein patterns of T-lymphocyte-derived cell lines accordingly showed similarities to the glycoprotein profiles of *in vitro* activated T lymphoblasts.

The "histiocytic" cell lines are biologically a heterogeneous group, which also was reflected in their diversified surface glycoprotein profiles (see Nilsson, this volume). Some of them showed glycoprotein patterns similar to those of blood monocytes (17).

Burkitt's lymphoma cell lines all had similar glycoprotein profiles, which were easily distinguishable from those of Epstein–Barr virus (EBV)-transformed lymphoblastoid cell lines of presumed nonneoplastic origin. We also noticed that Burkitt's lymphoma lines and three non-Burkitt lymphoma B lines, regardless of the presence or absence of EBV, had two characteristic closely spaced pairs of surface glycoproteins with apparent molecular weights of 87,000–85,000 and 71,000–69,000. These were not detected on normal B cells, B blasts, or lymphoblastoid cell lines (15).

Although the real nature of the gp69/71 and -85/87 on human cells is still unclear, they show suggestive similarities to the retrovirus-induced gp69/71 on murine cells. Yi Wang *et al.* recently identified apparently the same protein(s) on human leukemic cells with monoclonal antibodies (18).

2. Surface Glycoprotein Patterns of Cells Isolated from Patients with Leukemia or Lymphoma

Tumor cells were isolated from blood, bone marrow aspirates, and lymph nodes and used for surface labeling at a morphological uniformity of 95%. Sometimes further purification procedures such as density gradient centrifugation and/or velocity sedimentation at unit gravity were included to remove contaminating normal cells.

The fluorographic patterns of cells from four patients with ALL are shown in Fig. 6D–G. The cells run in slots D, E, and F were null cells according to surface marker analysis, whereas the case shown in Fig. 6G involved ALL T cells (sheep red blood cell rosette-positive). The ALL cells of non-B, non-T cell type are characterized by a distinct labeling of gp210, which is also found on null lymphocytes and B lymphocytes but not on mature cells. On the other hand, ALL cells with the ability to bind sheep erythrocytes did not express gp210 but instead some of the T-cell characteristic bands of gp160/200. Intermediate forms of differentiation toward T cells can also be seen, as shown in Fig. 6F. In this particular case there is expression of some of the T-cell bands in the upper-molecular-weight region. These cells were unable to bind sheep erythrocytes, but the clinical course was highly malignant. This finding indicates that, within the group of common or null ALLs, cases with incomplete T-cell differentiation can be observed. The heavy labeling of gp120/130 seems to be a common feature of undifferentiated leukemias of the lymphoblastic or myeloblastic type. Moreover, the distinct expression of gp210 coincided with the presence of gp42 (which is

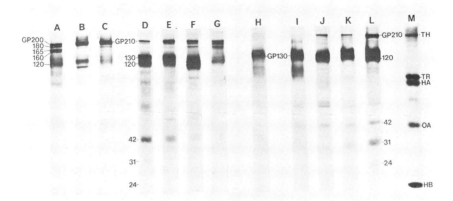

Fig. 6. Fluorography patterns of surface glycoproteins labeled after NE + GO treatment. (A) Normal blood T lymphocytes; (B) normal blood B lymphocytes; (C) normal non-T, non-B lymphocytes; (D and E) leukemic cells from patients with non-T, non-B ALL; (F) leukemic cells from a patient with T-ALL; (H) normal granulocytes; (I) leukemic cells from a patient with promyelocytic leukemia; (J–L) leukemic cells from patients with undifferentiated AML; (M) standard proteins as in Fig. 2.

the heavy chain of HLA) and gp31 and -24 (HLA-D). Based on our experience from extensive studies on ALL and acute myeloid leukemia (AML) cells we suggest that this represents the real null cell pattern (19).

The general surface glycoprotein patterns of cells obtained from patients with chronic lymphocytic leukemia (CLL) were clearly distinct from those of patients with ALL. Two types of CLL patterns were seen. In one type, the most prominent band was gp210. Moreover, gp42, -31, and -24 were clearly labeled, while the region of gp120 was weakly labeled. In the cells of the other CLL type, gp210 was usually absent and a prominent band was seen with an apparent molecular weight of 120,000 (19, 20).

Leukemic cells from patients with AML expressed the most strongly labeled proteins in the 120,000–130,000-molecular-weight region. The gp210 was labeled in some AML cells but was absent in cells showing promyelocytic differentiation. The gp42, -31, and -24 were usually seen on myeloid leukemia cells with a strong gp210. The cells from patients with CML showed basic glycoprotein patterns similar to those of normal granulocytes but with a more strongly labeled diffuse band in the 130,000-molecular-weight region (21).

The surface glycoprotein profiles of undifferentiated ALL and AML cells were rather similar. This indicates that both of these disorders are characterized by malignant cells at very early stages of hematopoietic differentiation apparently close to pluripotent stem cells. When the lymphocytic leukemia cells showed differentiated phenotypes, they gained a glycoprotein profile resembling that of

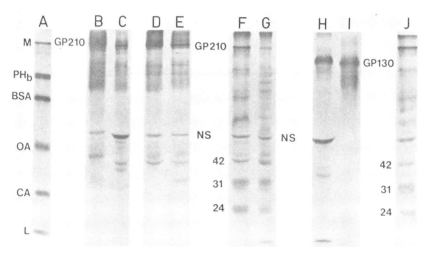

Fig. 7. Fluorography patterns of surface glycoproteins of cells from two patients with hairy cell leukemia. (A) ^{14}C-labeled standard proteins: M, myosin; PH_b, phosphocylase b; BSA, bovine serum albumin; OA, ovalbumin; CA, carbonic anhydrase; L, lysozyme; (B-C) cells from patient 1 labeled after treatment with NE + GO (B) and with PI (C); (D-E) cells from patient 2; (D) labeled as in (B) and (E) as in (C); (F-G) the hairy cell leukemia line JOK-1; (F) labeled after treatment with NE + GO and (G) after treatment with PI; (H) glycoprotein pattern of the promonocytic line U-937 labeled after NE + GO treatment; (I) glycoprotein pattern of granulocytes labeled as in (H); (J) glycoprotein pattern of the Burkitt's lymphoma line Raji labeled as in (H). (NS) Protein labeling directly with NaB^3H_4.

normal T or B cells. Myeloid leukemias showing cytological differentiation acquired glycoprotein patterns resembling those of normal granulocytes.

During the past few years the derivation of hairy cells has been widely discussed. These cells, which usually heavily infiltrate the bone marrow and spleen but rarely cause leukemic blood pictures, have phenotypical features compatible with both a monocyte–macrophage origin and a lymphoid (B-cell) origin. Since hairy cells have been found to synthesize immunoglobulins, most investigators favor a B-cell derivation.

The surface glycoprotein profiles of freshly isolated hairy cells also support a lymphoid derivation. They show similarities to the profiles of EBV-induced lymphoblastoid lines and of B lymphomas but are clearly different from those of monocytes and macrophages and also of monolytic leukemias (Fig. 7).

III. *In Vitro* Differentiation and Surface Glycoprotein Changes of Human Malignant Hematopoietic Cells

Specific changes in the surface glycoprotein profile were observed during thymocyte maturation to immunocompetent T cells and during *in vitro* induction of T lymphocytes to killer cells. Typical profiles of surface glycoprotein patterns corresponding to the degree of maturation of various leukemic cells freshly isolated from patients could also be demonstrated. To further study the differentiation-related membrane changes in human malignant hematopoietic cells we have used different *in vitro* models.

The promyelocytic leukemia line HL-60, obtained from R. Gallo's laboratory (Bethesda, Maryland), is inducible to terminal granulocytic differentiation when cultivated in the presence of dimethyl sulfoxide (DMSO) (22, 23). During differentiation the cell acquires phagocytic and chemotactic capacities (23).

The most strongly labeled glycoprotein of uninduced HL-60 cells had an apparent molecular weight of 160,000 (gp160). After culturing for 2 days in the presence of DMSO, the surface glycoprotein pattern changed, with a complete loss of gp160. Instead there appeared a strongly labeled gp130. At this stage very little label in other surface glycoproteins was seen. During subsequent growth in the presence of the inducer, the label in gp130 remained essentially unchanged but gp210 and -155 appeared.

Purified HL-60 blasts contained label almost only in gp160, whereas purified HL-60 differentiated cells had labeled gp155 and -130. Purified granulocytes from blood had a surface glycoprotein pattern similar to that of differentiated HL-60 cells, with a strong gp130 (23) (Fig. 8). The relationship between gp160 and -130 is still unclear. Their disappearance and appearance during induced differentiation suggests a precursor–product relationship. Analysis of the glycopeptides and oligosaccharides shows similar structures, but the polypeptide portions have not been characterized in detail.

An indirect indication of the functional involvement of gp130 was obtained with the observation that this protein was poorly labeled in granulocytes from patients with 7-monosomy (24). These granulocytes have normal mobility but do not respond to chemotactic stimuli (25). Chromosome 7 seems to be involved in the expression and/or glycosylation of this particular protein which might be involved in chemotaxis.

The K562 cell line established by Lozzio and Lozzio was originally reported to represent an early stage of the granulocytic lineage (26). During our study on a large panel of hematopoietic cell lines we observed that this cell line expressed a surface glycoprotein pattern which was not compatible with a myeloid or granulocytic origin (16). Instead, we noticed striking similarities to the glycoprotein profile of mature erythrocytes (27). An immune heteroantiserum prepared against this cell line and extensively adsorbed with other lymphoid lines still showed reactivity against the whole erythroid lineage of normal bone marrow. By monospecific anti-glycophorin A antiserum we could demonstrate that the K562 cell line expressed (27) and synthesized glycophorin A (28) which is the major sialoglycoprotein of normal erythrocytes. Subsequently we noticed that, on cultivation together with sodium butyrate, this cell line was inducible to erythroid maturation including benzidine positivity, hemoglobin synthesis, and

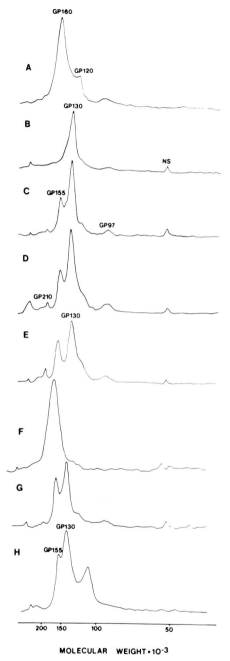

Fig. 8. Scanning patterns of surface glycoproteins of HL-60 cells labeled after NE + GO treatment. (A) Noninduced HL-60 cells; (B-E) HL-60 cells cultivated in the presence of 1.0% DMSO for 2 days (B), for 3 days (C), for 4 days (D), and for 5 days (E). (F) Purified HL-60 blasts; (G) purified HL-60 granulocytes; (H) normal blood granulocytes.

formation of erythrocyte-like particles (29). During differentiation the surface glycoprotein profile changed. The most striking change was the disappearance of the sharp gp105 band and the appearance of a diffuse gp115 band (Fig. 9).

One practical implication of these studies is that glycophorin A is an exclusive marker for the erythroid lineage which is expressed before the onset of hemoglobin synthesis during erythropoiesis (1). We have used anti-glycophorin A antiserum for the identification of leukemias which express early erythroid features. These studies have clearly shown that erythroid leukemia is much more common in humans than previously reported (30, 31).

We have recently established a continuous cell line from the blood of a patient with hairy cell leukemia. This cell line, called JOK-1, which has phenotypical

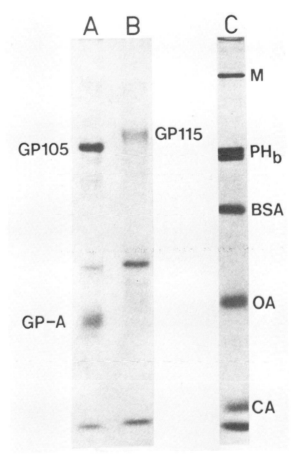

Fig. 9. The major surface glycoproteins of K562 cells labeled after PI treatment (A) and of K562 cells cultivated with 1 mM sodium butyrate for 4 days (B). Standard proteins (C) as in Fig. 7.

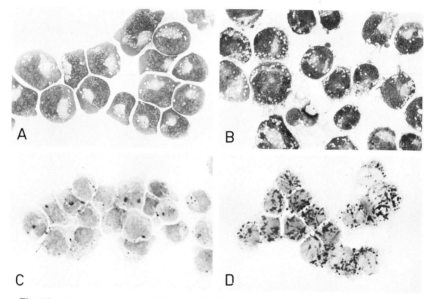

Fig. 10. Microphotographs of the JOK-1 cell line (A), and after cultivation in the presence of 2 mM sodium butyrate for 3 days (B). Tartrate-resistant (2.3×10^{-2} M) acid phosphatase activity in uninduced JOK-1 cells (C), and after sodium butyrate induction for 3 days (D).

features of an early B cell with intracytoplasmic μ chains, grows in suspension culture and has an abnormal karyotype with 48 chromosomes and only one chromosome 6. Its surface glycoprotein profile is similar to that of freshly isolated hairy cells. The cell line also shows weak acid phosphatase reactivity which cannot be inhibited by 2×10^{-2} M sodium tartrate (Fig. 10). This cell line can be induced to a "hairy" state by cultivation in the presence of 2 mM sodium butyrate for 3 days (Fig. 11). During this differentiation a small but significant change was observed in the surface glycoprotein profile (Fig. 12). "New" bands with apparent molecular weights of 57,000, 46,000, and 37,000 appeared. Moreover, this led to an increase in the acid phosphatase activity and disappearance of the intracytoplasmic immunoglobulin with subsequent expression of κ light chains on the cell surface.

IV. Molecular Basis for Changes in the Surface Glycoprotein Profile or the Expression of New Antigens during Hematopoietic Differentiation

The changes in the surface glycoprotein pattern observed during induced differentiation in normal and malignant hematopoietic cells are represented by

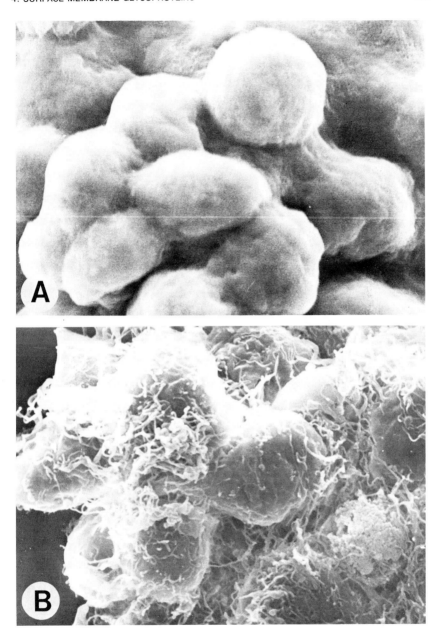

Fig. 11. Scanning electron micrographs of JOK-1 cells before (A) and after (B) induction for 3 days with 2 m*M* sodium butyrate.

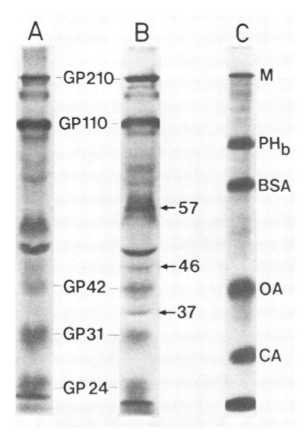

Fig. 12. Surface glycoprotein patterns of JOK-1 cells labeled after NE + GO treatment. (A) Uninduced cells, (B) cells treated with 2 m*M* sodium butyrate for 3 days, (C) standard proteins as in Fig. 7.

altered mobility on SDS gels of surface proteins or the occurrence of new bands. In several cases the disappearance of a specific band results in the simultaneous appearance of a new band. Although this suggests a precursor–product relationship, the real causes of these changes at the molecular level are still poorly understood. However, there are several observations indicating that the changes are primarily caused by differences in the glycosylation of the proteins, whereas the peptide portion of the glycoprotein remains constant.

We have previously reported that oligosaccharide components of the membrane glycoproteins on murine T and B lymphocytes are structurally different. The T lymphocytes are rich in alkali-labile *O*-glycosidic oligosaccharides and have a relatively low proportion of alkali-stable *N*-glycosidic oligosaccharides, whereas the opposite is true for B lymphocytes (32).

The reciprocal interrelationship of gp130 and -120 in the alloantigen-versus mitogen-activated T blasts suggests differences in the carbohydrate portion which induces different mobility on SDS gels. The finding that the gp130 in human killer T cells (and T145 in the mouse) selectively reacts with the blood group A-specific *Vicia villosa* lectin while gp120 is nonreactive (33) also indicates sugar differences. The switch from gp160 to -130 during granulocyte maturation also supports this assumption, especially since both proteins can be precipitated with the same heteroantiserum apparently reacting with the peptide backbone (23).

A further indication of the impact of the carbohydrates on the electrophoretic mobility and antigenicity of lymphocyte surface proteins was recently reported by Dunlap *et al.* (34) and Hoessli and Vassalli (35). They found apparent identity of the peptide portions of the antigenically different high-molecular-weight glycoproteins on mouse T and B cells.

Taken together, these observations indicate that changes in the glycosylation of the carbohydrate portions of surface glycoproteins may be of fundamental importance in cellular development and may constitute many of the differentiation antigens. Carbohydrate differences are apparently more easily detected with monoclonal antibodies than with conventional antisera which are difficult to make specific for subsets of cells unless their antigens express allotype-linked variations in the peptide portions. This might also indicate that the genetic information for surface alterations during cell differentiation is expressed through the regulation of carbohydrate transferases.

V. Concluding Remarks

During the past few years a panel of sophisticated tests has been employed for the characterization of cells in human hematopoietic malignancies. The improved classification of leukemias and lymphomas according to cellular phenotypes has not had any dramatic impact on the treatment and/or prognosis of these malignancies. The reason might be that surface marker analysis is usually carried out on the cell type accumulating during the disease, while possible precursor stages are overlooked. Continuous differentiation is a major feature of the hematopoietic system. During malignant transformation this capacity is more or less retained. A typical example is chronic granulocytic leukemia where the chromosomal marker, the Philadelphia chromosome, can be traced to stem cell level involving the erythroid and megakaryocytic lineages. The granulocytes accumulating during disease are progenitors of the uncontrolled granulopoiesis. Eventually the differentiation terminates in a blast crisis. Another example of differentiation during hematopoietic malignancies has been shown by Preud'homme and Seligmann (36) in plasmacytomas where the paraprotein idiotype can be followed to a B-lymphocyte-like precursor. In childhood non-T, non-B ALL, accumulating cells seem to be arrested at an early stage close to the pluripotent hematopoietic stem cells. This might provide an explanation for the good therapeutic results, since a low differentiation capacity might imply limited ability to give rise to therapy resistance. We have recently observed a few cases of relapsing childhood ALL where a phenotypical change in the malignant cells from non-T, non-B lymphoid to glycophorin A-expressing early erythroid occurs during the relapse (37). This phenomenon is compatible with the hypothesis that the therapy has selected for clones with early erythroid characteristics. The emergence of phenotypically altered subclones during the disease in solid lymphomas remains to be investigated.

Evaluation of the differentiation potential, i.e., the capacity of malignant cells to generate therapy-resistant clones, might turn out to be a more important parameter in the classification of leukemias and lymphomas than the current surface marker analysis.

Acknowledgments

This work was supported by the Finnish and Swedish Cancer Societies, the Academy of Finland, Finska Läkaresällskapet, the Association of Finnish Life Insurance Companies, and the National Institutes of Health, grant I ROI CA 26294-OIAI.

References

1. L. C. Andersson, K. Nilsson, and C. G. Gahmberg, *Int. J. Cancer* **23**, 143 (1979).
2. M. F. Greaves, G. Brown, N. Rapson, and T. A. Lister, *Clin. Immunol. Immunopathol.* **4**, 67 (1975).
3. G. Janossy, A. H. Goldstone, D. Capellaro, M. F. Greaves, J. Kulenkampff, M. Pippard, and K. Welsh, *Br. J. Haematol.* **37**, 391 (1977).
4. G. Köhler and C. Milstein, *Eur. J. Immunol.* **6**, 511 (1976).
5. C. G. Gahmberg, *in* "Dynamic Aspects of Cell Surface Organization" (G. Poste and G. L. Nicholson, eds.). Vol. 3, p. 371. North-Holland Publ., Amsterdam, 1976.
6. C. G. Gahmberg and L. C. Andersson, *J. Biol. Chem.* **252**, 5888 (1977).
7. C. G. Gahmberg and S. Hakomori, *J. Biol. Chem.* **248**, 4311 (1973).
8. W. M. Bonner and R. A. Laskey, *Eur. J. Biochem.* **46**, 83 (1974).
9. L. C. Andersson and C. G. Gahmberg, *Blood* **52**, 57 (1978).
10. L. C. Andersson, K. K. Karhi, C. G. Gahmberg, and H. Rodt, *Eur. J. Immunol.* **10**, 359 (1980).
11. C. G. Gahmberg, P. Häyry, and L. C. Andersson, *J. Cell Biol.* **68**, 642 (1976).
12. L. C. Andersson, C. G. Gahmberg, A. K. Kimura, and H. Wigzell, *Proc. Natl. Acad. Sci. U.S.A.* **75**, 3455 (1978).
13. A. K. Kimura and H. Wigzell, *J. Exp. Med.* **147**, 1418 (1978).
14. L. C. Andersson and C. G. Gahmberg, *Clin. Immunol. Immunopathol.* **10**, 41 (1978).
15. L. C. Andersson, C. G. Gahmberg, K. Nilsson, and H. Wigzell, *Int. J. Cancer* **20**, 702 (1977).
16. K. Nilsson, L. C. Andersson, C. G. Gahmberg, and H. Wigzell, *Int. J. Cancer* **20**, 708 (1977).

17. K. Nilsson, A. Kimura, L. Klareskog, L. C. Andersson, C. G. Gahmberg, S. Hammarström, P. Peterson, and H. Wigzell, *Leukemia Res.* **5,** 185 (1981).

18. C. Yi Wang, R. A. Good, P. Ammirati, G. Dymbort and R. L. Evans, *J. Exp. Med.* **151,** 1539 (1980).

19. L. C. Andersson, C. G. Gahmberg, M. A. Siimes, L. Teerenhovi, and P. Vuopio, *Int. J. Cancer* **23,** 306 (1979).

20. L. C. Andersson and C. G. Gahmberg, "Function and Structure of the Immune System," p. 623, Plenum, New York, 1979.

21. C. G. Gahmberg and L. C. Andersson, *Proc. 5th Meet. Eur. Assoc. Cancer Res.,* p. 200, Kugler Publ., Amsterdam, 1980.

22. S. J. Collins, R. C. Gallo, and R. E. Gallagher, *Nature (London)* **270,** 347 (1977).

23. C. G. Gahmberg, K. Nilsson, and L. C. Andersson, *Proc. Natl. Acad. Sci. U.S.A.* **76,** 4087 (1979).

24. C. G. Gahmberg, L. C. Andersson, P. Ruutu, T. Timonen, A. Hänninen, P. Vuopio, and A. de la Chapelle, *Blood* **54,** 401 (1979).

25. P. Ruutu, T. Ruutu, P. Vuopio, T. Kosunen, and A. de la Chapelle, *Nature (London)* **265,** 146 (1977).

26. C. B. Lozzio and B. B. Lozzio, *Blood* **45,** 321 (1975).

27. C. G. Gahmberg, M. Jokinen, and L. C. Andersson, *Blood* **52,** 379 (1978).

28. M. Jokinen, C. G. Gahmberg, and L. C. Andersson, *Nature (London)* **279,** 604 (1979).

29. L. C. Andersson, M. Jokinen, and C. G. Gahmberg, *Nature (London)* **278,** 364 (1979).

30. L. C. Andersson, C. G. Gahmberg, L. Teerenhovi, and P. Vuopio, *Int. J. Cancer* **23,** 717 (1979).

31. L. C. Andersson, E. von Willebrand, M. Jokinen, K. Karhi, and C. G. Gahmberg, *Haemato. Blood Transfus.* **26,** 338 (1981).

32. T. Krusius, J. Finne, L. C. Andersson, and C. G. Gahmberg, *Biochem. J.* **181,** 451 (1979).

33. A. Kimura, H. Wigzell, G. Holmquist, B. Ersson, and P. Carlsson, *J. Exp. Med.* **147,** 473 (1979).

34. B. Dunlap, P. F. Mixter, B. Koller, A. Watson, M. B. Widmer, and F. H. Bach, *J. Immunol.* **125,** 1829 (1980).

35. D. C. Hoessli and P. Vassalli, *J. Immunol.* **125,** 1758 (1980).

36. J. L. Preud'homme and M. Seligmann, *Proc. Natl. Acad. Sci. U.S.A.* **69,** 2132 (1972).

37. L. C. Andersson, R. Wegelius, G. Borgström, and C. G. Gahmberg, *Scand. J. Haematol.* **24,** 115 (1980).

5

Immunoglobulin Idiotype: A Tumor-Specific Antigen for Human B-Cell Lymphomas

RONALD LEVY, ADA HATZUBAI, SHERRI BROWN, DAVID MALONEY, AND JEANETTE DILLEY

I. Introduction

Human B-cell malignancies constitute greater than 75% of the cases of lymphoproliferative diseases in adults. Diseases in this category include chronic lymphocytic leukemia of the B-cell type (B-CLL), diffuse, well-differentiated lymphocytic lymphoma (DLWD), nodular, poorly differentiated lymphocytic lymphoma (NLPD), diffuse "histiocytic" lymphoma (DHL), Burkitt's lymphoma, hairy cell leukemia, Waldenstrom's macroglobulinemia, and multiple myeloma. With the exception of the last two disorders, these diseases are characterized by cells which have surface and/or cytoplasmic immunoglobulin (Ig) but which do not secrete appreciable amounts of these Ig products. The cell surface Ig of these neoplasms should provide a convenient target for immunodiagnosis and immunotherapy.

Because B-cell leukemias and lymphomas are monoclonal, each synthesizes an Ig with a unique idiotype. Therefore, the idiotype can be used as a tumor-specific marker. An antiidiotype raised against this marker could be used to monitor tumor growth and might also be useful as a tool in studying the immunobiology of the disease. Also, such an antiidiotype reagent might be exploitable as a therapeutic agent (1–5).

Stevenson *et al.* (1–3) raised an antiidiotype antiserum against a guinea pig B-cell leukemia and against human CLL cells. In their approach, limited papain digestion of leukemic cells released Fab fragments that were then coupled to a cellulose matrix and utilized as an immunogen.

We have recently found that secretion of Ig from nonsecreting malignant human B cells can be rescued by somatic cell hybridization with mouse myeloma cells (6). This provided an alternative approach for obtaining idiotype from the malignant clone. The monoclonal Ig rescued from the lymphoma cells of one patient was used as an immunogen to raise an antiidiotype antiserum as well as antiidiotype hybridoma antibodies. These antiidiotype antibodies were used, in turn, to develop sensitive assays to monitor the patient's malignancy.

II. Materials and Methods

A. Human Malignant Cells

Malignant lymphocytes from a patient (Ka) with nodular lymphoma were isolated from the peripheral blood and stored as previously described (7).

B. Preparation of Ka Idiotype-Bearing Immunoglobulin

Peripheral blood lymphocytes (PBLs) from Patient Ka were fused with the mouse myeloma line NS1/Ag4 as previously described (7,8). Clones resulting from this hybridization secreted human IgM λ chain that was idiotypically identical to the IgM found in the membrane of patient Ka's malignant cells. This Ig, Ka idiotype (Id-Ka), was isolated from culture fluids by affinity chromatography on a Sepharose-linked goat anti-human IgM column as previously described (7).

C. Production of Antiidiotype Antiserum

A New Zealand white rabbit was given repeated intradermal injections of 30 μg of the purified Ka protein in complete Freund's adjuvant and exsanguinated 3 weeks after the last injection.

To render the rabbit antiserum idiotype-specific, it was absorbed on a series of Sepharose columns containing covalently coupled (9) fetal calf serum (FCS), proteins, mouse Ig, normal human Ig, and a human $\mu\lambda$ myeloma protein. Then it was further absorbed on normal human PBLs. The antiidiotype antibodies were then purified by absorption to a Ka protein–Sepharose column and eluted with 0.1 M acetic acid.

D. Monoclonal Antibodies

A BALB/c mouse was immunized with Id-Ka (100 μg) in complete Freund's adjuvant intraperitoneally on day 0. On day 7 the mouse was boosted with 100 μg Id-Ka in phosphate-buffered saline (PBS) intravenously. The mouse spleen was removed on day 10. The spleen cells were fused with P3/X63/Ag8.653 cells (10) according to Kennett's fusion protocol (11).

Clones were examined for secretion of antibodies specific for human μ or λ chain and for Id-Ka by radioimmunoassay (RIA) (see below). Subcloning of clones secreting these antibodies was performed by limiting dilutions into wells containing normal mouse spleen cells as feeders.

E. Radioimmunoassay

1. *Radioimmunoassay for Testing for Specificity of Antibodies to Human μ or κ Chain and Id-Ka*

A solid-phase RIA was performed by using polyvinyl microtiter plates (Cooke Laboratory Products) coated by absorption with various human Ig's at a concentration of 10 μg/ml. After coating, the plates were washed with PBS–5% FCS. To the coated wells, 25 μl of test culture fluid samples was added. The plates were then incubated overnight at 4°C and washed four times with PBS–5% FCS, after which ^{125}I-labeled goat anti-mouse κ chain was added. The plates were then incubated for at least another 4 hours and washed. The wells were cut out with a hot-wire device and counted in a gamma counter.

2. *Radioimmunoassay for Detecting Id-Ka or Anti-Id-Ka Antibodies in Serum*

Plates (same as above) were coated with either Id-Ka or purified anti-Id-Ka antibodies. Binding of the complementary ^{125}I-labeled ligand (anti-Id-Ka in the first case and Id-Ka in the second case) was inhibited by test substances. The assay was performed in the following way: The standard solutions or the substances to be tested were added to the coated wells. The plates were then incubated for at least 2 hours at room temperature (longer incubations were carried out at 4° C) and washed four times; only then was the ^{125}I-labeled ligand added at a time when no free inhibitor was present. In this assay, Id-Ka and anti-Id-Ka could be distinguished from each other.

III. Results

A. Specificity of Antiidiotype Reagents

The absorbed rabbit anti-Id-Ka was tested for specificity against the Ka protein by RIA. In Fig. 1 it can be seen that the RIA had a sensitivity for detection of the Ka protein of $1\mu g/ml$ and that the antiserum showed no reactivity against an unrelated IgM (λ chain). The monoclonal antiidiotype used in this study (DM1) showed a similar specificity for the Ka protein. Further evidence of specificity of the antiidiotype reagents included indirect immunofluorescence, in which only the Ka tumor cells were stained by these antibodies and not lymphoma B cells from other patients or normal B cells from Patient Ka. Finally, immunoprecipitation was performed using radiolabeled membrane protein from Ka tumor cells. The antiidiotype reagents specifically immunoprecipitated the Ka protein from Ka tumor cells and did not react with labeled proteins from lymphoma B cells of other patients or normal B cells from Patient Ka (7).

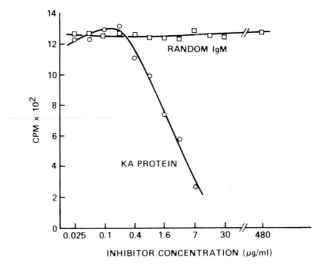

Fig. 1. Specificity of the antiidiotype antibody. Vinyl microtiter plates were coated with the purified antiidiotype antibody at a dilution of 1:800 in PBS. ^{125}I-Labeled Ka protein was added in the presence of either unlabeled Ka protein (○) or an unrelated human IgM (λ chain) (□).

B. Sensitive Detection of Tumor Cells in Blood using Antiidiotype Reagents

Because of the exquisite specificity of the antiidiotype antibodies, they could be used to detect small numbers of tumor cells by immunofluorescence. Artificial mixtures of tumor and nontumor cells were made and stained with antiidiotype antibodies. With the fluorescence microscope, tumor cells could be detected by this method when they were present at a frequency of 1/1000 (7).

C. Monitoring Tumor Burden by Detection of Tumor Cells in Blood

From 3/29/79 to 4/20/79, Patient Ka was treated on an experimental protocol with human leukocyte interferon. The details of this therapy are described elsewhere (12). During this time, indirect immunofluorescent staining with antiidiotype antibody was used to monitor tumor cells in his peripheral blood. The results are shown in Table I and Fig. 2. By 4/3/79, morphological examination of Patient Ka's peripheral blood showed no abnormal-appearing lymphocytes, yet immunofluorescent staining demonstrated that 18.9% of the cells were still idiotype-positive. At the end of treatment this number had fallen to 2.3%. One month after treatment, idiotype-positive cells had increased in the peripheral blood to 3.9%. Thus, the antiidiotype reagent could be used successfully to monitor the malignant B-cell clone.

D. Detection of Free Idiotype Protein in the Serum of the Patient

The patient's lymphoma (NLPD type) was not associated with a serum M component nor did the tumor cells from the patient secrete detectable amounts of

TABLE I

Percent Staining[a]

Cells	Antiidiotype	NRS	Specific staining[b]
Ka PBLs			
3/21/79	51.4	1.4	50.0
3/27/79	27.4	0.3	26.8
4/03/79	19.5	0.1	18.9
4/10/79	4.9	0.7	4.2
4/17/79	2.9	0.3	2.3
5/22/79	4.5	0.1	3.9
Normal PBLs	0.6	—	—

[a] Indirect immunofluorescence, analyzed by a fluorescence-activated cell sorter.
[b] Calculated by subtracting either NRS control or PBL control, whichever is larger.

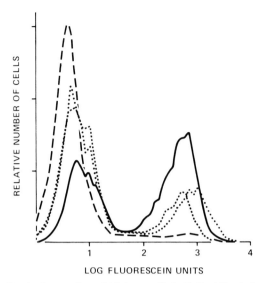

Fig. 2. Alteration in the number of idiotype cells in Patient Ka during treatment. Serial blood samples were obtained from the patient during therapy, and lymphocytes were purified by Ficoll–Hypaque sedimentation and stored frozen in dimethyl sulfoxide. Indirect immuno-fluorescence analysis and analysis with a fluorescence-activated cell sorter were performed on all samples in parallel. (——) 3/21/79; (- - - -) 3/27/79; (· · · ·) 4/03/79; (---) 4/18/79.

immunoglobulin *in vitro*. Nevertheless, a sensitive RIA was able to detect low levels of free idiotype protein in the serum of Patient Ka. As shown in Fig. 3, as much as 30 µg/ml of free idiotype was found in the serum at a time when the patient was in relapse. Furthermore, the level of idiotype varied with the tumor burden, falling in remission and rising in relapse. Serum idiotype was isolated for analysis. We found it to be a 19 S pentamer. Therefore, we conclude that it represented low-level secretion from the tumor cells rather than shedding of the 7 S membrane IgM.

E. Absence of an Antiidiotype Response by the Patient

We asked whether or not the patient makes an immune response against the idiotype on his tumor cells. This was done in two ways. First, a RIA was designed which could distinguish between the presence of free idiotype protein and the presence of antiidiotype antibody. When the patient's serum was examined at various times during the course of his disease, we never found antibody against the idiotype (Fig. 4B), whereas we could consistently find free idiotype (Fig. 4A).

Second, we looked for the presence of antiidiotype T cells in the patient. In order to determine whether a T-cell response to the idiotype of the tumor oc-

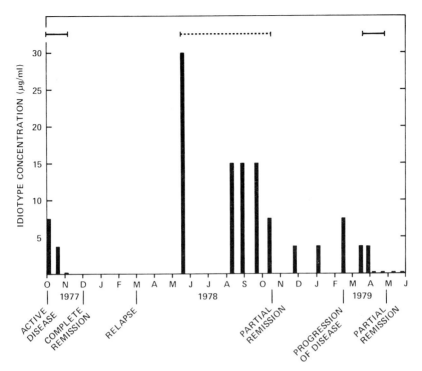

Fig. 3. Detection of free idiotype in the serum of patient Ka. Serum samples were collected from Patient Ka at various times and stored at −80°C. Determination of circulating idiotype was performed on all samples in parallel. Three periods of therapy are indicated: (——), human leukocyte interferon; (---), chemotherapy. The patient's clinical status at various points in time is also indicated.

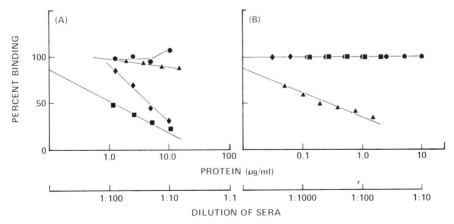

Fig. 4. Site consumption assay demonstrating inhibition of binding of ^{125}I-labeled Id-Ka-Ig to anti-Id-Ka-coated plate (A) and ^{125}I anti-Id-Ka to Id-Ka-Ig-coated plate (B) by anti-Id-Ka (▲), Id-Ka-Ig (■), Ka serum (♦), and normal human serum (●).

curred *in vivo,* Ka PBLs were doubled-stained for the presence on the same cell
of T-cell markers and Id-Ka. Peripheral blood leukocytes were incubated first
with a mixture of biotinylated monoclonal anti-Id-Ka and fluoresceinated
L17F12 (a general marker for all peripheral T cells). After washing,
rhodamine–avidin was added. In a typical sample taken during relapse, L17F12
stained 30% of the cells and anti-Id-Ka stained 55% of the cells. No double-
stained cells were detected among several thousand that were examined. This
result indicated that there were no Id-Ka-bearing T cells and probably indicated
that there were no T cells capable of binding Id-Ka. The latter conclusion is
inferred from the fact that there was circulating Id-Ka in the Ka serum. If there
were any T cells with receptors for Id-Ka, they would have been saturated with
Id-Ka from the serum and detected as double-stained by anti-Id-Ka and L17F12.

IV. Discussion

A tumor-specific antigen can be defined as an antigen present on tumor cells
but never found on normal cells. Despite a continuing search for such antigens in
humans, so far none have been found. However, certain types of normal cell
surface antigens can also be used as tumor markers. Most tumors represent the
clonal proliferation of a single cell (13) and, therefore, all the cells in this clone
may be antigenically similar. An antigen that is unique to this expanded clone
can serve as a tumor-specific marker even though its existence may be independent
of and predate tumorigenesis (14). The cell surface Ig of a B-cell lymphoma provides an excellent example of such a tumor-specific marker. In this case, the
idiotype of the cell surface Ig is a characteristic antigenic marker for the clone of
cells the tumor represents.

In this article secretion of Ig was rescued from a B-cell lymphoma by somatic
cell hybridization with a mouse myeloma cell. An antiidiotype antiserum and
antiidiotype hybridoma antibodies were made against the human Ig. Finally, the
antiidiotypes were used to monitor the malignant B-cell clone in the original
patient, demonstrating the usefulness of idiotype as a clonal marker.

Taking advantage of the specificity of the antiidiotype antibodies, we were
able to study a number of clinical issues. To begin with, the patient's disease was
monitored by following the percentage of Id-Ka-positive cells in his blood. The
percent of idiotype-positive cells was found to correlate well with the patient's
clinical condition (Fig. 2). Circulating Id-Ka-positive cells were found to increase at a time when the patient's disease was relapsing but prior to the time that
this relapse became clinically apparent. After treatment with chemotherapy, the
idiotype-bearing cells fell coincidentally with the clinical response. Second, the
antiidiotype was used to detect Id-Ka protein in the serum. This idiotype-bearing
Ig was found to be 19 S IgM and likely represented low-level secretion by

malignant cells rather than shedding 7 S protein from the membrane. Like the number of idiotype-positive cells, the concentration of idiotype changed in parallel with the patient's clinical status (Fig. 3). Both parameters rose during relapse and fell during response to therapy.

In principle, there is no reason why every patient with a B-cell lymphoma could not be monitored clinically in this manner. However, a specific antiidiotype reagent would need to be prepared for each individual—an effort that would be worth undertaking only if it resulted in improved patient survival. Improved monitoring of therapy or of remission status might improve current treatment regimens for B-cell lymphoma, although this is by no means clear (15,16). Alternatively, antiidiotype reagents might be employed to develop new approaches to therapy. Direct administration of antiidiotype antibodies to patients (17) or elimination of idiotype-bearing cells from bone marrow prior to autologous bone marrow transplantation deserve consideration. In the first case, circulating idiotype protein in the serum of patients presents a problem that would need to be addressed. Circulating idiotype would need to be removed if antiidiotype antibodies were to be expected to reach the tumor cells *in vivo*. Because 19 S IgM does not equilibrate rapidly between tissues and blood, it would be difficult to remove. On the other hand, bone marrow purging of idiotype-bearing cells presents less of a technical problem. This can be accomplished by complement-dependent cytotoxicity of idiotype-positive cells or by solid-phase absorption of idiotype-positive cells on antiidiotype-coated surfaces. Both procedures are extremely effective. The more difficult question involving autologous bone marrow transplantation is whether more aggressive therapy will successfully eliminate residual tumor in the patient prior to the transplant.

In addition to purely clinical considerations, antiidiotype antibodies allow a number of questions to be asked about the biology of B-cell lymphoma. The advantage of studying humans as opposed to animal models is that the disease can be studied in the original tumor-bearing host. The first question we addressed was whether evidence could be found for a host immune response against the tumor clone—that is, a host antiidiotype response. By several criteria we were able to conclude that the patient made no humoral antiidiotype response. No free or complexed antiidiotype could be found in the serum of the patient at any point during his disease. An attempt was then made to look for T cells with antiidiotype specificity. Total T cells were enumerated with a fluorescent anti-T-cell hybridoma reagent, and cells bearing or binding idiotype were enumerated by a second color of fluorescence. No double-staining cells were detected, even though the T cells were bathed *in vivo* in an excess of idiotype protein. Of course, one cannot conclude from the absence of demonstrable idiotype-binding T cells that T cells with antiidiotype specificity do not exist. They could have been below the limit of detection, they may have been sequestered in tissue compartments, or they may not bind antigen with sufficient avidity to be detectable by this method. One can at least conclude from the experiment that idiotype-*bearing* T cells do not exist in our patient with any detectable frequency. T cells bearing idiotype have been detected in patients with multiple myeloma or CLL by some (18–23), but not by other, investigators (24).

Does the host with B-cell lymphoma allow growth of his malignant clone because of his failure to respond to the specific idiotype? A test of this hypothesis might involve an attempt to induce an antiidiotype response in the lymphoma-bearing host. Cooper and colleagues (24) have proposed that B-cell malignancy actually represents the proliferation of pre-B cells, i.e., cells which do not express surface Ig or even light chains. How could pre-B cells exist which give rise to a tumor population uniformly expressing a specific idiotype and therefore a specific light chain? Such pre-B cells would have to have made a commitment to the use of a particular V_L gene even though they had not actually begun to express it. Somatic cell hybridization of pre-B cells with myeloma cells has failed to induce the expression of light chains by pre-B cells (25). Ultimately, a test of the hypothesis will require the use of light chain nucleic acid probes to determine if pre-B cells have, indeed, already rearranged their light-chain genes, therefore committing themselves to a specific V_L. If this does turn out to be the case, it might still be possible to regulate growth of the malignant clone through antiidiotype mechanisms, since pre-B cells not expressing surface idiotype may ultimately be eliminated as they differentiate into B cells expressing idiotype.

V. Summary

The Ig synthesized by nonsecreting human B-cell tumors can be obtained in large quantities by hybridizing the malignant human B cells with mouse myeloma cells. Stable human Ig-secreting hybrids can be derived, and the monoclonal human Ig can, in turn, be used as an immunogen for the production of antiidiotype reagents. We have produced both heterologous antisera and hybridoma antibodies against the idiotype of one such B-cell lymphoma patient. With these antiidiotype antibodies, we have explored a number of clinical and biological questions concerning the patient and his disease. For instance, we found both idiotype-positive cells as well as free idiotype protein in the blood of the patient. Moreover, the levels of both idiotype-positive cells and idiotype protein correlated with the tumor burden, rising in relapse and falling in remission. We found no evidence of antiidiotype response by the host, nor did we find idiotype-positive T cells in the host.

The antiidiotype antibodies can be used to deplete tumor cells selectively by solid-phase absorption or by C'-dependent cytolysis, raising the possibility of the use of these antibodies for autologous bone marrow transplantation. Other possible therapeutic uses of antiidiotype antibodies include their *in vivo* administration to lymphoma patients.

Acknowledgments

This work was supported in part by the American Cancer Society grant IM-114-B and Public Health Service grant CA-21223-04. Ronald Levy is an investigator of the Howard Hughes Medical Institute. David G. Maloney is a medical scientist trainee, Grant GM-06365, Public Health Service, from the National Institute of General Medical Sciences.

References

1. G. T. Stevenson, E. V. Elliott, and F. K. Stevenson, *Fed. Proc., Fed. Am. Soc. Exp. Biol.* **36**, 2268 (1977).
2. G. T. Stevenson and F. K. Stevenson, *Nature (London)* **254**, 714 (1975).
3. B. W. Hough, R. P. Eady, T. J. Hamblin, F. K. Stevenson, and G. T. Stevenson, *J. Exp. Med.* **144**, 960 (1976).
4. G. Haughton, L. L. Lanier, G. F. Babcock, and M. Lynes, *J. Immunol.* **121**, 2358 (1978).
5. K. A. Krolick, P. C. Isakson, J. W. Uhr, and E. S. Vitetta, *Immunol. Rev.* **48**, 81 (1979).
6. R. Levy and J. Dilley, *Proc. Natl. Acad. Sci. U.S.A.* **75**, 2411 (1978).
7. S. Brown, J. Dilley, and R. Levy, *J. Immunol.* **125**, 1037 (1980).
8. R. Levy, J. Dilley, and L. A. Lampson, *Curr. Top. Microbiol. Immunol.* **81**, 164 (1978).
9. R. Axén, J. Porath, and S. Ernback, *Nature (London)* **241**, 1302 (1967).
10. J. F. Kearney, A. Radbruch, B. Liesengange, and K. Rajewsky, *J. Immunol.* **123**, 1548 (1979).
11. R. H. Kennet, *in* "Methods in Enzymology" (W. G. Jakoby and I. H. Pastan, eds.), p. 345. Academic Press, New York, 1979.
12. T. C. Merigan, K. Sikora, J. H. Breeden, R. Levy, and S. Rosenberg, *N. Engl. J. Med.* **299**, 1449 (1978).
13. J. M. Friedman and P. G. Fialkow, *Transplant. Rev.* **28**, 2 (1976).
14. L. Lampson and R. Levy, *JNCI, J. Natl. Cancer Inst.* **62**, 217 (1973).
15. S. E. Jones, Z. Fuks, M. Bull, M. E. Kadin, R. F. Dorfman, H. S. Kaplan, S. A. Rosenberg, and H. Kim, *Cancer* **31**, 806 (1973).
16. R. I. Fisher, V. T. Devita, Jr., R. L. Johnson, R. Simon, and R. C. Young, *Am. J. Med.* **63**, 177 (1977).
17. T. J. Hamblin, A. K. Abdul-Ahad, J. Gordon, F. K. Stevenson, and G. T. Stevenson, *Br. J. Cancer* **42**, 495 (1980).
18. J. L. Preud'homme, M. Klein, S. Laboume, and M. Seligman, *Eur. J. Immunol.* **7**, 840 (1977).
19. T. Lea, Ø. T. Førre, T. E. Michaelsen, and J. B. Natvig, *J. Immunol.* **122**, 2413 (1979).
20. H. Binz and H. Wigzell, *Contemp. Top. Immunobiol.* **7**, 113 (1977).
21. S. J. Black, G. J. Hammerling, C. Berck, K. Rajewsky, and K. Eichmann, *J. Exp. Med.* **143**, 846 (1976).
22. K. Eichmann and K. Rajewsky, *Eur. J. Immunol.* **5**, 661 (1975).
23. G. Moller, *Immunol. Rev.* **34**, 1 (1977).
24. H. Kubagawa, L. B. Vogel, J. D. Capra, M. E. Conrad, A. R. Lawton, and M. D. Cooper, *J. Exp. Med.* **150**, 792 (1979).
25. P. Burrows, M. LeJeune, and J. F. Kearney, *Nature (London)* **280**, 838 (1979).

Expression of Normal Differentiation Antigens on Human Leukemia and Lymphoma Cells

LEE M. NADLER, PHILIP STASHENKO, ELLIS L. REINHERZ, JEROME RITZ, RUSSELL HARDY, AND STUART F. SCHLOSSMAN

I. Introduction

Leukemias and lymphomas, which previously were not distinguishable by either morphological or histochemical criteria, can now be subdivided into clinically and pathologically distinct subgroups by the use of a number of cell surface markers expressed on normal lymphocytes (1–3). For example, both normal and malignant B cells are defined by their expression of cell surface immunoglobulin (4,5). Other markers of the B-cell membrane, including receptors for the Fc portion of human immunoglobulin (Fc) (6), receptors for components of the complement system (C3) (7), and HLA-D-related Ia-like antigens (8,9) are less useful because they are not restricted to cells of B lineage and are also found on normal and malignant monocytes (10–12). In addition, Fc receptor-bound immunoglobulin may give spuriously positive results for cell surface immunoglobulin (13). Although T cells have been shown to be reactive with anti-T-cell antisera (14,15) and to form E rosettes with sheep erythrocytes (16), they too may express Fc or C3 receptors of Ia-like antigens (17–19). Finally, null cells, which lack the conventional markers of T and B cells (20), have also been shown to express C3, Fc, or Ia-like antigens (21–23). Given the extent of overlap of many of these cell surface markers, considerable attention has been directed toward defining unique cell surface antigens present on normal T, B, and null cells which can then be used to identify and classify leukemias and lymphomas.

With the advent of techniques for the production of antibodies against cell surface antigens, we have recently developed and characterized a series of hetero- and monoclonal antibodies which define cell surface antigens expressed on lymphocytes of T- and B-cell origin. Specifically, a number of anti-T-cell antibodies have been recently reported that are capable of dissecting normal intrathymic and extrathymic maturation (24–32). The identification of these antigens has permitted the division of human thymocytes into three major subpopulations (29). These stages of T-cell differentiation have been defined by the expression of distinct cell surface antigens which are either lost or acquired during T-cell maturation.

The observation that T-cell differentiation antigens exist has provided us with the impetus to develop monoclonal antibodies to antigens expressed uniquely on lymphocytes of B-cell lineage. To date, two monoclonal antibodies which define B-cell differentiation antigens have been described (33,34). The B1 antigen appears to be expressed on most stages of B-cell differentiation except the generally accepted terminal stage of B-cell ontogeny, the plasma cell. The B2 antigen, in contrast, appears to have a more restricted expression on B cells isolated from normal tissues and appears to be limited to the early stages of B-cell differentiation.

The ability of unique cell surface antigens to delineate specific stages of T- and B-cell differentiation has permitted us to further dissect the heterogeneity of leukemias and lymphomas of T, B, and null cell origin. In the studies described below, we demonstrated that these lymphoid malignancies reflected the same degree of heterogeneity and maturation as that seen in normal T- and B-cell ontogeny. This discussion will review the data obtained in our laboratory, and no attempt will be made to review the literature extensively.

II. Materials and Methods

A. Patients and Sample Preparation

All patients in this study were evaluated at the Sidney Farber Cancer Institute, the Children's Hospital Medical Center, the Brigham and Women's Hospital, the Beth Israel Hospital, and the Massachusetts General Hospital. The diagnosis of lymphoma or leukemia was made using standard clinical, morphological, and cytochemical criteria (35–37). Heparinized peripheral blood or bone marrow was collected from leukemic patients or from patients with circulating lymphomas (lymphosarcoma cell leukemias) prior to the administration of chemotherapeutic agents or blood products. Lymphocytes were separated from these specimens by Ficoll–Hypaque (Pharmacia Fine Chemicals, Piscataway, New Jersey) density gradient centrifugation as previously described (38). Tumor masses and lymphoid tissue from patients with lymphomas were gently teased, minced into single-cell suspensions, and passed through stainless steel mesh wire filters. Tumor cells were readily distinguishable from normal lymphocytes by Wright–Giemsa morphology, and all neoplastic preparations selected for this study had >75% abnormal cells. Isolated tumor cells were studied either fresh or cryopreserved in 10% dimethyl sulfoxide (DMSO) and 20% fetal calf serum (FCS) at $-196°C$ in the vapor phase of liquid nitrogen until the time of surface characterization.

B. Cell Surface Markers

The cellular lineage of tumor cells was determined by a number of cell surface markers. The definition of T-cell lineage was established by reactivity with a T-cell-specific heteroantiserum (14), monoclonal antibodies (15), and sheep erythrocytes (E rosettes), as previously described. All the T-cell leukemias and lymphomas were >75% reactive with the T-cell specific monoclonal antibodies and heteroantisera, and these tumor cells had variable E rosettes (0–90%) (39,40).

The B-cell derivation of the tumor cell was demonstrated by the expression of either monoclonal κ or λ light chains on the tumor cell surface. Monoclonal antibodies specific for κ or λ light chains were used in all studies (kindly provided by Victor A. Raso, Sidney Farber Cancer Institute, Boston, Massachusetts). In addition, a monoclonal antibody (I-2) (41), specific for the framework of the human HLA-D-related Ia-like antigen, was used to analyze all normal and malignant cells for reactivity. The Ia-like antigens have not been detected on the vast majority of T-cell leukemias and lymphomas but are expressed on most hematopoietic non-T-cell malignancies.

Non-T-cell leukemias were characterized using a monoclonal antibody (J-5) (42) shown to have the specificity of a previously described rabbit antisera against common acute lymphocytic leukemia antigen (CALLA) prepared in this laboratory.

C. Indirect Immunofluorescence Analysis of Normal and Malignant Cells with Monoclonal Antibodies

Normal or malignant cells were used fresh or thawed and washed extensively at the time of study; their viability exceeded 85% in all cases. In brief, $1-2 \times 10^6$ cells were treated with either 0.1 ml of a 1:500 dilution of the specific monoclonal antibody to be tested or 0.1 ml of a 1:500 dilution of an unreactive control antibody of a similar immunoglobulin isotype, incubated at 4°C for 30 minutes, and washed three times. These cells were then reacted with 0.1 ml of a 1:40 dilution of fluorescein-conjugated goat anti-mouse IgG (G/M FITC) (Meloy Laboratories, Springfield, Virginia), incubated at 4°C for 30 minutes, washed three times, and analyzed as previously described. The intensity of fluorescence was determined for 40,000 cells in each population on a fluorescence activated cell sorter (FACS-I) (Becton-Dickinson, Mountain View, California) and compared to the fluorescence of a control nonreactive ascites as previously described (43).

III. Results and Discussion

A. Antigens Dissecting Normal Intra- and Extrathymic Maturation

The importance of a thymic microenvironment in differentiation and functional maturation of T cells has been demonstrated in several species. It appears that precursor bone marrow cells (prothymocytes) migrate to the thymus gland where they are processed, become functionally competent, and are then exported into the peripheral lymphoid compartment. Moreover, profound changes in cell surface antigens mark the stages of T-cell ontogeny.

In humans the earliest lymphoid cells within the thymus bear antigens shared by some bone marrow cells, but these cells lack antigens expressed on mature T cells (44). This population accounts for approximately 10% of thymic lymphocytes and is reactive with two monoclonal antibodies, anti-T9 and anti-T10 (Fig. 1, stage I). These antigens are not T-lineage-restricted but are found on transformed cells as well. With maturation, thymocytes lose T9, retain T10, and acquire a thymocyte-distinct antigen (T6). Concurrently, these cells express antigens defined by anti-T4 and anti-T5 (stage II). The $T4^+$, $T5^+$, $T6^+$, and $T10^+$

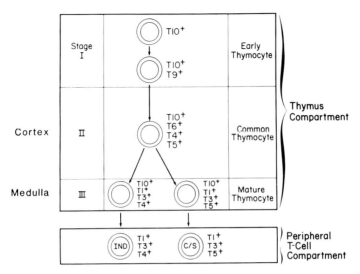

Fig. 1.   Stages of T-cell differentiation in humans. Three discrete stages of thymic differentiation can be defined on the basis of reactivity with monoclonal antibodies. These cell surface antigens expressed during T-cell ontogeny are shown.

thymocytes account for approximately 70% of the total thymic population and are primarily cortical in location (45). With further maturation, thymocytes lose the T6 antigen, acquire T1 and T3 antigens, and segregate into $T4^+$ and $T5^+$ subsets (stage III). The latter cells are found primarily in the medullary region of the thymus and account for approximately 10% of the thymic population (44,45). Immunological competence is acquired at this stage but is not fully developed until thymic lymphocytes are exported. Outside the thymus, the $T1^+$, $T3^+$, $T4^+$ and $T1^+$, $T3^+$, $T5^+$ subsets lack T10 and represent the circulating inducer (helper) and cytotoxic/suppressor populations, respectively (Fig. 1).

Unlike the majority of thymocytes, all circulating peripheral T cells are $T1^+$ and $T3^+$. The T4 antigen is expressed on approximately 55–65% of peripheral T cells, and the T5 antigen is present on 20–30%. These two subsets correspond to TH_2^- helper and TH_2^+ suppressor cells, respectively.

B. The Expression of T-Cell Antigens on Lymphomas and Leukemias of T-Cell Origin

The ability to define T-cell surface differentiation antigens has permitted us to begin to dissect further the heterogeneity of T-cell malignancies according to the state of differentiation of the malignant cell. Earlier studies employing the T-cell subset-specific heteroantiserum TH_2 permitted one of the first demonstrations of heterogeneity within T-cell lymphoblastic malignancies by serological methods (39,46,47). Specifically, it was found that tumor cells isolated from the majority of patients with T-cell acute lymphoblastic leukemia (T-ALL) were unreactive with TH_2 antiserum, whereas tumor cells isolated from patients with lymphoblastic lymphoma (LL) were TH_2-reactive. The expression of TH_2 antigen in these diseases suggested that the malignant lymphoblasts were derived from different T-cell populations. Furthermore, correlation of the TH_2 phenotype with the clinical presentation and disease course provided further confirmation that TH_2 antigen divided these diseases into clinically relevant subgroups. For example, T-ALL patients possessing predominantly TH_2^- tumor cells had a major tumor burden involving bone marrow, lymph node, and spleen. Although the majority of these patients had mediastinal masses, they tended to be smaller and did not lead to clinical symptoms. In contrast, patients with LL possessed predominantly TH_2^+ tumor cells and had respiratory symptoms due to markedly enlarged mediastinal masses and pleural effusions. A subgroup of patients with TH_2^+ T-ALL presented a different clinical picture. Unlike all other subgroups, these patients were primarily female children lacking a mediastinal mass and had very high white blood cell counts and severe anemia. More importantly, these preliminary studies suggested that the TH_2 phenotype of malignant lymphoblasts may correlate with response to therapy.

These studies with TH_2 heteroantiserum suggested that a more precise dissection of T-cell malignancies according to T-cell differentiative stages might further subdivide these diseases into clinically relevant subgroups. Recent studies have provided evidence that T-cell malignancies do, in fact, reflect the same degree of heterogeneity and maturation as is seen in normal T-cell ontogeny. In these studies, all T-cell leukemias tested were reactive with pan T-cell heteroantisera (A99) to human T cells, had a variable ability to form spontaneous rosettes with sheep erythrocytes, and lacked surface immunoglobulin and Ia-like antigen. In collaboration with Bernard and Boumsell (48,49), we have extended our earlier studies defining the T-cell phenotype of a larger number of patients with T-ALL and LL. As shown in Table I, most T-ALLs possessed antigens found on early thymocytes or prothymocytes (stage I). Approximately 20% of the T-ALLs expressed antigens found on stage II thymocytes and only rarely on stage III thymocytes. These observations confirmed earlier findings with a more limited group of T-ALL patients (29,39).

T-cell lymphoblastic lymphomas share many of the clinical features of T-ALLs in that they arise predominantly in adolescent males who often have a mediastinal mass. By definition, patients with T-cell malignant lymphoma have minimal bone marrow involvement ($<5\%$), whereas patients with T-ALL have extensive marrow and blood involvement. These diseases appear as two distinct clinical entities; however, as LL progresses, bone marrow and peripheral blood

TABLE I

Cell Surface Antigens Expressed on T-Cell-Derived Human Leukemias and Lymphomas

Stage of differentiation	T-Cell antigen expression	Malignant correlate
Stage I, prothymocyte	T9, T10	Majority of T-ALLs
Stage II, thymocyte	T6, T4, T5/8, T10	Majority of T-LLs
		Minority of T-ALLs
Stage III, thymocyte	T4, T5/8, T10, T1, T3	Minority of T-LLs
		Rare T-ALLs
Mature T, inducer	T1, T3, T4	All Sezary and MF tested
		Majority of T-CLLs
Mature T, cytotoxic or suppressor	T1, T3, T5/8	Rare T-CLLs

tumor infiltration frequently occur. Analysis of cell surface phenotypes of tumor cells from patients with LL demonstrates that in the majority of cases LL arises from stage II or III thymocytes.

Only a minority of patients with LL have tumor cells which arise from stage I thymocytes. These results suggest that T-ALL and LL are probably not different clinical stages of a single neoplastic process. The differences noted in clinical presentation, survival, and response to therapy may well result from the specific thymic pool, the differentiative stage, or the drug susceptibility of a distinct malignant T lymphoblast.

In addition to T-ALL and LL, several T-cell malignancies were studied to correlate these diseases with stages of T-cell differentiation (49,50). Patients with Sezary's syndrome and T-cell chronic lymphocytic lymphoma (CLL) are quite distinct, and every patient studied had a phenotype identical to a mature T-cell subset; i.e., either a T1, T3, T4 inducer cell or a T1, T3, T5/T8 cytotoxic/suppressor cell. As shown in Table I, all patients with Sezary's syndrome were T1, T3, T4, whereas patients with T-CLL were either T1, T3, T4 or T1, T3, T5/T8. It should be noted that these cells did not express or coexpress antigens associated with earlier stages of thymic maturation. Not shown are data indicating that some of these patients' cells also expressed Ia-like antigens (50). Although Ia antigen is commonly found on B cells, monocytes, and a fraction of null cells, its presence on activated T cells has now been well documented (51).

The studies described above support the conclusion that heterogeneity of T-cell malignancies, for the most part, reflects stages of normal T-cell differentiation. Anomalous expression of T-cell antigens on T-ALLs and LLs are also seen. Some cases bear both early and late antigens, but these represent a minority of the patients studied to date.

C. Monoclonal Antibodies Identifying B-Cell-Specific Antigens

In several previous reports, two human B-cell-specific antigens, designated B1 and B2, were identified and characterized with the use of monoclonal antibodies (33,34). B1 is present on >95% of B cells in peripheral blood and lymphoid organs and is absent from resting and activated T cells, monocytes, null cells, and granulocytes. This antigen was shown to be distinct from human immunoglobulin isotypes, Ia-like antigens, and Fc and C3 receptors. Functional studies demonstrated that removal of the B1 antigen-positive population from peripheral blood by cell sorting or complement-mediated lysis resulted in the elimination of B cells capable of being induced by pokeweed mitogen to differentiate into immunoglobulin-secreting cells.

A second human B-cell lymphocyte-specific antigen, B2, has also been identified (34). By indirect immunofluorescence and quantitative absorption, B2 was shown to be expressed exclusively on Ig^+ B cells isolated from peripheral blood and lymphoid tissues. In addition, B2 was not found on monocytes, resting or activated T cells, or granulocytes, nor was it found on cell lines of T-cell or myeloid origin. In contrast to B1 antigen, B2 antigen is weakly expressed on peripheral blood cells but is strongly expressed on B cells isolated from lymph node, tonsil, and spleen. Similar to the studies with B1 antigen, it was shown that B2 antigen was distinct from previously described B-cell surface determinants including surface immunoglobulin, Ia-like antigens, and Fc and C3 receptors. Immunoprecipitation of B1 and B2 antigens definitively confirmed that these antigens were distinct. Under reducing and nonreducing conditions B2 antigen precipitates a single band with a molecular weight of approximately 140K. In contrast, under similar conditions, B1 antigen precipitates a single band of approximately 30K molecular weight. Functional studies similar to those done for B1 demonstrated that only B2 antigen-positive splenocytes could be induced to differentiate into plasma cells under the stimulus of pokeweed mitogen, further confirming the B-cell specificity of B2.

D. The Expression of B1 and B2 on Leukemias and Lymphomas of B-Cell Origin

In recent studies (33,34,52), we have investigated the expression of B1 and B2 antigens on tumor cells isolated from patients with leukemias and lymphomas. As is seen in Table II, the tumor cells from all 24 patients with B-cell chronic lymphocytic leukemia (B-CLL) and 65 of 68 patients with B-cell lymphomas, all bearing κ or λ light chains, were reactive with the anti-B1 antibody. Anti-B1 was unreactive with acute T-cell leukemias and lymphomas and with tumor cells from patients with acute myeloblastic leukemia and a stable phase of chronic myelogenous leukemia. The expression of B1 on these tumors further confirms the B-cell specificity of the anti-B1 antibody. These observations

TABLE II

B-Cell Surface Antigen Expression on Leukemias and Lymphomas

Tumor	Number of patients	Number reactive with antisera		
		Ia	κ or λ	B1
Lymphomas				
B Cell	68	66	65	64
Null cell	5	4	0	2
T Cell	15	0	0	0
Leukemias				
CLL	24	24	24	24
ALL, non-T	41	41	0	21
ALL, T	17	0	0	0
CML, stable phase	6	4	0	0
CML, blast crisis	10	7	0	5
AML	16	15	0	0

suggest that anti-B1 adds to the repertoire of cell surface determinants which define B-cell tumors and, unlike Ia, Fc, and C3, it is restricted to this class of cells. More importantly, the presence of the B-cell antigen in conjunction with the expression of monoclonal light chains, either the κ or the λ type, provide additional criteria for the definition of a malignant B-cell clone.

Although anti-B1 was reactive with the vast majority of B-cell lymphomas and all B-CLLs, the non-T-ALLs were divided into several distinct entities. These tumor cells were strongly reactive with anti-Ia and anti-CALLA. Previous studies had shown that 95% of non-T-ALLs were Ia$^+$, whereas CALLA was coexpressed on approximately 80% of non-T-ALLs. These studies indicated that the majority of non-T-ALLs were CALLA$^+$, Ia$^+$, and a small group was CALLA$^-$, Ia$^+$.

We recently showed that approximately 50% of patients with non-T-ALL were reactive with anti-B1 (Table II) (52). More importantly, most of the CALLA$^+$, Ia$^+$ ALLs were anti-B1 reactive, whereas all the CALLA$^-$, Ia$^+$ ALLs were anti-B1-unreactive (Table III). Thus, non-T-ALLs can now be divided into three major subclasses: (1) CALLA$^+$, Ia$^+$, B1$^+$; (2) CALLA$^+$, IA$^+$, B1$^-$; and (3) CALLA$^-$, Ia$^+$, B1$^-$. These studies provide additional support for the view that a significant fraction of CALLA$^+$ ALLs are B-cell-derived. Other investigators have demonstrated that approximately 20–30% of CALLA$^+$ ALLs have the characteristics of pre-B cells in that they contain intracytoplasmic μ chains and lacked both surface and cytoplasmic light chains. The present study suggests that, in fact, the majority of CALLA$^+$, Ia$^+$ ALLs are B-cell-derived, since 75% were anti-B1$^+$. Whether B1 is expressed earlier than cytoplasmic immunoglobulin in B-cell differentiation or, alternatively, is a more sensitive marker of pre-B

TABLE III

Reactivity of Anti-B1 and Anti-B2 with CALLA-Positive and Negative Leukemic Cells

Tumor	Number of patients	Number reactive with antisera		
		Ia	B1	B2
Non-T ALL, CALLA$^+$	28	28	21	3
Non-T ALL, CALLA$^-$	13	13	0	0
CML, blast crisis, CALLA$^+$	7	6	5	0
CML, blast crisis, CALLA$^-$	3	1	0	0

cells, is yet to be resolved. The cellular derivation of the CALLA$^-$, Ia$^+$, B1$^-$ ALL is still not clear using presently available serological reagents.

Although all B-cell malignancies except myelomas expressed Ia-like antigens, κ or λ light chains, and B1 antigen, the expression of B2, as we have recently shown, appeared to be more restricted (Table IV) (34). Tumor cells from patients with myelomas, Waldenström's macroglobulinemia, Burkitt's lymphoma, nodular mixed lymphocytic lymphoma (N-H/L), and diffuse histiocytic lymphoma (DHL) (large cell-transformed lymphoma) did not express B2 antigen. Although all diffuse, poorly differentiated lymphocytic (D-PDL) and nodular, poorly differentiated lymphocytic (N-PDL) lymphomas were reactive with anti-κ or -λ, anti-B1, and anti-Ia, only a fraction (approximately 50%) were reactive with anti-B2. In contrast, all patients with undifferentiated lymphoma and almost all patients with CLL expressed B2. Interestingly, although approximately half (21 of 41) of the patients with non-T-ALL expressed B1, <10% expressed B2 (3 of

TABLE IV

Reactivities of Anti-B1 and Anti-B2 with B-Cell Malignances

Tumor	Number of patients	Number reactive with antisera			
		Ia	κ or λ	B1	B2
Myeloma	4	2	1	0	0
Waldenström's	4	4	4	4	0
Burkitt's	11	11	11	11	0
Nodular mixed (H/L)	4	4	4	4	0
Diffuse histiocytic (D/H)	11	11	11	11	2
Diffuse, PDL	26	26	26	26	13
Nodular, PDL	6	6	6	6	3
Undifferentiated	3	3	3	3	3
CLL	24	24	24	24	21

41). The presence of B2 antigen on only a fraction of the B-cell malignancies further supports the hypothesis that B1 and B2 antigens are distinct.

It has been hypothesized that B-cell non-Hodgkin's lymphomas represent a clonal proliferation of distinct stages of B-cell differentiation (53). Indeed, these tumor cells express either monoclonal κ or λ light chains, but not both. Examination of Table IV suggests that the B-cell tumors previously thought to correspond to the latter stages of differentiation (54) lack B2 antigen. Specifically, transformed or large-cell lymphomas (N-H/L and DHL), Waldenström's macroglobulinemia, and plasma cell myeloma are B2-negative. These tumors (N-H/L and DH) may correspond to the transformed B lymphocyte, and Waldenström's and myeloma to the cells of the secretory phase of B-cell differentiation (3). The precise stage of differentiation in which one places Burkitt's lymphoma is conjectural, since evidence exists for both an early and a late position (55). Increasing evidence has recently accumulated that B-CLL corresponds to an early stage of B-cell differentiation, since these cells express faint surface immunoglobulin (56), as do early B cells (57), and have receptors for monkey and murine erythrocytes (58,59). The observation that the tumor cells from 21 of 24 patients with B-CLL expressed B2 suggests that B2 may be present on these early B cells. In summary, the heterogeneity of reactivity within B-cell non-Hodgkin's lymphomas suggests that B2 is a differentiation antigen which may be expressed only at certain B-cell differentiation stages. The differential expression of B2 on normal B cells from different lymphoid organs may reflect the presence of B cells at varying stages of differentiation and, alternatively, may be related to the specific migratory potential of distinct subpopulations of B lymphocytes. In contrast, B1 appears to be a B-cell-specific differentiation antigen expressed throughout B-cell maturation excluding the plasma cells.

Because monoclonal antibodies are of extremely high titer and can be produced in unlimited quantities as compared to heteroantisera, the use of these markers can now be readily adopted in many laboratories studying leukemias and lymphomas. It is hoped that monoclonal antibodies defining unique cell surface differentiation antigens will provide the tools for a more precise classification of leukemias and lymphomas. The data presented in this article represent only a first step in the serological classification of lymphoid malignancies. Additional monoclonal antibodies will be required to further our understanding T- and B-cell differentiation. This approach may eventually permit a rapid and reproducible serological classification of T- and B-cell malignancies. Moreover, it is hoped that this method of classification will define clinically relevant subgroups upon which therapeutic decisions can be made.

Acknowledgments

The authors would like to thank the members of the Divisions of Hematology and Oncology and the Department of Surgery of the Sidney Farber Cancer Institute, the Brigham and Women's Hospital, the Beth Israel Hospital, and the Massachusetts General Hospital, Boston, Massachusetts, for their help in obtaining tissue specimens. We would also like to thank John Daley for technical assistance and Luci M. Grappi for secretarial assistance. Nadler is a recipient of a research fellowship from the Medical Foundation, Inc., Boston, Massachusetts. This work was supported by National Institutes of Health grants AI 12069, CA 19589, CA 06516, DE 04881, and RR 05526.

References

1. F. P. Siegal, *in* "The Immunopathology of Lymphoreticular Neoplasms" (J. J. Twomey and R. A. Good, eds.), p. 281. Plenum, New York, 1978.
2. J. C. Brouet and M. Seligmann, *Cancer* **42**, 817 (1978).
3. R. B. Mann, E. S. Jaffe, and C. W. Berard, *Am. J. Pathol.* **94**, 104 (1979).
4. S. Froland, J. B. Natvig, and P. Berdal, *Nature (London), New Biol.* **234**, 251 (1971).
5. A. C. Aisenberg and K. J. Bloch, *N. Engl. J. Med.* **287**, 272 (1972).
6. H. B. Dickler and H. G. Kunkel, *J. Exp. Med.* **136**, 191 (1972).
7. C. Bianco, R. Patrick, and V. Nussenzweig, *J. Exp. Med.* **132**, 702 (1970).
8. R. J. Winchester, S. M. Fu, P. Wernet, H. G. Kunkel, B. Dupont, and C. Jersild, *J. Exp. Med.* **141**, 924 (1975).
9. S. F. Schlossman, L. Chess, R. E. Humphreys, and J. L. Strominger, *Proc. Natl. Acad. Sci. U.S.A.* **73**, 1288 (1976).
10. H. Huber, S. D. Douglas, and H. H. Fudenberg, *Immunology* **17**, 7 (1969).
11. J. L. Preud'homme and G. Flandrin, *J. Immunol.* **113**, 1650 (1974).
12. E. S. Jaffe, E. M. Shevach, E. H. Sussman, M. Frank, I. Green, and C. W. Berard, *Br. J. Cancer* **31**, 107 (1975).
13. R. J. Winchester, S. M. Fu, and H. G. Kunkel, *J. Immunol.* **114**, 1210 (1975).
14. D. M. Pratt, S. F. Schlossman, and J. L. Strominger, *J. Immunol.* **124**, 1449 (1980).
15. E. L. Reinherz and S. F. Schlossman, *Cell* **19**, 821 (1980).
16. N. F. Mendes, M. E. A. Tolnai, N. P. A. Silveira, R. B. Gilbertsen, and R. S. Metzgar, *J. Immunol.* **111**, 860 (1973).
17. G. D. Ross, E. M. Rabellino, M. C. Polley, and H. M. Grey, *J. Clin. Invest.* **52**, 377 (1973).
18. L. Moretta, M. Ferrarini, M. C. Mingari, A. Moretta, and S. R. Webb, *J. Immunol.* **117**, 2171 (1977).
19. R. L. Evans, T. J. Faldetta, R. E. Humphreys, D. M. Pratt, E. J. Yunis, and S. F. Schlossman, *J. Exp. Med.* **148**, 1440 (1977).
20. R. P. MacDermott, L. Chess, and S. F. Schlossman, *Clin. Immunol. Immunopathol.* **4**, 415 (1975).
21. L. Chess, H. Levine, R. P. MacDermott, and S. F. Schlossman, *J. Immunol.* **115**, 1483 (1975).
22. L. Chess and S. F. Schlossman, *in* "Advances in Immunology" (F. J. Dixon and H. G. Kunkel, eds.), p. 213. Academic Press, New York, 1977.
23. L. Chess, R. L. Evans, R. E. Humphreys, J. L. Strominger, and S. F. Schlossman, *J. Exp. Med.* **144**, 113 (1976).
24. R. L. Evans, H. Lazarus, A. C. Penta, and S. F. Schlossman, *J. Immunol.* **120**, 1423 (1978).
25. E. L. Reinherz and S. F. Schlossman, *J. Immunol.* **122**, 1335 (1979).
26. E. L. Reinherz, A. J. Strelkauskas, C. O'Brien, and S. F. Schlossman, *J. Immunol.* **123**, 83 (1979).
27. E. L. Reinherz, P. C. Kung, G. Goldstein, and S. F. Schlossman, *Proc. Natl. Acad. Sci. U.S.A.* **76**, 4061 (1979).
28. E. L. Reinherz, P. C. Kung, G. Goldstein, and S. F. Schlossman, *J. Immunol.* **123**, 2894 (1979).
29. E. L. Reinherz, P. C. Kung, G. Goldstein, R. H. Levey, and S. F. Schlossman, *Proc. Natl. Acad. Sci. U.S.A.* **77**, 1588 (1980).

30. E. L. Reinherz, P. C. Kung, G. Goldstein, and S. F. Schlossman, *J. Immunol.* **124,** 1301 (1980).
31. E. L. Reinherz, P. C. Kung, G. Goldstein, and S. F. Schlossman, *J. Immunol.* **123,** 1312 (1979).
32. E. L. Reinherz and S. F. Schlossman, *in* "Regulatory T Cells" (B. Pernis and H. J. Vogel, eds.), p. 345. Academic Press, New York, 1980.
33. P. Stashenko, L. M. Nadler, R. Hardy, and S. F. Schlossman, *J. Immunol.* **125,** 1678 (1980).
34. L. M. Nadler, P. Stashenko, R. Hardy, A. van Agthoven, C. Terhorst, and S. F. Schlossman, *J. Immunol.* **126,** 1941 (1981).
35. J. M. Bennett, D. Catovsky, M. T. Daniel, G. Flandrin, D. A. G. Galton, H. R. Gralnick, *et al., Br. J. Haematol.* **33,** 451 (1976).
36. F. G. J. Hayhoe, M. Quagliano, and R. Doll, HM Stationery Office, London, 1964.
37. F. G. J. Hayhoe and R. J. Flemans, "An Atlas of Haematological Cytology," p. 110. Wiley (Interscience), New York, 1970.
38. A. Boyum, *Scand. J. Clin. Lab. Invest.* **21,** 51 (1968).
39. E. L. Reinherz, L. M. Nadler, S. E. Sallan, and S. F. Schlossman, *J. Clin. Invest.* **64,** 392 (1979).
40. S. Melvin, *Blood* **54,** 210 (1979).
41. L. M. Nadler, P. Stashenko, R. Hardy, J. M. Pesando, E. J. Yunis, and S. F. Schlossman, *Hum. Immunol.* **1,** 77 (1981).
42. J. Ritz, J. M. Pesando, J. Notis-McConarty, H. Lazarus, and S. F. Schlossman, *Nature (London)* **283,** 583 (1980).
43. L. M. Nadler, P. Stashenko, R. Hardy, and S. F. Schlossman, *J. Immunol.* **125,** 570 (1980).
44. E. L. Reinherz and S. F. Schlossman, *N. Engl. J. Med.* **303,** 370 (1980).
45. A. K. Bhan, E. L. Reinherz, S. Poppema, R. McCluskey, and S. F. Schlossman, *J. Exp. Med.* **152,** 771 (1980).
46. L. M. Nadler, E. L. Reinherz, H. J. Weinstein, C. J. D'Orsi, and S. F. Schlossman, *Blood* **55,** 806 (1980).
47. L. M. Nadler, E. L. Reinherz, and S. F. Schlossman, *Cancer Chemother. Pharmacol.* **4,** 11 (1980).
48. L. Boumsell, A. Bernard, E. L. Reinherz, L. M. Nadler, J. Ritz, H. Coppin, Y. Richard, L. Dubertret, L. Degos, J. Lemerle, G. Flandrin, J. Dausset, and S. F. Schlossman, *Blood* **57,** 526 (1981).
49. A. Bernard, L. Boumsell, E. L. Reinherz, L. M. Nadler, J. Ritz, H. Coppin, Y. Richard, F. Valensi, J. Dausset, G. Flandrin, J. Lemerle, and S. F. Schlossman, *Blood* **57,** 1105 (1981).
50. E. L. Reinherz, L. M. Nadler, D. S. Rosenthal, W. C. Moloney, and S. F. Schlossman, *Blood* **53,** 1066 (1979).
51. E. L. Reinherz, P. C. Kung, J. M. Pesando, J. Ritz, G. Goldstein, and S. F. Schlossman, *J. Exp. Med.* **150,** 1472 (1979).
52. L. M. Nadler, P. Stashenko, J. Ritz, R. Hardy, J. M. Pesando, and S. F. Schlossman, *J. Clin. Invest.* **67,** 134 (1981).
53. S. E. Salmon and M. Seligmann, *Lancet* **2,** 1230 (1974).
54. R. S. Stein, J. Cousar, J. M. Flexner, and R. D. Collin, *Semin. Oncol.* **12,** 244 (1980).
55. E. S. Jaffe and I. Green, *in* "Mechanism of Tumor Immunity" (I. Green, S. Cohen, and R. T. McCluskey, eds.), p. 251. Wiley, New York, 1979.
56. A. C. Aisenberg, K. J. Bloch, and J. Long, *Am. J. Med.* **55,** 184 (1973).
57. M. D. Cooper and A. R. Lawton, *in* "The Immunopathology of Lymphoreticular Neoplasms" (J. J. Twomey and R. A. Good, eds.), p. 9. Plenum, New York, 1978.
58. S. Gupta and M. H. Grieco, *Int. Arch. Allergy Appl. Immunol.* **49,** 734 (1975).
59. M. A. Pellegrino, S. Ferrone, and A. N. Theofilopoulos, *J. Immunol.* **115,** 1065 (1975).

7

The Impact of Phenotypic Heterogeneity of Malignant Tumors on Tumor-Related Monoclonal Antibodies

LENNART OLSSON

I. Introduction

Phenotypic characteristics such as morphology, proliferation rate, cell surface antigens, and *in vitro* culture properties have individually or in combination been considered criteria of malignancy (1–3). Although each of these characteristics has proven to be of some value in the phenotypic description of malignant cells, none has been demonstrated to be essential for the neoplastic behavior of cells *in vivo*. Implicitly, each individual malignant tumor may have a number of characteristics that are not necessarily expressed by another morphologically indistinguishable tumor; malignancy can accordingly be expressed by different combinations of cell biological functions found in normal cells. The question therefore arises whether the malignant cell population of a given tumor is phenotypically heterogeneous, as this affects not only the interpretation of cell kinetic, biochemical, and immunological studies on such tumors but also the outcome of clinical treatment trials.

II. Heterogeneity in Relation to Etiology

The etiology of malignant tumors is traditionally ascribed to spontaneous somatic mutation, an oncogenic virus, a chemical carcinogen, or a combination of two or more of these phenomena. The process leading to malignant transformation may involve several independent events (steps) of which the mutation, virus, or carcinogen is the transformation-determining step (4), but each step may determine part of the acquired transformation phenotype. When a known carcinogen is a determining step, multicellular origin of a tumor can come about in at least two ways: (a) A relatively large number of cells may be affected (transformed) simultaneously by the carcinogen, or (b) the carcinogen may initially alter only a single cell, and this alteration subsequently may lead to recruitment to the tumor of hitherto normal neighboring cells (e.g., through activation and release of an oncogenic factor). However, the etiology of most human spontaneous tumors is unknown and, until otherwise proven, is ascribed to somatic mutations. Somatic mutations are often considered rare, randomly occurring events (5), and tumors arising in relation to such mutations are therefore considered of monoclonal origin. However, the most frequent human tumors emerge at very discrete sites in the total cell mass of an organism in which a somatic mutation can occur, thus indicating that the cells at such discrete sites have a high tendency to undergo spontaneous mutations, and a multicellular origin of such tumors is a distinct possibility.

Phenotypic variation within a malignant tumor cell mass is particularly illustrated by the metastasis phenomenon. Pathologists have recognized for years that the morphology of tumor cells from metastases may differ from that of cells from the primary tumor. The extensive work by Fidler and co-workers on the murine B16-melanoma system (6,7) indicates that cells with metastatic potential can be detected in small numbers in the primary tumor cell mass. These cells selectively give rise to metastatic tumor cell masses that seem to have a stable phenotype as far as metastatic potential is concerned. However, these results do not unambiguously demonstrate whether the phenotype of the metastatic cell occurs as a result of selection *and* adaptation or solely because of selection. That adaptation may be involved in some tumor systems is suggested by our recent experiments with the murine Lewis lung tumor system (8). This experimental tumor system is a transplantable, subcutaneously growing tumor in the $C57BL_6$ strain with rather extensive metastatic potential, especially to the lungs. We have been able to establish malignant cell lines from the primary tumor site and from a lung metastatic focus (Table I). We have generated a mouse monoclonal antibody that

TABLE I

Some Phenotypic Characteristics of Cloned Lewis Lung Tumor Cells

Parameter	CIPT14	CIPT28	CIM28
Morphology	Round, mononuclear cell; variable cytoplasmic nuclear ratio	Round, mono-nuclear cell; variable cyto-plasmic nuclear ratio	Round, mononuclear cell; variable cytoplasmic nuclear ratio
Size (μm)	15–30	15–30	15–30
Cloning efficiency in agarose (%)[a]	18 (15–21)	20 (16–22)	18 (14–21)
Doubling time in RPMI-1640 medium with 15% fetal calf serum (hours)[b]	28	26	30
Number of lung metastases 3 weeks after injec-tion of 10^5 cells (6 mice per group)	9 ± 2	6 ± 3	43 ± 11
Neoantigen as detected by a murine mono-clonal antibody (M36D3)	–	–	+

[a] The values are the mean and the range of five experiments.
[b] Determined in the exponential growth phase of the tumor cells.

reacts with almost all tumor cells from metastatic foci but with none of the tumor cells from the primary tumor site. The metastatic cells seem thus to have acquired an antigen during their metastatic spread and growth. The cells of the primary tumor seem during the metastatic process to acquire new characteristics that may be related to adaptation to their new microenvironment. This further implies the possibility that the phenotype of the malignant cells continues to change in relation to perturbations in the microenvironment that inevitably take place dur-ing the metastatic process.

The concept of tumor progression proposed by Foulds about 25 years ago (9) seems thus to have pertinent value. During tumor progression, tumor cells may undergo independent changes in such phenotypic traits as karyotype, immunogenicity, drug resistance, hormone dependence, metastatic potential, and *in vitro* growth properties. Thus a tumor cannot be regarded simply as a homogeneous population of malignant cells. Instead, it is a dynamically evolving population; the inherent instability [probably mostly genetic (10)] of the malignant phenotype continuously results in new variants with a selective growth advantage. The result is a slow but inexorable evolution toward an increasingly malignant and autonomously growing tumor cell population.

III. Antigenic Heterogeneity of Tumors

Prehn provided the first indication of immunological heterogeneity of tumors by demonstrating in a methylcholantrene-induced mouse sarcoma that antigenically different sublines of malignant cells could be isolated from the same tumor (11). This antigenic heterogeneity was lost after serial transplantation of the tumor in mice. The importance of immunological heterogeneity in relation to immunological approaches to the treatment of experimental lymphomas was demonstrated by experiments with specific active immunotherapy in the AKR mouse lymphoma system (12). Attempts were made to prevent the growth of AKR mouse thymic lymphomas by repeatedly injecting young AKR mice with irradiated (10,000 rads) AKR lymphoma cells (first passage) after the recipients had been injected with untreated cells from primary AKR thymomas. The procedure was generally unsuccessful, and about 70% of the treated mice developed thymomas. However, it was found that the lymphomas arising in mice treated with irradiated cells differed immunologically as assessed by antibody and cytotoxic T-lymphocyte assays. After initially analyzing 14 individual thymomas, it was concluded that AKR thymomas were immunologically heterogeneous and consisted of at least four different subtypes (A, B, C, and D) which we were able to isolate and expand (Table II). The expanded clones were used to generate murine monoclonal antibodies with a specificity for one of the clones; we successfully established hybridoma clones producing specific antibodies against three of the four clones. The fourth clone (type D) was nonimmunogenic in AKR mice, and we were unsuccessful in our attempts to generate a specific antibody against it. The three monoclonal antibodies (all IgG_{2a}) were used to treat primary AKR lymphomas (Table III). Administration of only one monoclonal antibody had little or no effect on AKR lymphomas cell growth. It was only by the combined administration of all three antibodies that any significant effect was obtained. The fact that the dominant clone (clone A) was immunogenic in the autologous host suggests that variants based on immunological selection seem not to be important in this lymphoma model. It is also of interest that the dominant clone had the same immunological phenotype in all 14 spontaneous AKR thymomas studies, which indicates that emergence of the various immunologically distinguishable clones was not a random process.

TABLE II

Characteristics of Subtypes of Cells in Spontaneous AKR Lymphomas

AKR lymphoma cell subtype	Relative abundance in spontaneous AKR thymomas (%)	Immunogenicity in AKR mice	Monoclonal antibody against non-viral antigen
A	~97	+	+
B	1.0–1.5	+	+
C	<1	+	+
D	<1	−	−

Such animal experiments clearly indicate that the immunological approach to the diagnosis and therapy of naturally occurring tumors in human beings may be more complex than previously anticipated. Controversy persists as to whether naturally occurring tumors are at all immunogenic in the autologous host (13,14). The antigenic properties of human neoplasms have until recently been studied with very insensitive and insufficiently specific methods. This difficulty may have been overcome now that the monoclonal antibody technique has been developed (15). Fusion of antibody-producing lymphocytes with myeloma cells to yield somatic cell hybrids capable of producing the same antibody as the parental lymphocyte should in principle make it possible in cancer patients to detect lymphocytes primed against the autologous tumor mass. This approach

TABLE III

Therapeutic Effect of Murine Monoclonal Antibodies on AKR Lymphoma Transplantation

Antibody[a]	No. of mice[b]	Prevention of tumor growth (%)	Type of AKR lymphoma clone emerging in lymphoma-positive mice
Anti-A	25	12	B,C,D
Anti-B	25	0	A,C,D
Anti-C	25	0	A,B,D
Anti-A plus anti-B	25	24	C,D
Anti-B plus anti-C	25	0	A,D
Anti-A plus anti-B plus anti-C	25	84	D

[a] The mice were injected intraperitoneally with 400 μg antibody per mouse once a week for a total of 6 weeks. Injections were started 7 days after the lymphoma cell challenge.

[b] The mice were injected with 10^6 AKR thymoma cells intravenously.

has been tried by fusing human lymphocytes with a mouse myeloma cell line, but such mixed hybrids are karyotypically unstable. Our recent development of a mutant cell line of human origin with which human B cells may be fused to produce human–human monoclonal antibodies (16) opens the way to the systematic exploration of this approach aimed at the detection of tumor-associated antigens in human malignant neoplasms.

However, even with notable success in obtaining antibodies with tumor specificity, it is not evident that such antibodies will be successful in diagnostic and therapeutic applications. The idea of tumor progression with a constant emergence of variants indicates that antigenic variants may occur with high probability in the clonogenic part of the malignant cell population. Cloning of spontaneous tumors has been described in some human tumor systems, normally with a cloning efficiency below 1% (17), but the general applicability of these

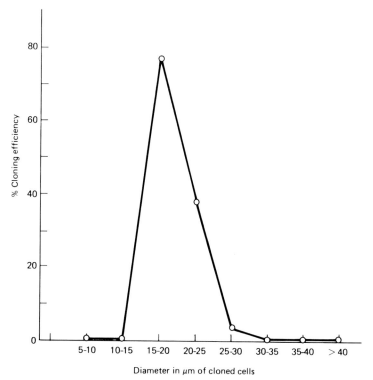

Fig. 1. Cloning efficiency of SU-HD-1 cells in 0.3% soft agar in relation to cell size. The cells were size-separated by centrifugal elutriation and seeded out in agar; clones were recorded 10 days after seeding. Only clones with more than 20 cells were counted. The values indicated are mean values of two separate experiments. Nonfractionated HD-1 cells were used.

methods to a broad range of human tumors has hitherto not been worked out as well as the relationship between *in vitro* and *in vivo* clonogenicity. Loss of clonogenicity implies loss of malignancy, but no data are available on changes in the immunological phenotype related to clonogenicity changes. Antibody reactivity against a majority of cells in a given tumor cell population does not implicitly indicate reactivity against the clonogenic (truly) malignant cells. In an attempt to increase the number of clonogenic cells, we used centrifugal elutriation (18) on an established human tumor cell line (type not yet determined). Figure 1 shows that the method, at least in this particular system, results in a cell population highly enriched in the clonogenic part of the tumor cell population. This method may be useful in enriching for clonogenic tumor cells in order to improve isolation and characterization of this part of the tumor cell population that we consider crucial for an appropriate evaluation of relevant monoclonal antibodies related to malignant tumors. An antibody toxic to a malignant cell population will, according to the tumor progression concept, result in a selection of tumor cell variants that do not express the corresponding antigen. Administration of cytotoxic monoclonal antibodies will therefore result in antigen-negative variants if the antibody does not eradicate all clonogenic tumor cells within a relatively short time period. *In vitro* experiments with murine monoclonal antibodies suggest that such antigenic modulation may take place within hours after antibody exposure (19), but that the antigen is reexpressed rapidly if the cells are

TABLE IV

Modulation of Metastatic Lewis Lung Tumor-Associated Antigen with a Monoclonal Antibody (M36D3)[a]

	Time for incubation of M28 cells with excess M36D3 antibody (hours)						
	0	½	1	1½	2	4	8
No. of viable cells after CDC	0–5	0–5	0–5	0–5	26 ± 13	31 ± 11	34 ± 5
Cloning efficiency after CDC (%)	0	0	3 ± 2	6 ± 2	12 ± 5	10 ± 6	11 ± 4
Percentage of total amount of clonogenic cells	0	0	16	33	66	56	62

[a] The cells were incubated at 37°C with 70 μg/ml antibody for various time periods, washed, and then tested for antigen presentation in a complement-dependent cytotoxicity (CDC) assay followed by cloning of viable cells in soft agar.

not exposed to the antibody. However, our experiments with the Lewis lung tumor model indicate that antigen modulation may vary in the clonogenic part of the tumor cell population in a different pattern as compared to the rest of the cell population. Table IV shows that significant antigen modulation occurred in the clonogenic part of the cell population as soon as 1 hour after incubation of the tumor cells with the specific antibody, whereas no antigen modulation was observed in the nonclonogenic tumor cell population 1 hour after incubation with the antibody. We will therefore have to generate for each tumor type complementary antibodies in line with our studies on the AKR leukemia model if the antigen-modulation phenomenon is shown to be valid for a broader range of monoclonal antibodies of both murine and human origin.

IV. Conclusion

The phenotype of malignant cells, including antigenicity, may change continuously during tumor progression as a result of environmental selection and genetic instability of the genome of the malignant cell, and this may have a significant impact on diagnositc and therapeutical approaches.

The monoclonal antibody technique, and in particular the use of human monoclonal antibodies, makes it feasible to identify and characterize the antigenic phenotype of human neoplasms as recognized by the autologous host, thereby possibly resulting in the generation of antibodies with high specificity for a given type of malignant cells. However, in order to evaluate properly the clinical usefulness of such antibodies, their reactivity pattern should be assessed in recognition of the possible antigenic heterogeneity of the tumor cell population as such, and of the clonogenic part of this population in particular.

References

1. J. C. Robbins and G. L. Nicholson, *in* "Cancer: A Comprehensive Treatise" (F. Becker, ed.), Vol. 4. p. 3. Plenum, New York, 1975.
2. L. Weiss, *Front. Biol.* **7**, 289 (1967).
3. M. H. Gail and C. W. Boone, *Exp. Cell Res.* **64**, 156 (1971).
4. A. Whittemore, *Adv. Cancer Res.* **27**, 55 (1978).
5. F. M. Burnet, *Adv. Cancer Res.* **28**, 1 (1978).
6. I. J. Fidler, *Cancer Res.* **38**, 2651 (1978).
7. I. J. Fidler, D. M. Gersten, and I. R. Hart, *Adv. Cancer Res.* **28**, 149 (1978).
8. L. Olsson, N. Kiger, and H. Kronström, *Cancer Res.* (in press).
9. L. Foulds, *JNCI, J. Natl. Cancer Inst.* **45**, 1039 (1970).
10. R. Nowell, *Science* **194**, 23 (1976).
11. R. T. Prehn, *JNCI, J. Natl. Cancer Inst.* **17**, 701 (1956).
12. L. Olsson and P. Ebbesen, *JNCI, J. Natl. Cancer Inst.* **62**, 623 (1979).

13. H. B. Hewitt, *Adv. Cancer Res.* **27**, 149 (1977).
14. G. Klein and E. Klein, *Proc. Natl. Acad. Sci. U.S.A.* **74**, 2121 (1977).
15. G. Köhler and C. Milstein, *Nature (London)* **256**, 495 (1975).
16. L. Olsson and H. S. Kaplan, *Proc. Natl. Acad. Sci. U.S.A.* **77**, 5429 (1980).
17. Z. P. Pavelic, H. K. Slocum, Y. M. Rustum, P. J. Creaven, N. J. Nowak, C. Karakousis, H. Takita, and A. Mittelman, *Cancer Res.* **40**, 4151 (1980).
18. C. R. McEwen, R. W. Stollard, and E. T. Juhos, *Anal. Biochem.* **23**, 369 (1968).
19. L. M. Nadler, P. Stashenko, R. Hardy, W. D. Kaplan, L. N. Button, D. W. Kufe, K. H. Autman, and S. F. Schlossman, *Cancer Res.* **40**, 3147 (1980).

Tumor Antigen–Antibody Interactions in Murine Lymphomas: Possible Implications for Human Lymphomas

I. WEISSMAN, E. PILLEMER, D. KOOISTRA, A. TSUKAMOTO,
L. JERABEK, D. HUMPHREY, R. COFFMAN, M. MCGRATH, S. NORD,
AND R. ELLIS

In Memory of Dr. David Pressman

I. Introduction

The search for tumor-associated and tumor-specific antigens *in vitro* and *in vivo* requires precise and reproducible immunological assays for these cell surface components, as well as model systems permitting analysis of the number of possible antigens expressed at the cell surface. For several years we have been analyzing various types of molecules on the surface of retrovirus-induced murine T-cell lymphomas with the expectation that knowledge gained from these systems will be transferable to the study of human lymphomas *in vitro* and *in vivo* (1–9).

We chose to study lymphoma cell surface antigens using direct antibody-binding techniques rather than an indirect technique such as cytolysis or complement fixation. Because one is studying the interaction of a labeled protein and a cell surface it is important to realize that such interactions may occur via the antibody-combining site, or via other cell surface receptors for other portions of the immunoglobulin molecule, and that one must simultaneously test tumors for binding activity and the normal cellular counterpart of such tumors—in this case thymocytes and T cells (2).

The initial insight that tumor-binding radioimmunoassays contain the potential for both precise definition of tumor antigens and for eliminating artifacts was made by Pressman and his colleagues. To define and distinguish fact from artifact they developed a paired radiolabel cell-binding assay utilizing both normal and neoplastic cells as targets (10, 11). Much of our work derives from their initial insight, both from a reading of their published papers and through direct, extensive, and helpful discussions with David Pressman. We dedicate this article to the memory of the late David Pressman.

II. A Model System for Studying Tumor Antigens on Lymphoma Cells *in Vitro* and *in Vivo*

Most murine lymphocytic leukemias begin as thymic lymphomas (12, 13). Such lymphomas are induced by or produce a class of lymphomagenic retroviruses which on their own can accelerate or induce the disease in otherwise untreated hosts (12). The shortest interval between injection of the most highly leukemogenic of these viral isolates and the appearance of a frank lymphoma is 2–3 months, as compared to the very short latent period (1–2 weeks) when sarcomagenic viruses such as murine sarcoma virus (MSV) and avian sarcoma virus (ASV) are used (14). Lymphomagenic viruses are also known as slowly transforming retroviruses, while sarcomagenic viruses belong to a class of rapidly transforming retroviruses. All rapidly transforming retroviruses analyzed thus far contain and transmit genes coding for the transformed state. These virus-transforming genes show sequence homology with endogenous cellular genes (15–18), which are presumably involved in the control of replication of subsets of normal cells. In contrast, the genome of slowly transforming retroviruses has not yet been found to contain genes which, when transcribed and translated, code directly for the transformed state. Rapidly transforming retroviruses act on many potential target cells and can effect transformation *in vitro*, whereas slowly transforming retroviruses have an as yet undefined target cell, presumably of low frequency, and are not transforming for normal cells of any type *in vitro* (14). The mechanism of transformation by these slowly transforming retroviruses is still a mystery, and several potential models have been proposed (14, 19–22). Nevertheless, the proteins coded for by viral genes may be expressed in the cell normally to effect viral replication and budding, or in some cases abnormally as cell surface proteins uninvolved in the budding process (23, 24). Several viral genes are involved in the production of proteins which may be virion structural proteins and virion-specified tumor antigens. The *gag* gene codes for a protein which forms the core of the virus, beginning as a 67,000-molecular-weight cytoplasmic protein synthesized on free polysomes and subsequently proteolytically cleaved to form four major core proteins, p30, p15, p12, and p10 (25). In many lymphomas proteolytic cleavage is efficient, and these proteins are produced and utilized rapidly in the formation of virions which bud through the cell surface and spread to other cells (26, 27). In some lymphomas, notably of the AKR and RadLV series, the precursor polyprotein (pr67) is associated with the rough endoplasmic reticulum and, following glycosylation, appears as cell surface *gag* glycoproteins (8, 23–25). These are not utilized in the budding cycle and may be prominent tumor antigens (18). The *env* gene codes for the envelope proteins of the virus and is initially translated also as a polyprotein, associated with the rough endoplasmic reticulum (26–29). Here an 80,000- to 90,000-molecular-weight protein is synthesized and simultaneously glycosylated within the rough endoplasmic reticulum (29). This polyprotein contains two (perhaps three) distinct proteins which are liberated by proteolytic cleavage in the cellular membranes (27). The polyprotein precursor contains an intrachain disulfide bond which, following one of the proteolytic cleavages, maintains itself as an interchain disulfide bond between the glycoprotein (gp70) and the hydrophobic membrane protein (p15E) (27). A third putative protein from this polyprotein complex is called R, and its exact location and involvement in the virus budding cycle is still unknown (30). The p15E-gp70 heterodimer appears on the cell membrane in massive excess and is utilized by the separately synthesized and assembled core (*gag* proteins plus a diploid copy of the viral RNA) at a nucleation site on the underside of the cell membrane, leading to virion budding (29). Thus both *gag* and *env* gene products may appear in large quantities on the cell surface as potential tumor antigens. We wished to study the extent to which virion protein antigens proved to be lymphoma cell surface antigens in a host bearing such tumors. To do so, we initially studied a Moloney lymphoma (LSTRA) with the paired radiolabeled antibody technique.

III. The Paired Radiolabeled Cell-Binding Antibody Technique

The basics of this technique are shown in Fig. 1. Animals which later rejected Moloney tumors were used to prepare both preimmune and immune IgGs by standard salt precipitation and chromatographic techniques. The preimmune im-

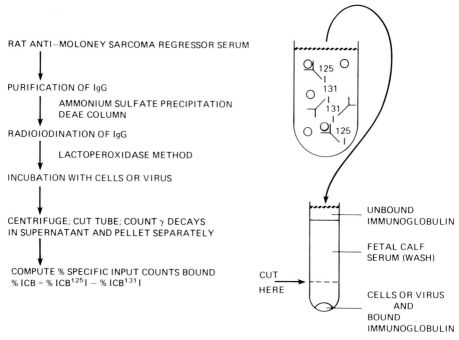

RAT ANTI—MOLONEY SARCOMA REGRESSOR SERUM

↓

PURIFICATION OF IgG

AMMONIUM SULFATE PRECIPITATION
DEAE COLUMN

↓

RADIOIODINATION OF IgG

LACTOPEROXIDASE METHOD

↓

INCUBATION WITH CELLS OR VIRUS

↓

CENTRIFUGE; CUT TUBE; COUNT γ DECAYS
IN SUPERNATANT AND PELLET SEPARATELY

↓

COMPUTE % SPECIFIC INPUT COUNTS BOUND
% ICB = % ICB^{125}I − % ICB^{131}I

CUT →
HERE

UNBOUND
IMMUNOGLOBULIN

FETAL CALF
SERUM (WASH)

CELLS OR VIRUS
AND
BOUND
IMMUNOGLOBULIN

Fig. 1. The paired radiolabeled cell-binding antibody technique for the detection of specific anti-tumor antibody.

munoglobulin (NγG) was labeled with ^{131}I using lactoperoxidase-catalyzed iodination, and the immune IgG similarly labeled with ^{125}I. The specific labeled proteins were then cleared of denatured complexes following labeling by passage through the bloodstream of a normal BALB/c mouse (4). This was necessary both to remove denatured molecules and to provide a high concentration of unlabeled immunoglobulin to block Fc receptor-mediated binding of both NγG and the anti-Moloney IgG antibodies (2). The radiolabeled immunoglobulins in mouse serum were then incubated with lymphoma cells at various concentrations, and the percentage of specific binding determined by subtracting ^{131}I counts bound from ^{125}I counts bound. Since only a portion of the immune host's immunoglobulin was specific for the tumor cell antigens (the rest being immunoglobulins whose formation was induced by other types of antigens such as intestinal bacteria), the first task was to develop a cell-binding quantitative assay which would define the amount of ^{125}I-labeled immunoglobulin which was antibody-specific for the tumor cell surface. To do so we titrated a fixed small amount of paired radiolabeled immunoglobulins against increasing numbers of LSTRA lymphoma or normal thymocyte cell populations. Figure 2 demonstrates diagrammatically that at a great cell excess all the immunoglobulins directed against lymphoma cells should reach their equilibrium binding capacities with lymphoma cells, leaving little or no specific antibody in the unbound (supernatant) fraction. Assuming these interactions were in fact roughly representative of antigen–antibody interactions in solution we demonstrated that the percentage of input counts bound/cell concentration ratio should vary linearly with the percentage of input counts bound (3). Thus we could plot on the ordinate the percentage of input counts bound/cell concentration ratio versus the percentage of input counts bound on the abscissa and obtain a plot which, at infinite cell concentration, would indicate the percentage of labeled immunoglobulin which was specific for the tumor cell surface antigens. In this case, testing a total of either 5 or 10 ng of labeled immunoglobulin, the extrapolated percentage of specific antibody was on the order of 5%, as shown in Fig. 3. Thus, even with the crude antiserum, we could detect precisely the binding activity on the order of 200–250 pg of labeled immunoglobulin. This observation will be discussed later in this article in connection with a very sensitive radioimmunoassay for the *in vivo* detection of occult tumor.

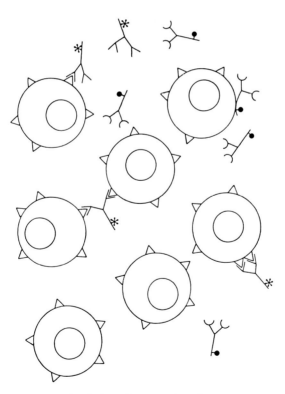

Fig. 2.   Cell-binding assay in cell excess.

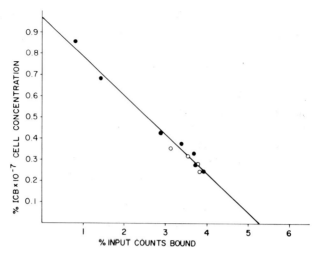

Fig. 3. Percent input counts bound (% ICB) plotted versus % ICB/CC for ^{125}I-αMo. A constant amount of either 5 ng (○) or 10 ng (●) of ^{125}I-αMo plus the equivalent amount of ^{131}I-NγG was added to increasing concentrations of LSTRA cells in 50% NRS. The average % ICB at each cell concentration was determined for both the αMo and the NγG. The results are plotted as % ICB versus % ICB/CC for ^{131}I-αMo after subtraction of ^{131}I-NγG binding (3).

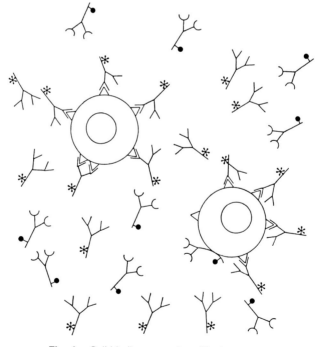

Fig. 4. Cell-binding assay in antibody excess.

One can also quantitate the number of antigenic determinants on the lymphoma cell surface by titrating a fixed number of cells with increasing amounts of paired radiolabeled immunoglobulin mixtures. Figure 4 demonstrates that, at great antibody excess levels, every cell surface antigenic determinant is likely to be bound by an antibody-combining site. Figure 5 shows a sample titration of such radiolabeled immunoglobulins, and Fig. 6 shows another type of equilibrium equation wherein the nanograms of antibody bound per total nanograms of antibody added is plotted versus the nanograms of bound antibody (3). In this case, approximately 58 ng of antibody are bound per 4×10^6 cells, or about 55,000 antibody molecules per cell.

In one example where we used this sensitive paired radiolabeled antibody binding assay to compare LSTRA cell surface and Moloney virion surface antigens we first determined the amount of antibody bound to a great excess of purified virions (Fig. 7) and then tested both the preabsorption and absorbed immunoglobulin mixture against LSTRA cells themselves (Fig. 8). Approximately one-third of the cell-binding antibodies also bound and were removed by the intact virions, whereas the other two-thirds of the labeled immunoglobulins, which would not bind to the virus surface, still bound to the cell surface (8). Thus there appeared to be antigens other than virion surface-accessible env gene products on the lymphoma cell surface. To test that these were virion proteins we isolated virions, extracted their proteins, immobilized those proteins by covalent

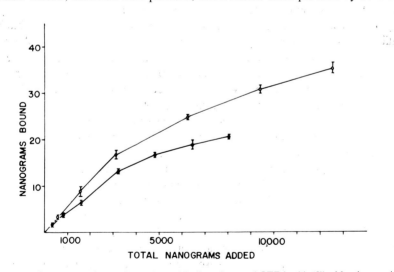

Fig. 5. Saturation of specific antibody-binding sites on LSTRA with ^{125}I-αMo. Increasing amounts of ^{125}I-labeled NγG or αMo plus ^{131}I-bovine serum albumin (BSA) in 0.22-ml 50% NRS were added to a small and constant number of LSTRA cells (4.1 $\times$ 10^6 cells/tube). The results are plotted as the total number of ng antibody added to the reaction mixture versus the mean and range of the number of ng αMo specifically bound to the cells (after subtraction of NγG binding). $\bigcirc$ = ^{125}I-αMo 1.3 I/γG; $\bullet$ = ^{125}I-αMo 0.0021 I/γG (3).

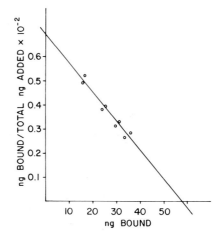

Fig. 6. Saturation of specific antibody binding sites on LSTRA cells. Plot of ng bound versus total ng added for αMo (1.31/γG) bound to LSTRA cells. Increasing amounts of ^{125}I/[127]I-labeled αMo or NγG plus ^{131}I BSA were added to a small, constant number of LSTRA cells (4.1 $\times$ 10^6 cells/tube) in 0.22 ml of 50% NRS. The ng bound for αMo was corrected by subtracting ng bound for NγG (3).

bonding on solid Sepharose bead supports, and used such protein-coated beads to absorb the same paired radiolabeled antibody mixture prior to testing on lymphoma cell surfaces. To our surprise, as shown in Fig. 9, most of the cell-binding antibodies were absorbed by these virion protein preparations (8). An even greater surprise was found when we tried to identify the virion proteins detected on the cell surface by these and other antibodies. Virtually all the proteins precipitated by such antibodies were *env* and not *gag* gene products (8), although nearly two-thirds of the virion antigens were not revealed until the virion was disrupted, presumably revealing *gag* (as well as some *env*) gene products for the first time. To verify that *env* gene products were quantitatively present on LSTRA cells in excess of *gag* gene products we prepared monospecific antibodies to the gp70 and the p30 viral proteins, prepared F(ab)$_2$ fragments from such antibodies to avoid Fc receptor binding, and used these antibodies in a fluorescence-activated cell sorter analysis to detect quantitatively the relative expression of these two proteins on the lymphoma cell surface (8). Figure 10 shows that gp70 antigens are indeed present well in excess of p30 antigens on the lymphoma cell surface, and neither antigen is expressed at detectable levels on normal thymocytes (Fig. 11). Thus we had to conclude that *env* gene products provided the major cell surface antigens detected by Moloney regressor antisera and that only a fraction of such antigenic determinants were accessible on the viral surface—perhaps because of the close packing array of envelope proteins on these extremely dense viral particles. However, this proved to be true only of the

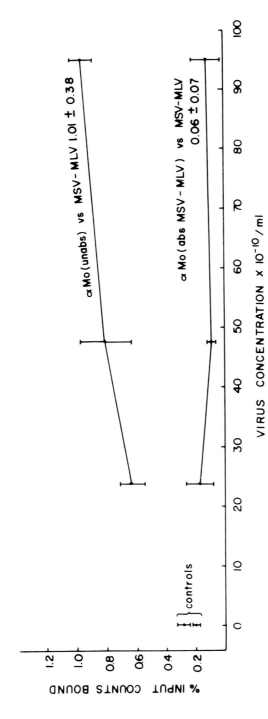

Fig. 7. Binding assays of αMo to intact virus (MSV-M-MuLV) which has (abs) or has not been preabsorbed (unabs). The immunoglobulin is labeled with radioactive iodine and the binding is shown as % ICB. In these and other assays, each incubation contained 200 μl of medium containing cells or virus, and 20 μl of radiolabeled immunoglobulin solution containing 2–20 ng of ^{125}I-αMo and 5–50 ng of ^{131}I-NγG (~10^4 cpm of each isotope). Each point represents triplicate incubations, and error bars are standard deviations from the mean (8).

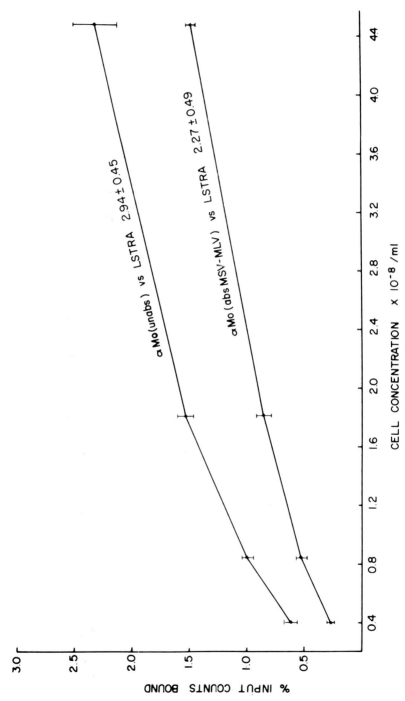

Fig. 8. Binding assays of αMo to LSTRA by using αMo which has (abs) or has not (unabs) been preabsorbed with MSV-M-MuLV. See Fig. 7 for conditions of the assays (8).

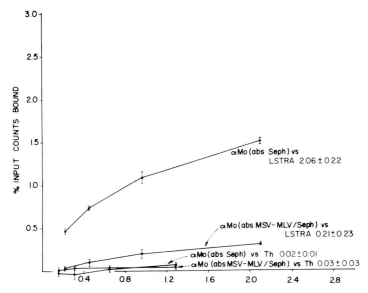

Fig. 9. Binding assays of αMo to Moloney lymphoma cells (LSTRA) and to BALB/c thymocytes (Th). αMo has been absorbed with BALB/c thymocytes (abs Th) or with Moloney lymphoma cells (abs LSTRA), or has not been absorbed. See Fig. 7 for conditions of assays (8).

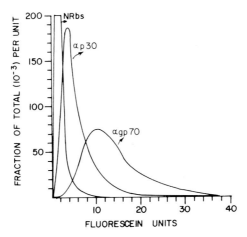

Fig. 10. FACS determined fluorescence-intensity profile of LSTRA cells with various F(ab)₂ rabbit sera. The fraction of the total sample is recorded on the vertical axis versus the relative fluorescence intensity per cell on the horizontal axis (8).

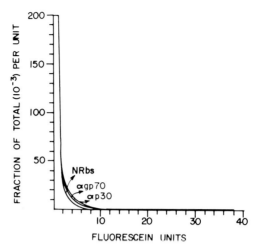

Fig. 11. FACS determined fluorescence-intensity profile of BALB/c thymocytes with various F(ab)₂ rabbit sera. The fraction of the total sample is recorded on the vertical axis versus the relative fluorescence intensity per cell on the horizontal axis (8).

Moloney lymphomas we examined. Every spontaneous AKR lymphoma examined showed profiles similar to the one demonstrated in Fig. 12; p30 antigens were present in abundance greater than gp70 antigens on these tumors, and this proved to be a property determined by the virus type itself rather than the host cell which is infected (8). The small residuum of nonviral cell surface antigens

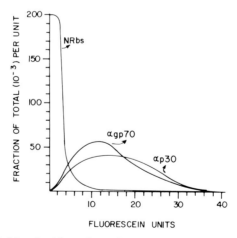

Fig. 12. FACS determined intensity profiles of KKT-2 cells (a spontaneous AKR lymphoma) with various F(ab)₂ rabbit sera. The fraction of the total sample is recorded on the vertical axis versus the relative fluorescence intensity per cell on the horizontal axis (8).

revealed in Fig. 10 was not adequately examined until monoclonal antibody technology was utilized (see below).

The ability to quantitate tumor antigens by such precise radiolabeled antibody techniques led us to propose and develop a new technique for the *in vivo* diagnosis of tumor antigens, no matter how or where these antigens are distributed.

IV. The *in Vivo* Antibody Disappearance Assay for the Analysis of Occult Tumors

The standard current methodology used to detect occult tumors requires the tumor antigen to be isolated in pure form for competitive radioimmunoassay and is best exemplified by several techniques for detecting human carcinoembryonic antigen (CEA) of the colon or primitive liver tumor α-fetoproteins (AFPs) in primary hepatomas (31–35). However, tumor antigen isolation is a long, laborious task, and there is strong evidence that such tumor antigens may not be constant from one tumor to another even with the given histological type, as exemplified by the tremendous polymorphism of tumor antigens on chemical carcinogen-induced tumors (36–38). An alternative is to use an assay such as Pressman's paired radiolabeled antibody-binding assay to detect tumor antigens which one cannot rapidly and unequivocally isolate for competitive radioimmunoassays. A second point is relevant here: Both CEA and AFP assays require that the tumor antigen be shed from the tumor cell into the circulation such that a sample of serum will be sufficient to detect tumor antigens above background levels (33–35). There is no guarantee that all such tumor antigens will behave in this way and that one can therefore sample the serum for the appearance or reappearance of tumor. We decided to establish a sensitive *in vivo* based radioimmunoassay which could be used initially to detect tumor antigens no matter how dispersed in the body, with the eventual hope of using such techniques to localize micrometastases for diagnosis and/or therapy (1, 5). Paired radiolabeled immunoglobulins are injected into the bloodstream of a mouse already bearing or subsequently injected with LSTRA lymphoma cells. Microsamples from the blood are withdrawn at defined intervals, and the clearance of specific LSTRA-binding antibodies is detected by analyzing their absence in the unbound form in the bloodstream. Such an absence is detected using the techniques first shown in Figs. 2 and 3, wherein the percentage of radiolabeled immunoglobulin specific for the tumor cells is defined by titrating against an excess of tumor cells. Figure 13 shows the disappearance of radiolabeled antibodies after the injection of tumor cells at hour 50; by hour 58 animals receiving 86 million cells showed a specific loss of tumor-binding antibody, and by hour 120 animals receiving as little as 350,000 tumor cells showed a specific and significant decrease in tumor-binding antibody. Since the doubling time of tumor

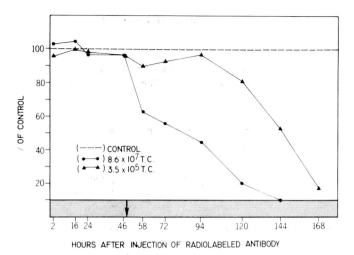

Fig. 13. *In vitro* detection of the removal of specific αMo antibody from the sera of mice injected with LSTRA cells. At t = 0, animals received intravenous injections of paired labeled mixtures of ^{125}I-αMo and ^{131}I-NγG. At t = 51 hours, control animals ($\bigcirc$) received no cells, and experimental animals ($\bullet$) received 1.7 $\times$ 10^6 LSTRA cells intravenously. Aliquots of radioactive sera were obtained at various times, frozen at $-70°C$, and later assayed *in vitro* for their ability to bind to LSTRA cells. The shaded area with a central line represents mean and range of % ICB for ^{131}I-NγG (5).

cells in this strain of mice is approximately 10–12 hours, this crude initial assay detected on the order of 10^7 cells maximally. When animals were injected with tumor cells 13 hours prior to the injection of radiolabeled antibodies, rapid disappearance of specific binding antibody was again seen (Fig. 14). In this case, 1.4×10^5 tumor cells led to a significant reduction in tumor-binding antibody at the 73-hour time point, whereas a significant increase in lymphoblasts in the blood of these hosts was not detected until hour 117. That this technique could detect tumor limited to intradermal or subcutaneous sites is shown in Fig. 15. As can be noted from Figs. 14 and 15, this particular assay was carried out with an immunoglobulin preparation of which only 1–2% was specific antibody. Thus the opportunity for a high signal/noise ratio was blunted considerably by the low percentage of specific antibody. Sensitive and specific *in vivo* clearance assays of this sort require that a high proportion of labeled immunoglobulins be directed specifically against tumor cell antigens. Sensitive imaging and radiotherapy with radiolabeled immunoglobulins also require a much better signal/noise ratio. Therefore, although these early studies show the power of such an *in vivo* antibody removal technique, its significant application in animals with much reduced tumor cell loads required the development of antibodies almost exclusively directed against tumor antigens. This became possible with the develop-

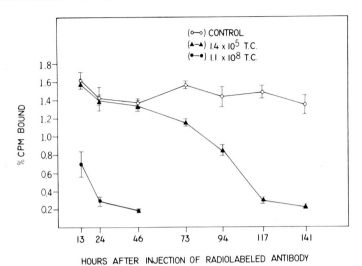

Fig. 14. Detection of "occult" tumors. (○) Control group; (▲) animals receiving 1.4 × 10^5 tumor cells, (T.C.); and (●) animals receiving 1.1 × 10^8 LSTRA cells 24 hours before paired radiolabeled antibody injection (5).

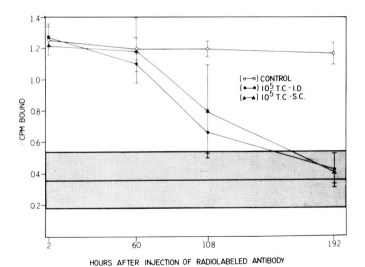

Fig. 15. Detection of extravascular tumor foci. (○) Control animals, no tumor cells (T.C.) before antibody injection; (●) animals receiving 10^5 ML cells intradermally 53 hours before antibody injection; (▲) animals receiving 10^5 ML cells subcutaneously 53 hours before antibody. The shaded area with a central line represents mean and range of % ICB for ^{131}I-NγG (5).

ment of the hybridoma technique of monoclonal antibody preparation, detailed previously by several other contributors to this volume. Another point should be emphasized here: The detection of micrometastases and the immunotherapeutic approaches of using radiolabeled antibodies would best be served by the demonstration of a new class of tumor cell antigens which remain tightly adherent to the tumor cell surface and are not shed into the circulation. If tumor antigens are present in the circulation at the time radiolabeled antibodies are injected into the blood, the major result will be the formation of radiolabeled antigen–antibody complexes, most of which would be filtered out on vascular basement membranes such as the glomerular basement membranes (5). This leads to the accumulation of potentially radiotoxic and certainly inflammation-inducing deposits in these basement membranes. Such deposits could cause significant immunopathology, would certainly be falsely detected as tumor deposits by imaging techniques, and as an antigen "sink" might prevent radiolabeled antibodies from reaching tumor cell foci. Such a class of tumor cell antigens was detected in various lymphoma and leukemia cells induced by both rapidly transforming and slowly transforming retroviruses.

V. Demonstration of a New Class of Tumor Cell Antigens

The first set of monoclonal antibodies which detect antigens expressed on the surface of retrovirus-induced tumor cells, but not present in detectable quantities on or in these virions, came from an immunization of Lewis rats with the AKR thymic lymphoma KKT-2. Screening of several antibodies from this fusion led to the isolation of two clones, 43-13 and 43-17, both of which detect primarily cell surface antigens present on neoplastic but not normal cells (39–41). While 43-17 did not bind to viruses isolated from the KKT-2 lymphoma, 43-13 showed low but significant binding to disrupted, but not intact, virions (Table I). Table II demonstrates that 43-13 is specific for cell surface antigens and virion antigens derived from AKR mice: Superinfection of the antigen-negative L-691 lymphoma line by AKR virus, by the KKT-2 virus (K), and by the AKR recombinant duotropic virus MCF-247 led to the cell surface expression of 43-13 antigenic targets. L-691 cells alone, or superinfected with Moloney (M), Gross (G), or LSTRA–Moloney virions did not lead to expression of the 43-13 target but led to infection and replication of each of the aforementioned virions. Thus the surface expression of 43-13 antigens is dependent upon infection by an AKR virus. The expression of 43-17 antigens is somewhat more widespread, in that the RadLV-induced tumor VL-3, all AKR virus-superinfected L-691 cells, and Gross virus-superinfected L-691 cells also express on their surface this antigenic determinant. 43-17 antibodies detect no antigenic target in any of the intact or disrupted virions. The fact that 43-17 antibodies detect only cell surface antigens, and no detectable or surface accessible virion internal antigens, makes them prime can-

TABLE I

Lymphoma Cell Surface Antigens Detected by Labeled Antibodies

		Cpm bound per 2.5×10^5 cells		
Cell line	Infecting virus	43–13	43–17	Control
L691	—	98	136	178
KKT$_2$	—	2102	1401	78
L691/K	KKT$_2$ SL virus	1751	1092	126
L691/B	LSTRA virus	96	135	92
L691/MCF	MCF 247	1433	790	133
L691/G	Gross passage A	93	376	89
L691/A	Cloned AKR ecotropic	1669	1061	157
L691/M	Moloney clone 2	102	130	116

didates for *in vitro* and *in vivo* tumor cell-binding assays, as described above. Because 43-17 antibody is easily isolated from hybridoma tissue culture supernatants by $(NH_4)_2SO_4$ precipitation followed by ion-exchange chromatography on DE-52 solid-state adsorbents, studies on the *in vivo* and *in vitro* effectiveness of this antibody for tumor diagnosis and localization have been initiated.

What antigen targets do these two monoclonal antibodies detect on the lymphoma cell surface? Surprisingly, both 43-13 and 43-17 antibodies precipitate the cell surface glycosylated *gag* polyproteins gp85 and gp95 (41). In addition, they precipitate a prominent band at 50,000–55,000 molecular weight (p55). With the use of supersaturating concentrations of these two antibodies and antibodies to any of the *gag* components (anti-p30, anti-p12, anti-p15) the amount of gp85 and gp95 precipitated is approximately 10-fold greater than the amount precipitated from the same aliquot of cells by 43-13 and 43-17. Anti-p10 precipitates only gp95, as reported by Ledbetter *et al.* (24). Thus it appeared that 43-13 and 43-17

TABLE II

Virus Antigens Detected by Labeled Antibodies

	Cpm bound per well		
Virus	43–13	43–17	Control
KKT$_2$ (AKR SL)	870	113	74
KKT$_4$ (AKR SL)	486	111	101
MCF 247 (AKR recombinant)	411	65	71
RadLV/VL$_3$	63	69	53
Moloney NIH clone 2	62	60	66
Rat C58NTD	74	96	54

detected only a subset of glycosylated *gag* antigens, but in addition detected another cell surface moiety. Figure 16 demonstrates that all the glycosylated *gag* antigens detected by 43-13 and 43-17 are molecules which contain p30 antigenic determinants: Lactoperoxidase-catalyzed iodination of KKT-2 cell membranes, followed by solubilization and first-stage immunoprecipitation with anti-p30 removed all soluble glycosylated *gag* antigens detectable by 43-13 and 43-17 antibodies but did not remove p55 molecules. The relative intensity of bands precipitated with 43-17 and 43-13 as shown in this figure does not reflect their actual representation on the cell surface, because the number of counts precipitated with each of these antibodies was increased prior to electrophoresis to demonstrate the extent to which anti-p30 removed such antigens. Figure 17 demonstrates that 43-17 clears most 43-17 antigenic targets from these soluble lysates but does not quantitatively remove 43-13 antigenic targets, and vice versa. Thus we have the curious situation that 43-13 and 43-17 each detect sets of glycosylated *gag* antigens largely independent of each other but both sharing other *gag* determinants such as p30. This phenomenon is not due to coinfection of these cells with two or more AKR-related virions, as cells infected with cloned AKR ecotropic viruses also behave the same way.

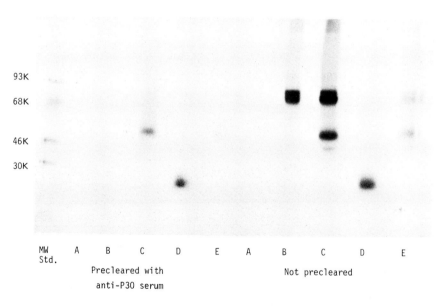

Fig. 16. Immunoprecipitation of solubilized surface-^{125}I-labeled KKT-2 cells. (A) Control, normal rat serum plus *Staphylococcus* A coated with rabbit anti-rat serum. (B) Rabbit anti-p30 plus *Staphylococcus* A. (C) 43-17 antibody plus *Staphylococcus* A coated with rabbit anti-rat serum. (D) 31-11 (anti-Thy 1) antibody plus *Staphylococcus* A coated with rabbit anti-rat serum. (E) 43-13 antibody plus *Staphylococcus* A coated with rabbit anti-rat serum.

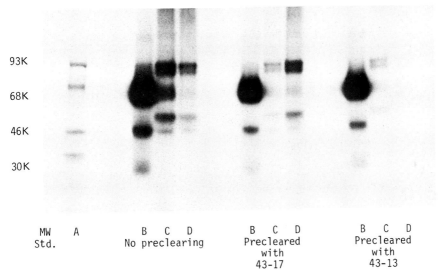

Fig. 17. Sequential immunoprecipitation of solubilized L691/AKR cells with gp69 (B), 43-17 (C), and 43-13 (D) after preclearing with nothing, 43-17, or 43-13. (A) Control, labeled material immunoprecipitated by normal rat serum.

Preliminary experiments with [³H]leucine- and [³²P]orthophosphate-labeled KKT-2 cells indicate that 43-13 may recognize p55 and viral p12 antigenic determinants. 43-17 immunoprecipitates only the 85-95 glycosylated *gag* polyproteins (no nonglycosylated *gag* precursors) and p55 antigenic targets from [³H]leucine- and [³²P]orthophosphate-labeled cells (Figs. 18 and 19).

Initial studies indicated that 43-17 and 43-13 antigenic determinants were located on the p55 protein(s) and that p55-glycosylated *gag* polyprotein association was sensitive to reducing agents, implying that they are disulfide-bonded to each other. This conclusion is difficult to reconcile with subsequent experiments showing that both 43-13 and 43-17 can precipitate gp85 and gp95 eluted from gels. Thus it is still important to determine whether 43-17 and 43-13 recognize an antigenic complex of p55 disulfide-bonded to a subpopulation of glycosylated *gag* polyproteins or whether the sensitivity of certain antigenic determinants to the reduction and alkylation procedure has some other basis. We take these experiments as evidence that a cluster of antigens (p55, gp85, gp95) exists with polymorphic determinants even within a cloned lymphoma line (KKT-2). These proteins are tumor-specific antigens in that they are expressed nowhere in detectable quantities on the surface of normal cells.

Another line of research begun in our laboratory and carried out in collaboration with Varda Rotter in David Baltimore's laboratory appears to confirm this as a more general phonomenon. We raised rat monoclonal antibodies against Abel-

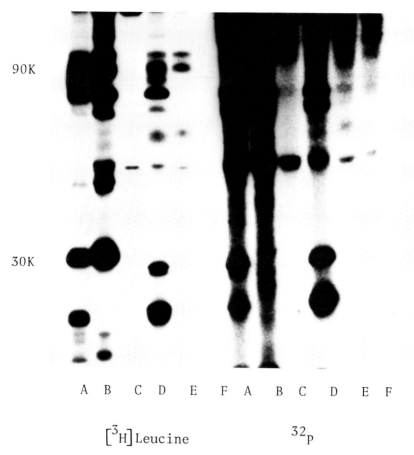

90K

30K

A   B   C   D   E   F   A   B   C   D   E   F

$[^3H]$ Leucine ^{32}P

Fig. 18. Sodium dodecyl sulfate polyacrylamide electrophoresis of KKT-2 cells labeled for 4 hours with either [^{3}H]leucine or $^{32}PO_4^{-3}$ followed by immunoprecipitation with goat anti-Moloney virus (A), rabbit anti-p30 (B), normal rabbit serum (C), 43-17 (D), 43-13 (E), and 31-11 (anti-Thy 1) (F).

son virus-induced pre-B-cell leukemias in order to analyze differentiation antigens characteristic of the pre-B-cell stage of B-cell differentiation (42, 43). One such antibody which detected both pre-B- cells and B cells in normal mice was called 2C2 (42). On an independent screening (by V. Rotter, O. Witte, and D. Baltimore) for virion- and tumor-specific antigens of Abelson lymphomas, 2C2 was seen to precipitate a major cellular protein of ~50,000 molecular weight (44). By peptide mapping this p50 appeared to be the same as the nonviral T antigen found in association with SV40 T antigens in the nucleus of SV40-transformed mouse cells (45), and the 50,000-molecular-weight protein precipitated from a methylcholanthrene-induced fibrosarcoma by a syngeneic antitumor antiserum (46, 47). 2C2 stains the nucleus of SV40-transformed cells (R. Carroll and A. Levine, personal communication). Similarly, 2C2 does not stain the surface of mouse thymocytes but precipitates an actively synthesized protein of ~50,000 molecular weight from normal thymocytes (44). We have recently found that 2C2 precipitates p50 as well as two other proteins, p35 and p11, in Abelson lymphomas. We are currently studying the relationship between molecules precipitated by 2C2, by 43-17, and by 43-13. In any case, this solidifies the possibility that a new class of tumor antigens may emerge which are normal cytoplasmic components in some cells (and perhaps cell surface components in others) but are universally present as tumor antigens in virus-transformed and even in chemical

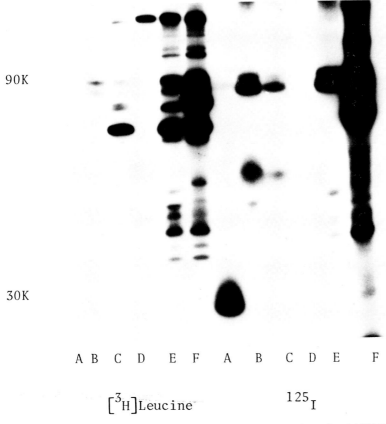

90K

30K

A B C D E F A B C D E F

$[^3H]$Leucine ^{125}I

Fig. 19. Sodium dodecyl sulfate polyacrylamide gel electrophoresis of KKT-2 cells labeled for 20 minutes with [³H]leucine or surface-labeled with ¹²⁵I followed by immunoprecipitation with 31-11 (anti-Thy 1) (A), 43-17 (B), 43-13 (C), normal rabbit serum (D), rabbit anti-p30 (E), and goat anti-Moloney (F).

carcinogen-transformed cells. Although we do not yet know the relationship of these proteins to cell surface fetal antigens, we believe that they shall prove to be both interesting biologically and important immunologically as markers of cells in the transformed state.

Finally, we should mention another set of lymphoma surface determinants which may prove to be tumor antigens. We have characterized a set of T lymphoma cell surface receptors specific for murine leukemia virus envelope determinants. Because this latter set of receptors appears to be involved in both virus binding and lymphoma cell proliferation (40), monoclonal antibodies might be developed which inhibit lymphoma cell proliferation *in vitro* and *in vivo*. A model for such action has been published elsewhere (40).

Acknowledgments

The experiments described herein cover a span of 10 years support by the American Cancer Society (IM-56), for which we are grateful. Several of the authors (E. P., M. M., and S. N.) were also supported by the Stanford Medical Scientist Program, GM1922. I. W. was a Faculty Research Awardee of the American Cancer Society during much of this work.

References

1. I. L. Weissman, S. Nord, and S. Baird, *Front. Radiat. Ther. Oncol.* **7**, 161 (1972).
2. S. Nord and I. L. Weissman, *JNCI, J. Natl. Cancer Inst.* **53**, 117 (1974).
3. S. Nord and I. L. Weissman, *JNCI, J. Natl. Cancer Inst.* **53**, 125 (1974).
4. S. Nord and I. L. Weissman, *JNCI, J. Natl. Cancer Inst.* **53**, 959 (1974).
5. I. L. Weissman, S. Nord, and R. L. Ellis, *in* "Interaction of Radiation and Host Immune Mechanisms in Malignancy," (E. Cronkite, ed.), Brookhaven Natl. Lab. Press, p. 379, New York, 1974.
6. R. I. Fox and I. L. Weissman, *J. Immunol.* **122**, 1698 (1979).
7. R. I. Fox and I. L. Weissman, *J. Immunol.* **123**, 1736 (1979).
8. D. Humphrey, A. Tsukamoto-Adey, O. N. Witte, R. Fox, L. Jerabek, and I. L. Weissman, *J. Immunol.* **123**, 412 (1979).
9. I. L. Weissman, *Prog. Exp. Tumor Res.* **25**, 193 (1980).
10. D. Pressman, E. D. Day, and M. Blau, *Cancer Res.* **17**, 845 (1957).
11. N. Tanigaki, Y. Yagi, and D. Pressman, *J. Immunol.* **98**, 274 (1967).
12. H. S. Kaplan, *Cancer Res.* **27**, 1325 (1967).
13. D. P. McEndy, M. C. Boon, and J. Furth, *Cancer Res.* **7**, 377 (1944).
14. I. L. Weissman and S. Baird, *Life Sci. Res. Rep.* **7**, 135 (1977).
15. H. E. Varmus, D. H. Spector, C. T. Deng, T. Padget, J. M. Bishop, D. Stehelin, and E. Stubblefield, *in* "Origins of Human Cancer," p. 1159. Cold Spring Harbor Press, Cold Spring Harbor, New York, New York, 1977.
16. T. Graf, N. Ade, and H. Beug, *Nature (London)* **275**, 496 (1978).
17. O. N. Witte, N. Rosenberg, and D. Baltimore, *Nature (London)* **281**, 396 (1979).
18. A. Shields, S. Goff, M. Paskind, and D. Baltimore, *Cell* **18**, 955 (1979).

19. M. S. McGrath and I. L. Weissman, *Cold Spring Harbor Conf. Cell Proliferation* **5,** 577–589 (1978).
20. I. L. Weissman, *Immunogenet. Anim. Viruses, ICN–UCLA Symp. Anim. Virus Genet., 1980,* p. 821, Academic Press, New York, 1980.
21. S. Manteuil-Brutlag, S. -L. Liu, and H. S. Kaplan, *Cell* **19,** 643 (1980).
22. H. L. Robinson, M. N. Pearson, D. W. DeSimone, P. N. Tsichlis, and J. M. Coffin, *Cold Spring Harbor Symp. Quant. Biol.* **44,** 1133 (1979).
23. J. -S. Tung, T. Yoshiki, and E. Fleissner, *Cell* **9,** 573 (1976).
24. J. Ledbetter, R. C. Nowinski, and S. Emery, *J. Virol.* **22,** 65 (1977).
25. R. N. Eisenman and V. M. Vogt, *Biochim. Biophys. Acta* **473,** 187 (1978).
26. O. N. Witte and I. L. Weissman, *Virology* **61,** 575 (1974).
27. O. N. Witte, A. Tsukamoto-Adey, and I. L. Weissman, *Virology* **76,** 539 (1977).
28. R. A. Knight, N. A. Mitchison, and G. R. Shellam, *Int. J. Cancer* **15,** 417 (1975).
29. O. N. Witte and I. L. Weissman, *Virology* **69,** 464 (1976).
30. J. G. Sutcliff, T. M. Shinnick, N. Green, F.-T. Liu, H. L. Niman, and R. A. Lerner, *Nature (London)* **287,** 801 (1980).
31. P. Alexander, *Nature (London)* **235,** 137 (1972).
32. P. Gold and S. O. Freedman, *J. Exp. Med.* **122,** 467 (1965).
33. J. E. Shively and C. W. Todd, *Scand. J. Immunol.* **7,** Suppl. 6, 19 (1978).
34. W. D. Terry, P. A. Henkart, J. E. Coligan, and C. W. Todd, *Transplant. Rev.* **20,** 100 (1974).
35. S. Sell and H. Skelly, *JNCI J. Natl. Cancer Inst.* **56,** 645 (1976).
36. R. T. Prehn and J. M. Main, *JNCI, J. Natl. Cancer Inst.* **18,** 769 (1957).
37. M. J. Embleton and C. Heidelberger, *Int. J. Cancer* **9,** 8 (1972).
38. M. A. Basombrio and R. T. Prehn, *Int. J. Cancer* **10,** 1 (1972).
39. E. Pillemer, D. Kooistra, and I. L. Weissman, in preparation.
40. M. McGrath, E. Pillemer, and I. L. Weissman, *Nature (London)* **285,** 259 (1980).
41. D. Kooistra, E. Pillemer, and I. L. Weissman, in preparation.
42. R. Coffman and I. L. Weissman, *J. Exp. Med.* **153,** 269 (1981).
43. R. Coffman and I. L. Weissman, *Nature (London)* **289,** 681 (1981).
44. V. Rotter, O. N. Witte, R. L. Coffman, and D. Baltimore, *J. Virol.* **36,** 547 (1980).
45. D. I. H. Linzer and A. J. Levine, *Cell* **17,** 43 (1979).
46. A. B. DeLeo, H. Shiku, T. Takahashi, M. John, and L. J. Old, *J. Exp. Med.* **146,** 720 (1977).
47. A. B. DeLeo, G. Jay, E. Appella, G. C. Dubois, L. W. Law, and L. J. Old, *Proc. Natl. Acad. Sci. U.S.A.* **76,** 2420 (1979).

The Role of Epstein–Barr Virus in the Etiology of Burkitt's Lymphoma and Nasopharyngeal Carcinoma

GEORGE KLEIN

I. Basic Biological Properties of the Virus

Epstein–Barr virus (EBV) is a lymphotropic herpesvirus of humans. A great deal has been learned about its biological and molecular properties during the last few years. Most of the available information can be found in two recent books (1, 2), and the main points can be briefly summarized as follows.

The known host cell range of the virus is extraordinarily restricted. Under experimental conditions, only human and some nonhuman primate B lymphocytes are found to be infectible. This restriction appears to be determined at the receptor level. Epstein–Barr virus receptors are either identical to or closely associated with one of the lymphocyte C3 receptors, probably the C3d receptor (3–5). Receptor bypass by microinjection (6) or membrane transplantation (7) makes a wide variety of cells susceptible to EBV infection. Surprisingly, nonnatural host cells turn out to be much more permissive to the viral cycle than the natural host, the human B lymphocyte. Infection of the latter leads to induction of Epstein–Barr nuclear antigen (EBNA) (8) but not to expression of the early antigen (EA) or late antigen (VCA) associated with the viral cycle. The appearance of EBNA is followed by blast transformation, DNA synthesis, cell division, and growth, in that order (9,10). So far, EBNA has been found to be expressed in all EBV DNA-carrying cells known, *in vitro* and *in vivo*.

Established EBV-carrying, normal, lymphocyte-derived lines designated lymphoblastoid cell lines (LCs) are polyclonal and have a series of well-defined phenotypic characteristics that distinguish them from malignant lymphoma-derived lines including EBV-carrying EBNA-positive Burkitt's lymphoma (BL) lines (11). Both types of lines carry multiple viral genomes, with a few integrated copies and a majority of free episomes (12–14). The relationship between the integrated and the free genomes is not known.

Lymphoblastoid and lymphoma lines carrying EBV can be virus producers or nonproducers. In producer lines, a relatively small number of cells switch on the viral cycle with a frequency that varies from line to line. The process can be facilitated by certain chemical inducers. Interestingly, all known inducers are agents that can interfere with the expression of differentiated characteristics in one system or another. Mutagens and carcinogens do not function as inducers (12). Known inducers include the halogenated pyrimidines 5-bromodeoxyuridine (BUDR) and 5-iododeoxyuridine (IUDR) (15–17), the tumor-promoting phorbol ester, 12-O-tetradecanoylphorbol-13-acetate (TPA) (18), sodium butyrate (19), antibodies that combine with the surface immunoglobulin of the target cell (20), and 5-azacytidine (20a), known to interfere with DNA methylation. All inducible lines appear to have a low rate of spontaneous production.

Nonproducer lines are also noninducible; they carry smaller numbers of viral genomes than inducible producer lines, as a rule.

These facts suggest that the virus utilizes some differentiated property of the B lymphocyte to secure its prolonged latency. This is also supported by somatic hybridization experiments showing that producer status and inducibility behave like differentiated properties (21).

The important question whether epithelial cells carry EBV receptors has not been answered, largely for technical reasons.

II. Does Epstein–Barr Virus Induce Lymphoproliferative Disease *in Vivo?*

A. Experimental Evidence

Since the known transforming effect is restricted to human and nonhuman primate B lymphocytes, experimentation has been possible only on nonhuman primates. The situation is further complicated by the fact that large apes and Old World monkeys carry viruses closely related to EBV (10, 22–26). In the best studied species, such as the chimpanzee, the orangutan, and the baboon, the indigenous lymphotropic herpesviruses show various degrees of DNA sequence homology with EBV, and their antigens cross-react with the corresponding antigens of the EBV system. The interaction of these viruses with the B lymphocyte of the host species is closely analogous to the interaction of EBV with the human lymphocyte; permanent virus-carrying lines can be established and are quite similar to their human counterparts. There are certain differences in producer status and in the quantity and specificity of the nuclear antigen (22–26). Neutralizing antibodies are present in all Old World monkey sera that fully cross-react with EBV, however. It is therefore hardly surprising that experiments to induce experimental disease have consistently failed in these species.

In New World monkeys, the situation is quite different. The species so far studied do not have EBV-related viruses. Some of them, such as the squirrel monkey and the spider monkey, carry lymphotropic viruses of their own (*H. saimiri* and *H. ateles*). The properties of their viruses and particularly their ability to transform T lymphocytes is an area of great interest in itself (for review, see Ref. 27). However, these viruses are entirely unrelated to EBV. There is thus no cross-neutralization against EBV. New and Old World monkeys separated approximately 50 million years ago; the evolution of EBV-like viruses is thus of a later date.

Epstein–Barr virus was found to induce progressive lymphoproliferative disease in the best studied New World species, the marmoset monkey (10). While often fatal, the disease is quite different from the EBV-carrying human BL. It is polyclonal and thus more akin to fatal infectious mononucleosis (IM). In all likelihood, the EBV-transformed B lymphocyte grows progressively in the immunologically naive host species as a result of the unavailability of established host defense mechanisms rather than as the result of specific cellular changes (other than EBV transformation).

The ability of EBV-transformed (immortalized) but otherwise normal B lymphocytes to grow progressively *in vivo* under immunologically privileged conditions is also emphasized by the inoculation of EBV-transformed LCLs of normal human origin into nude mice (28, 29). As long as the cells remain diploid, they fail to grow in the subcutaneous space of the T-cell-deficient adult nude mouse but can nevertheless grow progressively in the brain of the nude (but not of the wild-type) mouse and also in the subcutaneous space of the newborn nude mouse. The histology of the brain-grown lesion resembles that of EBV-induced lymphoproliferative disease in the marmoset and the lesions seen in fatal mononucleosis.

The effectors that restrict LCL proliferation in the subcutaneous space of the adult nude mouse are not known; natural killer (NK) cells or antispecies antibodies, alone or together with lymphocyte effectors, represent some of the possibilities. There is no reason to assume, however, that the effectors of this artificial system are akin to the immune effectors in the normal, EBV-carrying human host.

It must be noted that BL cells can grow progressively at the subcutaneous sites of the adult nude mouse at the earliest stage after establishment *in vitro* and even after inoculation of the tumor biopsy (30). This indicates that LCL and BL cells differ in their sensitivity to a relevant immune effector.

B. Clinical Evidence

The lack of experimental evidence on the corresponding human conditions has been richly compensated for by a variety of clinical situations that represent "experiments of nature." First, it was discovered (31) that EBV was the causative agent of IM. Although the precise pathogenesis and course of this disease still remain to be clarified in many ways, certain details are quite clear. It is due to the primary EBV infection of EBV-seronegative persons, usually adolescents or young adults. During the acute phase, a relatively small fraction of the peripheral B-lymphocyte pool (1–2%) becomes EBNA-positive (32). Recently, it was shown (33) that the EBNA-positive cells could divide in the peripheral blood. Since EBNA is a chromosomal protein (8), the dividing, antigen-positive cells could be readily identified. The peripheral lymphocyte pool does not give a true picture of the frequency of EBNA-positive cells in the tissues, as indicated by the EBV DNA positivity of the bone marrow in some mononucleosis patients (12) and by the extensive invasion of lymphoid tissues with EBNA-positive cells in a fatal case where death was due to respiratory complications rather than immune failure (34).

In contrast to the relatively small frequency of EBNA-positive B cells in the peripheral blood of acute IM patients, the majority of the atypical blasts have T-cell characteristics (35–39). Svedmyr and Jondal found (40) that the T-cell fraction of acute IM blood had a powerful and apparently preferential killing effect on EBV-carrying target cells, acting in a non-HLA-restricted fashion. They are thus clearly different from EBV-specific, HLA-restricted memory T cells, derived from the circulation of healthy EBV-seropositive donors (where the acute IM-type killers are never found), that appear only after an *in vitro* step of sensitization with autologous, EBV-carrying B cells (41–43). Since specific killer T cells are major histocompatibility complex (MHC)-restricted in both human and murine systems, as a rule, it is conceivable that the killer cells in acute IM represent a first line of defense, perhaps akin to interferon-activated natural killer (IAK) cells known to kill EBV-carrying B cells of both normal and lymphoma origin with high efficiency (44). They belong to the T-cell series and show no MHC restriction. If this is correct, one could envisage at least two main phases in the T-lineage-mediated response against EBV-carrying cells: a prompt but relatively blunt (i.e., not rigorously specific) NK or IAK reaction, and a more delayed but more specific (restricted) cytotoxicity.

About one-half of the primary EBV infections in adolescents and young adults and most primary infections in young children pass without symptoms of mononucleosis, probably as "silent" infections. The reasons for this age-related difference are unknown. It could be due to a difference in the severity of the acute (rejection-like) reaction that may in itself be responsible for many of the symptoms. As another alternative, one may recall the age-related difference in the virus producer status of EBV-transformed lymphoblastoid cell lines (45). Lines from children under the age of 10 are more frequently virus nonproducers than LCLs from teenagers or adults. If a similar difference prevails with regard to activation of the viral cycle *in vivo*, it might be responsible for differences in the degree of virally induced killer cell activation.

It follows from what has been said so far that EBV must be a potentially dangerous agent in immunologically unprepared hosts. It may be recalled that EBV is the most powerful transforming virus known, superior to all other known transforming viruses with regard to transforming efficiency per virus particle (10,14). Since the virus is ubiquitous, i.e., succeeds in infecting most individuals in all human populations and must have been living with our species for a very long time, as shown by the simian evidence, it can be expected that a wide variety of effector mechanisms participate in protecting the human host against the growth of EBV-transformed cells. Two cell-mediated mechanisms, based on effectors of the T-cell lineage, have already been mentioned. In addition, there is also evidence that antibody-dependent cellular cytoxicity (ADCC), the antibody-dependent lymphocytotoxicity (ADLC) reaction against membrane-associated EBV antigens (46,47), and humoral antibodies by themselves may also play a certain protective role (48, 49).

Can a massive breakdown of immune defenses cause EBV-carrying lympho-proliferative disease in humans? The positive answer to this question stems largely from the pioneering work of Purtilo (50). He described the familiar occurrence of a disease complex, now known as the X-linked lymphoproliferative syndrome (XLP), and postulated, mainly on the basis of its histological similarity to the pleiotropic picture of fatal mononucleosis and immunoblastic sarcoma, that it was due to the unrestrained proliferation of EBV-transformed B cells. At first glance, this appeared unlikely, because EBV antibodies were not prevalent. However, the patients invariably had hypo- or agammaglobulinemia as well. Recently, with Purtilo, we have found multiple EBV genomes in six of six studied cases of XLP (51), in seven of seven "lymphomas" arising in renal transplant patients (52), and in one lymphoma that developed in a Turkish child with ataxia telangiectasia (53).

Recently, we initiated a comparison of effector mechanisms in patients with a high EBV load and various degrees of immunodeficiencies with and without EBV-carrying lymphoproliferative disease (54, 55). The diseased group included two cases of chronic mononucleosis and four cases of XLP. Effectors studied included NK cells in short-term cytotoxicity tests, IAK killing, the full spectrum of EBV antibodies, and ADLC. We also included a newly developed EBV-specific lymphocyte migration inhibition test (56–58). A special advantage of this test lies in the fact that sensitization of the patient's lymphocytes to different EBV-associated antigens, such as EBNA, the lymphocyte-defined membrane antigen (LYDMA), and the viral cycle-associated EA–VCA antigen complex can be tested separately.

As the relatively immunodefective group with a high EBV load but without EBV-carrying lymphoproliferative disease we have chosen Hodgkin's and non-Hodgkin's lymphoma patients in remission with extraordinarily high EBV antibody titers (IgG anti-VCA > 10,000), indicating a high virus load. The preliminary results (54, 55) indicate that patients with EBV-carrying lymphoproliferative disease have a more polyvalent and quantitatively more serious immunosuppression than patients who hold their EBV-transformed cells under control. It seems that normal (i.e., genetically unchanged) EBV-carrying cells cause disease only under conditions of multiple and very heavy immunosuppression. Apparently, the system is buffered by a rich variety of alternative, compensatory mechanisms.

An interesting special situation is represented by the high frequency of lymphomas that arise in renal transplant recipients with a primary localization in the central nervous system (CNS) (59). More than 40% of the transplant patient lymphomas originate in the CNS, in contrast to 2% of the lymphomas arising in the general population. The possible relationship between this observation and the preferential ability of normal diploid, EBV-transformed lymphoblastoid cells to grow in the nude mouse brain (29) is intriguing.

Continued studies on progressive lymphoproliferative disease in immunosuppressed patients will be interesting for several reasons. The information that will be gained about the role of EBV in these lesions is one of them. It will be important to know whether the EBV genomes detected by nucleic acid hybridization are mainly or exclusively carried by virus-transformed by non-virus-producing (EBNA-positive, EA–VCA-negative) cells or partly also by cells with replicative viral DNA synthesis. Simultaneous multiple marker tests will have to be developed to determine whether EBNA-positive cells are engaged in monoclonal or polyclonal proliferation. Moreover, multiple effector analyses for patients with EBV-carrying lymphoproliferative disease will elucidate the relative role of different immune mechanisms in keeping the proliferation of EBV-transformed cells under control.

Polyclonal EBV-carrying lymphoproliferative disease represents an interesting contrast to BL and must be clearly distinguished from it. The latter arises in immunocompetent patients, is always monoclonal, and shows a regular chromosomal change. The relationship between the two disease types is reminiscent of the distinction between conditioned and autonomous neoplasms (60). The former grow mainly (although not necessarily exclusively) as a result of the breakdown of some critically important host control mechanism. Both the overproduction of positive and the defective generation of negative feedback signals can be responsible. Both are known to occur in relation to EBV. Viral immortalization provides the positive driving force, whereas immune breakdown corresponds to abolition of the negative feedback. In contrast, BL is apparently due to a specific genetic change in a single cell, as discussed in the following section.

III. Burkitt's Lymphoma

The disease and its relationship to EBV have been reviewed frequently (see, e.g., Refs. 1, 2, 12, 61). It may be sufficient to recapitulate some of the most important facts.

Burkitt's lymphoma is a well-defined histopathological or clinical entity (62). The BL cell is a low-differentiated B lymphocyte. Only one other disease, B-cell-derived acute lymphatic leukemia (B-ALL), sometimes designated Burkitt's leukemia, shows analogous cytological features. It also has an identical cytogenetic marker, as will be discussed below.

Cells of BL are less differentiated than those of EBV-transformed LCLs of normal origin (11). In contrast to the latter, they have mainly surface, but little or no secretory immunoglobulin. They are frequently surface IgM-positive but are virtually always negative for surface IgD, whereas LCLs can be positive for both (63,64). This, by itself, could "place" the BL cell to the left (less differentiated) or to the right (more differentiated) side of the "IgD-positive window" in B-cell development. However, the absence of secretory immunoglobulin and the low concentration of insulin receptors, contrasting with the strong expression of both markers in EBV-transformed LCLs (65), clearly indicate that the BL cell is on the less differentiated side. One further important difference between BL cells and LCLs lies in the high agarose clonability of the former, as contrasted to the very low clonability of the latter (28, 66). Clonability in soft agar is usually regarded as the *in vitro* parameter that shows the closest correlation with tumorigenicity.

Studies on the EBV DNA- and EBNA-carrying status of African BL, performed at different laboratories, are in close agreement, showing that 97–98% of the cases are EBV-carrying tumors (67–71).

Cells of BL are quite similar to those of LCLs with regard to the number of viral genome copies, the occurrence of integrated versus free episomal viral DNA, the antigenic specificity of EBNA, and the latency and inducibility of the viral cycle. Attempts to detect DNA sequence differences between BL-associated EBV, on the one hand, and normal LCL- or IM-associated virus, on the other, failed to reveal any disease-related difference; the variations appear to reflect the properties of the individual isolates (for review, see Ref. 12,14). Taken together with the marked phenotypic differences between LCL and BL cells, this suggests that the malignant behavior of the BL cell is not determined at the level of the virus–cell interaction but at the level of the cell–host relationship. This is even more strongly emphasized by the chromosomal studies discussed in Section II,C.

A. Epstein–Barr Virus-Negative Burkitt Lymphomas

Approximately 3% of the African BLs studied did not carry the EBV genome (68). One of them (BJAB) that has been established in culture shows a variety of atypical features, described below. Outside the highly endemic African regions, BL occurs at a much lower frequency and in a sporadic fashion, without any evidence of time–space clustering (72). Only limited material has been studied for EBV genomes; these data suggest that about 20% are EBV-carrying, whereas 80% are EBV-negative (73).

As discussed below, sporadic BL cases from nonendemic regions, EBV-negative forms included, were found to carry the same type of chromosomal marker as the BLs of the highly endemic regions.

Two EBV-negative BLs, the American Ramos and the African BJAB, have been established as continuous, EBV-negative lines in culture (74–76). Like other normal and malignant B cells, they carry EBV receptors and can be infected with the virus *in vitro*. Permanently EBV-converted, EBV DNA,-positive and EBNA-positive sublines were established from both (77,78). The availability of EBV-negative and EBV-carrying sublines, derived from the same monoclonal tumor, provides otherwise unparallelled opportunities to study the effects of the viral genome on the cellular phenotype. Such studies have shown that EBV conversion increases the resistance of the cells to saturation conditions *in vitro,* decreases their serum dependence, obviates a requirement for a dialyzable serum factor, reduces the lateral mobility (capping) of various surface components, increases the ability of the cells to activate the alternate complement pathway, and increases their agarose clonability (79–85). Taken together, these changes are reminiscent of the phenotypic effects of viral transformation in quite different systems, e.g., the transformation of fibroblast monolayers by a variety of oncogenic RNA and DNA viruses. This suggests the existence of some common denominator in the transforming action of widely different agents, such as a human lymphotropic herpesvirus, EBV, and the smaller experimental oncoviruses, and in relation to very different cell types. The capability for progressive *in vitro* growth without a continuous supply of specific growth stimuli, i.e., immortality may represent the common phenotypic basis.

B. Are There Intermediate Levels of Transformation?

This question arises mainly from studies on a single lymphoma line, BJAB. As already mentioned above, BJAB is exceptional in several respects. It has been derived from what has been diagnosed as a somewhat atypical BL in an African child (74,75). Although a lymphoma line by phenotypic criteria (11), BJAB has a variety of unusual features. Alone among the known African BL-derived lines, it is EBV DNA- and EBNA-negative (74). It is also unique in lacking the 14q+ chromosomal marker. Unlike typical BL lines, it has low agarose clonability and it fails to grow in nude mice (85a).

Gahmberg *et al.* (86) have described a glycoprotein (gp69/71) double band present on all the BL-derived lines *except* BJAB, but not on LCLs of normal origin. It, therefore, appears as a phenotypic marker associated with the BL cell type.

Recently, we found that all BL-associated phenotypic characteristics, except the chromosomal marker, could be induced in the EBV-negative BJAB line by superinfection with the transforming (B95-8) strain of EBV (86a). The phenotypic changes included increased agarose clonability, progressive growth in the subcutaneous space of adult nude mice, and the gp69/71 double band. It is unlikely that EBV codes for any of these properties, since all of them can be found in other EBV-negative BL lines, e.g., the Ramos line that carries the typical BL-associated 14q+ marker, arising from a reciprocal 8;14 translocation. Nevertheless, EBV appears to be capable of inducing a pleiotropic "quantum jump" as far as expression of the transformed (tumorigenic) phenotype of BJAB is concerned. This suggests that the presence of the viral genome and specific genetic changes in the cell, particularly those resulting from the nonrandom chromosomal change associated with this tumor, may converge in their effect; i.e., their interaction can lead to a fully transformed, tumorigenic phenotype. The underlying concept, stepwise transformation, has been documented in numerous other systems. One may regard the various steps as reflecting different levels of cellular independence. Viral transformation and/or genetic changes can push the cell to a higher level.

C. Chromosomal Studies

Manolov and Manolova (87) first reported that BL biopsies and derived lines regularly contained a 14q+ marker carrying an extra band at the distal end of one of the two homologous chromosomes 14. Subsequently, Zech et al. (88) found that the marker arose by a reciprocal translocation between chromosomes 8 and 14. Recently, Manolova et al. (89) defined the breaking points on chromosomes 8 and 14 by the high-resolution prophase banding technique and showed that it was very constant in different individual tumors. While other types of human hemo- and lymphopoietic neoplasias were quite frequently found to carry 14q+ markers, these were different from the BL-associated reciprocal 8:14 translocation: The donor chromosome of the extra band was variable, and so was the breaking point on chromosome 14 itself (90,91). B-Cell-derived ALL is the only exception: it contains the BL-type 8:14 reciprocal translocation (92). Interestingly, this leukemia is believed to originate from the same target cell as BL (62).

Since EBV-negative and EBV-positive BLs and EBV-negative B-ALL all contain the 8:14 translocation, it is most unlikely that EBV is involved in generating this marker. This is further emphasized by the fact that EBV-transformed CLCs of normal origin are purely diploid, as a rule, for several months up to a year after their establishment and do not contain the marker. They tend to become aneuploid later, but without any specific pattern (88). Manolov et al. (93) recently examined 10 LCLs of normal origin by banding. Two of the 10 EBV-transformed lines contained a 14q+ marker in a low frequency of the cells (2 and 9%). By means of the high-resolution "mesome–prosome" analysis of the G-band patterns of these markers, it was established that the additional chromosome segments of these two 14q+ markers came from chromosomes 3 and 5, respectively, and not from chromosome 8 as in the 14q+ marker of BL. Chromosome 8 was not involved in any changes in the 10 cell lines studied.

A variety of mechanisms were discussed to explain the origin of the BL marker, including DNA homology between appropriate segments on chromosomes 8 and 14, particular closeness of the two chromosomes during some phase of cell kinetics, and transposable genetic elements (90,91). Until evidence becomes available to the contrary, we favor the simplest explanation: a random event, occurring by chance, in persistent, EBV-carrying, latently infected B cells that are urged to divide but cannot differentiate properly because of the presence of the viral genome. Division may be stimulated by an environmental cofactor, possibly chronic holo- or hyperendemic malaria, as discussed below.

There are some interesting parallels between the human 8:14 translocation in BL and the murine plasmacytoma-associated 12:15 translocation, as recently analyzed by our cytogenetic group (94). The basis of this statement is the following.

There is much recent evidence indicating that the distal part of murine chromosome 15 is involved in the genesis of both T- and B-cell leukemias in the mouse. The predominating nonrandom chromosomal change in murine T-cell leukemias of diverse etiologies is 15-trisomy (95, 96). B-Cell leukemias have not been analyzed to an equal extent, but there is evidence indicating that 15-trisomy is involved there as well (97). Leukemias induced in Robertsonian translocation mice, carrying large chromosome markers derived from the centromeric fusion of chromosome 15 and another autosome, have provided further important evidence on the significance of 15-trisomy (98). In virally and chemically induced T-cell leukemias, the entire translocation element has been duplicated. Since the chromosome attached by centromeric fusion is thus compelled to become a "fellow traveler," this excludes the possibility that 15-trisomic cells are the sole survivors among all possible trisomies and strongly suggests that 15-trisomy plays a primary (causal) role in the genesis of these leukemias. Studies on T6 (14;15) translocation mice and in SJL mice have shown, moreover, that the gene(s) that must be duplicated in the course of T-cell leukemogenesis are localized in the distal part of chromosome 15 (99, 100).

During the development of mineral oil-induced IgA-producing plasmacytoma in BALB/C mice, the distal portion of chromosome 15 is translocated to chromosome 12 (94). The translocation site is in the same major area as the heavy-chain immunoglobulin locus, but the precise relationship remains to be studied. In kappa (but not lambda)-producing plasmacytomas there is another translocation present, reciprocal 6:14 (94, 101). This is remarkable in view of the fact that chromosome 6 is known to carry the kappa gene of the mouse.

These findings suggest that a gene or a cluster of genes that influences the normal growth and differentiation of a given cell series (such as the lymphocyte–plasmacyte series) may favor neoplastic development if translocated to another chromosomal region that is particularly active in the target cell.

In humans, the heavy-chain immunoglobulin locus has been recently localized to chromosome 14 (102). This raises the question whether the BL-associated 8:14 translocation is analogous to the 12:15 translocation of the murine plasmacytoma. By inference, it follows that the distal segment of human chromosome 8 may contain a region that is of importance for the normal function of the human B lymphocyte. Based on this hypothesis, the translocation of 8, rather than the breakage or translocation of 14, is the crucial event in the genesis of BL. This speculation has received striking and unexpected support from three independently described "variant" cases of BL (103–107). The three cases arose in low endemic regions (France, Belgium, Japan). All three showed translocation of the same distal segment of chromosome 8 as the usual cases, but to chromosomes other than 14 (chromosome 22 in two cases, and chromosome 2 in one case). In addition to emphasizing the role of chromosome 8, these findings are also of great interest in view of the obvious analogy with the classic (9;22) and variant forms of the Philadelphia chromosome.

On the basis of this reasoning, one would also expect to find 8-trisomies in human leukemia, by analogy with the role of 15-trisomy in murine lymphoma. The recent extensive survey of the literature by Mitelman and Levan (108, 109) actually shows that trisomy of chromosome 8 is *the* most common trisomy in human leukemia.

D. Etiology of Burkitt's Lymphoma

As far as the most common form of BL, the EBV-carrying lymphoma of the highly endemic African regions is concerned, we have previously suggested (110) that the tumor develops in three phases, as detailed below.

Phase 1: Primary EBV infection. In the African pre-BL child this event is probably quite similar to the corresponding event in healthy brothers and sisters who never develop BL, except in one respect. The prospective study of de Thé *et al.* has shown (111) that the EBV antibody titers of pre-BL children are higher, on a statistical basis, than those of normal controls. This suggests that pre-BL children have a relatively higher virus load. This is not a sufficient explanation for BL, however, since the difference is merely one of statistical distribution, with much overlapping. High antibody titers are by themselves neither necessary nor sufficient for the development of BL.

Phase 2. This phase must be related to the environmental cofactor. On the basis of geographic and epidemiological evidence, Burkitt has suggested that the cofactor is holo- or hyperendemic malaria (112). In what ways could such a cofactor act?

We know from studies on established LCLs that EBV-transformed B cells are not only immortal but are also relatively frozen in their differentiation. Under the influence of certain inducers, they can make certain limited differentiation steps, but they cannot go all the way to the plasma cell stage. It is reasonable to assume that EBV-carrying B lymphocytes have similar intrinsic properties *in vivo,* although their proliferative capacity is held in check by some type of immunological or nonimmunological host control. This means that they are stimulated to divide when normal B cells divide and perhaps even more often, at times when the immunological growth control fails or is less efficient. But while activated normal B cells differentiate toward the end stage of the plasma cell and thereby disappear from the B-cell pool, the EBV-carrying B cells linger on and can accumulate genetic damage in direct proportion to the number of cell divisions.

Chronic, heavy malaria infections exert a continuous growth-stimulating effect on the lymphatic system. It might be expected that the EBV-infected B-cell lineage is urged to proliferate as well, albeit under control. The number of cell divisions per infected B cell will be obviously very large in comparison to the frequency of BL cell division. This becomes particularly apparent if we consider the fact that BL is a relatively rare disease, even in the areas with the highest incidence (approximately 5 per 100,000 of the risk age per year), and the fact that virtually all children are infected, many of them with a high virus load, as indicated by their antibody titers. One can therefore allow for a large variety of nonspecific genetic damage before the crucial cytogenetic change arises, representing the third step.

Phase 3: The specific chromosomal change. We regard the translocation of the distal part of chromosome 8 to 14 (or to another chromosome, as in the variants) as the crucial event in the triggering of autonomous growth. The mechanism of its action is obscure, but this is also true for other nonrandom tumor-associated chromosomal changes, including the Philadelphia chromosome. Gene dosage effects may be considered, particularly since overproduction of normal cellular constituents appears to be the crucial change in many types of viral oncogenesis (for review, see Ref. 113). Switching crucially important regulatory factors on or off is another plausible alternative. Clarification will have to await the collection of more information on the molecular biology of mammalian cells, with particular focus on the specific chromosomal regions involved. Experiments are presently available for determining whether the *deletion* of chromosome 8, the *translocation* of the deleted piece to certain other chromosomes, or both, represent the crucial requirement for progressive growth. Somatic hybridization–segregation experiments, coupled with tumorigenicity tests, represent one possible approach.

In the EBV-negative form of *nonendemic BL,* the course of events must be different. The final change, the chromosomal translocation, is the same, however. Its postulated significance is greatly enhanced by the fact that the regularly EBV-negative B-cell-derived form of acute lymphatic leukemia, believed to originate from the same target cell as BL, carries the typical BL-type translocation, in contrast to other leukemias (92). This also supports our concept of convergence in tumor evolution (110), i.e., the notion that neoplasms arising from the same target cell may be generated by the same specific cytogenetic change, irrespective of the initiating (etiological) agent.

On the basis of this hypothesis, the 8:14 translocation, if arising by chance in a previously intact lymphoid tissue, ought to be able to create BL by itself. This may be actually the reason for at least some of the nonendemic cases, always a great rarity. It cannot be excluded, however, that other viral or nonviral agents play an initiating, immortalizing role similar to that of EBV in BL. One can also think of growth-promoting cofactors analogous to malaria. In the absence of any evidence, all these ideas must remain highly speculative at this time.

IV. Nasopharyngeal Carcinoma

Much less is known about the genesis of nasopharyngeal carcinoma (NPC) than about BL. One reason lies in the unavailability of appropriate experimental materials. The carcinoma cells of NPC have not been successfully propagated in culture. Normal epithelial cells could not be infected or transformed by EBV in the experimental systems so far tested. Nevertheless, the association between the virus and the tumor is equally or even more stringent than in BL. The less differentiated or anaplastic form of NPC was found to carry the viral genome in 100% of the critically studied cases, where histological examination and nucleic acid hybridization tests have been made on the same specimen to ascertain the presence of viable tumor tissue and proper histological type (114,115). The association between EBV and NPC is independent of geography, ethnic origin of the donors, and the incidence rate of the tumor in the population. As long as the tumor is of the proper histological type, the carcinoma cells carry multiple EBV genomes, no matter whether they have been derived from the high-incidence southern Chinese population or from one of the rare Western cases. Other nasopharynx-localized tumors, including both lymphoid and epithelial malignancies, do not carry EBV genomes. This further stresses the special significance of the relationship between the virus and the carcinoma cells (for review, see Ref. 116).

If it is assumed that EBV plays a causal role in the etiology of NPC, one has to face the same dilemma as in the case of BL, posed by the ubiquity of the virus, as contrasted to the relative rarity of the tumor. Possible cofactors must be considered here as well. The situation is different from that of BL, however, where the cofactor(s) are believed to be purely environmental. Nasopharyngeal carcinoma shows great ethnic variations among different human populations (117–124). It has been suggested that both genetic and environmental factors contribute to its etiology. Its frequency is remarkably high in certain areas of southern China, the Kwang-tung Province in particular. First-generation immigrants of southern Chinese origin maintain a high frequency of NPC (121,125). In Singapore, different Chinese dialect groups show frequencies that correspond to their points of origin in China (126,127). Later generations of Chinese Americans show a decline in NPC mortality, but it is not clear whether this is due to their changed environment or to the intermarriage of different Chinese ethnic subgroups with differing incidences of NPC.

Caucasians have a low incidence of NPC. Offspring of mixed marriages between southern Chinese and non-Chinese groups show an intermediate frequency (117,126,127). This prompted the suggestion that genetic factors play an important role. Since the disease is rare in northern China and in Japan, there is obviously no association between high risk and the mongoloid race as such. Several reports speak of familial aggregation of NPC (120,124,128,129). Males have a higher frequency of NPC than females, irrespective of race and geography.

While it is thus perfectly possible that the pertinent cofactors in NPC are genetic in nature, it must be remembered that cultural factors can easily mimic genetic influences in human populations. In this connection, a recent report of Hirayama and Ito is of considerable interest (130). They have found a certain relationship between the use of two tumor promoters (croton oil) containing Chinese herbal drugs and the highly endemic regions of NPC. In view of the fact that tumor-promoting phorbol esters are potent inducers of the EBV cycle and also have a profound influence on a variety of carcinogenic processes, this finding may be significant, but more detailed and extensive epidemiological evidence will be required to establish its validity.

V. Epilogue

While the causative role of EBV in mononucleosis is generally accepted, its relationship to BL and NPC is often discussed in more ambiguous terms. It is often said that an association has been established but that its meaning is uncertain. Sometimes it is implied that the decisive experiments still remain to be done, but the nature of such experiments is either not defined or, if defined, it is hard to see how they could give decisive evidence.

Implicit in this argumentation is the concept that oncogenic viruses cause tumors in nature by a direct transforming action, more or less like that of an ordinary infectious agent. Elsewhere, we have referred to this notion as the "illusion of direct oncogenicity" (113). Viruses rarely cause tumors by a direct transforming action under natural circumstances. The epizootic chicken lymphomatosis, Marek's disease, is the major exception. It is caused by another lymphotropic herpesvirus (MDV) that acts on a genetically largely unprotected species in a way that is reminiscent of what has been discussed above for the EBV–marmoset combination. Unless the oncogenic virus is of relatively recent origin or has recently spread through unprotected species from isolated reservoirs, as in the case of Marek's disease, the situation is quite different, however. As a rule, the virus and its natural host succeed in establishing a mutually protective relationship where tumor development is a great rarity, if it occurs at all, and must always be considered a biological accident. It appears quite certain that BL represents such an accident; NPC may be another accident, but its natural history is much less well understood, particularly since consequences of the virus–cell association remain unknown in the absence of appropriate *in vitro* systems. With this reservation about NPC, we argue that the involvement of EBV in these two human neoplastic diseases, particularly BL, is probably as direct and causative as the involvement of viruses in tumors is ever likely to be in natural outbred species studied in their original habitats.

Acknowledgments

The work of the author and his co-workers has been supported (in part) by Contract N01 CP 33316 from the Division of Cancer Cause and Prevention, National Cancer Institute, by grant 1 R01 CA 30264-01 awarded by the National Cancer Institute, DHEW, the Swedish Cancer Society, and the King Gustaf V Jubilee Fund.

References

1. M. A. Epstein and B. G. Achong, eds., "The Epstein-Barr Virus." Springer-Verlag, Berlin and New York, 1979.
2. G. Klein, "Viral Oncology," Raven, New York, 1980.
3. E. Yefenof, G. Klein, M. Jondal, and M. B. A. Oldstone, *Int. J. Cancer* **17**, 693 (1976).
4. M. Jondal, G. Klein, M. B. A. Oldstone, V. Bokisy, and E. Yefenof, *Scand. J. Immunol.* **5**, 401 (1976).
5. G. Klein, E. Yefenof, K. Falk, and A. Westman, *Int. J. Cancer* **21**, 552 (1978).
6. A. Graessmann, H. Wolf, and G. W. Bornkamm, *Proc. Natl. Acad. Sci. U.S.A.* **77**, 433 (1980).
7. D. J. Volsky, I. M. Shapiro, and G. Klein, *Proc. Natl. Acad. Sci. U.S.A.* **77**, 5453 (1980).
8. B. M. Reedman and G. Klein, *Int. J. Cancer* **11**, 499 (1973).
9. L. Einhorn and I. Ernberg, *Int. J. Cancer* **21**, 157 (1978).
10. G. Miller, *in* "Viral Oncology" (G. Klein, ed.), p. 713. Raven, New York, 1980.
11. K. Nilsson and J. Pontén, *Int. J. Cancer* **15**, 321 (1975).
12. H. zur Hausen, *Biochim. Biophys. Acta* **417**, 25 (1975).
13. A. Adams and T. Lindahl, *Proc. Natl. Acad. Sci. U.S.A.* **72**, 1477 (1975).
14. A. Adams, *in* "Viral Oncology" (G. Klein, ed.), p. 683. Raven, New York, 1980.
15. G. Klein, L. Dombos, and B. Gothoskar, *Int. J. Cancer* **10**, 44 (1972).
16. P. Gerber, *Proc. Natl. Acad. Sci. U.S.A.* **69**, 83 (1972).
17. B. Hampar, J. G. Derge, L. M. Martos, and J. L. Walker, *Proc. Natl. Acad. Sci. U.S.A.* **69**, 78 (1972).
18. N. Yamamoto and H. zur Hausen, *Nature (London)* **280**, 244 (1979).
19. J. Luka, B. Kallin, and G. Klein, *Virology* **94**, 228 (1979).
20. M. C. Tovey, G. Lenoir, and J. Bergnon-Lours, *Nature (London)* **276**, 270 (1978).
20a. S. Ben-Sasson and G. Klein, *Int. J. Cancer* **28**, 131 (1981).
21. J. Zeuthen and G. Klein, *in* "Transfer of Cell Constituents into Eukaryotic Cells" (J. E. Celis, A. Graessman, and A. Loyter, eds.), p. 235. Plenum, New York, 1980.
22. R. H. Neubauer, H. Rabin, B. C. Strnad, M. Nonoyama, and W. A. Nelson-Rees, *J. Virol.* **31**, 845 (1979).
23. H. Rabin, R. H. Neubauer, and R. F. Hopkins, *IARC Sci. Publ.* **24**, Part II (1978).
24. S. Ohno, J. Luka, L. A. Falk, and G. Klein, *Eur. J. Cancer* **14**, 955 (1978).
25. A. L. Falk, G. Henle, W. Henle, F. Deinhardt, and A. Schudel, *Int. J. Cancer* **20**, 219 (1977).
26. L. Falk, T. Lindahl, and G. Klein, *IARC Sci. Publ.* **24**, (1978).
27. B. Fleckenstein and C. Mulder, *in* "Viral Oncology" (G. Klein, ed.), p. 799. Raven, New York, 1980.
28. K. Nilsson, B. C. Giovanella, J. S. Stehlin, and G. Klein, *Int. J. Cancer* **19**, 337 (1977).
29. B. C. Giovanella, K. Nilsson, L. Zech, O. Yim, and G. Klein, *Int. J. Cancer* **24**, 103 (1979).
30. C. O. Povlsen, P. J. Fialkow, E. Klein, G. Klein, J. Rygaard, and F. Wiener, *Int. J. Cancer* **11**, 30 (1973).

31. G. Henle, W. Henle, and V. Diehl, *Proc. Natl. Acad. Sci. U.S.A.* **59**, 94 (1968).
32. G. Klein, E. Svedmyr, M. Jondal, and P. O. Persson, *Int. J. Cancer* **17**, 21 (1976).
33. J. Robinson, D. Smith, and J. Niederman, *Nature (London)* **287**, 334 (1980).
34. S. Britton, M. Andersson-Anvret, P. Gergely, W. Henle, M. Jondal, G. Klein, B. Sandstedt, and E. Svedmyr, *N. Engl. J. Med.* **298**. 89 (1978).
35. E. Svedmyr, M. Jondal, W. Henle, O. Weiland, L. Rombo, and G. Klein, *J. Clin. Lab. Immunol.* **1**, 225 (1978).
36. P. K. Pattengale, R. W. Smith, and E. Perline, *N. Engl. J. Med.* **291**, 1145 (1974).
37. V. J. Giulano, H. A. Jasin, and M. Ziff, *Clin. Immunol. Immunopathol.* **3**, 90 (1974).
38. R. N. Ernberg, B. J. Eberle, and C. R. Williams, Jr., *J. Infect. Dis.* **130**, 104 (1974).
39. P. J. Sheldon, M. Papamichael, E. H. Hemsted, and E. J. Holborow, *Lancet* **1**, 1153 (1973).
40. E. Svedmyr and M. Jondal, *Proc. Natl. Acad. Sci. U.S.A.* **72**, 1622 (1975).
41. A. B. Rickinson, D. J. Moss, and J. H. Pope, *Int. J. Cancer* **23**, 610 (1979).
42. D. J. Moss, A. B. Rickinson, and J. H. Pope. *Int. J. Cancer* **23**, 618 (1979).
43. D. J. Moss, A. B. Rickinson, and J. H. Pope, *Int. J. Cancer* **23**, 662 (1978).
44. M. G. Masucci, G. Masucci, E. Klein, and W. Berthold, *Proc. Natl. Acad. Sci. U.S.A.* **77**, 3620 (1980).
45. P. Gerber, IARC Sci Publ. **11**, (1975).
46. G. Pearson, B. Johansson, and G. Klein, *Int. J. Cancer* **22**, 120 (1978).
47. G. Pearson, L. F. Qualtiere, G. Klein, T. Norin, and I. S. Bal, *Int. J. Cancer* **24**, 402 (1979).
48. T. Mukojima, P. Gunvén, and G. Klein, *JNCI, J. Natl. Cancer Inst.* **51**, 1319 (1973).
49. P. Gunvén, G. Klein, P. Clifford, and S. Singh, *Proc. Natl. Acad. Sci. U.S.A.* **71**, 1422 (1974).
50. D. T. Purtilo, *Lancet* **8163**, 300 (1980).
51. A. K. Saemundsen, D. T. Purtilo, K. Sakamoto, J. Sullivan, A. C. Synnerholm, D. Hanto, R. Simmons, M. Anvret, R. Collins, and G. Klein, *Cancer Res.* (in press).
52. D. W. Hanto, G. Frizzera, D. T. Purtilo, K. Sakamoto, J. Sullivan, A. K. Saemundsen, G. Klein, R. Simmons, and J. S. Najarian, *Cancer Res.* (in press).
53. A. K. Saemundsen, A. I. Berkel, W. Henle, G. Henle, M. Anvret, Ö. Sanal, F. Ersoy, M. Caglar, and G. Klein, *Br. Med. J.* **282**, 425 (1981).
54. M. G. Masucci, R. Szigeti, I. Ernberg, G. Masucci, G. Klein, J. Pritchard, C. Sieff, S. Lie, A Glomstein, L. Businco, W. Henle, G. Henle, G. Pearson, K. Sakamoto, and D. Purtilo, *Cancer Res.* (in press).
55. M. G. Masucci, R. Szigeti, I. Ernberg, M. Björkholm, H. Mellstedt, G. Henle, W. Henle, G. Pearson, G. Masucci, E. Svedmyr, J. Johansson, and G. Klein, *Cancer Res.* (in press).
56. R. Szigeti, J. Luka, and G. Klein, *Cell. Immunol.* **58**, 269 (1981).
57. R. Szigeti, M. G. Masucci, W. Henle, G. Henle, D. Purtilo, and G. Klein, *Cancer Res.* (in press).
58. R. Szigeti, D. J. Volsky, J. Luka, and G. Klein, *J. Immunol.* **126**, 1676 (1981).
59. I. Penn, *Adv. Cancer Res.* **28**, 32 (1978).
60. J. Furth, *Cancer Res.* **13**, 477 (1953).
61. G. Klein, *N. Engl. J. Med.* **293**, 1353 (1975).
62. K. Lennert, "Malignant Lymphomas," Springer-Verlag, Berlin and New York, 1978.
63. P. Gunvén, G. Klein, E. Klein, T. Norio, and S. Singh, *Int. J. Cancer* **29**, 711 (1980).
64. J. A. van Boxel and D. N. Buell, *Nature (London)* **251**, 443 (1974).
65. G. Spira, P. Áman, N. Koide, G. Lundin, G. Klein, and K. Hall, *J. Immunol.* **126**, 122 (1981).
66. M. Zerbini and I. Ernberg, *J. Gen. Virol.* (in press).
67. Ch. L. M. Olweny, I. Atine, A. Kaddu-Mukasa, R. Owor, M. Andersson-Anvret, G. Klein, W. Henle, and G. de Thé, *JNCI, J. Natl. Cancer Inst.* **58**, 1191 (1977).
68. G. Klein, *Cold Spring Harbor Symp. Quant. Biol.* **39**, 783 (1975.

69. T. Lindahl, G. Klein, B. M. Reedman, B. Johansson, and S. Singh, *Int. J. Cancer* **13**, 764 (1974).
70. H. zur Hausen and H. Schulte-Holthausen, *Nature (London)* **227**, 245 (1970).
71. M. Nonoyama, C. H. Huang, J. S. Pagano, G. Klein, and S. Singh, *Proc. Natl. Acad. Sci. U.S.A.* **70**, 3265 (1973).
72. G. de Thé, *in* "Viral Oncology" (G. Klein, ed.), pp. 769–797. Raven, New York, 1980.
73. M. Andersson, G. Klein, J. Ziegler, and W. Henle, *Nature (London)* **260**, 357 (1976).
74. G. Klein, T. Lindahl, M. Jondal, W. Leibold, J. Menezes, K. Nilsson, and C. Sundström, *Proc. Natl. Acad. Sci.* **71**, 3283 (1974).
75. J. Menezes, W. Leibold, G. Klein, and G. Clements, *Biomedicine* **22**, 276 (1975).
76. G. Klein, B. Giovanella, A. Westman, J. Stehlin, and D. Mumford, *Intervirology* **5**, 319 (1976).
77. G. Klein, J. Zeuthen, P. Terasaki, R. Honig, R. Billing, M. Jondal, A. Westman, and G. Clements, *Int. J. Cancer* **18**, 639 (1976).
78. K. G. Fresen and H. zur Hausen, *Int. J. Cancer* **17**, 161 (1976).
79. L. Montaignier and J. Gruest, *Int. J. Cancer* **23**, 71 (1979).
80. M. Steinitz and G. Klein, *Proc. Natl. Acad. Sci. U.S.A.* **72**, 3518 (1975).
81. M. Steinitz and G. Klein, *Virology* **70**, 570 (1976).
82. M. Steinitz and G. Klein, *Eur. J. Cancer* **15**, 217 (1979).
83. E. Yefenof, G. Klein, H. Ben-Bassat, and L. Lundin, *Exp. Cell Res.* **108**, 185 (1977).
84. E. Yefenof and G. Klein, *Exp. Cell Res.* **99**, 175 (1976).
85. I. McConnell, G. Klein, T. F. Lint, and P. J. Lachmann, *Eur. J. Immunol.* **8**, 453 (1978).
85a. I. Ernberg, K. Nilsson, B. Giovanella, and G. Klein, submitted for publication.
86. C. G. Gahmberg, K. Nilsson, and L. C. Andersson, *IARC Sci. Publ.* **24**, 649 (1978).
86a. N. Koide, A. Wells, G. Klein, and I. Ernberg, *Intervirol.* (in press).
87. G. Manolov and Y. Manolova, *Nature (London)* **237**, 33 (1972).
88. L. Zech, U. Haglund, K. Nilsson, and G. Klein, *Int. J. Cancer* **17**, 47 (1976).
89. Y. Manolova, G. Manolov, J. Kieler, A. Levan, and G. Klein, *Hereditas* **90**, 5 (1979).
90. S. Fukuhara, J. D. Rowley, D. Variakojis, and H. M. Golomb, *Cancer Res.* **39**, 3119 (1979).
91. S. Fukuhara and J. D. Rowley, *Int. J. Cancer* **22**, 14 (1978).
92. F. Mitelman, M. Andersson-Anvret, L. Brandt, D. Catovsky, G. Klein, G. Manolov, Y. Manolova, E. Mark-Vendel, and P. G. Nilsson, *Int. J. Cancer* **24**, 27 (1979).
93. G. Manolov, Y. Manolova, G. Klein, A. Levan, and J. Kieler, *Cancer Gen. Cytogen.* (in press).
94. S. Ohno, M. Babonits, F. Wiener, J. Spira, G. Klein, and M. Potter, *Cell* **18**, 1001 (1979).
95. F. Wiener, S. Ohno, J. Spira, N. Haran-Ghera, and G. Klein, *JNCI, J. Natl. Cancer Inst.* **61**, 227 (1978).
96. F. Wiener, J. Spira, S. Ohno, N. Haran-Ghera, and G. Klein, *Int. J. Cancer* **22**, 447 (1978).
97. F. Wiener, M. Babonits, J. Spira, U. Bregula, G. Klein, R. M. Merwin, R. Asofsky, M. Lynes, and G. Haughton, *Int. J. Cancer* **27**, 51 (1981).
98. J. Spira, F. Wiener, S. Ohno, and G. Klein, *Proc. Natl. Acad. Sci. U.S.A.* **76**, 6619 (1979).
99. F. Wiener, S. Ohno, J. Spira, N. Haran-Ghera, and G. Klein, *Nature (London)* **275**, 658 (1978).
100. J. Spira, M. Babonits, F. Wiener, S. Ohno, Z. Wirschubsky, N. Haran-Ghera, and G. Klein, *Cancer Res.* **40**, 2609 (1980).
101. F. Wiener, M. Babonits, J. Spira, G. Klein, and M. Potter, *Somatic Cell Genet.* **6**, 731 (1980).
102. C. M. Croce, M. Shander, J. Martinis, L. Cicurel, G. G. D'Ancona, T. W. Dolby, and M. Koprowski, *Proc. Natl. Acad. Sci. U.S.A.* **76**, 3416 (1979).
103. R. Berger, A. Bernheim, H. J. Weh, G. Flandrin, M. T. Daniel, J.-C. Brouet, and N. Colbert, *Hum. Genet.* **53**, 111 (1979).

104. R. Berger, A. Bernheim, G. Flandrin, M. T. Daniel, G. Schaison, J.-C. Brouet, and J. Bernard, *Nouv. Presse Med.* **8,** 181 (1979).
105. R. Berger, A. Bernheim, J.-C. Brouet, M. T. Daniel, and G. Flandrin, *Br. J. Haemtol.* **43,** 87 (1979).
106. I. Miyoshi, S. Hiraki, I. Kimura, K. Miyamoto, and I. Sato, *Experientia* **35,** 742 (1979).
107. H. van den Berghe, C. Parloir, S. Gosseye, V. Englebienne, G. Cornu, and G. Sokal, *Cancer Genet. Cytogenet.* **1,** 9 (1979).
108. F. Mitelman and G. Levan, *Hereditas* **89,** 207 (1978).
109. F. Mitelman and G. Levan, *Hereditas* **95,** 79 (1981).
110. G. Klein, *Proc. Natl. Acad. Sci. U.S.A.* **76,** 2442 (1979).
111. G. de Thé, A. Geser, N. E. Day, P. M. Tukei, E. H. Williams, D. P. Beri, P. G. Smith, A. G. Dean, G. W. Bornkamm, P. Feorino, and W. Henle, *Nature (London)* **274,** 756 (1978).
112. D. P. Burkitt, *JNCI, J. Natl. Cancer Inst.* **42,** 19 (1969).
113. G. Klein, *in* 1980 Proc. Int. Symp. Cancer, p. 81, Grune and Stratton, New York, 1981.
114. M. Andersson-Anvret, N. Forsby, and G. Klein, *Prog. Exp. Tumor Res.* **21,** 100 (1978).
115. M. Andersson-Anvret, N. Forsby, G. Klein, W. Henle, and A. Björklund, *Int. J. Cancer* **23,** 762 (1979).
116. G. Klein, *in* "The Epstein-Barr Virus" (M. A. Epstein and B. G. Achong, eds.), p. 339. Springer-Verlag, Berlin and New York, 1979.
117. C. S. Muir, *Int. J. Cancer* **8,** 351 (1971).
118. C. S. Muir, *JAMA, J. Am. Med. Assoc.* **220,** 393 (1972).
119. C. S. Muir, *Bull. Cancer* **62,** 261 (1975).
120. H. C. Ho, *Adv. Cancer Res.* **15,** 57 (1972).
121. H. C. Hoe, *J. R. Coll. Surg. Edinburgh* **20,** 223 (1975).
122. C. S. Muir and K. Shanmugaratnam, "Cancer of the Nasopharynx." Munksgaard, Copenhagen, 1967.
123. P. Clifford, *Int. J. Cancer* **5,** 287 (1970).
124. K. Shanmugaratnam, *Int. Rev. Exp. Pathol.* **10,** 361 (1971).
125. P. Buell, *Cancer Res.* **34,** 1189 (1974).
126. K. Shanmugaratnam and C. S. Muir, *in* "Cancer of the Nasopharynx" (C. S. Muir and K. Shanmugaratnam, eds.), p. 47. Munksgaard, Copenhagen, 1967.
127. K. Shanmugaratnam and C. S. Muir, *in* "Cancer of the Nasopharynx" (C. S. Muir and K. Shanmugaratnam, eds.), p. 153. Munksgaard, Copenhagen, 1967.
128. S. Nevo, W. Meyer, and M. Altman, *Cancer* **28,** 807 (1971).
129. E. H. Williams and G. de Thé, *Lancet* **2,** 295 (1974).
130. T. Hirayama and Y. Ito, submitted for publication.

10

Feline Lymphomas and Leukemias as Models for Human Neoplasia

M. ESSEX

I. Introduction

Progress toward understanding the etiology of many human diseases has been hastened by the availability of appropriate animal models. For many questions of either a theoretical or practical nature small laboratory rodents represented a logical choice.

Concerning the etiology of human lymphoma and/or lymphoid leukemia, an initial wave of optimism concerning the possibility that RNA tumor viruses might be etiologically involved was followed by pessimism concerning this possibility. The pessimism is probably closely tied to the skepticism voiced about the new ''human'' tumor viruses. Although several such recently described putative human candidate viruses (see Gallo *et al.* and Goodenow *et al.*, this volume) clearly deserve experimental attention, we must also recognize that several earlier ''human'' isolates represented ''false alarms'' where a retrovirus of murine or feline origin was apparently growing in human cells (1,2). Such

MALIGNANT LYMPHOMAS

results induced many virologists to avoid direct questions about human agents and instead to concentrate their efforts on the molecular biology of retroviruses known to cause cancer in selected strains of mice or chickens and/or known to transform cells *in vitro*. An inevitable result was the tendency to shelf or over-look questions about the actions of the virus at the level of the host and/or the outbred population. Yet, in at least one model species, the cat, we are in a position where theoretical questions can be addressed at both the *in vitro* and the population levels.

Cats are desirable as experimental animals for numerous reasons. They are outbred, as are humans, they live in the same environment, and they have the same general type of diet. Individual animals are large enough so that adequate amounts of tissue can be obtained, yet small enough so they can be accommodated with limited space and expense. They adapt well to handling and breed well in laboratory environments.

For more than a decade it has been widely accepted that most cases of naturally occurring feline lymphoma are caused by the horizontally transmitted feline leukemia virus (FeLV). We have a reasonably thorough understanding of the epidemiology and pathobiology of the agent and the disease, but we know very little about how FeLV causes lymphoma at the cell and molecular levels. However, an intriguing epidemiological association has also been found between exposure to FeLV and the development of lymphoma or leukemia in "virus-negative" (VN) cats, suggesting that the virus may sometimes cause lymphoma in a "hit-and-run" manner (3,4). If we could understand how FeLV functions at the cellular and molecular level in both the virus-positive and VN forms of feline lymphoma, we would probably be in a better position to propose experiments for the examination of human tumor materials.

II. Pathobiology of Feline Lymphoma

Different forms of leukemia and lymphoma are associated with FeLV. These include both myeloid and lymphoid forms of true leukemia, as well as lymphoma. Most lymphomas originate at primary sites such as the thymus, lymph nodes, spleen, gut wall, and kidney capsule. However, a small proportion originate as isolated tumors in tissues such as the skin and the central nervous system. The vast majority of lymphomas and lymphoid leukemias are tumors of T cells, but a few appear to have originated in B or null cells (5). Some, but not all, are positive for terminal deoxynucleotidyl transferase (6). Hypoplastic anemia is also seen in some cats as a distinct entity caused by FeLV (7,8). There appears to be some geographical variation in the relative incidence of the specific forms of lymphoma and lymphoid leukemia. In Glasgow, for example, the most common form of lymphoma appears to be alimentary and true leukemias are rare, while in

Boston true leukemias represent a significant proportion of the total and among the lymphomas the thymic form is most prevalent (9).

III. Epidemiology and Infectious Origin

Feline leukemia virus is transmitted from cat to cat in saliva (10). Infectious FeLV is not present in significant levels in urine or feces, and the levels in saliva are generally even higher than the blood levels in viremic cats. Most cats probably become infected when they lick or groom each other. Thus FeLV spreads most efficiently among cats that are in close contact and in confinement, and especially among cats that are familiar to each other. One very effective mechanism for transmission is by maternal grooming, when an infected dam carries the virus to her nursing kittens. Under such circumstances cats appear to receive larger doses of virus and themselves become persistently infected more often than would occur if the first exposure occurred while roaming at postweaning ages. It is clear, however, that persistent infections can become established in some when they are first exposed to FeLV as adults. Since the distribution of FeLV among cats occurs much more efficiently when close contact is present, this occasionally results in "clusters" of leukemia or lymphoma (10,11). Such clusters are rare, however, and in fact sufficiently rare so that they were not interpreted as evidence of causation by a transmissible virus until this could be established on the basis of seroepidemiology (11–13).

Following acquisition of FeLV by mouth, limited replication occurs in the epithelium of the oropharynx and in local lymph nodes and salivary glands. This is apparently followed by growth in bone marrow and subsequently by persistent viremia (14). If FeLV is inoculated parenterally, a large proportion of the animals develop persistent viremia (15,16). If cats are naturally exposed, however, especially in adulthood, most will not develop persistent viremia but will only experience transient infections that may leave them in an immune state (17).

When cats become persistently infected with FeLV under natural conditions, they clearly have a very high risk for developing leukemia. The induction period is normally a year or more in duration and highly variable (18,19). This obviously makes it difficult to coordinate the time of exposure in a retrospective sense after the disease is recognized by a clinician. During the prolonged induction period most cats remain healthy, and such animals represent the major source of excreted FeLV for maintaining the virus in a population. Persistently viremic cats are also immunosuppressed, however, and at great risk for development of various other infectious diseases which, when they result, may kill the animal before the induction period for leukemia or lymphoma is completed (20). Various immune complex diseases such as glomerulonephritis also occur in cats that are persistently infected with FeLV (19).

An interesting group of lymphomas and leukemias are those that occur in VN cats, because they also occur at a much higher frequency following exposure to FeLV and there is strong suspicion that they may also be caused by this agent (3,4). Virus-negative cases occur within all the pathological forms, although there is general agreement that the alimentary form is more often VN and the thymic form is usually FeLV-positive (3,21,22). Most preparations from VN tumors lack detectable levels of all the major virion structural proteins (3,23), but a minority of the VN cases appear to have some virus structural proteins circulating in the blood (24). The proportion of cases that are VN varies with age at time of diagnosis (3,21,25). Both forms of leukemia and lymphoma are seen more frequently in younger animals, and older cats appear to develop almost exclusively the VN form (21).

IV. General Properties of the Virus

FeLV is a typical retrovirus. It has three genes, *gag, pol,* and *env,* situated in that order starting from the 5'-end of the single-stranded RNA (26). The genome is terminally redundant, as in all retroviruses, and about 8.5 kilobases in length (27). It replicates by forming a double-stranded DNA provirus which becomes integrated into the genome of the cell. Normal cat cells have complete copies of an unrelated nononcogenic retrovirus, designated RD-114, but uninfected animals do not have complete copies of FeLV. Incomplete sequences related to FeLV are present in normal cat cells (28,29). The *gag* gene encodes for a polyprotein that undergoes cleavage to form the peptides of the virion core. The products of the polyprotein are designated p15c, p12, p30, and p10, with the analogous information in the RNA situated in that order (30). The *pol* gene codes for reverse transcriptase, and the other associated nucleic acid enzymes involved in genome replication. The *env* gene encodes for pg70, a glycoprotein, and p15e. Both of the latter proteins occur in the envelope of the virion. All the virus structural proteins are immunogenic in cats. Tests for several of these proteins and/or the antibodies directed against them have provided valuable seroepidemiological tools. Most of the proteins have several antigenic determinants. Some of the determinants are group-specific in that they are common for all FeLVs; some are interspecies-specific in that they cross-react with other retroviruses, especially murine viruses; and some are subgroup-specific in that they react only with certain subclasses of FeLV (31).

The classification of FeLV into subgroups was based on the biological activity of the virion envelope glycoprotein gp70 (31,32). Such properties as host cell attachment interference and neutralization of infectivity allowed the division of FeLV into three subgroups, designated A, B, and C. Early studies suggested that the designated subgroups also had distinct host ranges, at least *in vitro*. While subgroup A appeared to grow easily only in feline cells, subgroups B and C grew equally well in nonfeline cells, with some selective differences between the two (32,33). Distinct differences can be observed in the composition of the RNA genomes as detected by oligonucleotide RNase T1 mapping (34). However, distinct "strain" differences can also be found for several isolates of one subgroup using this same technique, and recent serological studies tend to support this observation (35).

Since retroviruses bud from the cell surface and acquire host cell carbohydrates as part of the virion envelope glycoprotein molecule, it was not surprising to find that virus particles could be neutralized to some extent using antiserum directed only against the host cell of origin (36). However, recent work with bovine leukemia virus has demonstrated that the carbohydrate portion of the virion envelope glycoprotein is the major target for neutralizing antibody produced following natural infection (37). This is in contrast to the activity of the major antibody type produced by goats or rabbits following artificial immunization. It opens up the possibility that antibodies directed against the carbohydrate portion and/or some epitope present only when the carbohydrate is joined to the protein in its native, "unpurified" state may be the most relevant in the sense of natural immunity.

Cells that replicate FeLV appear to express one or more antigenic determinants of essentially all the major structural proteins (p15c, p12, p30, p10, gp70, and p15e) at the cell surface (38,39). Thus, even though the *gag* peptides do not serve as targets for virolytic antibody, they could, at least in theory, serve as targets for cytotoxic antibodies.

Since most feline lymphomas occur in T cells, we examined the possibility that T cells might be more sensitive to infection with FeLV than B cells. This was apparently true for cultured human B and T cells from the same individual (40). Similarly, when peripheral lymphoid cells from persistently viremic cats were examined for replicating FeLV, most of the virus was found to be replicating from T cells rather than B cells (41).

No clear correlation has been established between the subgroup characteristics of FeLVs and pathogenic activity. It is accepted that all animals with replicating FeLV (whether cancerous or not) have subgroup A (42). Some also have B and/or C, but B and C are never isolated alone. This would lead to the obvious interpretation that C and/or B are defective and dependent on A for replication and/or transmission, were it not for the fact that both cultures and animals can be readily infected with B and C alone in the laboratory (43). Epidemiological studies suggest that the presence of B might aid the horizontal transmission cycle, since populations having animals infected with A and B generally have a higher proportion of animals that are persistently viremic (44). Although rarely isolated at all, a surprising number of cats have antibodies against subgroup C FeLV, including many cases of VN leukemia or lymphoma (42). This observation has caused speculation about the possibility that subgroup C FeLV represents an endogenous form of FeLV or FeLV-related sequences that are sometimes activated.

Virus-negative lymphoma cells, which usually lack all FeLV structural proteins (3,23), have also been examined for the possible activation of unexpressed FeLV using various techniques. This question was recently investigated using transfected DNA from VN lymphoma cells, but no FeLV could be rescued (45). However, in the same study a "new" type of FeLV was rescued using DNA from virus-producing tumor cells. The newer form of FeLV detected in this manner exhibited a host range that had not previously been documented for replicating strains of FeLV.

A set of defective retroviruses that are closely related to FeLVs, feline sarcoma viruses (FeSVs), have been isolated from cats with fibrosarcoma (for review, see Ref. 26). These agents have a genome that contains the same 5'- and 3'-termini as FeLVs but have lost all of the *pol* gene and large portions of the *gag* and *env* genes (27). As a result, they can only replicate in the presence of FeLV or a related helper virus which can provide the missing functions. A portion of the FeLV genome sequences that are absent in FeSVs have been replaced by a newly acquired sequence which apparently represents a cellular gene involved in differentiation or growth regulation. This new gene apparently gives FeSVs the ability to transform cultured fibroblasts and to induce polyclonal tumors *in vivo* with very brief induction periods.

The only class of protein product thus far identified for the FeSV genome is designated *gag*-x (23, 46–48). It represents a fusion polyprotein containing the FeLV-related p15c and p12 peptides linked to a new protein designated "x", which is present as a cell membrane protein in transformed cells and fibrosarcoma cells where it apparently serves as a target for the immune response (49). The x portion of the *gag*-x protein also shares a cross-reacting antigenic determinant with feline lymphoma cells, including VN lymphoma cells that lack p12 and p15c (50). The antigen expressed on lymphoma cells has been designated the feline oncornavirus-associated cell membrane antigen (FOCMA). FOCMA has been identified in a protein of approximately 68,000 daltons in leukemia cells, where it occurs free of p15c, p12, and other virus structural proteins (51,52). Neither FOCMA nor *gag*-x protein are found in feline retrovirus particles, but when FeSV is rescued with certain unrelated helper viruses, such as murine amphotropic agents, very small amounts of this protein can be found in the virions (53).

The FeSV-related *gag*-x protein is expressed coordinately with the malignant phenotype in distinctly different types of tumors. Using antisera directed only against the x fragment, we showed that the protein was present in tumor cells from FeSV-induced melanomas or fibrosarcomas which originate from different embryonic germ layers (50,54). The protein is also expressed in transformed cat cells, as well as in the transformed cells from distant species, and from both

FeLV producer and nonproducer cells (54). The feline antiserum directed specifically against the x fragment also reacts with FOCMA on lymphoma cells, supporting earlier observations that the antigens on lymphoma cells and on FeSV-transformed fibroblasts shared at least one determinant (23,55,56).

V. Role of the Immune Response

Early studies indicated that cats inoculated with FeSV that resisted the development of progressing fibrosarcomas regularly developed high levels of circulating antibodies against FOCMA (for review, see Ref. 26). Similar studies with FeLV-inoculated cats and cats naturally exposed to FeLV revealed that resistance to the development of lymphoma was also related to an efficient humoral antibody response to FOCMA (26).

Although all the other virus structural proteins were immunogenic in cats, the immune response to them was not necessarily correlated with resistance to tumor development (26). The immune response to FeLV gp70 was, however, quite important in that it could prevent the establishment of persistent viremia. Cats with detectable levels of antibodies against FeLV gp70 regularly lacked detectable levels of virus proteins and infectious virus in the circulation (57). Additionally, it appears that antisera to gp70 (and perhaps to other virus structural proteins) is lytic for cells that produce FeLV; whether these cells are malignant or normal, such antibodies can cause termination of the virus infection and, at least in the case of fibrosarcoma, tumor regression (16,58).

The mechanism by which the immune response to FOCMA prevents the development of leukemia and lymphoma appears to be complement-mediated antibody lysis (59,60). Such antibodies are highly lytic for cultured lymphoma cells in the presence of cat complement (60). It seems possible in fact that complement deficiencies, rather than a lack of anti-FOCMA, cause lymphoma development in a small proportion of the FeLV-infected cats that develop lymphoma.

We recently proposed an immunoselection hypothesis as a theoretical explanation of how VN forms of leukemia and lymphoma emerge (26). If, for example, an adequate immune response to gp70 occurred in the absence of an effective immune response to FOCMA, perhaps only lymphoma cells that were VN could "sneak through," while FeLV producer cells and free FeLV would be lysed. Preliminary evidence in support of this hypothesis has been obtained in the case of FeSV-induced fibrosarcomas (61).

VI. Conclusions

Several conclusions can be established concerning the feline model. First, the disease is pathologically similar to several forms of lymphoma and/or leukemia that occur in humans. Second, the disease is caused by a transmissible agent that is primarily excreted in saliva. Third, only a small proportion of cats that are exposed to FeLV actually develop leukemia or lymphoma, and when they do it is only after a long and variable induction period. Fourth, an active immune response plays a role in both the prevention of persistent viremia and the prevention of tumor development. Fifth, the target for the antitumor immune response appears to be a tumor cell membrane antigen (FOCMA) shared by both lymphoma and fibrosarcoma cells.

Epidemiological evidence strongly supports the hypothesis that FeLV, or a defective variant, may also cause VN lymphoma in cats (3,4). With serological and nucleic acid technologies now available it should be possible to provide a direct answer to this question in the near future. If this question is answered in the affirmative, the information developed should provide leads concerning the type of agent(s) we should seek as possible cause(s) of human lymphoma.

References

1. E. S. Priori, L. Dmochowski, B. Myers, and J. R. Wilbur, *Nature (London), New Biol.* **232**, 61 (1972).
2. R. M. McAllister, M. Nicolson, M. B. Gardner, R. W. Rongey, S. Rasheed, P. S. Sarma, R. J. Huebner, M. Hatanaka, S. Oroszlan, R. V. Gilden, A. Kabigting, and L. Vernon, *Nature (London), New Biol.* **235**, 3 (1972).
3. W. D. Hardy, Jr., A. J. McClelland, E. E. Zuckerman, H. W. Snyder, Jr., E. G. MacEwen, D. Francis, and M. Essex, *Nature (London)* **288**, 90 (1980).
4. D. P. Francis, M. Essex, S. M. Cotter, N. Gutensohn, R. Jakowski, and W. D. Hardy, Jr., *Cancer Lett.* **12**, 37 (1981).
5. W. D. Hardy, Jr., E. E. Zuckerman, E. G. MacEwen, A. A. Hayes, and M. Essex, *Nature (London)* **270**, 249 (1977).
6. R. McCaffrey and S. Cotter, personal communication.
7. L. Mackey, W. Jarrett, O. Jarrett, and H. Laird, *JNCI, J. Natl. Cancer Inst.* **54**, 209 (1975).
8. E. A. Hoover, G. J. Kociba, W. D. Hardy, Jr., and D. S. Yohn, *JNCI, J. Natl. Cancer Inst.* **53**, 1271 (1974).
9. M. Essex, S. M. Cotter, W. D. Hardy, Jr., P. Hess, W. Jarrett, O. Jarrett, L. Mackey, H. Laird, L. Perryman, R. G. Olsen, and D. S. Yohn, *JNCI, J. Natl. Cancer Inst.* **55**, 463 (1975).
10. S. M. Cotter, M. Essex, and W. D. Hardy, Jr., *Cancer Res.* **34**, 1061 (1974).
11. M. Essex, R. M. Jakowski, W. D. Hardy, Jr., S. M. Cotter, P. Hess, and A. Sliski, *JNCI, J. Natl. Cancer Inst.* **54**, 637 (1975).
12. W. D. Hardy, Jr., L. J. Old, P. W. Hess, M. Essex, and S. M. Cotter, *Nature (London)* **244**, 266 (1973).
13. M. Essex, A. Sliski, S. M. Cotter, R. M. Jakowski, and W. D. Hardy, Jr., *Science* **190**, 790 (1975).
14. J. L. Rojko, E. A. Hoover, L. E. Mathes, R. G. Olsen, and J. P. Schaller, *JNCI, J. Natl. Cancer Inst.* **63**, 759 (1979).
15. E. A. Hoover, R. G. Olsen, W. D. Hardy, Jr., J. P. Schaller, and L. E. Mathes, *JNCI, J. Natl. Cancer Inst.* **58**, 365 (1976).
16. F. de Noronha, F. Schafer, M. Essex, and D. P. Bolognesi, *Virology* **85**, 617 (1978).

17. C. K. Grant, M. Essex, M. B. Gardner, and W. D. Hardy, Jr., *Cancer Res.* **40**, 823 (1980).
18. D. P. Francis, M. Essex, S. M. Cotter, R. M. Jakowski, and W. D. Hardy, Jr., *Leuk. Res.* **3**, 435 (1979).
19. D. P. Francis, M. Essex, R. M. Jakowski, S. M. Cotter, T. J. Lerer, and W. D. Hardy, Jr., *Am. J. Epidemiol.* **11**, 337 (1980).
20. M. Essex, W. D. Hardy, Jr., S. M. Cotter, R. M. Jakowski, and A. Sliski, *Infect. Immunol.* **11**, 470 (1975).
21. D. P. Francis, S. M. Cotter, W. D. Hardy, Jr., and M. Essex, *Cancer Res.* **39**, 3866 (1979).
22. W. Jarrett, M. Essex, L. Mackey, O. Jarrett, and H. Laird, *JNCI, J. Natl. Cancer Inst.* **51**, 261 (1973).
23. J. R. Stephenson, A. S. Khan, A. H. Sliski, and M. Essex, *Proc. Natl. Acad. Sci. U.S.A.* **74**, 5608 (1977).
24. C. Saxinger, M. Essex, W. D. Hardy, Jr., and R. Gallo, *in* "Feline Leukemia and Sarcoma Viruses" (W. D. Hardy, Jr., M. Essex, and A. J. McClelland, eds.), p. 489. Elsevier/North-Holland Biomedical Press, Amsterdam and New York, 1980.
25. M. B. Gardner, S. Rasheed, R. W. Rongey, H. W. Charman, B. Alena, R. V. Gilden, and R. J. Huebner, *Int. J. Cancer* **14**, 97 (1974).
26. M. Essex, *in* "Viral Oncology" (G. Klein, ed.), p. 205. Raven, New York, 1980.
27. C. J. Sherr, L. A. Federle, M. Oskarsson, J. Maizel, and G. Vande Woude, *J. Virol.* **34**, 200 (1980).
28. R. Levin, S. K. Ruscetti, W. P. Parks, and E. M. Scolnick, *Int. J. Cancer* **18**, 661 (1976).
29. R. Koshy, F. Wong-Staal, R. C. Gallo, W. D. Hardy, Jr., and M. Essex, *Virology* **99**, 135 (1979).
30. A. S. Khan and J. R. Stephenson, *J. Virol.* **23**, 599 (1977).
31. P. S. Sarma and T. Log, *Virology* **54**, 160 (1973).
32. O. Jarrett, H. M. Laird, and D. Hay, *Nature (London)* **238**, 220 (1972).
33. P. S. Sarma, T. Log, J. Damine, P. R. Hill, and R. Huebner, *Virology* **64**, 438 (1975).
34. Z. F. Rosenberg, F. S. Pedersen, and W. A. Haseltine, *J. Virol.* **35**, 542 (1980).
35. P. H. Russell and O. Jarrett, *Int. J. Cancer* **21**, 768 (1978).
36. J. Azocar and M. Essex, *Cancer Res.* **39**, 3388 (1979).
37. D. Portetelle, C. Bruick, M. Mammerick, and A. Burny, *Virology* **105**, 223 (1980).
38. M. Essex, A. H. Sliski, W. D. Hardy, Jr., S. M. Cotter, and F. De Noronha, *Adv. Comp. Leuk. Res., Proc. Int. Symp., 8th, 1977* p. 337 (1978).
39. T. H. Lee and M. Essex, in preparation.
40. J. Azocar and M. Essex, *JNCI, J. Natl. Cancer Inst.* **63**, 1179 (1979).
41. J. Azocar and M. Essex, *in* "Virus-Lymphocyte Interactions: Implications for Disease" (M. Proffitt, ed.), p. 179. Elsevier/North-Holland Biomedical Press, Amsterdam and New York, 1979.
42. O. Jarrett, W. D. Hardy, Jr., M. C. Golder, and D. Hay, *Int. J. Cancer* **21**, 334 (1978).
43. O. Jarrett and P. H. Russell, *Int. J. Cancer* **21**, 466 (1978).
44. O. Jarrett, P. H. Russell, and W. D. Hardy, Jr., *Adv. Comp. Leuk. Res., Proc. Int. Symp., 8th, 1977* p. 25 (1978).
45. Z. F. Rosenberg, R. L. Crowther, M. Essex, O. Jarrett, and W. A. Haseltine, *Virology* **115**, 203 (1981).
46. M. Barbacid, A. V. Lauver, and S. G. Devare, *J. Virol.* **33**, 196 (1980).
47. W. J. M. Van de Ven, A. S. Khan, F. H. Reynolds, K. T. Mason, and J. R. Stephenson, *J. Virol.* **33**, 1034 (1980).
48. S. K. Ruscetti, L. P. Turek, and C. J. Sherr, *J. Virol.* **35**, 259 (1980).
49. M. Essex, A. H. Sliski, M. Worley, C. K. Grant, H. Snyder, Jr., W. D. Hardy, Jr., and L. B. Chen, *in* "Viruses in Naturally Occurring Cancers" (M. Essex, G. J. Todaro, and H. zur Hausen, eds.), p. 589. Cold Spring Harbor Press, Cold Spring Harbor, New York, 1980.

50. A. P. Chen, M. Essex, T. Mikami, D. Albert, J. Y. Niederkorn, and J. P. Shadduck, *in* "Feline Leukemia and Sarcoma Viruses" (W. D. Hardy, Jr., M. Essex, and A. J. McClelland, eds.), p. 441. Elsevier/North-Holland Biomedical Press, Amsterdam and New York, 1980.

51. H. W. Snyder, Jr., W. D. Hardy, Jr., E. E. Zuckerman, and E. Fleissner, *Nature (London)* **275,** 656 (1978).

52. M. Worley and M. Essex, *in* "Feline Leukemia and Sarcoma Viruses" (W. D. Hardy, Jr., M. Essex, and A. J. McClelland, eds.), p. 431. Elsevier/North-Holland Biomedical Press, Amsterdam and New York, 1980.

53. C. J. Sherr, A. Sen, G. T. Todaro, A. Sliski, and M. Essex, *Proc. Natl. Acad. Sci. U.S.A.* **75,** 1505 (1978).

54. A. P. Chen, M. Essex, F. de Noronha, J. A. Shadduck, J. Y. Niederkorn, and D. Albert, *Proc. Natl. Acad. Sci. U.S.A.* **78,** 3915 (1981).

55. A. H. Sliski, M. Essex, C. Meyer, and G. T. Todaro, *Science* **196,** 1336 (1977).

56. A. H. Sliski and M. Essex, *Virology* **95,** 581 (1979).

57. J. R. Stephenson, M. Essex, S. Hino, S. A. Aaronson, and W. D. Hardy, Jr., *Proc. Natl. Acad. Sci. U.S.A.* **74,** 1219 (1977).

58. F. de Noronha, R. Baggs, W. Schafer, and D. P. Bolognesi, *Nature (London)* **267,** 54 (1977).

59. C. K. Grant, D. J. De Boer, M. Essex, M. B. Worley, and J. Higgins, *J. Immunol.* **119,** 401 (1977).

60. C. K. Grant, C. Ramaika, B. R. Madewell, D. K. Pickard, and M. Essex, *Cancer Res.* **39,** 75 (1979).

61. M. Essex, C. K. Grant, S. M. Cotter, A. H. Sliski, and W. D. Hardy, Jr., *Haematol. Blut-transfus.* **23,** 453 (1979).

11

Expression of C-Type RNA Viral Proteins by a Human Lymphoma Cell Line

ROBERT S. GOODENOW, SAI-LING LIU, KIRK E. FRY,
RONALD LEVY, AND HENRY S. KAPLAN

I. Introduction

C-type RNA retroviruses have been demonstrated to cause leukemia and lymphomas in a number of species including subhuman primates (cf. Ref. 1). The apparent ubiquity of these etiological agents has stimulated interest in determining whether retroviruses are also the causative agents of the corresponding human malignant neoplasms.

A number of reports have cited evidence for the existence of retroviral components in primary human tumor material (2–8). C-type RNA viruses contain a unique enzyme, reverse transcriptase, which is responsible for transcribing the high-molecular-weight RNA genome into a proviral DNA copy which is then integrated into the host genome. The intracellular detection of reverse transcriptase-like enzymatic activity, measured by the incorporation of labeled precursors into a DNA product still hybridized with the RNA template, provided a screening procedure known as the simultaneous detection assay (2). When used to examine primary tumor specimens, such assays revealed apparent 70 S viral RNA and/or associated reverse transcriptase-like activity in the majority of human leukemia and lymphoma cells tested (3–7). Moreover, DNA probes synthesized from the viral RNA genome of a murine leukemia virus (MuLV) reportedly detected sequence homology in the genomic DNA of some human tumor tissues (8). However, the observed sequence homology may have been spurious, because of hybridization of the probes with normal cellular sequences as a result of contamination of the viral RNA templates with cellular rRNA.

The first reported isolation of a putative human C-type RNA virus was from a human acute myeloid leukemia (9). This virus, designated HL23V, was isolated from cultures of human leukemic cells grown on a human embryonic feeder layer. The accidental loss of the embryonic cell strain necessitated propagating the virus in other cell lines (10), and it is this derivative virus that has been extensively characterized. The HL23V virus is apparently indistinguishable from two unrelated subhuman primate viruses, baboon endogenous virus (BaEV) and the woolly monkey sarcoma virus complex (SSV-1/SSAV), with respect to nucleic acid sequence homology and the immunological properties of the virion structural proteins (11, 12).

In the last several years, there has been a dramatic increase in the number of human lymphoma cell lines permanently established in culture. Of the cell lines screened for retrovirus production, at least two have given evidence of the expression of C-type RNA viruses. The first such report involved the detection of particles with reverse transcriptase activity and a density of 1.15 gm/ml (13) in the supernatant culture fluid of a human diffuse histiocytic lymphoma cell line, SU-DHL-1, previously established and characterized by Epstein and Kaplan (14). Recently, Gallo and his associates have reported the isolation of a putative human C-type RNA virus from a recently established human T-cell lymphoma cell line (15). Some of the virus-like protein components detected in each of these cell lines have now been partially characterized.

The proteins produced by the SU-DHL-1 cell line which have been most extensively studied are a polymerase resembling reverse transcriptase and a 28,000-dalton (p28) component analogous to the major core-associated structural protein of C-type RNA viruses. The polymerase has been shown to possess a significant relatedness to the reverse transcriptases of the subhuman primate viruses based on its enzymatic, structural, and immunological properties (16–18). That the SU-DHL-1 enzyme and the reverse transcriptase of SSV-1/SSAV share antigenic determinants was indicated by cross-reaction of the SSV-1/SSAV reverse transcriptase with a monoclonal hybridoma antibody to the SU-DHL-1 polymerase (18). The p28 protein produced by the SU-DHL-1 cell line has been less extensively studied. A monoclonal hybridoma antibody prepared against this protein also cross-reacted with SSV-1/SSAV p28 (18). However, the SU-DHL- does the reverse transcriptase, based on the binding of monoclonal antibodies to virion proteins in radioimmunoassays (RIAs).

The proteins of the virus produced by the human T-cell lymphoma cell line (15) appear to be less closely related to those of SSV-1/SSAV than the SU-DHL-1 viral proteins. Both the polymerase and the major core-associated antigen cross-react minimally with reagents specific for the subhuman primate virion proteins (15).

In this article, we present further evidence that a monoclonal antibody to the SU-DHL-1 p28 recognizes a protein with antigenic determinants shared by the p28 of SSV-1/SSAV. Specifically, evidence is presented for the cross-reaction of a monoclonal antibody to the SU-DHL-1 p28 with the *in vitro* translation product of the SSV-1/SSAV *gag* gene.

II. Materials and Methods

A. Cells

The SU-DHL-1 cell line was established in our laboratory from the malignant pleural effusion of a 10-year-old Caucasian boy with diffuse histiocytic lymphoma (14). The cultured tumor cells were readily distinguishable from lymphoblastoid cells by their aneuploid karyotypes, histochemical features, lack of lymphocyte surface markers, and absence of the Epstein–Barr virus (EBV) nuclear antigen (EBNA). The human lymphoblastoid cell line SU-LB-8 was established in our laboratory as previously described (16).

B. Viruses

The Moloney murine leukemia virus (M-MuLV) was propagated in the rat cell line 78A-1 and purified on sucrose density gradients. Gibbon ape leukemia virus (GaLV) and SSV-1/SSAV grown on HF (marmoset lung), CCL-88 (bat lung), and NC37 or A204 (human) cells; feline leukemia virus (FeLV) grown on FL64 (feline) cells; RD114 endogenous feline virus propagated on RD (human) cells;

Mason–Pfizer mammary virus (MPMV); and BaEV grown on BKCT or canine thymus cells, all doubly banded in sucrose density gradients, were supplied by Pfizer, Inc., through the Resources and Logistics Program of the National Cancer Institute.

C. Hybridoma Antibodies

The preparation of hybridoma antibodies to the SU-DHL-1 polymerase and p28 has been previously described (18). Briefly, spleen cells from a BALB/c mouse immunized with SU-DHL-1 culture fluids concentrated by ion-exchange chromatography (17) were fused with the NS-1 nonsecreting mouse myeloma cell line, as described by Levy and Dilley (19). Hybrids were selected by growth in hypoxanthine–aminopterin–thymidine (HAT) medium. Subcloning of hybrids was performed by plating cells at limiting dilution in microtiter wells in the presence of normal thymus cells.

Supernatants from hybrid clones were assayed for the presence of antibody directed against SU-DHL-1 viral proteins by a solid-phase RIA. SSV-1/SSAV polymerase purified by affinity chromatography on poly rC–agarose (17) was used to coat polyvinyl chloride (PVC) flexible microtiter plates at a concentration of 10 μg/ml for 18 hours at room temperature. Plates were washed with 5% fetal calf serum (FCS) or 1.0 mg/ml bovine serum albumin (BSA) in phosphate-buffered saline (PBS), and hybridoma culture fluids were added. After a further 2-hour incubation, the plates were washed again, and bound antibody was detected with radioiodinated goat anti-mouse κ light chain.

For competition RIAs, dilutions of spent culture fluids were incubated for at least 18 hours prior to assay with dilutions of viral lysates in 0.01% Triton X-100 in PBS.

D. *In Vitro* Translation

SSV-1/SSAV viral RNA was purified using sodium dodecyl sulfate (SDS) lysis and poly dT-cellulose affinity chromatography (20). Total cellular RNA was extracted from SSV-1/SSAV-infected and uninfected CCL-88 cells by a modification of the procedure of Chirgwin *et al.* (21), as communicated to us by N. Davidson. Briefly, $2\text{--}4 \times 10^8$ cells were trypsinized, washed, and lysed by resuspension in 25 ml of filtered 4 M guanidinium thiocyanate (Tridom-Fluka Chemical Company), 50 mM sodium acetate, pH 5.0, and 1 mM EDTA. After homogenization with several strokes of a loose-fitting Dounce homogenizer, 25 gm of solid cesium chloride (CsCl) was added and dissolved. This solution was then loaded into a heat-sealable Beckman Ti 60 centrifuge tube and underlaid with enough 1.82 gm/cm^3 CsCl in 50 mM sodium acetate, 1 mM EDTA, pH 5.0, to fill the tube (about 10 ml). Centrifugation was carried out for 48–72 hours. The fractions containing the RNA were located by fluorography of 0.001-ml samples from each fraction placed on a 1% agarose plate containing 1.0 μg/ml ethidium bromide and 0.5 M ammonium acetate at pH 5.0. Under these conditions, the RNA fractions migrated about one-half to two-thirds the length of the gradient. The fractions containing the RNA were combined with 2 parts water and 6 parts ethanol, and the precipitate collected by centrifugation. Following poly A selection (22), the RNA was size-fractionated by neutral velocity sedimentation. *In vitro* translation of 2.0 μg of RNA from each of the velocity gradient fractions or viral RNA was carried out in accordance with the directions which accompanied the rabbit reticulocyte translation kit.

E. Immunoprecipitation and Gel Electrophoresis

The procedures used for immunoprecipitation of viral proteins using monoclonal hybridoma antibodies have been described elsewhere (18). For the immunoprecipitation of *in vitro* translation products, a slightly modified version of the procedure of Dobberstein *et al.* (23) was used. Immunoprecipitates were analyzed on sodium dodecyl sulfate (SDS)-polyacrylamide gels using the buffer system described by Laemmli (24). Slab gels were subjected to fluorographic analysis using sodium salicylate (25).

F. Reagents

Isotopes and the rabbit reticulocyte translation kits were obtained from New England Nuclear Corporation. Heterologous antisera to mouse immunoglobulins were purchased from Cappel or Bionetics Laboratories; radioiodinated *Staphylococcus aureus* was obtained from Amersham.

III. Results

A. Specificities of the Monoclonal Hybridoma Antibodies for the SU-DHL-1 Proteins

Two murine monoclonal hybridoma antibodies to SU-DHL-1 viral proteins, produced as outlined in Section II, have been studied in some detail. When tested by solid phase RIA, the culture fluids of the hybridoma clone designated 3H4 demonstrated significant binding to a partially purified preparation of SSV-1/SSAV reverse transcriptase, whereas the culture fluids of the clone designated 3D7 bound to SU-DHL-1 viral protein and to lysates of SSV-1/SSAV. Both 3H4 and 3D7(2B9), a subclone of 3D7, were shown to produce monoclonal IgG_1 (Fig. 1).

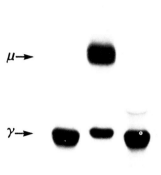

Fig. 1. Electrophoretic analysis of the 3D7 and 3H4 hybridoma immunoglobulins. The immunoglobulins produced by each cell line were analyzed on 10% acrylamide–SDS gels as previously described (18). The positions of the μ, γ, and light (L$_{1-4}$) chains are indicated on the left. The NS-1 parental myeloma light chain is designated L$_1$. Shown from left to right are a known monoclonal IgG, biclonal 3D7 containing IgM and IgG, and monoclonal 3H4 immunoglobulin. Subcloning of the 3D7 cell line yielded subclone 3D7(2B9) which produced only the γ heavy chain (not shown).

The 3H4 antibody was tested for its ability to neutralize the enzymatic activity of viral reverse transcriptase and to immunoprecipitate radioiodinated viral proteins of the appropriate molecular weight. The 3H4 antibody effectively neutralized the SU-DHL-1 polymerase and the reverse transcriptases of the subhuman primate viruses (Fig. 2). It also immunoprecipitated proteins of the appropriate molecular weight for reverse transcriptase from preparations of SU-DHL-1 virus, SSV-1/SSAV, and BaEV, but not more distantly related viral enzymes such as that of MPMV (Fig. 3).

The immunoglobulin produced by subclone 3D7(2B9) bound to and immuno-precipitated a core protein of 28,000 molecular weight (p28) from lysates of SSV-1/SSAV, and a protein of similar molecular weight from concentrated supernates of SU-DHL-1 culture fluids (Fig. 4). The 3D7(2B9) antibody cross-reacted predominantly with SSV-1/SSAV and only to a limited extent with BaEV (Fig. 5). In competition RIAs SSV-1/SSAV preparations competed with the SU-DHL-1 p28 for binding to the 3D7(2B9) antibody, but with a different slope than that observed with the homologous antigen (Fig. 6). This may indicate that the SSV-1/SSAV antigenic site with which this antibody cross-reacts is only

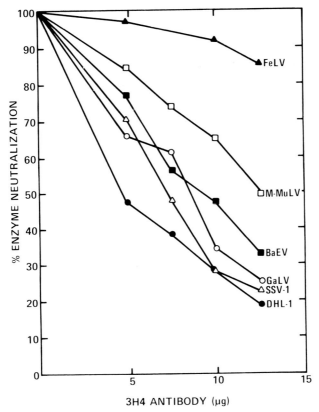

Fig. 2. Neutralization of the reverse transcriptase activities of various C-type RNA viruses by the 3H4 monoclonal antibody. Enzyme neutralization assays were carried out as previously described (18). Poly rA-, oligo dT-stimulated polymerase activity was measured in the presence of increasing amounts of 3H4 immunoglobulin and control myeloma IgG totaling 15 μg per reaction. Enzyme activities ranged between 7000 and 50,000 cpm of ^{3}H-TMP incorporation per hour in the presence of 15 μg myeloma IgG.

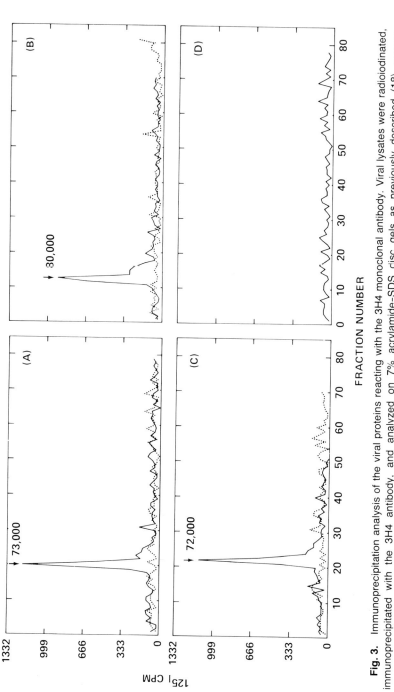

Fig. 3. Immunoprecipitation analysis of the viral proteins reacting with the 3H4 monoclonal antibody. Viral lysates were radioiodinated, immunoprecipitated with the 3H4 antibody, and analyzed on 7% acrylamide–SDS disc gels as previously described (18). ——, 3H4 immunoprecipitates; ·····, preclear precipitates. (A) SSV-1/SSAV; (B) SU-DHL-1; (C) BaEV; (D) MPMV, MuLV, lymphoblastoid cellular proteins, or FCS.

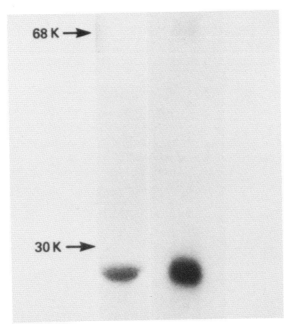

Fig. 4. Immunoprecipitation of SU-DHL-1 and SSV-1/SSAV proteins with the 3D7(2B9) monoclonal antibody. Radioiodinated proteins were analyzed on 20-cm 20% acrylamide-SDS slab gels as previously described (18).

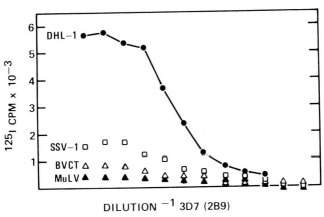

Fig. 5. Radioimmunoassay of viral proteins using the 3D7(2B9) monoclonal antibody. The reaction of viral proteins with 3D7(2B9) immunoglobulin was measured as described in Section II.

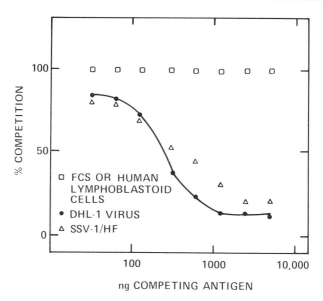

Fig. 6. Competition RIA of the SU-DHL-1 p28 using the 3D7(2B9) monoclonal antibody. The binding of 3D7(2B9) IgG to the SU-DHL-1 viral preparation used for immunization of mice for hybridoma antibody production (18) was measured following preincubation of the antibody with dilutions of the competing antigens. The antigens (in 20-μl aliquots) were serially diluted in 20 μl of the 3D7(2B9) hybridoma fluids and incubated at 4°C for 18 hours. The solid-phase RIA was then carried out as usual. The percentage competition was calculated relative to the antibody binding measured with PBS as the competing substance.

partially homologous with the antigenic site on the SU-DHL-1 viral p28. If the difference in slope or the less avid reaction of the 3D7(2B9) antibody with SSV-1/SSAV (Fig. 6) were due to the antigenic site being present in reduced numbers on the SSV-1/SSAV p28 as compared with the SU-DHL-1 p28, then the competition curve for SSV-1 would have been expected to have the same slope but to be shifted to the right.

When a heterologous monospecific antiserum to SSV-1/SSAV p28 (Fig. 7) was used to block the binding of the 3D7(2B9) antibody to SSV-1/SSAV p28, competition was observed out to dilutions of the antiserum corresponding with those of the end point for binding to the homologous antigen (Fig. 8). Conversely, the 3D7(2B9) antibody was ineffective in blocking or reducing the binding of the heterologous antibody to SSV-1/SSAV p28 even at high dilutions of the anti-SSV-1/SSAV reagent (data not shown). These results are consistent with the interpretation that the 3D7(2B9) monoclonal antibody cross-reacts with only a single antigenic site and is thus unable to block the binding of the heterologous antibody to its multiple antigenic sites.

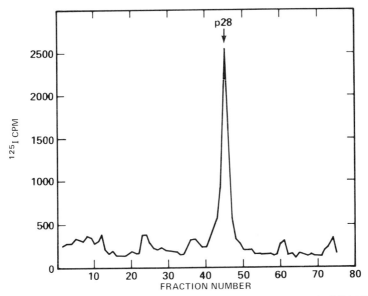

Fig. 7. Specificity of goat heterologous antiserum for SSV-1/SSAV p28. An SSV-1/SSAV viral lysate (100 μg) was electrophoresed on a 10% acrylamide disc gel as previously described (18), and 1-mm slices of the gel were treated with 0.5 ml 0.01% SDS at 25°C and tested by solid-phase RIA for reactivity with the heterologous antiserum (generously supplied by the Logistics and Resources Program, NCI) using radioiodinated *Staphylococcus aureus* as the secondary detector.

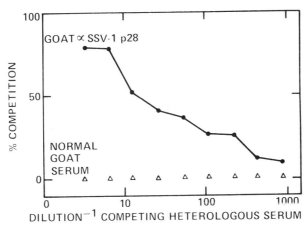

Fig. 8. Competition of heterologous antiserum to SSV-1 p28 with the 3D7(2B9) monoclonal antibody. Dilutions of the heterologous antiserum used in the experiment depicted in the legend for Fig. 7 and normal goat serum were incubated in flexible microtiter wells coated with SSV-1/SSAV viral protein. Following a 2-hour incubation, the binding of 3D7(2B9) IgG was measured using radioiodinated rabbit antibody to mouse IgG_1 which was known not to cross-react with goat IgG. The percentage competition was calculated relative to the binding of the 3D7(2B9) antibody to SSV-1/SSAV viral protein preincubated with PBS.

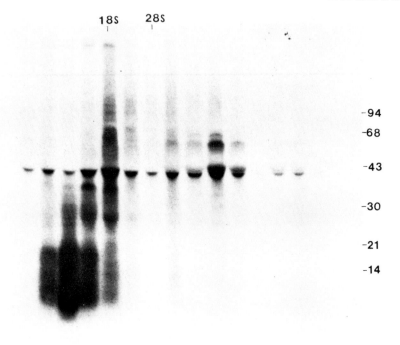

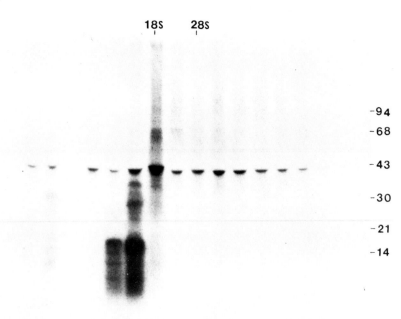

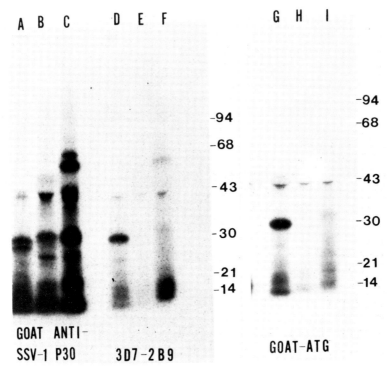

Fig. 10. Immunoprecipitation of *in vitro* translation products of GaLV and SSV-1/SSAV viral RNAs. *In vitro* translation products of vesicular stomatitis virus control RNA (tracks A, D and E), GaLV viral RNA (tracks B, E and H), and SSV-1/SSAV viral RNA (tracks C, F and I) were immunoprecipitated by the three indicated reagents. 3D7(2B9) is a monoclonal antibody whose specificity is explained in the text, and goat ATG is a heterologous antibody directed against human T lymphocytes. The ^{35}S-labeled translation products were analyzed as described in the legend for Fig. 9.

Fig. 9. Immunoprecipitation of *in vitro* translation products of RNA from SSV-1/SSAV-infected and uninfected CCL-88 cells. Poly A-selected mRNA was sized on velocity gradients. Samples from each gradient fraction were translated and immunoprecipitated with goat anti-SSV-1/SSAV p28. The upper channels were from infected and the lower from uninfected cells. Tracks to the left contain products translated from the slowest sedimenting RNA. The 18 and 28 S markers denote the sizes of the RNA used for the translation of the indicated tracks. The ^{35}S-labeled translation products were analyzed on 10% SDS–polyacrylamide gels and visualized by autoradiography. Protein size standards are indicated.

B. Reaction of the *in Vitro* Translation Products of SSV-1/SSAV RNA with Heterologous and Hybridoma Antibodies

To confirm that the 3D7(2B9) antibody cross-reacts with the SSV-1/SSAV *gag* gene product, we translated SSV-1/SSAV *in vitro* and immunoprecipitated the [^{35}S]methionine-labeled product(s) with the monoclonal reagent. Poly A-selected mRNA was isolated from cells infected with SSV-1/SSAV and from uninfected control cells, fractionated by velocity gradient sedimentation, and translated in a rabbit reticulocyte lysate. Figure 9 shows that the monospecific heterologous antiserum to SSV-1/SSAV p28 precipitates two proteins in the 60,000–65,000 dalton range which are translated from mRNA of approximately 30–35 S in SSV-1/SSAV infected cells. Similarly immunoprecipitable translation products are not observed with the mRNA from uninfected cells. Pulse-chase labeling experiments (26) and *in vitro* translation studies with other viral genomes (27, 28) have shown that virion structural proteins are first synthesized as polypeptide precursors and subsequently cleaved into their individual components. The direct precursor of MuLV p30 has been demonstrated to be a 65,000-dalton protein (Pr65^{gag}) which is synthesized from the 35 S viral RNA (27, 29–31) and is immunoprecipitable with antibodies to MuLV p30. By analogy, the antibody to the SSV-1/SSAV p28 probably recognizes a 65,000-dalton *gag* polyprotein translated from SSV-1/SSAV RNA.

When SSV-1/SSAV viral RNA was translated and the translation products immunoprecipitated, a result similar to that for the translation products of mRNA from virus-infected CCL-88 cells was obtained (Fig. 10). However, the heterologous antibody again precipitated both 65,000- and 60,000-dalton products, whereas the monoclonal antibody to the SU-DHL-1 viral p28 precipitated only the 65,000-dalton translation product of SSV-1/SSAV.

IV. Discussion

We previously reported the production of two monoclonal hybridoma antibodies to SU-DHL-1 viral proteins with the characteristics of a reverse transcriptase and p28 (18). These monoclonal reagents appeared to cross-react with the analogous proteins of the subhuman primate virus complex, SSV-1/SSAV. These proteins have been isolated from SU-DHL-1 culture supernatants, from SSV-1/SSAV virus harvests, and from cells infected with this subhuman primate virus complex and have been characterized immunologically and biochemically in order to assess their relatedness.

The 3H4 monoclonal antibody against the reverse transcriptase isolated from SU-DHL-1 also bound to and neutralized the enzymatic activity of the SSV-1/SSAV reverse transcriptase (18). It also immunoprecipitated proteins of appropriate molecular weight for mammalian C-type viral reverse transcriptases (75,000 daltons) from SU-DHL-1 virus, SSV-1/SSAV, and BaEV but not from unrelated viruses (MPMV, MuLV) or fetal calf serum (FCS). It has also been shown that the tryptic digest peptide map of the SU-DHL-1 viral enzyme is similar, but not identical, to those of SSV-1/SSAV, GaLV, and BaEV (17).

In this article we have also presented further evidence that the 3D7(2B9) monoclonal antibody recognizes an antigenic determinant on the p28 and also on the *gag* gene translation product of SSV-1/SSAV. A heterologous antibody monospecific for the SSV-1/SSAV p28 effectively competed against the binding of the 3D7(2B9) antibody to SSV-1/SSAV protein (Fig. 8). The 3D7(2B9) monoclonal antibody also immunoprecipitated a 65,000-dalton protein which appeared to be the SSV-1/SSAV *gag* gene translation product, since its translation was viral message-dependent, i.e., it was translated *in vitro* from 30–35 S mRNA isolated from SSV-1/SSAV-infected but not from uninfected cells (Fig. 9). A similar product was translated from SSV-1/SSAV virion RNA (Fig. 10). Translation products from either form of the viral RNA were also specifically immunoprecipitated by the heterologous antibody to the SSV-1/SSAV p28 and not by secondary precipitating reagents (Fig. 10). These results argue that the antigenic determinant recognized by the 3D7(2B9) monoclonal antibody on these 28,000- and 65,000-dalton proteins is encoded by the SSV-1/SSAV viral genome, and thus by analogy that the SU-DHL-1 p28 is also of viral origin. Demonstration of base sequence homologies of their mRNAs, or of amino acid sequence homologies of the antigenic determinants recognized by the 3H4 and 3D7(2B9) monoclonal antibodies, will be necessary to establish this conclusion more firmly.

Acknowledgments

This investigation was supported (in part) by research contract N01 CP 91044 and by grant CA-09302 from the National Cancer Institute, NIH.

References

1. H. S. Kaplan, *Ser. Haematol.* **7,** 94 (1974).
2. J. Schlom and S. Spiegelman, *Science* **174,** 840 (1971).
3. W. Baxt, R. Hehlmann, and S. Spiegelman, *Nature (London), New Biol.* **240,** 72 (1972).
4. R. C. Gallo, N. R. Miller, W. C. Saxinger, and D. Gillespie, *Proc. Natl. Acad. Sci. U.S.A.* **70,** 3219 (1972).
5. S. S. Witkin, T. Ohno, and S. Spiegelman, *Proc. Natl. Acad. Sci. U.S.A.* **72,** 4133 (1975).
6. C. Chezzi, D. Dettori, V. Manzari, S. M. Agliano, and S. Sanna, *Proc. Natl. Sci. U.S.A.* **73,** 4649 (1976).

7. K. Nooter, S. M. Aarssen, P. Bentvelzen, F. G. deGroot, and F. G. van Peet, *Nature (London)* **256**, 595 (1975).

8. G. S. Aulakh and R. C. Gallo, *Proc. Natl. Acad. Sci. U.S.A.* **74**, 353 (1977).

9. R. E. Gallagher and R. C. Gallo. *Science* **187**, 350 (1975).

10. N. M. Teich, R. A. Weiss, S. F. Salahuddin, R. E. Gallagher, D. H. Gillespie, and R. C. Gallo, *Nature (London)* **256**, 551 (1975).

11. E. Chan, W. P. Peters, R. W. Sweet, T. Ohno, D. W. Keefe, S. Spiegelman, R. C. Gallo, and R. E. Gallagher, *Nature (London)* **260**, 266 (1976).

12. H. Okabe, R. V. Gilden, M. Hatanaka, J. R. Stephenson, R. E. Gallagher, R. C. Gallo, and R. E. Gallagher, *Nature (London)* **260**, 264 (1976).

13. H. S. Kaplan, R. S. Goodenow, A. L. Epstein, S. Gartner, A. Declève, and P. N. Rosenthal, *Proc. Natl. Acad. Sci. U.S.A.* **74**, 2564 (1977).

14. A. L. Epstein and H. S. Kaplan, *Cancer* **34**, 1851 (1974).

15. B. J. Poiesz, F. W. Ruscetti, A. F. Gazdar, P. A. Bunn, J. D. Minna, and R. C. Gallo, *Proc. Natl. Acad. Sci. U.S.A.* **77**, 7415 (1980).

16. H. S. Kaplan, R. S. Goodenow, S. Gartner, and M. M. Bieber, *Cancer* **43**, 1 (1979).

17. R. S. Goodenow and H. S. Kaplan, *Proc. Natl. Acad. Sci. U.S.A.* **76**, 4971 (1979).

18. R. S. Goodenow, S. Brown, R. Levy, and H. S. Kaplan, *in* "Viruses in Naturally Occurring Cancers" (M. Essex, G. Todaro, and H. zur Hausen, eds.), p. 737. Cold Spring Harbor Lab., Cold Spring Harbor, New York, 1980.

19. R. Levy and J. Dilley, *Proc. Natl. Acad. Sci. U.S.A.* **75**, 2411 (1978).

20. R. G. Smith, L. Donehower, R. C. Gallo, and D. H. Gillespie, *J. Virol.* **17**, 287 (1976).

21. J. M. Chirgwin, A. E. Przybyla, R. L. MacDonald, and W. J. Rutter, *Biochemistry* **18**, 5294 (1979).

22. H. Aviv and P. Leder, *Proc. Natl. Acad. Sci. U.S.A.* **69**, 1408 (1972).

23. B. Dobberstein, H. Garoff, and G. Warren, *Cell* **17**, 759 (1979).

24. V. K. Laemmli, *Nature (London)* **227**, 680 (1970).

25. J. P. Chamberlin, *Anal. Biochem.* **98**, 132 (1979).

26. R. B. Naso, L. J. Arcement, and R. B. Arlinghaus, *Cell* **4**, 31 (1975).

27. I. M. Kerr, V. Olshevsky, H. F. Lodish, and D. Baltimore, *J. Virol.* **18**, 627 (1976).

28. M. Salden, F. Asselbergs, and H. Bloemendal, *Nature (London)* **259**, 696 (1976).

29. A. L. J. Gielkens, D. Van Zaane, H. P. J. Bloemers, and H. Bloemendal, *Proc. Natl. Acad. Sci. U.S.A.* **73**, 356 (1976).

30. M. Barbacid, J. R. Stephenson, and S. A. Aaronson, *Nature (London)* **262**, 554 (1976).

31. J. R. Stephenson, R. K. Reynolds, S. G. Devare, and F. H. Reynolds, *J. Biol. Chem.* **252**, 7818 (1977).

12

Regulation of Human T-Cell Proliferation: T-Cell Growth Factor, T-Cell Leukemias and Lymphomas, and Isolation of a New C-Type Retrovirus

ROBERT C. GALLO

I. Introduction

A. Objectives

In this article I will briefly comment on some general features of the class of viruses (retroviruses) which cause naturally occurring leukemias and lymphomas in several animal species. This is followed by some remarks on human leukemogenesis, and finally a more thorough description of relatively new results which focus on the control of proliferation of normal and neoplastic human T cells and the recent isolation of a new group of retroviruses from some new T-cell lymphomas and leukemia cell lines.

B. Background on Retroviruses

Retroviruses (oncornaviruses, RNA tumor viruses) are known to be involved in the natural cause of leukemia and lymphomas of chickens, wild mice, cats, cows, and gibbon apes (see ref. 1 for recent summary). The spectrum of disease type includes most if not all forms seen in humans, but perhaps the most prevalent virus-induced blood cell neoplasias are leukemias and lymphomas of T cells. Therefore, they have long been sought in association with the corresponding diseases in humans (1). An additional interest in retroviruses has come about from the realization that they may be unusually useful tools for understanding neoplastic transformation even when the transformation is not virus-induced. This is for two reasons. First, some retroviruses (those which transform cells *in vitro* and induce disease relatively acutely *in vivo*) carry a gene which directly transforms cells, and this transforming gene was derived from normal host cell DNA in the past, apparently by a process of recombination between viral and host DNA. These genes (*src, onc, leuk,* etc.) must be important for growth control and, since their counterparts are present in normal host cell DNA, they may be important in abnormal growth (e.g., by being switched on when they should be inactive) due to various causes such as chemical, radiation, or spontaneous neoplastic transformation. Since some retroviruses carry these genes, it is possible to isolate them, subject them to detailed analysis, and determine the nature of the gene product. Moreover, these genes have been conserved during evolution, and there is every reason to believe they will be present in human DNA. In fact, the results I am aware of are already consistent with this assumption. Thus, it is possible that, by studying these genes carried by acutely transforming retroviruses, we may learn more information which will subsequently be useful in human cancer. Second, and in striking contrast to acutely transforming viruses, the retroviruses which cause most naturally occurring leukemias may not cause transformation directly by coding for a transforming protein. Instead, some viruses (which require relatively long periods for induction of neoplasia and have no transforming activity *in vitro*) may induce disease by providing gene promoter sequences which induce growth only because they switch on certain cell genes when they should not be expressed. These viruses may lead us to the identification of these cell genes and an understanding of their regulation. It could be that the cell genes turned on are the analogues of the directly transforming genes carried by the previously alluded to acutely transforming retroviruses.

The molecular biology and biochemistry of retroviruses are now understood in much of their detail. The reader is referred to a recently published book edited by G. Klein (2a) which includes several chapters on this subject. Here I will only very briefly outline some general features which may be useful to the nonspecialist in the subsequent discussion of new viruses from human cells.

The genome of retroviruses consists of 35 S RNA subunits which (going from 5′ to 3′) code for structural proteins, polymerase (reverse transcriptase), and the envelope of the virus. Some defective retroviruses lack one or more of these genes; e.g., when the genome contains a directly transforming gene, this gene usually replaces a portion or all of one or more of the above replicative genes. The gene products undergo considerable cleavage maturation, so that mature virions contain several different structural proteins named according to their molecular size. One of these (p24/30) is the major internal core protein which also provides the major internal antigenic determinant of a retrovirus. The size of this nonglycosylated protein varies among different viruses (about 24,000–30,000). The reverse transcriptase (varying in size from about 60,000 to 120,000) is responsible for catalyzing the conversion of viral RNA to the DNA provirus. This process occurs after the virus enters the cell; the DNA provirus is then integrated into the host cell DNA. After integration the viral DNA may be completely, incompletely, or not transcribed. This and subsequent steps (RNA and protein maturation, assembly, and release mechanisms) determine if a cell will produce virus or not and in part whether or not this will lead to cell transformation.

C. General Comments on Human Leukemogenesis

Most epidemiological studies relating to human leukemia and lymphoma do not indicate that these are diseases commonly involving radiation, chemical carcinogens, or clearly defined inherited traits. In the same regard they also suggest that these diseases are not the result of acute infections directly transmitted from patients. However, none of these studies rule out transmissible agents in the cause of the disease, because epidemiological patterns can be confused by long latency periods, vertical transmission of virus, and/or requirements for additional factors. In fact, these complications sometimes occur in virus-caused leukemias and lymphomas of animals. For example, the species closest to humans for which an animal model of leukemia is available is the gibbon ape. The leukemia of this animal is due to a C-type retrovirus, and the virus may take a few years to induce the disease. Moreover, factors other than virus must also be involved in determining the outcome, since newborns are more susceptible than adults in almost all species studied and since many animals may carry a leukemia virus but only a fraction of these acquire leukemia.

Different results over the past several years suggested that retrovirus proteins and nucleic acids may sometimes be found in human leukemia or lymphoma, and in a few instances recognizable virus particles (see Refs. 1 and 2 for reviews). However, these viruses were shown to be closely related to known primate C-type viruses carried in laboratories and therefore cannot be distinguished from laboratory contaminants. Also related to a primate retrovirus, but showing significant differences, are the interesting viral particles described in diffuse histiocytic lymphomas by Kaplan and his co-workers (3,4 and see Goodenow and Kaplan *et al.*, this volume).

Because animal RNA tumor viruses often cause leukemias and lymphomas of T cells and because isolation of virus is usually obtainable only after successful culture conditions have been developed, methods for the continuous propagation of human T cells were obviously needed. A successful system for T-cell propagation also has many other potentially interesting uses. In the remaining portion of this article I will summarize the system developed in our laboratory about 5 years ago, which allows for growth of normal or neoplastic T cells in liquid suspension culture for long periods. The system is based on the use of a growth factor, termed T-cell growth factor (TCGF); its use led to the growth in culture of several new neoplastic T-cell lines which in turn led to the recent isolation of a new group of C-type retroviruses [human T-cell leukemia (lymphoma) viruses, HTLVs].

II. Growth of Normal Human T Cells

Continuously growing T lymphocytes, capable of long-term growth in culture while retaining functional specificity, have been obtained (5–7). Nylon column-purified normal human mononuclear cells pooled from several donors are treated with phytohemoagglutinin (PHA) for 2–3 days, and the lymphocyte conditioned medium obtained. Some T cells release TCGF into the medium after PHA treatment. Thus, the conditioned medium is a crude starting material for TCGF purification. Subsequently, when other blood or bone marrow samples are treated with PHA, they can be maintained as growing T-lymphoblast cultures by addition of the previously obtained TCGF every 3–4 days. The properties of the cultured cells after many months in culture are summarized in Table I, an outline of this system is illustrated below, and a portion of it schematically shown in Fig. 1.

TABLE I

Characteristics of Normal Cells Grown with TCGF for Long Periods

Source of cells	Normal blood or bone marrow
Morphology	Lymphoblast
Test for B lymphoblast	Negative for immunoglobulins and for EBV
Histochemistry	Negative for myeloid (myeloperoxidase, chloroacetate esterase) and monocyte–macrophage (NSE) markers
Tests for T-cell markers	Positive for E-rosette and functional mature T-cell assays (cytotoxic and helper T-cell activity); terminal transferase-negative
Initiation of growth	Requires PHA or antigen; TCGF cannot initiate
Maintenance of growth	Requires TCGF
Karyotype	Remains normal diploid even after growth over 1 year

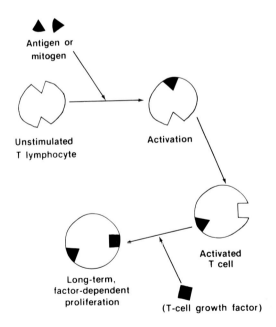

Fig. 1. Simplified scheme for normal T-cell proliferation in response to an antigen.

1. Antigen or lectin	+	receptor-specific T Cells	→	activated T lymphoblast with newly made TCGF receptor
2. Antigen or lectin	+	Adherent cell and T-cell precursor of TCGF producer	→	TCGF-producing T cell
3. Activated T lymphoblast	+	TCGF from producer T cell	→	T-cell proliferation

It is clear from the characteristics listed in Table I that the responding cells are T cells. It is also evident that TCGF is the direct mitogenic stimulus but only on normal T cells which have been activated by antigen or by PHA to develop TCGF receptors. The basic discovery described above has now been confirmed in numerous laboratories, and many fundamental concepts have emerged, especially in the murine system, notably from work of Smith (see Ref. 8).

III. Purification of TCGF

The purification of human TCGF from PHA–lymphocyte serum-free conditioned medium has been reported (9,10). The procedure involves $(NH_4)_2SO_4$ precipitation followed by a series of conventional column chromatographic steps and preparative sodium dodecyl sulfate polyacrylamide gel electrophoresis (SDS-PAGE). Some biochemical and biological properties of this polypeptide are listed in Tables II and III, respectively. The purification is a minimum of 800-fold over the TCGF in the starting serum-free medium.

TABLE II

Biochemical Properties of Human TCGF

Sensitivity to:	
Boiling	+
RNase	−
DNase	−
Trypsin	+
Freezing[a]	−
N-Ethylmaleimide	−
Dithiothreitol	−
HgCl$_2$	−
Stabilized by:	
Polethylene glycol	+
Albumin	+
Glycerol	−
Molecular weight	12,000–13,000 (SDS-PAGE)
pI	6.8
Tests for glycosyl moiety	−

[a] Stable with polyethylene glycol.

TABLE III

Summary of Biological Properties of Human TCGF

Origin	Released from a subset of T cells but also requires macrophage in this process
Target cell	Activated T cells (helper, suppressor, cytotoxic)
Biological effect	Promotes growth of activated T cells after binding to membrane
Species specificity	Very little; human TCGF active on other primates, cows, cats, rodents, chickens

IV. Growth of Neoplastic Human T Cells

A. Direct Response to TCGF

TCGF was tested for its effects on T cells obtained from patients with a variety of T-cell neoplasias. Tumor cells from patients with leukemias and lymphomas involving mature T cells grew directly with TCGF (11). They did not require prior *in vitro* activation by lectin or antigen, in contrast to normal T cells. This suggests that these cells are chronically antigenically stimulated *in vivo*, that a cryptic receptor for TCGF is exposed during the process of neoplastic transformation, or that there is a very small number of T cells which normally contain TCGF receptors but are not detectable in the larger normal cell population and that these are target cells for some T-cell neoplasias. In any case it appears that such cells have TCGF receptors. Transformed T cells responding in this manner have characteristics of more mature T cells in that they are negative for terminal transferase but contain receptors for sheep erythrocytes (E-rosette-positive assay). Leukemias and lymphomas of mature T cells include a small fraction of chronic lymphocytic leukemia (CLL) and acute lymphoblastic leukemia (ALL) cases and all of the Sezary and mycosis fungoides patients (cutaneous T-cell leukemias and lymphomas).* We obtained clinical specimens from blood and bone marrow of patients with different T-cell neoplasias. Most studies were performed on material from patients with cutaneous T-cell leukemia (the Sezary syndrome) and lymphoma (mycosis fungoides) and a few with T-cell ALL (Table IV). When crude TCGF was used, growth was only obtained for 3–6 weeks. However, with more highly purified TCGF long-term growth of neoplastic T cells was often obtained.

---

*Other leukemias and lymphomas of mature T lymphocytes that we have subsequently studied include peripheral T-cell lymphoma, acute lymphosarcoma T-cell leukemia, and Japanese adult T-cell leukemia.

TABLE IV

Comparative Properties of Continuously Cultured Human T Cells

Source of cells	Requirements for growth			Morphology	TdT[a]	EBV, IgG[b]	E Rosette	Acid phosphatase	NSE	Chromosomes
	No additions	TCGF alone	TCGF and PHA initiation							
Normal	–	–	+	Normal lymphoblasts	–	–	+	+, mild granular cytoplasmic	–	Normal diploid
T-Cell ALL	– (rarely +)	+	+	Homogeneous lymphoblasts—sometimes with multiple nucleoli in nucleus	–	–	+	++, concentrated in Golgi region	–	Variable and like primary cells
CTCL[c]	– (rarely +)	+	+	Heterogeneous giant multinucleated cells and other smaller lymphoblasts, mono- or binucleated; some with convoluted nuclei	–	–	+	+++, diffuse, intense reaction	Diffuse, intense reaction in a few cells; majority are small paranuclear cytoplasmic granules	Variable and like primary cells

[a] TdT, Terminal deoxyribonucleotidyl transferase.

[b] Tests for EBV were by assays for the EBV-specific nuclear antigen; IgG refers to tests for surface immunoglobulins.

[c] CTCL, Cutaneous T-cell leukemia or lymphoma (Sezary or mycosis fungoides).

B. Characteristics of Cultured Cells

Several findings indicate that the cultured cells are derived from the neoplastic cells of the primary tumor (Table V). We are most impressed by their abnormal morphology. As shown in Fig. 2, some cells (1–15% of the Sezary leukemia cultures) are giant multinucleated cells. Others show fine projectile filaments which resemble hairy cells. The majority of cells are mono- or binucleated lymphoblasts (Fig. 2). Electron micrographs of some lymphoblasts show the convoluted nuclei characteristics of Sezary cells (Fig. 3). Most of the cells are E-rosette-positive, negative for B-cell and myeloid cell markers, and positive for nonspecific esterase (NSE) (11). The response to TCGF, the derivation from T-cell neoplasias, and the E-rosetting are indicative of the T-cell nature of these cells. Normal T cells and T-cell ALLs when grown in culture or assayed fresh are NSE-negative. We interpret the positive NSE results with the cultured Sezary cells as an abnormal expression of a gene in a transformed cell or as indicating that the target cell in these diseases is a population of NSE-positive T cells.

C. Release of Biologically Active Materials by Cultured Neoplastic T Cells

An interesting feature of some of these cell lines is their release of hematopoietic growth factors and other activities (12). For instance, colony-stimulating activity for granulocyte–macrophages, burst-promoting activity, interferon, and TCGF are produced by one or more lines. These findings could be due to an *in vitro* artifact with no physiological relevance. However, the results are consistent with the idea that T cells are involved in the regulation of proliferation of other

TABLE V

Characteristics of T Cells Cultured from Patients with Mature T Cell Leukemias and Lymphomas Indicative of Neoplastic Origin

Morphology	Some giant multinucleated cells; some cells with markedly convoluted nuclei (Sezary cells)
Karyotype	Same in each case as primary tumor
Response to TCGF	Direct (no lectin or antigen *in vitro* activation required)
Histochemistry[a]	In the case of cutaneous T-cell leukemias and lymphomas, NSE-positive
Virus	Three lines release a C-type retrovirus (HTLV) not found in any normal T-cell line
TCGF-Independent growth	Some lines become TCGF-independent and produce their own TCGF

[a] Normal T cells and those from patients with ALL fresh or grown in culture are NSE-negative.

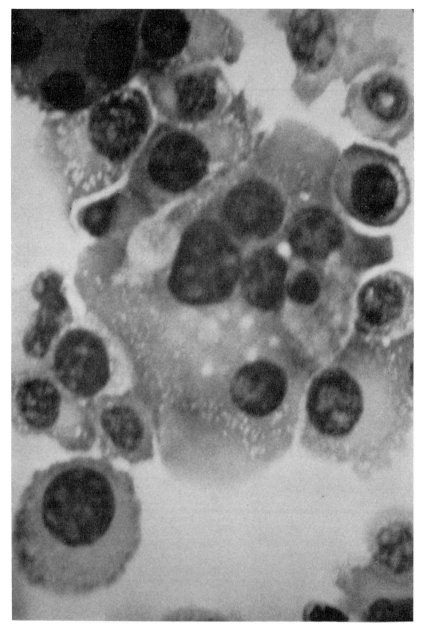

Fig. 2. Light microscopy of cultured cells (CTCL-2) established as a cell line from a patient with Sezary cutaneous T-cell leukemia. The origin of the sample was leukemic cells from peripheral blood. The figure shows one of the multinucleated giant cells which make up about 10% of the cell population.

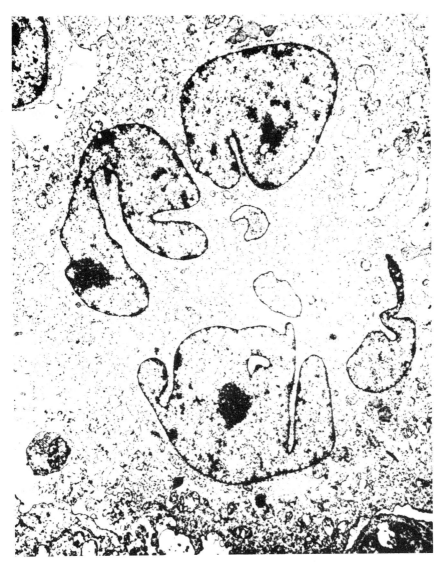

Fig. 3. Electron micrograph of a giant multinucleated cell showing convoluted nuclei. Some cells show more extremely convoluted nuclei, characteristic of the Sezary cell. The cells are from the same culture as shown in Fig. 1.

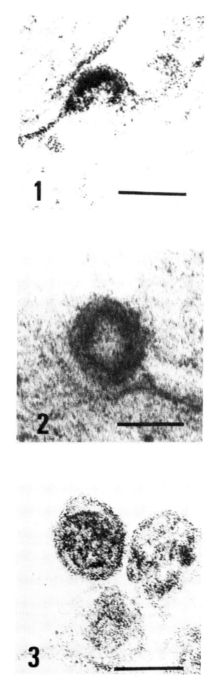

Fig. 4. Electron micrograph of the C-type retrovirus, HTLV, from CTCL-2 cells, the cell line described in Fig. 2. Note the formation of a typical virus bud in (A), the early formed virus in (B), and the mature released virions in (C). The virus size is variable but approximates 1000 Å.

TABLE VI

Isolations of Type-C Retroviruses (HTLV) from Human Cutaneous T-Cell Lymphoma and Leukemia

Diagnosis	Source of specimen	Cell line	IDU Induction needed	Constitutive virus producer	Requirement for exogenous TCGF
Mycosis fungoides	Lymph nodes	HUT-102	Passages 4–50	—	±
		HUT-102	No	Passage 56 on	—
	Blood leukocytes	None (fresh lymphocytes)[a]	No	Yes, immediately	+
	Blood leukocytes	CTCL-3	No	Yes, immediately	+
Sezary	Blood leukocytes	CTCL-2	No	Yes, immediately	—

[a] No attempt has been made to keep these cells continuously in culture.

Note added in proof: Subsequent to these studies, HTLV has also been identified in cultured mature neoplastic T cells from patients with other T-cell leukemias and lymphomas, e.g., peripheral T-cell lymphoma, Japanese adult T-cell leukemia, acute lymphosarcoma T-cell leukemia, and T-cell variant of hairy cell leukemia.

hematopoietic cells. Moreover, the release of TCGF by some of the lines is of particular interest because all the lines were initiated with TCGF. The lines which subsequently released TCGF became independent of exogenous TCGF, presumably because they make and are stimulated by their own TCGF. Some of these cells also release virus (see below).

V. Isolation of a New C-Type RNA Tumor Virus

As noted above, some of the cultured T cells from patients with cutaneous T-cell leukemia or lymphoma become independent of TCGF, apparently because they are constitutive TCGF producers. In some of these cultures we noted release of a C-type RNA tumor virus (13–16). The first isolate, called HTLV strain CR (HTLV$_{CR}$), obtained from a patient with mycosis fungoides, has been studied most extensively in a collaboration with John Minna and his colleagues, A. Gazdar and P. Bunn, of the NCI-VA Clinical Oncology Branch. The cells were obtained from an inguinal lymph node biopsy. Subsequently, independent clinical specimens were obtained (blood samples) from which T cells were grown and HTLV$_{CR}$ again identified. About the same time we received a blood sample from J. Rosenthal (Downstate Medical Center, New York) obtained from a patient with Sezary leukemia. We established a cell line and again identified a C-type virus termed HTLV$_{MB}$ (Fig. 4). Analyses of HTLV$_{CR}$ and HTLV$_{MB}$ have revealed that they are closely related to each other but distinct from previously isolated animal retroviruses (16–18). The history of the various HTLV isolates is summarized in Table VI. We have distinguished the HTLV isolates from other viruses by three sets of tests: (a) The reverse transcriptase of HTLV was antigenically unrelated to the reverse transcriptase of animal retroviruses by enzyme neutralization tests (16); (b) the p24 (major internal core protein) of HTLV was distinguished from the major core proteins of animal retroviruses by competition radioimmune assay (17); (c) the nucleotide sequences of HTLV were not significantly related to nucleotide sequences of other viruses by liquid molecular hybridization (18).

VI. Origin of HTLV and the Possible Role of TCGF and HTLV in the Pathogenesis of Lymphomas and Leukemias of Mature T Cells

HTLV was chiefly found in cells which also release TCGF. It appears from cell cloning studies carried out by M. Maeda in our laboratory that leukemic cells which release TCGF also respond to it. This seems different from the normal situation where most observations suggest that one subset of T cells releases TCGF while a separate set responds to it. This suggested the following model (Fig. 5). In this model the HTLV envelope protein interacts with a very specific group

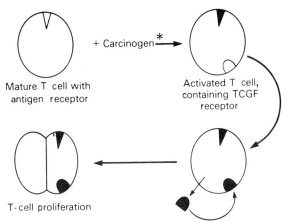

+ Carcinogen *——→

Mature T cell with
antigen receptor

Activated T cell,
containing TCGF
receptor

T-cell proliferation

Fig. 5. A schematic and simple model for the first stage of T-cell leukemic transformation. We propose that the target cell is a mature T cell with an antigen receptor site, which in the case of a proposed virus-induced disease recognizes an envelope protein of HTLV. This leads to the recently known antigen effect of inducing the availability of receptors for TCGF. Concomitantly, nucleic acid sequences contained in the HTLV genome which are integrated into the host cell DNA include sequences which can act as promoters for the expression of certain cell genes. (Much evidence suggests that this may be the case in animal models with animal retroviruses.) We suggest that this leads to an abnormal expression of the gene for TCGF. We think the available data indicate that separate subsets of T cells usually make and respond to TCGF under normal circumstances. The above model of a cell both making and responding to TCGF may lead to uncontrolled proliferation. In turn, this may subsequently lead to an increase in the likelihood of mutational events which "fix" the transformed state. Later in the progression of leukemogenesis, cells which express virus may be selected against by immune mechanisms, making their location rare and difficult by the time of frank disease. *Model may be limited to viral transformation.

of T cells (those which have receptors for the envelope). This mimics an antigen stimulation of blastogenesis. The T cell is one normally designed to develop TCGF receptors and does so. It is proposed that promoter-like nucleotide sequences contained in the HTLV provirus are integrated "upstream" from the TCGF gene and trigger derepression of the TCGF gene, leading to TCGF release and autostimulation. Subsequently, the increase in proliferation leads to an increased incidence of mutation with fixation of the transformed state. Virus-expressing cells are selected against by immune mechanisms, so that one may only rarely identify virus by the time overt leukemia occurs. Other initiators (nonviral) may be involved in the early stages of other forms of T-cell lymphomas and leukemias, but even in these cases abnormalities in TCGF production or response may be central to the pathogenesis of these diseases.

The natural reservoir of HTLV is unknown. It is not a ubiquious endogenous (germ line-transmitted) virus of humans, because no homologous sequences can be found in DNA from normal humans (18). However, it is possible that it is endogenous within select families, i.e., families with a predisposition for these

TABLE VII

Specificity of Natural Antibodies from Serum of Patients with Cutaneous T-Cell Lymphoma Against HTLV: Competition in Radioimmunoprecipitation and ELISA Assays

	Test of competing antigen								
		Proteins from viruses[b]			Proteins from human cell lysates				
Patient source of serum antibody[a]	FCS	BSA	HTLV$_{CR}$	HTLV$_{MB}$	Numerous animal retroviruses	HUT-102[c]	CTCL-2[c]	Normal T-cells	B-Cell lines	Normal transformed T-cell lines not producing HTLV
CTCL-CR	–	–	+	+	–	+	+	–	–	–
CTCL-4	–	–	+	+	–	+	+	–	–	–

[a] CTCL-CR is the patient from whom cell line HUT-102 was established. The virus HTLV$_{CR}$ was first isolated from these cells. CTCL-4 is another patient with a similar stage of disease as patient CTCL-CR.

[b] FCS, Fetal calf serum; BSA, bovine serum albumin.

[c] Cell lines producing HTLV.

diseases. This can be tested. If it is germ line-transmitted in these families, we should find sequences in the DNA of normal cells from the mother or father of a patient whose neoplastic cells yield HTLV. We should also find nucleotide sequences of HTLV in the DNA of normal cells of the same patient. Neither experiment has been done.*

Specific antibodies to HTLV were recently found in the sera of some patients with cutaneous T-cell lymphomas and in ALL (19,20). One positive result was with serum from C.R., the first patient from whom HTLV was isolated. These antibodies were detected by both enzyme-linked immunoabsorbent assay (ELISA) and radioimmunoprecipitation (RIP) assays, and in both cases competition assays showed remarkable specificity (see summary of specificity data in Table VII). The presence of antibodies is more suggestive of an exogenous entry of HTLV, i.e., by some kind of a poorly understood infection. However, antibodies to endogenous viruses can occur, so the question of its origin must remain open.* It will be important to look carefully for clusters of patients with these types of leukemias and lymphomas. A careful study of disease clusters and of family studies combined with information generated from molecular biological studies with HTLV reagents may lead to a better understanding of the origin of these diseases.

VII. Summary

Human normal and neoplastic T cells can be grown in liquid suspension culture for long periods by using a protein growth promoter called TCGF. Normal T cells must first be activated by lectin or antigen before they respond. This appears to result in the development of TCGF receptors. Cells from patients with leukemias and lymphomas of relatively mature T cells respond directly to TCGF, suggesting that these cells already have TCGF receptors. Cell cultures from some cases of cutaneous T-cell lymphoma and leukemia (the Sezary syndrome) release a C-type retrovirus (called HTLV) which is not significantly related to animal retroviruses. Antibody specifically reactive with HTLV proteins has been found in sera of some patients with these diseases.

Acknowledgments

Many of the studies described here were carried out by colleagues in our laboratory. Notably, Dr. B. Poiesz, a former postdoctoral research associate in our laboratory made important contributions to the growth of the neoplastic T cells and to the early detection of HTLV. My present co-worker, Dr. F. Ruscetti, made significant contributions to the biological work on TCGF and to growth of the T cells,

*Studies of normal cells from patient CR have now been completed. In contrast to the HTLV provirus positive neoplastic T cells, the normal cells were negative. This clearly shows that HTLV entered by infection (not endogenous).

Dr. J. Mier, formerly a postdoctoral research associate with us, to the purification of TCGF, and Drs. M. Guroff and L. Posner to the serum antibody studies. Several colleagues have contributed to the analysis of HTLV, especially Dr. M. Reitz, Dr. H. Rho, and Dr. V. Kalyanaraman. In addition, as mentioned in the text, a portion of the work in the first virus isolate involving patient C.R. and the cell line established from that patient, as well as all clinical serum samples, were in collaboration with Drs. J. Minna, P. Bunn, and A. Gazdar of the NCI-VA Oncology Branch.

References

1. F. Wong-Staal and R. C. Gallo, in "Retroviruses and Leukemia" (F. Gunz and E. Henderson, eds.). Grune & Stratton, New York (in press).
2. R. C. Gallo, F. Wong-Staal, P. D. Markham, F. Ruscetti, V. S. Kalyanaraman, L. Ceccherini-Nelli, R. Dalla Favera, S. Josephs, N. Miller, and M. S. Reitz, Jr., in "Viruses in Naturally Occurring Cancer" (G. Todaro, M. Essex, and H. zur Hausen, eds.). Cold Spring Harbor Lab., Cold Spring Harbor, New York, Vol. 7, p. 753, 1980.
2a. G. Klein (ed.), "Viral Oncology." Raven, New York, 1980.
3. H. S. Kaplan, R. S. Goodenow, A. L. Epstein, S. Gartner, A. Decleve, and P. N. Rosenthal, Proc. Natl. Acad. Sci. U.S.A. **74**, 2564 (1977).
4. R. S. Goodenow and H. S. Kaplan, Proc. Natl. Acad. Sci. U.S.A. **76**, 4691 (1978).
5. D. A. Morgan, F. W. Ruscetti, and R. C. Gallo, Science **193**, 1007 (1976).
6. F. W. Ruscetti, D. A. Morgan, R. C. Gallo, J. Immunol. **119**, 131 (1977).
7. F. W. Ruscetti and R. C. Gallo, Blood (Editorial Review) **57**, 379 (1981).
8. K. Smith, Proc. Natl. Acad. Sci. U.S.A. (in press).
9. J. W. Mier and R. C. Gallo, Proc. Natl. Acad. Sci. U.S.A. **77**, 6134 (1980).
10. J. W. Mier and R. C. Gallo, J. Immunol. (in press).
11. B. J. Poiesz, F. W. Ruscetti, J. W. Mier, A. M. Woods, and R. C. Gallo, Proc. Natl. Acad. Sci. U.S.A. **77**, 6815 (1980).
12. C. Tarella, F. Ruscetti, B. Poiesz, A. Woods, and R. C. Gallo, in preparation.
13. B. J. Poiesz, F. W. Ruscetti, A. F. Gazdar, P. A. Bunn, J. D. Minna, and R. C. Gallo, Proc. Natl. Acad. Sci. U.S.A. **77**, 7415 (1980).
14. B. J. Poiesz, F. W. Ruscetti, M. S. Reitz, V. S. Kalyanaraman, and R. C. Gallo, Nature (London) **294**, 268 (1981).
15. R. C. Gallo, B. J. Poiesz, and F. W. Ruscetti, in "Modern Trends in Human Leukemia IV" (R. Neth, R. C. Gallo, T. Graf, K. Mannweiler, and K. Winkler, eds.). Springer-Verlag, Berlin and New York, p. 502, 1981.
16. H. M. Rho, B. Poiesz, F. W. Ruscetti, and R. C. Gallo, Virology **112**, 355 (1981).
17. V. S. Kalyanaraman, M. G. Sarnagadharan, B. Poiesz, F. W. Ruscetti, and R. C. Gallo, J. Virol. **38**, 906 (1981).
18. M. S. Reitz, Jr., B. J. Poiesz, F. W. Ruscetti, and R. C. Gallo, Proc. Natl. Acad. Sci. U.S.A. **78**, 1887 (1981).
19. L. E. Posner, M. Robert-Guroff, V. S. Kalyanaraman, B. J. Poiesz, F. W. Ruscetti, B. Fossieck, P. A. Bunn, Jr., J. D. Minna, and R. C. Gallo, J. Exp. Med. **154**, 333 (1981).
20. V. S. Kalyanaraman, M. G. Sarngadharan, Y. Nakao, Y. Ito, and R. C. Gallo, Proc. Natl. Acad. Sci. U.S.A. (in press).

13

Lymphoma in Cyclosporin A-Treated Nonhuman Primate Allograft Recipients

CHARLES P. BIEBER, JOHN L. PENNOCK, AND BRUCE A. REITZ

I. Introduction

Cyclosporin A is a new immunosuppressive agent whose use in initial clinical trials has been associated with a favorable maintenance of allograft function and with the prevention of graft-versus-host disease (1, 2). The administration of cyclosporin A does not produce the leukopenia or lymphopenia one sees in association with the use of antimetabolic and antilymphocytic agents and appears to have none of the deleterious metabolic effects associated with the use of

MALIGNANT LYMPHOMAS

corticosteroids. These features combine to make cyclosporin A a desirable agent for prophylactic control of the immune response in transplant recipients.

Cyclosporin A is a water-insoluble cyclic polypeptide composed of 11 amino acids, which can be extracted from several species of fungus (3). The drug is not digested in the gut and may be administered by mouth to cognizant or cooperative patients. In nonhuman primates treated with cyclosporin A, the agent is usually administered intramuscularly in an oil base. The efficiency of absorption from either route is currently unknown, as methodology for measurement of serum levels of the agent has only recently become available (4). By both routes of administration, absorption appears sufficient for the agent's pharmacological properties to become manifest. A clear disadvantage of administration by the intramuscular route is the marked inflammatory response induced by the oil base.

The pharmacological action of cyclosporin A includes inhibition of host antibody responses to T-cell dependent antigens but not to B-cell dependent lipopolysaccharide antigens (5), and inhibition of proliferative responses of peripheral blood lymphocytes to mitogenic and allogeneic stimuli (6). Cyclosporin A inhibits the development of lymphocytotoxic effector and suppressor lymphocyte functions normally generated in mixed lymphocyte reactions. Cytolytic effector functions of responder cells can be inhibited at drug concentrations of $0.064-1.0$ μg/ml. Suppressor functions are inhibited only at drug concentrations greater than 1.0 μg/ml. This latter evidence suggests that a therapeutic ratio relevant to allograft adaptation may be obtained if drug doses sufficient to inhibit recipient cytotoxic response but too low to affect suppressor activation could be achieved. The mechanism by which the functions of lymphocytes might be affected by cyclosporin A are reported to be blockage of resting T-cell responses to T-cell growth factors (7). Action of this sort would greatly reduce the magnitude of rejection by effectively blocking the recruitment phase of the immune response.

Adverse effects associated with the chronic use of cyclosporin A include mild hepatorenal dysfunction, neurological changes, and the development of lymphoma (1, 8). This latter complication is not uniquely associated with the use of cyclosporin A, as an increased incidence of lymphoma in immunosuppressed transplant recipients is well documented (9). In this report we describe the incidence of lymphoma in nonhuman primate allograft recipients treated with various immunosuppressive agents including cyclosporin A.

II. Materials and Methods

A. Animals

Ninety-seven nonhuman primate cardiac or heart–lung allograft recipients not succumbing during the first 2 weeks following transplantation surgery were considered at risk for lymphoma onset. The primate population included 3 rhesus (*Macaca mullata*) and 94 cynomolgus (*Macaca fasicularis*) species. Rhesus primates were obtained from the Stanford University and the University of Washington primate colonies. Cynomolgus species were obtained from Primate Imports, New York, New York.

B. Treatment

Immunosuppressive agents were used either singly or in various combinations for prophylactic prevention and maintenance control of rejection responses. Rejection was usually manifest by graft failure. Augmentative immunosuppressive treatment for suspected rejection crises was not generally given. The agents used were cyclosporin A in miglyol 812 (an oil base), 25 mg/kg given intramuscularly for 14 consecutive days and then every other day thereafter, or 17 mg/kg per day continuously; azathioprine, 2 mg/kg per day for 14 days or continuously;

TABLE I

Summary of Treatment of Macaques Developing Posttransplant Lymphoma

Monkey no.[a]	Allograft[b]	Treatment[c]	Lymphoma diagnosis (days)	Lymphoma location, gross	Survival
347	OH	CyA25, I	66	Kidneys	66
339	OH	CyA25, I	122	Inguinal nodes, heart	122
330	OH	CyA25, I	123	Kidneys, iliac nodes	123
27	OHL	CyA25, I	128	Kidneys, iliac nodes, thigh, heart	144
273	HH	CyA25, I, M, ATG	148	Spleen, liver	148
323	HH	CyA25, I, M, ATG	92	Spleen, liver	92
379	OH	CyA17	454	Kidney, iliac nodes, thigh, heart	454
354	HH	CyA25, ATG	319	Pelvic mass	319
399	OH	CyA17, TLI (1800 rads)	76	Kidneys, iliac nodes, heart	76
394	OH	CyA17, TLI (600 rads)	109	Kidney, iliac nodes, heart	128
405	OH	CyA17, TLI (1800 rads)	113	Iliac nodes, spleen	173
433	OHL	CyA30-10	97	Kidneys, iliac nodes, spleen, heart	97

[a] All macaques were cynomolgus except no. 27, a rhesus.

[b] OH, Orthotopic heart; HH, heterotopic heart; HL, heart–lung replacement.

[c] CyA25, Cyclosporin A, 25 mg/kg per day intramuscularly (thigh) for 14 days and then qod thereafter; CYA17, 17 mg/kg per day intramuscularly; CyA30-10, 30 mg/kg reduced to 10 mg/kg; I, azathioprine, 2 mg/kg per day; M, methyl prednisolone, 14 mg/kg per week; ATG, antithymocyte globulin, 10 mg/kg per day for 7 days; TLI, total lymphoid irradiation.

TABLE II

Malignant Lymphomas in Immunosuppressed Nonhuman Primate Allograft Recipients

Treatment[a]	No.	Mean survival (days)	Cumulative risk (years)	Lymphoma (no.)	Lymphomas/year risk (%)
Cyclosporin A-treated					
All	55	83 ± 10	12.4	12	97
CyA alone	16	52 ± 7	2.3	2	88
CyA, I	9	173 ± 39	4.3	4	94
CyA, ATG	6	76 ± 38	1.2	1	79
CyA, ATG, I, M	13	60 ± 13	2.1	2	93
CyA, TLI	11	82 ± 13	2.5	3	120
Non-cyclosporin A-treated					
All	42	50 ± 5	5.8	0	0
I, M	10	43 ± 15	1.2	0	0
I, M, ATG	23	54 ± 11	3.4	0	0
I, ATG, TLI	9	48 ± 12	1.2	0	0

[a] CyA, Cyclosporin A, 25 mg/kg daily for 2 weeks then q.o.d. or 17 mg/kg q.d. all given intramuscularly in oil base; I, Imuran, 2 mg/kg per day, continuous; ATG, antithymocyte globulin of rabbit origin, 10 mg/kg daily for 6 days; M, methylprednisolone, 14 mg/kg once weekly s.q.; TLI, total lymphoid irradiation, 100 rads/day for a total of 600–1800 rads prior to the operation.

cyte globulin (to rhesus thymocytes), 10 mg/kg per day given intramuscularly daily on postoperative days 0–7; and total lymphoid irradiation (TLI) given in 100 rads/day fractions preoperatively for a total dose of 600–1800 rads. Treatments for given animals and groups of animals are listed in Tables I and II.

C. Diagnosis of Lymphoma

When lymphoma was suspected, biopsies of the lesion were taken or, in the case of moribund primates, the animal was sacrificed and autopsied. In all but two instances where lymphoma was detected, tissue was obtained either fresh or within 1 hour of death. In all cases representative tissue samples were fixed in 10% buffered Formalin and processed routinely. In eight instances fresh tissue samples were fixed in glutaraldehyde and processed for electron microscopy. Selected tissue and serum samples were submitted to the Southwest Foundation for Research in San Antonio, Texas, for viral studies.

D. Laboratory Studies

Complete blood counts were performed for all transplant recipients twice weekly. In addition, T-cell counts as defined by the ability of the peripheral blood lymphocytes to form rosettes with sheep erythrocytes were performed on selected primates. In primates receiving cyclosporin A renal and hepatic function was assessed monthly by measurement of blood urea nitrogen (BUN) and serum creatinine levels. Hepatic function was assessed monthly by measurement of serum enzyme levels of glutamic-oxalo and -pyruvic transaminase, alkaline phosphatase, lactic dehydrogenase, and creatinine phosphokinase. Analysis of data, comparison of allograft survival, and instance of lymphoma in animals methylprednisolone, 14 mg/kg given subcutaneously once weekly; antithymo-treated with cyclosporin A or conventional immunosuppressive therapy were determined by the method of Kaplan and Meier (10). The significance of the difference in survival and lymphoma onset in these two groups was assessed by the method of Gehan (11).

III. Results

A. Allograft Survival and Lymphoma Onset

Allograft survival in animals receiving cyclosporin A was significantly greater than in those treated with other forms of immunosuppression ($p < .02$, Fig. 1). Sixteen (35%) animals not receiving cyclosporin A had not experienced transplant failure and remained at risk for lymphoma onset after the 60th postoperative day. Only one (2%) remained at risk after 110 postoperative days. In contrast, 27 (60%) animals receiving cyclosporin A were at risk after 60 postoperative days and 15 (35%) at risk after 110 days. All lymphomas occurred in cyclosporin A-treated animals and were diagnosed between the 66th and 454th postoperative days. The mode onset date was 112 days. The tumor-related onset in cyclosporin A-treated primates relative to that of the more conventionally treated group was

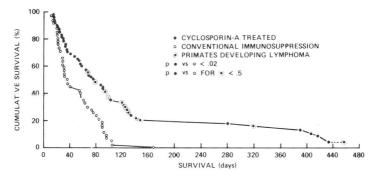

Fig. 1. Cumulative survival in macaque cardiac allograft recipients whose treatment included the use of cyclosporin A or more conventional immunosuppression.

not statistically significant ($p < .5$). The difference in the incidence of lymphoma in subgroups of animals receiving cyclosporin A alone or cyclosporin A in combination with other therapeutic agents was not significant (Table II).

Indications of the presence of disease were generally present 1–2 weeks prior to death. In three instances disease was suspected upon occurrence of leukomoid reactions to greater than 30,000 cells/ml 1–6 weeks prior to death. In another three instances disease was manifested as rapidly growing pelvic, inguinal, or lower-extremity soft tissue masses. In the remaining six cases disease was heralded by scrotal edema occurring 1–3 weeks prior to death. The appearance of scrotal edema in posttransplant recipients was in every instance associated with lymphoma.

B. Laboratory Studies

None of the fluctuations observed in the laboratory parameters could be attributed to the use of cyclosporin A. Specifically, in no instance was leukopenia, platelet depression, or anemia more severe in cyclosporin A-treated animals than in those treated with other forms of immunosuppression. In contrast to animals receiving conventional immunosuppressive therapy, there was no generalized depression of circulating lymphocyte levels and particularly no depression of the T-lymphocyte fraction in cyclosporin A-treated animals. Renal function in cyclosporin A-treated animals, as assessed by BUN and serum creatinine levels, was at no time abnormal. Enzyme levels in the primates were generally high compared to human values but did not differ significantly from their preoperative control values.

C. Description of Tumors

Twelve of 97 animals at risk 2 weeks or more after transplantation developed lymphoproliferative lesions. All were among 55 animals who had received cyclosporin A either as a single agent or in combination with other immunosuppressive agents. The anatomical extent of gross disease found at autopsy had a similar pattern in most instances. The most common area of gross involvement was the inguinal-pelvic and lower abdominal retroperitoneal lymph nodes (9/12 cases). Tumor masses in this region were generally large, and in one instance the tumor mass achieved a diameter of 8 cm. Mediastinal lymph nodes were as frequently involved (10–12 cases), however, often by microscopic rather than gross involvement. The spleen was involved in 7/12 instances. Outside the lymphoid system the kidney was the most common site of gross involvement (7/12 cases), and in 6 of the 7 instances the lesions were bilateral. Renal lesions were frequently quite large, reaching up to 5 cm in diameter. Gross involvement of the liver was apparent in two instances. Microscopic infiltration of the allograft was generally apparent. Three patterns of allograft involvement were noted. These included subendocardial infiltration by tumor cells (seen in recipients whose initial manifestation had been a leukomoid reaction), pericardial infiltration, and multiple diffuse nodular lesions within the myocardium.

Similarities could be seen in the histological appearance of the 12 tumors. Normal lymph node architecture was effaced by a mononuclear cell type with scanty cytoplasm, large vesicular nuclei, centrally located nucleoli, and clumped chromatin at the border of the nucleus (Fig. 2). Three to four mitotic figures per 100 cells were commonly seen. In many of the tumors an occasional cell with abundant cytoplasm containing phagocytosed red cells or other particles imparted a "starry-sky" appearance to the lymph node histology. The likely B-cell lymphoid origin of the predominant tumor cell type was evident from their ultrastructure. These studies demonstrated that many of the tumor cells possessed a well-developed and frequently stacked endoplasmic reticulum characteristic of plasmacytoid development (Fig. 3). Viral particles were noted within the endoplasmic reticulum of plasmacytoid cells in seven of the eight cases examined. These particles, although small (40 nm), were easily recognized by their accumulation in crystalline arrays. The particles did not appear to be enveloped, and no evidence of budding into the endoplasmic reticulum was seen. No particles were found within the nuclei of tumor cells, nor were they seen in extralymphoid

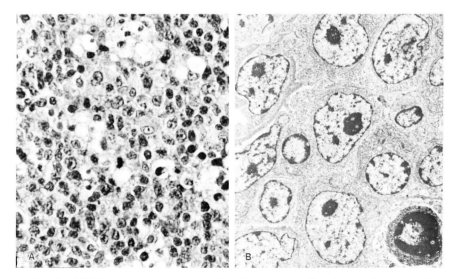

Fig. 2. (A) Histological appearance of lymphomatous proliferation of primate no. 339 within iliac lymph nodes. Cells are monotypic, many with prominent nucleoli. Hematoxylin–eosin. (B) Electron microscope appearance of a tumor illustrating well-developed endoplasmic reticulum in most cells. Original magnification ×4440.

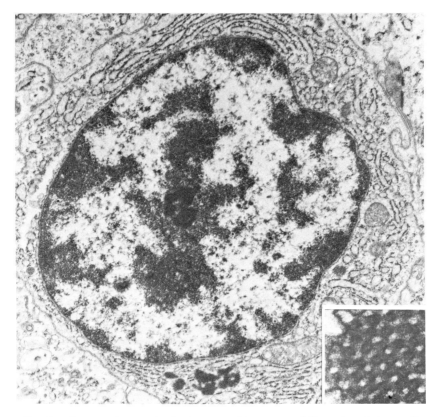

Fig. 3. Electron micrograph of primate no. 339 tumor cell illustrating viral crystalline arrays in endoplasmic reticulum. ×14,269. Inset: Higher magnification of particles. ×132,176.

sections of heart, lung, or hepatic specimens. Virus identification from culture and antibody studies is in progress.

IV. Discussion

The lesions described in this study meet criteria for diagnosis as lymphoma. Initially, we classified these lesions as histiocytic lymphoma based on nuclear morphology and the appearance of phagocytic cells within the tumor nodules; however, the plasmacytoid appearance of noncleaved cells might be considered more characteristic of immunoblastic sarcoma as described by Lukes (12). The malignant behavior of the disease is confirmed by the rapidly developing and widespread involvement of the lymphoid and visceral organs.

The consistent presence of virus particles within the tumor cells examined in our series suggests their participation in the pathogenesis of disease. Several criteria remain to be met, however, in order to establish any etiological role for these virus particles. Although we suspect the observed particles are nonenveloped nucleocapsids, the resolution we have been able to obtain in ultrastructural studies has not been sufficient to exclude the presence of a viral envelope. The 40-nm nucleocapsid size would be consistent with smaller types of either RNA or DNA viruses but not with the larger herpesviruses. Viral serological studies and attempts to establish the tumor cell as a line in culture are currently in progress.

Viral association with the development of lymphoproliferative disease has also been suspected in human allograft recipients treated with cyclosporin A. Crawford et al. (13) reported an undifferentiated large-cell tumor developing in the groin of a renal recipient who was among 18 treated with 17 mg/kg of cyclosporin A daily. On the basis of surface markers the tumor was considered to be consistent with B immunoblastic lymphoma. Immunofluorescent studies demonstrated the presence of the Epstein–Barr virus (EBV) nuclear antigen in tumor cells. In another series Nagington and Gray (14) reported rising titers to the EBV capsid antigen in 10 of 21 cyclosporin A-treated allograft recipients from whom he obtained pretransplant and 6-months posttransplant sera. Three patients in this series who developed lymphoma were among the 10 with rising titers of antibody to EBV.

Viruses closely associated with EBV have been found in chimpanzees, baboons, and orangutans, among Old World primates, but not in macaques (15). The oncogenic potential of these viruses has not yet been described. In New World primates, viruses which are oncogenic and analogous to EBV have been reported. Marmosets inoculated with human EBV have been reported to develop lymphoma (16).

Lymphoma is a serious general complication of transplantation which appears to be associated with immunosuppression given to maintain allograft function (17). Within our cardiac transplant unit, where a high degree of immunosuppression is required to ensure continuous graft function, a 5.5% instance of lymphoma has been observed. This is higher than the 0.8% instance of lymphoma reported from a large renal transplant series (18) but lower than the 7.6% incidence derived from reported series of allograft recipients treated with cyclosporin A (1, 13). Neither the incidence of lymphoma reported from our institution nor that reported from any other institution including those using cyclosporin A, however, is as high as that seen in the macaques reported on here.

The incidence of spontaneous hematopoietic neoplasms in nonhuman primates is generally considered to be low; however, outbreaks of lymphoma among macaques have been reported. Terrell et al. (19) reported an apparent epidemic of lymphoma in macaques housed at the California Primate Research Center

(CPRC). Forty-five lymphomas, 42 in rhesus and 3 in stump-tailed macaques (*Macaca arctoides*), developed in a colony of 1200 predominantly rhesus macaques housed at the CPRC. The outbreak began in 1969, peaked between 1971 and 1973, and subsided thereafter. The last reported case was in 1977. A variety of non-Hodgkin's histiological patterns were described including lymphocytic, histiocytic, and mixed histiocytic-lymphocytic lymphoma. No etiology common to all affected animals was described, but evidence regarding common housing and mother-to-offspring occurrence suggested both vertical and horizontal transmission of disease. Reduced immunological tolerance was suggested as a necessary condition for disease. This particular study bears importantly upon the observed incidence of lymphoma in macaque allograft recipients treated with cyclosporin A at Stanford. Our initial primate colony was established from rhesus primates obtained from the CPRC between 1977 and 1978. Although none of the CPRC animals we received developed recognizable disease and none were used in the study reported here, some were eventually used as organ and blood donors for later experiments, such that horizontal transmission of any agent which might relate to disease occurrence cannot be excluded. Additionally, since the establishment of our primate colony in 1977, both rhesus and cynomolgus primates have been continuously housed in common rooms.

The suspicion that macaques studied in our series might have been predisposed to the development of lymphoma requires that the incidence of lymphoma in cyclosporin A and non-cyclosporin A-immunosuppressed recipients be compared if one is to conclude that cyclosporin A immunosuppression specifically predisposes to lymphoma development. The animals treated with more conventional forms of immunosuppression in our series generally failed to survive or were not treated beyond the period of greatest observed risk for lymphoma diagnosis. For this reason, the difference in the incidence of disease between cyclosporin A-treated and nontreated groups did not achieve statistical significance. Given the aforementioned character of lymphoma in macaques, it seems reasonable to ask whether the incidence of lymphoma in our conventionally treated primates would have been different had it continued into the period of greatest risk observed for the cyclosporin A-treated group. Our data do not resolve this question.

It would also be important to know whether the frequency of lymphoma in cyclosporin A-treated primates reflects that which may be expected in humans treated in a similar fashion. The appearance of four lymphomas in 54 humans receiving cyclosporin A that have been reported to date indicates that a significant but lower instance of disease will be observed. Whether the incidence, behavior, and response of these induced lymphoproliferative disorders will increase the risk of use of cyclosporin A to a point where its beneficial effect is offset at present appears unlikely. However, at this time, data are insufficient to draw this conclusion.

Acknowledgments

The authors wish to express their gratitude to Roger Warnke and Marilyn Masek of the Stanford Pathology Department for valuable professional assistance. This study was supported in part by NHLBI research grant HL 13108.

References

1. R. Y. Calne, K. Rolles, S. Thiru, *et al., Lancet* **2,** 1033 (1979).
2. R. L. Powles, A. J. Barrett, H. Klink, *et al., Lancet* **1,** 1327 (1980).
3. M. Dreyfus, E. Hgerri, H. Hotman, *et al., Eur. J. Appl. Microbiol.* **3,** 125 (1976).
4. W. Niederberger, P. Schaub, and T. Beveridge, *J. Chromatogr.* **182,** 454 (1980).
5. J. F. Borel, *Immunology* **31,** 631 (1976).
6. A. D. Hess and P. J. Tutschka, *J. Immunol.* **124,** 2601 (1980).
7. E. Larsson, *J. Immunol.* **124,** 2828 (1980).
8. C. Bieber, B. A. Reitz, S. W. Jamieson, *et al., Lancet* **1,** 43 (1980).
9. I. Penn, ''Malignant Tumors in Organ Transplant Recipients.'' Springer-Verlag, Berlin and New York, 1970.
10. E. Kaplan and M. Meier, *J. Am. Stat. Assoc.* **53,** 457 (1958).
11. E. Gerhan, *Biometrika* **52,** 203 (1965).
12. R. Lukes and R. Collins, *Cancer* **34,** 1488 (1974).
13. D. H. Crawford, J. Thomas, G. Janossy, *et al., Lancet* **1,** 1356 (1980).
14. J. Nagington and I. Gray, *Lancet* **1,** 536 (1980).
15. H. Rabin, ''Primates and Human Cancer,'' DHEW Publ. No. (NIH) 79 1889, p. 117. US-DHEW, Washington, D.C., 1979.
16. T. Shope, D. Dechairo, and G. Miller, *Proc. Natl. Acad. Sci. U.S.A.* **70,** 2487 (1973).
17. I. Penn, *Cancer (Philadelphia)* **34,** 1474 (1974).
18. A. Sheil, *Transplant. Proc.* **9,** 1133 (1977).
19. T. Terrell, D. Gribble, and B. Osburn, *JNCI, J. Natl. Cancer Inst.* **64,** 561 (1980).

14

Lymphomas in Cardiac Transplant Recipients: Immunological Phenotype

ROGER A. WARNKE

I. Introduction

At Stanford University Medical Center, 182 patients underwent 199 cardiac transplants from January 1968 to January 1980. The number of patients surviving at 5 years following transplantation increased from $18 \pm 5\%$ in 1974 to $45 \pm 5\%$ in 1980 [1]. This improvement in survival has been largely attributed to the recognition and treatment of complications in the first three postoperative months [1]. The incidence of fatal complications occurring after the third postoperative month has remained relatively constant; the spectrum of these later complications and their incidence have been recently summarized [1]. Especially those patients who survive more than 2 years following cardiac transplantation are at increased risk of developing malignant neoplasms [1, 2]. The incidence and types of malignant neoplasms observed in cardiac allograft recipients have been similar to the incidence and spectrum seen in noncardiac allograft recipients (2). Of particular interest have been the large number of lymphomas seen in allograft recipients, the marked predominance of non-Hodgkin's lymphoma in such patients, and the unusual localization to the central nervous system at presentation in a high percentage of such patients (3).

Furthermore, a number of lymphomas in the setting of organ transplantation have been reported to be polyclonal B-cell proliferations based on immunoglobulin light-chain staining (4, 5). We have noted that transplant lymphomas are often associated with extensive necrosis, perhaps as a consequence of ongoing immunosuppressive therapy which commonly compromises the obtaining of satisfactory cell suspensions for immunoglobulin staining. Thus many of the transplant lymphomas which have been reported to be polyclonal have been studied with methods applied to routinely fixed and paraffin-embedded lymphoma tissue (4, 5). Erroneous polyclonal staining patterns which may result from studies on fixed lymphoma tissues have been reviewed recently (6). We have reported frozen section methods which allow accurate assessment of partially necrotic lymphomas and have reported nontransplant lymphomas to be monoclonal B-cell proliferations (7–9) in agreement with numerous studies performed on viable cells in suspension (10–15). The purpose of this article is to summarize frozen section staining of four lymphomas from three cardiac allograft recipients with hybridoma monoclonal antibodies detected by an antibody–biotin–avidin–horseradish peroxidase method.

II. Materials and Methods

A. Tissue Specimens

We examined specimens at the time of surgical removal. Representative 1-mm cross sections were divided and placed in embedding medium in airtight plastic capsules which were frozen in a mixture of isopentane and dry ice and stored at $-50°C$ until sectioned.

The eight patients who developed lymphoma after cardiac transplanation during the period from January 1968 to January of 1980 are the subject of a more detailed report (16). Preliminary immunological characterization of two of the lymphomas has been reported previously (9). The lymphomas from the three patients which form the basis of this report arose in the following clinical settings:

1. Two years following a second cardiac allograft a 20-year-old male patient with a history of end-stage cardiomyopathy developed large-cell lymphoma in the right anterior thigh at the site of antithymocyte globulin injections. The patient had no other evidence of disease and was treated with local radiotherapy.

TABLE I

Hybridoma Antibodies

Hybridoma clone	Designation	Tentative reactivity
L203[a]	HLA-DR (Ia)	B cells, macrophages, thymic epithelium, some T cells, etc.
L17F12[a]	Leu-1	All peripheral blood T cells
SK-1[b]	Leu-2a	Suppressor or cytotoxic T cells
SK-3[b]	Leu-3a	Inducer or helper T cells

[a] Applied in collaboration with Ronald Levy.
[b] A gift of Robert Evans.

A chest wall lesion was resected 8 months later, and the patient died with widespread lymphoma shortly thereafter. The initial thigh lesion and the chest wall recurrence were both studied.

2. Four years after cardiac transplantation for end-stage cardiomyopathy, a 26-year-old man developed a large-cell lymphoma of the right lung which was treated by surgical excision. He died 8 months later of coronary artery disease with no evidence of lymphoma at autopsy.

3. A year and a half after a second cardiac transplant a 44-year-old physician with a history of severe coronary artery disease underwent biopsy of a cerebral mass which showed large-cell lymphoma. Following radiotherapy, this patient is alive without any evidence of disease 10 months later.

All three patients were treated with prednisone, azathioprine, and antithymocyte globulin.

B. Hybridoma Monoclonal Antibodies

A summary of the hybridoma monoclonal antibodies we utilized in this study is presented in Table I. The approach used in immunizing mice with human cells, in fusing spleen cells with the myeloma cells, in culturing, in cloning, and in screening for desired reactivities has been previously described (17). The characterization of these antibodies has also been reported (18–20). These particular monoclonal antibodies are available from a commercial source (Becton-Dickinson, Sunnyvale, California).

C. Immunohistochemical Staining Procedure

Cryostat sections 4–6 μm thick were fixed in acetone (less than 5 seconds) prior to storage at $-20°C$. Before staining, the frozen sections were fixed in acetone for 10 minutes at $4°C$. Sections then were incubated with phosphate-buffered saline for 10 minutes at $20°C$. Appropriate dilutions of monoclonal antibodies

TABLE II

Antibody Staining of Lymphomas Following Cardiac Allografts in Three Patients[a]

Site	HLA-DR (Ia)	Leu-1[b]	Leu-2a[b]	Leu-3a[b]
Thigh (1978)	+	−	−	−
Chest wall (1979)	+	−	−	−
Lung	+	−	−	−
Brain	+	−	−	−

[a] These lymphomas were previously shown not to stain for immunoglobulin light chains or heavy chains or with α-naphthylbutyrate esterase as a marker of monocytes and macrophages.

[b] Although the lymphoma cells did not react with these antibodies, an estimated 5–10% of associated cells did stain, which were generally of the phenotype Leu-1[+], Leu-2a[+], Leu-3a[−].

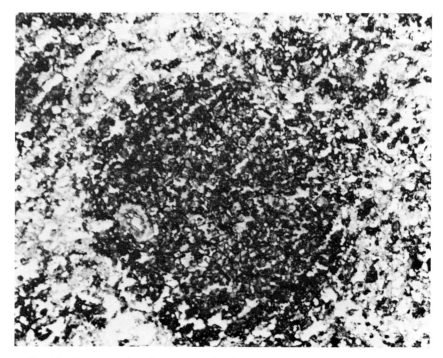

Fig. 1A. Frozen section of a posttransplant large-cell lymphoma of the brain stained for HLA-DR (Ia). The lymphoma cells around the vessel and in the adjacent areas of necrosis stain darkly.

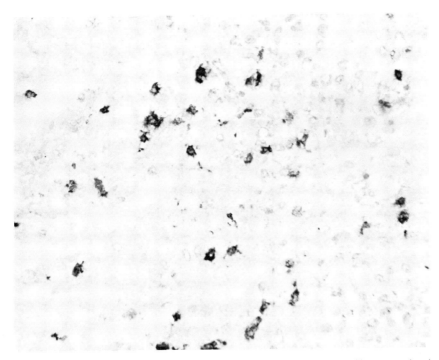

Fig. 1B. A frozen section from the same case stained for Leu-2a. Note occasional suppressor or cytotoxic T cells predominantly localized to the necrotic zones.

were placed on the sections for 15 minutes. After washing and incubation with PBS for 5 minutes, biotinylated goat anti-mouse antibody was placed on the sections for 15 minutes. A mixture of purified goat anti-mouse heavy-chain antibodies was obtained from a commercial source (Tago, Inc., Burlingame, California) and conjugated with biotin succinimide ester (Biosearch, San Rafael, California) as previously described (21). After a PBS wash, the sections were incubated for 15 minutes with avidin conjugated to horseradish peroxidase (Vector Laboratories, Inc., Burlingame, California). After two PBS washes the sections were incubated with 1 mg/ml 3,3-diaminobenzidine in 0.01% H_2O_2 in PBS. After two washes in PBS, sections were incubated with a 0.5% solution of $CuSO_4$ in normal saline (22). Prior to mounting, sections were counterstained with methylene blue.

III. Results

A summary of the results of staining these transplant lymphomas for HLA-DR, Leu-1, Leu-2a, and Leu-3a, is presented in Table II. Cells from two of these lymphomas were previously shown not to stain for immunoglobulin light chains and heavy chains or for α-naphthylbutyrate esterase as a marker for monocytes and macrophages (9). The central nervous system (CNS) lymphoma likewise did not stain for immunoglobulin light chains or heavy chains or for α-naphthylbutyrate esterase. The lymphoma cells from all three cases did stain for HLA-DR but not for the three T-cell antigens. Staining of a frozen section of the large-cell lymphoma of the CNS for Ia is illustrated in Fig. 1A. All the lymphoma cells around the vessel stained for Ia. The nonstaining areas represent necrotic zones which are extremely common in posttransplant lymphomas. Figure 1B shows that occasional cytotoxic or suppressor T cells were seen around nodules of lymphoma despite ongoing immunosuppressive therapy with prednisone and azathioprine. An estimated 5–10% of the cells stained for Leu-1 in all four specimens studied; these cells were predominantly of the phenotype Leu-$2a^+$, Leu-$3a^-$.

IV. Discussion

The lymphomas that arise following renal transplantation and after thymic implants in patients with severe combined immunodeficiency have been reported to be polyclonal (4, 5). The lymphomas of the three patients reported here did not bear immunoglobulin, and the clonality therefore cannot be determined. A number of the previously reported cases have been studied with immunohistochemical methods applied to fixed tissue which can result in erroneous polyclonal staining patterns (6). Even if frozen sections or viable cells from such cases are available for study, it may be necessary to use f(ab')$_2$ antibody fragments to circumvent spurious polyclonal staining due to nonspecific Fc adherence (9). Furthermore it is possible that some of these previous cases were in fact polyclonal virus-associated lymphoid proliferations which simulated nontransplant malignant lymphoma.

Immunological studies do not indicate the nature of the neoplastic cells in our lymphomas. The cells from our three cases did not stain for immunoglobulin, for three T-cell antigens, or for α-naphthylbutyrate esterase. Whether these lymphomas arise from the B-cell lineage at a stage prior to immunoglobulin production or arise from some other cell type such as NK cells remains to be determined. Whatever their nature, Ia provides evidence of an hematolymphoid origin. Ia has been shown to stain many of the large-cell lymphomas which do not bear other conventional surface markers (9, 23, 24). Another question is whether these lymphomas are of host or donor origin. The three cases reported in the literature all appeared to have been of host origin (25).

The possible role of Epstein–Barr virus (EBV) or other herpesviruses such as cytomegalovirus (CMV) in the pathogenesis of these lymphomas is also of interest (26, 27). Marker *et al.* have described a 19-year-old renal allograft recipient who was exposed to infectious mononucleosis prior to transplantation. Approximately 2 weeks after transplantation, the patient developed generalized adenopathy, a polyclonal elevation in immunoglobulins, and rising titers to EBV (28). Lymph node biopsy sections were felt to show malignant lymphoma (immunoblastic sarcoma). This patient eventually succumbed to a rapidly progressive lymphoproliferative process thought to be lymphoma or an overwhelming viral infection. The plasmacytoid cells which made up the neoplasm were said to stain for gamma, alpha, mu, kappa, and lambda chains. Such a staining profile suggests Fc binding. This particular case and others like it are probably more akin clinically, pathologically, and immunologically to fatal infectious mononucleosis rather than to lymphoma. Whether such cases should be regarded as fatal uncontrolled infectious disease in the setting of persistent antigenic stimulation (an allograft) and impaired immunity (immunosuppressive therapy) or lymphoma is open to question (26, 27). It is also known that virus-associated histiocytic proliferations occur in the setting of transplantation, which simulate histiocytic malignancy (29).

We suspect transplant patients are at risk of more conventional lymphomas (asymptomatic, extranodal, and treatable) as well as these lymphoma-like lymphoid proliferations. We are hopeful of studying our cases for EBV antigens. If such antigens are present, they will provide a link to the virus-associated lymphoid proliferations; if EBV antigens are absent, our cases will be more similar to spontaneous large-cell lymphomas which have not been associated with EBV (30).

Acknowledgment

Supported in part by grants from the National Institutes of Health (AI-11313 and CA-05838).

References

1. C. P. Bieber, S. A. Hunt, D. A. Schwinn, S. A. Jamieson, B. A. Reitz, P. E. Oyer, N. E. Shumway, and E. B. Stinson, *Transplant Proc.* **13**, 207 (1981).
2. J. G. Krikorian, J. L. Anderson, C. P. Bieber, I. Penn, and E. B. Stinson, *JAMA, J. Am. Med. Assoc.* **240**, 639 (1978).
3. I. Penn, *Transplant. Proc.* **9**, 1121 (1977).
4. B. F. Hertel, J. Rosai, L. P. Dehner, and R. L. Simmons, *Lab. Invest.* **36**, 340 (1977).
5. M. S. Borzy, P. Hong, S. D. Horowitz, E. Gilbert, D. Kaufman, W. DeMendonca, V. Oxelius, M. Dictor, and L. Pachman, *N. Engl. J. Med.* **301**, 565 (1979).
6. D. Y. Mason and P. Biberfeld, *J. Histochem. Cytochem.* **28**, 731 (1980).
7. R. Levy, R. Warnke, R. F. Dorfman, and J. Haimovich, *J. Exp. Med.* **145**, 1014 (1977).
8. R. Warnke and R. Levy, *N. Engl. J. Med.* **298**, 481 (1978).

9. R. Warnke, R. Miller, T. Grogan, M. Pederson, J. Dilley, and R. Levy, *N. Engl. J. Med.* **303,** 293 (1980).

10. K. J. Gajl-Peczalska, C. D. Bloomfield, P. F. Coccia, H. Sosin, R. D. Brunning, and J. H. Kersey, *Am. J. Med.* **59,** 674 (1975).

11. J. H. Leech, A. D. Glick, J. A. Waldron, J. M. Flexner, R. G. Horn, and R. D. Collins, *JNCI, J. Natl. Cancer Inst.* **54,** 11 (1975).

12. G. S. Pinkus and J. W. Said, *Am. J. Pathol.* **9,** 349 (1978).

13. D. A. Filippa, P. H. Lieberman, R. A. Erlandson, B. Koziner, F. P. Siegal, A. Turnbull, A. Zimring, and R. A. Good, *Am. J. Med.* **64,** 259 (1978).

14. C. W. Berard, E. S. Jaffe, R. C. Braylan, R. B. Mann, and K. Nanba, *Cancer (Philadelphia)* **42,** 911 (1978).

15. A. C. Aisenberg, B. M. Wilkes, J. C. Long, and N. L. Harris, *Am. J. Med.* **68,** 206 (1980).

16. J. Weintraub, R. Levy, and R. Warnke, *Transplantation* (in press).

17. R. Levy, J. Dilley, and L. A. Lampson, *Curr. Top. Microbiol. Immunol.* **81,** 164 (1978).

18. L. Lampson and R. Levy, *J. Immunol.* **125,** 293 (1980).

19. E. G. Engleman, R. Warnke, R. I. Fox, and R. Levy, *Proc. Natl. Acad. Sci. U.S.A.* **78,** 1791 (1981).

20. J. A. Ledbetter, R. L. Evans, M. L. Lipinski, C. Cunningham-Rundles, R. A. Good, and L. A. Herzenberg, *J. Exp. Med.* **153,** 310 (1981).

21. R. Warnke and R. Levy, *J. Histochem. Cytochem.* **28,** 771 (1980).

22. J. S. Hanker, W. W. Ambrose, C. J. James, J. Mandelkorn, P. E. Yates, S. A. Gall, E. H. Bossen, J. W. Fay, J. Laszlo, and J. O. Moore, *Cancer Res.* **39,** 1635 (1979).

23. M. E. Kadin, *Arch. Pathol. Lab. Med.* **104,** 503 (1980).

24. J. P. Halper, D. M. Knowles, II, and C. Y. Wang, *Blood* **55,** 373 (1980).

25. I. Penn, *Transplantation* **27,** 214 (1979).

26. S. Louie and R. S. Schwartz, *Semin. Hematol.* **15,** 117 (1978).

27. A. J. Matas, B. F. Hertel, J. Rosai, R. L. Simmons, J. S. Najarian, *Am. J. Med.* **61,** 716 (1976).

28. S. C. Marker, N. L. Ascher, J. M. Kalis, R. L. Simmons, J. S. Najarian, and H. H. Balfour, *Surgery* **85,** 433 (1979).

29. R. J. Risdall, R. W. McKenna, M. E. Nesbit, W. Krivit, H. H. Balfour, Jr., R. L. Simmons, and R. D. Brunning, *Cancer (Philadelphia)* **44,** 993 (1979).

30. A. L. Epstein, R. Levy, H. Kim, W. Henle, and H. S. Kaplan, *Cancer (Philadelphia)* **42,** 2379 (1978).

15

Studies on the Oncogenicity of Procarbazine and Other Compounds in Nonhuman Primates

R. H. ADAMSON AND S. M. SIEBER

I. Introduction

There is increasing evidence that various groups of cancer patients successfully treated with chemotherapy, with or without irradiation, are at high risk of developing a second primary malignancy (1). Some of these patient groups have been identified for several years and include multiple myeloma patients treated with melphalan (2–8) and long-term survivors of Hodgkin's disease receiving therapy with the nitrogen mustard–vincristine–procarbazine–prednisone (MOPP) regimen (9–14). A possible increased risk in other groups of patients, including those receiving alkylating agent therapy for breast (15–17) or ovarian carcinomas (18–24) and nitrosoureas for central nervous system (CNS) tumors (25), has more

MALIGNANT LYMPHOMAS
ISBN 0-12-597120-6

239

recently been recognized. It appears that acute myelogenous leukemia (AML) is the most frequently occurring second malignant tumor in such patients (26).

There is also evidence that patients receiving long-term immunosuppressive therapy (particularly with azathioprine) for nonmalignant conditions such as renal or cardiac homografts are at risk for tumor development (27–29). Unlike the AML developing in cancer patients receiving chemotherapy, however, the tumors developing in kidney transplant recipients are predominantly lymphomas (28).

The role of chemotherapeutic agents in the etiology of AML in cancer patients and lymphomas in immunosuppressed patients requires clarification. Thus it has been suggested that AML might be part of the natural history of Hodgkin's disease and multiple myeloma which is only becoming apparent because of the increases in survival attributable to chemotherapy (30); furthermore, it has been suggested that the lymphomas in renal homograft recipients might arise indirectly through an azathioprine-induced impairment of the immune surveillance system or from the presence of continuous antigenic stimulation combined with immunosuppression, rather than through a direct carcinogenic effect of azathioprine (1). The issue is a complex one and is confounded because many cancer patients and homograft recipients receive irradiation, a known carcinogen in humans (31–33), in addition to one or more chemotherapeutic agents.

However, the mutagenic effects of most of the clinically useful antitumor agents have been demonstrated both in *in vitro* assay systems such as the Ames test (34) and in the *in vivo* dominant lethal test in rodents (35). Many of these agents have been shown to be carcinogens in standard rodent bioassays (36, 37) and in other experimental situations as well (38, 39). We are evaluating the potential carcinogenicity of selected antitumor and immunosuppressive agents in nonhuman primates, a species of experimental animal relatively close to humans on the phylogenetic scale. The agents under study are procarbazine, 1-methylnitrosourea (MNU), adriamycin, melphalan, azathioprine, and cyclophosphamide, and some of the drugs have been under test for 10 years or longer. An interim report on these ongoing studies is presented below.

II. Methods

A. Animals

The present colony consists of approximately 545 animals, 54 of which are adult breeders which supply the newborn animals for experimental studies. One group of 119 animals is currently being used to evaluate the carcinogenic potential of antitumor agents, and the remaining 372 monkeys are employed in studies on the carcinogenicity of a variety of other chemicals. The monkeys in the former group represent three species (Table I): approximately 50% are *Macaca mulatta* (rhesus), 43% are *Macaca fascicularis* (cynomolgus), and 7% are *Cercopithecus*

TABLE I

Composition of Control Colony and the Group of Monkeys Receiving Antitumor Agents

Group	Number of monkeys[a]				Females (%)
	Rhesus	Cynomolgus	African greens	Total	
Control[b]	91 (41.6)	83 (37.9)	45 (20.5)	219	62
Experimental	93 (49.7)	81 (43.3)	13 (7.0)	187	48

[a] Percentage is indicated in parentheses.
[b] Includes untreated animals, breeders, and vehicle-treated controls.

aethiops (African green) monkeys; 48% of the monkeys are females. Details of maintenance and management procedures, and the method used to rear neonates, have been described elsewhere (40). Newborns produced by the breeding colony are taken within 12 hours of birth to the nursery which is staffed on a 24-hour basis. They receive Similac formula until the age of 6 months and are then maintained on a diet of Purina monkey chow supplemented by half an apple and a vitamin sandwich each day. The vitamin sandwich consists of powdered milk, Parvo (a folic acid supplement obtained from Fox Company, Inc., Broadway, Virginia), Cecon (a vitamin C supplement obtained from Abbott Laboratories, North Chicago, Illinois), and molasses.

The monkeys are housed individually, and various clinical, hematological, and biochemical parameters are monitored to evaluate their general health. Tuberculin skin testing is done at bimonthly intervals. Blood is collected at weekly or biweekly intervals from a femoral vein into heparinized tubes. Routine hematological examinations (hematocrit, red blood cell counts, white blood cell counts, platelet counts, hemoglobin levels, and differential counts) and other clinical tests including those for alkaline phosphatase, total bilirubin, serum glutamic-pyruvic transaminase and serum glutamine-oxaloacetic transaminase are performed in treated and control monkeys. Surgical procedures are performed under phencyclidine hydrochloride, ketamine, or sodium pentobarbital anesthesia. All animals which die or are sacrificed are carefully necropsied, and their tissues subjected to histopathological examination.

The control population is composed of 219 untreated animals, breeders and vehicle-treated monkeys (Table I). They range in age from neonates to older than 18 years. Forty-two percent of the control monkeys are rhesus, 38% are cynomolgus, and 20% African greens; 62% of the monkeys are females.

B. Administration of Test Compounds

Procarbazine hydrochloride was obtained from Hoffman-La Roche, Inc., Nutley, New Jersey, and was used as obtained without further purification. All doses were calculated on the basis of the hydrochloride salt. The drug was kept under refrigeration until immediately prior to use. It was dissolved in distilled water and administered once every week in a volume of 1.0 ml/kg [for subcutaneous (sc) injections], 0.2 ml/kg [for intraperitoneal (ip) injections], or 0.4 ml/kg [for intravenous (iv) injections]; oral (po) doses were incorporated into a vitamin sandwich and given 5 days every week. Dosing with procarbazine began within 1–5 months of birth.

1-Methylnitrosourea was purchased from K & K Laboratories, Plainview, New York, and used as obtained without further purification. It was stored inside a desiccator at $-10°C$ until immediately before use. When given orally, it was mixed with Karo syrup and put on a vitamin sandwich that was immediately fed to the monkeys. The MNU was given orally on a schedule of five consecutive daily doses per week at 10 mg/kg (120 mg/m^2), 20 mg/kg (240 mg/m^2), or 40 mg/kg (480 mg/m^2) with two exceptions. In one case, a monkey received weekly iv injections of MNU (5 mg/kg, 60 mg/m^2) for 57 months and then was given the drug orally (10 mg/kg, 120 mg/m^2) 5 days a week for 30 months. In the other case, the animal received weekly iv (5 mg/kg, 60 mg/m^2) injections of the drug for 58 months and then weekly intraperitoneal (5 mg/kg, 60 mg/m^2) injections for 4 weeks. When injected intraperitoneally or intravenously, MNU was dissolved in isotonic saline. The administration of MNU began within 1 week of birth.

Adriamycin hydrochloride (Adria Laboratories, Inc., Wilmington, Delaware) was dissolved in sterile distilled water immediately before dosing and was injected at doses of 0.2 mg/kg (2.4 mg/m^2), 0.4 mg/kg (4.8 mg/m^2), 1 mg/kg (12 mg/m^2) in a volume of 0.5 ml/kg. The monkeys received monthly iv injections of adriamycin beginning at 2 months of age.

Melphalan was obtained from the Drug Synthesis and Chemistry Branch, Division of Cancer Treatment, National Cancer Institute, NIH, Bethesda, Maryland, and was stored at $-70°C$ until use. Dose solutions were prepared by dissolving the drug in dimethylsulfoxide (DMSO) and were administered by oral intubation immediately after preparation. Melphalan was given at a dose of 0.1 mg/kg (1.2 mg/m^2) daily 5 days every week to monkeys beginning at 2 months of age.

Azathioprine was the gift of Burroughs Wellcome Company, Research Triangle Park, North Carolina, and was used as obtained without further purification. It was suspended in 0.3% hydroxypropyl cellulose and was given to the monkeys daily 5 days every week in prunes. Dosing with azathioprine, at 2.0 mg/kg (24 mg/m^2) and 5.0 mg/kg (60 mg/m^2), began at 2 months after birth.

Cyclophosphamide was supplied by the Drug Synthesis and Chemistry Branch, Division of Cancer Treatment, National Cancer Institute, NIH, Bethesda, Maryland. It was dissolved in distilled water and injected into prunes which were given to the monkeys daily 5 days every week. Monkeys received the first dose of cyclophosphamide (3 mg/kg, 36 mg/m^2) when they were 6–7 months of age, and the dose was increased to 6 mg/kg (72 mg/m^2) when they were 1 year old.

III. Results

Our control colony numbers 219 animals and includes untreated animals, breeder monkeys, and vehicle-treated controls. Ninety of these animals have been necropsied and seven malignant tumors diagnosed, yielding an overall spontaneous tumor incidence of 3.2%. All seven tumors arose in breeder monkeys and included three cases of malignant lymphoma or reticulum cell sarcoma developing in African green monkeys, a gallbladder carcinoma in a 10-year-old rhesus female, a rhabdomyosarcoma in a rhesus female, and two cases of adenocarcinoma of the liver or bile ducts in a rhesus and a cynomolgus monkey, respectively (Table II).

It has long been known that procarbazine is a potent carcinogen in mice and rats (36, 41, 42). Procarbazine is also carcinogenic in nonhuman primates: We reported recently that 11 of 50 monkeys receiving long-term treatment with procarbazine developed malignant neoplasms (43). Since that report was published, an additional 2 monkeys have been diagnosed with tumors, yielding an overall tumor incidence in this group of 26% (Table III). Six of the 13 neoplasms induced by procarbazine were solid tumors, and 7 were acute leukemias. Table IV lists the procarbazine-induced solid tumors, which include 2 hemangioendothelial sarcomas, 1 lymphocytic lymphoma, and 3 osteogenic sarcomas. These tumors developed in monkeys receiving an average cumulative procarbazine dose of 19.82 gm/kg (237.9 gm/m^2), with a range of 8.28–53.6 mg/kg (99.4–

TABLE II

Histological Diagnosis of Tumors in Control Colony

Monkey no.	Species	Sex	Estimated age at diagnosis (years)	Histological diagnosis
378T	African green	M	8	Reticulum cell sarcoma
100X	Rhesus	F	10	Carcinoma, gall bladder
516T	African green	M	12	Diffuse malignant lymphoma
379T	African green	F	13	Diffuse histiocytic lymphoma
413K	Rhesus	F	13	Adenocarcinoma, liver
140T	Rhesus	F	17	Rhabdomyosarcoma
510T	Cynomolgus	M	18	Adenocarcinoma, bile duct

TABLE III

Summary of Control and Procarbazine-Treated Monkeys, 1961–1980

| Group | Alive | Number dead | | Total |
		Without tumor	With tumor[a]	
Procarbazine	9	28	13 (26)	50
Control[b]	129	83	7 (3.2)	219

[a] Percentage is indicated in parentheses.
[b] Includes nontreated animals, breeders, and vehicle-treated controls.

643.2 gm/m^2); they were diagnosed after latent periods ranging from 71 to 148 months (average 98 months).

Table V shows the seven cases of acute leukemia noted after prolonged treatment with procarbazine. Six of the seven leukemias were myelogenous, and one was undifferentiated. The monkeys developing acute leukemia had received a cumulative procarbazine dose averaging 15.81 gm/kg (189.7 gm/m^2), with a range of 0.92–36.0 gm/kg (11.0–432.0 gm/m^2); the latent period for leukemia development (averaging 77 months) was highly variable, ranging between 16 and 143 months. We have not been able to find a correlation between the type of tumor induced and the cumulative dose of procarbazine given or the duration of treatment with this drug. There also does not appear to be a difference in sensitivity between the sexes or among the species.

The chronic nature of the procarbazine study has given us the opportunity to evaluate other long-term adverse effects of this drug in monkeys in addition to oncogenicity (Table VI). The most striking adverse effect noted in the monkeys necropsied after receiving treatment with procarbazine for longer than 1 year has been related to the reproductive system. Thus 68% of the monkeys necropsied to date have shown severe gonadal damage. This damage has been more marked in the males, 86% of which have had the "Sertoli-only syndrome" in which the seminiferous tubules are devoid of spermatogenesis but are lined with normal-appearing Sertoli cells. Gonadal damage in the females has been manifested chiefly as atrophic ovaries containing few, if any, developing follicles. In addition to damage to the reproductive system, 52% of the necropsied animals (excluding those with leukemia) have been found to have bone marrow lesions, such as decreased marrow cellularity and erythromyeloid hyperplasia. The respiratory system was affected in 48% of the animals, with pneumonia and pulmonary edema or hemorrhage being the most frequently noted lesions; approximately one-third of the necropsied animals have had lymphoid depletion of major proportions, and 27% have shown liver damage such as fatty degeneration and centrolobular necrosis.

TABLE IV

Solid Tumors Induced in Monkeys by Procarbazine

Monkey no.	Species	Sex	Dose, route, and months dosed[a]	Total dose (gm/m²)[b]	Latent period (months)[c]	Tumor diagnosed
734I	Rhesus	M	120–240 mg/m² ip (62 months), then 5 months po	99.4	71	Hemangioendothelial sarcoma, kidney
731I	Rhesus	F	120–240 mg/m² ip (63 months), then 5 months po	100.9	68	Osteosarcoma, humerus
314E	Cynomolgus	F	60–600 mg/m² sc (35 months), then 62 months po	137.0	97	Hemangiosarcoma, spleen
315E	Cynomolgus	M	60–600 mg/m² sc (35 months), then 63 months po	209.1	98	Lymphocytic lymphoma
333E	Cynomolgus	F	120–600 mg/m² sc (33 months), then 70 months po	237.7	103	Osteosarcoma, jaw
557G	Cynomolgus	F	120–600 mg/m² sc (7 months), then 140 months po	643.2	148	Osteosarcoma, humerus

[a] The sc and ip doses were given once a week; po doses (120 mg/m²) were given daily 5 days/week.
[b] The average total dose was 237.0 gm/m².
[c] The latent period was the number of months from the first dose to the diagnosis of tumor. The average latent period was 98 months.

TABLE V

Acute Leukemias Induced in Monkeys by Procarbazine

Monkey no.	Species	Sex	Dose, route, and months dosed[a]	Total dose (gm/m²)[b]	Latent period (months)[c]	Type of leukemia
267D	Rhesus	F	600 mg/m² sc (15 months), then 1 month po	11.0	16	Myelogenous
733I	Cynomolgus	M	240 mg/m² ip (57 months)	30.4	57	Undifferentiated
726I	Cynomolgus	M	240 mg/m² ip (68 months)	67.7	68	Myelogenous
313E	Rhesus	F	60–600 mg/m² sc (35 months), then 33 months po	155.2	68	Myelogenous
567G	Rhesus	F	120–300 mg/m² sc (6 months), then 71 months po	208.3	77	Myelogenous
13T	Rhesus	M	300–600 mg/m² sc (36 months), then 73 months po	423.5	109	Myelogenous
336E	Rhesus	F	120–600 mg/m² sc (33 months), then 110 months po	432.0	143	Myelogenous

[a] The sc and ip doses were given once a week; po doses (120 mg/m²) were given daily 5 days/week.
[b] The average total dose was 189.7 gm/m².
[c] The latent period was the number of months from the first dose to the diagnosis of leukemia. The average latent period was 77 months.

TABLE VI

Necropsy Findings in Monkeys Treated with Procarbazine[a]

Organ or tissue	Monkeys affected (%)	Example
Gonads	68	Sertoli cell-only syndrome, atrophic ovaries
Bone marrow	52	Erythromyeloid hyperplasia and/or atrophy
Lungs	48	Bronchopneumonia, interstitial fibrosis
Lymphoid	32	Lymphocytes absent from germinal centers
Liver	27	Centrolobular necrosis, fatty degeneration

[a] Surviving longer than 6 months after the first dose of procarbazine; monkeys were treated for periods up to 12 years and received total doses of procarbazine ranging from 0.6 to 59.2 gm/kg (7.3–710.1 gm/m²).

Nine monkeys are currently being treated with procarbazine (10 mg/kg, 120 mg/m², 5 days every week) by the oral route. All monkeys have received total doses of procarbazine exceeding the average total dose ingested by the 13 monkeys developing malignant neoplasms. None of the animals have developed clinical signs of illness, although 3 of the monkeys have been anemic (hemoglobin < 10 gm%, hematocrit < 34 ml%) and/or leukopenic (white blood cell count <4000 cells/mm³) for prolonged periods.

1-Methylnitrosourea is a potent carcinogen in several species of laboratory animals (44–47), and we recently reported that this compound induced squamous cell carcinomas of the esophagus in 5 of a total of 43 monkeys treated by the oral route (48). Since that report was published, 4 additional monkeys have developed malignant tumors (Table VII), yielding an overall tumor incidence of 20.9%. All the tumors induced by MNU have been squamous cell carcinomas (Table VIII), and in every case the tumor has been located at one or more sites along the esophagus. In addition, some of the monkeys have developed squamous cell carcinomas at other locations in the upper digestive tract such as the pharynx, soft palate, tongue, and buccal mucosa, as well as squamous metaplasia and squamous papillomas of the tongue and buccal mucosa. The clinical manifestations of the esophageal tumors included difficulty in swallowing, frequent vomiting and subsequent weight loss, and sialorrhea; regurgitation, aspiration, sepsis, and hemorrhage were frequently encountered complications of tumor growth.

A rough parallel has been observed between the cumulative MNU dose ingested and the degree of esophageal damage found at necropsy of the treated

TABLE VII

Summary of Control and 1-Methylnitrosourea-treated Monkeys, 1961–1980

| | | Number dead | | |
| | | | | |
Group	Alive	Without tumor	With tumor[a]	Total
MNU	25	9	9 (20.9)	43
Control[b]	129	83	7 (3.2)	219

[a] Percentage is indicated in parentheses.
[b] Includes nontreated animals, breeders, and vehicle-treated controls.

monkeys (Table IX). No esophageal lesions were found in two monkeys that had ingested an average of 5.32 gm/kg (63.8 gm/m^2) MNU for a period averaging 26 months, whereas esophagitis accompanied by candidiasis and chronic inflammatory infiltrates was noted in the esophageal mucosa of two monkeys receiving an average of 6.9 gm/kg (82.9 gm/m^2) of MNU for an average of 58 months. In five monkeys that were necropsied after having ingested an average of 16.46 gm/kg (197.5 gm/m^2) of MNU for an average of 54 months, esophageal lesions were more severe and included esophageal epithelial atrophy, hyper- or dyskeratosis, and dysplasia. The nine monkeys with squamous cell carcinomas of the esophagus had received MNU for an average of 93 months (range 63–133 months); during this period they had ingested an average cumulative MNU dose of 41.67 gm/kg (500 gm/m^2), with a range of 18.48–62.72 gm/kg (221.7–752.7 gm/m^2). Only one monkey receiving in excess of 18.48 gm/kg of MNU was found at necropsy to be without a carcinoma; this monkey had ingested 69.93 gm/kg (839.2 gm/m^2) of MNU over the course of 124 months, and histopathological examination of sections of esophagus revealed chronic esophagitis and extensive esophageal dysplasia.

Twenty-five monkeys continue to receive oral doses of MNU (10 mg/kg, 120 mg/m^2) 5 days every week. The monkeys are observed daily and weighed every week. When lesions of the tongue, cheek pouch, or buccal mucosa are noted, they are biopsied. If clinical evidence of tumor becomes apparent, the upper digestive tract is examined radiographically following a barium swallow. Recently attempts have been initiated to treat the MNU-induced lesions and/or tumors of the upper digestive tract with bleomycin and other agents, but these attempts have met with limited success.

An evaluation of the carcinogenic potential of adriamycin was initiated approximately 6 years ago in a group of 10 monkeys. It was originally planned to administer 30 doses of adriamycin at 1 mg/kg (12 mg/m^2) to a cumulative dose of 30 mg/kg (360 mg/m^2); when this total dose was attained, the monkeys were to be held under observation for the remainder of their lives. However, a monkey died with acute clinical signs of congestive heart failure (ascites, periorbital edema, and rapid and labored respiration) after receiving 26 doses of adriamycin (26 mg/kg, 312 mg/m^2). Dosing of all monkeys in this group was terminated approximately 1 month later, but in the following 2 months 5 more monkeys developed congestive heart failure and died, and 2 additional monkeys died 3 and 4 months later, respectively. Necropsy of all 8 animals revealed similar cardiac changes. Grossly, the hearts of these monkeys were enlarged and flabby, and

TABLE VIII

Tumors in Monkeys Receiving 1-Methylnitrosourea by the Oral Route[a]

Monkey no.	Species	Sex	Total dose (gm/m^2)	Latent period (months)[b]	Histological diagnosis[c]
617H	Cynomolgus	M	221.7	63	SCA, pharynx and esophagus with invasion of mediastinal lymph nodes; squamous metaplasia, trachea
622H	Rhesus	F	273.9	57	SCA, soft palate, tongue, and esophagus with invasion into stomach
539G	Rhesus	F	450.6	72	SCA, mouth; SCA in situ, pharynx; squamous papillomas, tongue, pharynx, and esophagus; dyskeratosis, esophageal mucosa
540G	Rhesus	M	538.7	83	SCA, mouth and esophagus; squamous papilloma and hyperkeratosis, buccal mucosa; SCA, esophagus
627H	Rhesus	M	541.3	133	SCA, esophagus
538H	Rhesus	M	557.5	72	SCA, mouth, pharynx, and esophagus; multiple squamous papillomas, pharynx and esophagus
569G	African green	M	571.7	124	SCA, mouth, pharynx, and esophagus
624H	Rhesus	F	593.0	129	SCA, gingiva and esophagus
579G	Rhesus	M	752.7	107	SCA, mouth and esophagus

[a] MNU (10–20 mg/kg, 120–240 mg/m^2) was incorporated into a vitamin sandwich and given daily five times every week; dosing was initiated within 1 week of birth.

[b] The latent period was the time in months from the first dose of MNU until the clinical diagnosis of tumor.

[c] SCA, Squamous cell carcinoma.

TABLE IX

Esophageal Lesions Found at Necropsy in Nonhuman Primates Given
1-Methylnitrosourea[a]

Number of monkeys	Average total dose (gm/m²)	Months dosed	Esophageal pathology
2	63.8	26	None
2	82.9	58	Esophagitis, candidiasis
5	197.5	54	Hyper- or dyskeratosis
9	500.0	93	Squamous cell carcinoma

[a] MNU (10–20 mg/kg, 120–240 mg/m²) was given orally 5 days/week.

pericardial and pleural effusions were present. Histologically, sections of myocardium showed extensive microvacuolar degeneration of myocardial fibers with marked nuclear hypertrophy. The myocardial lesions were characterized by focal degeneration of myocardial fibers, edema, and interstitial fibrosis. These monkeys had received an average cumulative adriamycin dose of 25.8 mg/kg (310 mg/m²) divided over 23–27 monthly doses (Table X). Another monkey was sacrificed because of marked weight loss and anorexia of approximately 5 weeks duration. Although no specific abnormalities were noted at necropsy of this monkey except for enlarged mesenteric lymph nodes, histological examination of sections of bone marrow showed that it was almost completely replaced by anaplastic cells with scanty cytoplasm and irregular nuclei, some of which appeared to be differentiating toward the granulocytic series. The histological appearance of the marrow was consistent with a diagnosis of acute myeloblastic leukemia. This animal had received a cumulative adriamycin dose of 27 mg/kg (324 mg/m²), and the leukemia was diagnosed 2 months after the last dose of adriamycin. The tenth monkey in this series is alive and without evidence of

TABLE X

Effects of Adriamycin in Monkeys–Summary of First Study[a]

Number of monkeys	Number of doses	Average total dose (mg/m²)[b]	Cause of death
8	23–27	310 (276–336)	Congestive heart failure
1	27	324	Acute myeloblastic leukemia
1	25	300	Alive

[a] Monkeys were given monthly iv doses of adriamycin (1 mg/kg, 12 mg/m²) beginning at 2 months of age.
[b] Range is indicated in parentheses.

TABLE XI

Summary of Monkeys Currently Receiving Adriamycin[a]

Number of monkeys	Dose (mg/m²)	Months dosed	Average total dose (mg/m²)
10	2.4	21	110
10	4.8	14	132

[a] As of 8/80. Monkeys are given monthly iv injections of adriamycin beginning at 2 months of age.

illness; it received 25 injections of adriamycin (25 mg/kg, 300 mg/m²), the last of which was administered 38 months ago (49).

We are currently repeating this study, using two groups of 10 monkeys each (Table XI); the monkeys are receiving monthly intravenous injections of adriamycin at 0.2 mg/kg (2.4 mg/m²) and 0.4 mg/kg (4.8 mg/m²), and dosing will be terminated when they have received a cumulative adriamycin dose of 20 mg/kg (240 mg/m²). To date, the monkeys receiving adriamycin at 2.4 and 4.8 mg/m² have been given cumulative drug doses of 9.2 mg/kg (110 mg/m²) and 11 mg/kg (132 mg/m²), respectively. None of the monkeys have as yet developed signs of congestive heart failure or other indications of ill health.

The carcinogenic potential of melphalan is being evaluated in 20 monkeys receiving the drug at a dose of 0.1 mg/kg (1.2 mg/m²) orally, 5 days every week (Table XII). The first group of 10 monkeys was put on test 64 months ago and since that time have ingested an average cumulative melphalan dose of 4.96 gm/kg (59.5 gm/m²). The second group of 10 monkeys was put on test 10 months later, and the average cumulative melphalan dose ingested by this group is 4.38 gm/kg (52.6 gm/m²). None of the 20 monkeys receiving melphalan have as yet died, and none have as yet demonstrated any clinical signs of ill health.

Two groups of monkeys are being given azathioprine orally, 5 days every week (Table XIII). A group of 14 monkeys has been receiving the compound at

TABLE XII

Summary of Melphalan-Treated Monkeys[a]

Number of monkeys	Months dosed	Average total dose (gm)	Average total dose (gm/m²)
10	54	4.38	52.6
10	64	4.96	59.5

[a] As of 8/80. Monkeys are dosed with melphalan (0.1 mg/kg, 1.2 mg/m²) orally, 5 days every week.

TABLE XIII

Summary of Azathioprine-Treated Monkeys[a]

Dose (mg/m^2)	Number of monkeys	Average total dose (gm/m^2)[b]	Average months dosed[b]
24	14	18.24 (4.32–20.64)	38 (9–43)
60	10	33.60 (30.0–34.80)	28 (25–29)

[a] As of 8/80. Monkeys are dosed with azathioprine orally, 5 days every week.
[b] Range is indicated in parentheses.

2.0 mg/kg (24 mg/m^2) for an average of 38 months (range 9–43 months); during this period they have received a cumulative azathioprine dose averaging 18.24 gm/m^2 (range 4.32–20.64 gm/m^2). A second group of 10 monkeys began receiving azathioprine (5.0 mg/kg, 60 mg/m^2) an average of 28 months ago (range 25–29 months); these monkeys have ingested to date an average of 33.6 gm/m^2 of azathioprine (range 30.0–34.8 gm/m^2). None of the monkeys at the 60-mg/m^2 dose have been necropsied. One monkey receiving the 24-mg/m^2 dose died after having received a total of 0.24 gm of azathioprine over the course of 4 months and is not included in Table XIII. No specific abnormalities were found at necropsy of this animal, although histopathological examination of tissue revealed moderate fatty changes in the liver. The remaining monkeys receiving azathioprine appear healthy and are without clinical signs of ill health.

A study of the potential carcinogenicity of cyclophosphamide was recently initiated (Table XIV). A group of 20 monkeys are receiving cyclophosphamide orally 5 days every week. Dosing (at 3 mg/kg, 36 mg/m^2) begins when the monkeys are 6 months old, and the dose is increased to 6 mg/kg (72 mg/m^2) when the monkeys are 1 year old. The study has been underway for an average of only 4 months; during this period an average cumulative cyclophosphamide dose

TABLE XIV

Summary of Cyclophosphamide-Treated Monkeys[a]

Number of monkeys	Average total dose (gm/m^2)[b]	Average months dosed[b,c]
20	3.24 (0.18–9.36)	4 (0.25–9)

[a] Monkeys are dosed with cyclophosphamide orally, 5 days every week. Dosing (3 mg/kg, 36 mg/m^2) begins at 6 months of age; at 12 months of age, the dose is increased to 6 mg/kg (72 mg/m^2).
[b] Range is indicated in parentheses.
[c] As of 10/80.

of 3.24 gm/m² (range 0.18–9.36 gm/m²) has been administered. Thus far, none of the monkeys have died, and there is no evidence of toxicity on this dosage schedule.

IV. Discussion

Antineoplastic agents are being used with progressively increasing success in treating human cancer; indeed, in some types of malignancies such as Hodgkin's disease, childhood acute lymphoblastic leukemia, Burkitt's lymphoma, choriocarcinoma and Ewing's sarcoma, modern therapy has produced apparent "cures" in a significant proportion of patients. Antitumor and immunosuppressive agents also appear to be attaining a role in the treatment of nonmalignant conditions including chronic glomerulonephritis, rheumatoid arthritis, and psoriasis, and they are being used to treat these disorders with increasing frequency. Therefore, as the survival of cancer patients is extended and as the tendency to use antitumor agents in nonmalignant conditions increases, our understanding of the long-term adverse effects of these drugs will also increase. One such effect which has been recognized relatively recently is the potential carcinogenicity of antineoplastic and immunosuppressive agents (1).

Most of the clinically useful cancer chemotherapeutic agents are mutagenic *in vivo* (35, 50) and *in vitro* (34) and are carcinogenic in the rodent bioassay (36, 50). However, results from rodent carcinogenesis studies are difficult to extrapolate to the human situation for a number of reasons, not the least of which is the high incidence of spontaneous tumors in rodent populations used in such testing (36). Yet information on the carcinogenic potential of antineoplastic and immunosuppressive agents in humans is urgently needed, because of the apparent increased risk of second malignant primary tumors in successfully treated cancer patients and because of the increasing use of such drugs in nonmalignant conditions and as adjuvants to surgery in forms of cancer potentially curable by surgery alone.

We are evaluating the long-term toxic effects of several of these drugs, including their carcinogenicity. Our studies are being carried out in nonhuman primates because of their phylogenetic proximity to humans, their longer lifespans, and their low spontaneous tumor incidence. The choice of nonhuman primates as the test species was fortuitous, since their relatively large size has enabled us to carry out various serial clinical tests and procedures (e.g., endoscopy, diagnostic radiography, biopsies of bone marrow and other tissue, and hematological examinations) which would be difficult to perform in smaller animals. The relatively long lifespan of the nonhuman primate has also allowed the administration of test chemicals at doses and according to schedules that are encountered clinically, and with the exception of procarbazine all the drugs have been tested under conditions which parallel human exposures. However, cancer patients frequently receive combinations of drugs with or without irradiation, whereas in the present study we have chosen to evaluate the potential carcinogenicity of individual agents.

Our study of procarbazine has indicated that the drug is both leukemogenic and oncogenic in monkeys. About one-half of the malignancies produced by procarbazine were AML, a finding which may be relevant to the relatively high risk for acute leukemia noted in Hodgkin's disease patients treated successfully with the MOPP regimen (9–14). However, the relationship between acute leukemia and treatment with the MOPP regimen is not clear-cut. Other components of the MOPP regimen, particularly nitrogen mustard, may also have leukemogenic potential. It should be noted that Hodgkin's disease patients frequently receive intensive radiotherapy, a known leukemogen in humans (31, 32), in addition to chemotherapeutic agents. That one-half of the solid tumors induced by procarbazine were osteogenic sarcomas is of interest. To our knowledge, there is only one case report in which procarbazine exposure was associated with the development of osteosarcoma. In this case the patient received several single chemotherapeutic agents, including procarbazine, and multiple courses of radiotherapy for Hodgkin's disease; 10 years after therapy for Hodgkin's disease was instituted, acute myeloblastic leukemia and osteogenic sarcoma were diagnosed, both within a period of 6 months (51). The cumulative procarbazine dose ingested by the patient was approximately 111 gm/m^2; as a point of comparison, the three osteogenic sarcomas noted in the present study developed after cumulative procarbazine doses of 100.9, 237.7, and 643.2 gm/m^2, respectively. Although the total dose of procarbazine ingested by the monkeys developing malignancies in this study was generally higher than that likely to be given a Hodgkin's disease patient receiving MOPP therapy, nevertheless it is clear that procarbazine is carcinogenic in nonhuman primates and that it may be responsible for inducing second malignant tumors in Hodgkin's disease patients.

1-Methylnitrosourea is also a carcinogen in nonhuman primates; when given orally it produced a relatively high incidence of squamous cell carcinoma of the esophagus, pharynx, and oral cavity. Although not currently employed as a cancer chemotherapeutic agent in the United States, clinical tests in the USSR indicate that it has activity against Hodgkin's disease and lung tumors (52). In addition, treatment with the nitrosoureas 1-(2-chloroethyl)-3-cyclohexyl-1-nitrosourea (CCNU) and methyl-CCNU has been associated with the development of acute leukemia in two patients with brain tumors (25). The results of the present study indicate that nitrosoureas as a class may be potential carcinogens in humans.

The results of our first study on the carcinogenicity of adriamycin provided some preliminary evidence for the leukemogenicity of this drug (49). One out of a total of 10 monkeys developed acute myeloblastic leukemia. Since 8 of the monkeys died of congestive heart failure before the end of the dosing period, a marked carcinogenic effect of the drug would have been obscured by the shortened survival of the animals. The study is therefore being repeated using a lower, and presumably noncardiotoxic, dose. Although adriamycin is carcinogenic in rats, the tumors it induces in this species are primarily mammary fibroadenomas and adenocarcinomas (53). To date, there has been only one instance in which adriamycin therapy was associated with the development of a second malignant neoplasm in humans. A patient received a cumulative adriamycin dose of 450 mg/m^2 as treatment for endometrial carcinoma and subsequently developed AML (54). However, the relationship between adriamycin and the development of leukemia was not clear-cut, as the patient had also received pelvic irradiation and a total of 12.6 gm of cyclophosphamide.

None of the remaining drugs under test have as yet shown any evidence of carcinogenicity. Melphalan increases the incidence of pulmonary tumors in mice (37), raises the number of lung tumor nodules per mouse from a control level of 0.5 to 4.5 (55), and produces peritoneal sarcomas in the CD rat (36). However, none of the monkeys in the present study have developed a malignancy despite their having received a cumulative drug dose ranging between 52 and 60 gm/m^2. By way of comparison, women receiving prophylactic melphalan therapy for ovarian carcinoma would ingest in the prescribed 18-month dosing period a total dose of 660 mg/m^2 (56), a dose some 100-fold lower than that already ingested by these monkeys. Thus it appears that if melphalan is a carcinogen in monkeys, the latent period required for its carcinogenic effects to become manifest is in excess of 5 years.

Similarly, both azathioprine (38) and cyclophosphamide (36, 37, 55) have demonstrated carcinogenic effects in rodents. Treatment with these drugs has not as yet resulted in the development of malignant neoplasms in nonhuman primates, although the drugs have been under test for a relatively short time. The azathioprine study has been underway for only about 3 years, and the cyclophosphamide study was initiated less than a year ago. Since the latent period for tumor induction by procarbazine and MNU has averaged 86 and 93 months, respectively, it is too early to assess the carcinogenic potential of either azathioprine or cyclophosphamide in nonhuman primates.

In conclusion, studies on the carcinogenic potential of clinically useful antineoplastic and immunosuppressive agents are imperative. This need arises not only because of epidemiological findings that point to an elevated risk for second malignant neoplasms in some groups of successfully treated cancer patients but also because of the increasing use of these agents as adjuvants to surgery in forms of cancer potentially curable by surgery alone, as well as in various nonmalignant conditions. Carcinogenesis studies in rodents are useful, but the results are difficult to extrapolate to humans. Nonhuman primate carcinogenesis studies are expensive and time-consuming, and the drugs studied in this system should be chosen with care. However, monkeys are phylogenetically closer to humans than rodents; their longer life-span and greater size make it possible to mimic human exposures and to carry out useful clinical tests and procedures. Based on the results of our studies with procarbazine, an observation of great potential significance is that nonhuman primates appear to resemble humans in the type of tumor that develops following exposure to a carcinogen.

Even if epidemiological surveys and carcinogenesis studies such as ours implicate an antitumor agent as being a human carcinogen, the clinician should not be dissuaded from using the drug in patients with cancer. However, this information should be used to caution physicians against employing antitumor agents for treating diseases in which, without the drug, survival would be relatively normal; furthermore, it should stimulate the search for antineoplastic agents with equal efficacy but diminished carcinogenic potential.

References

1. S. M. Sieber and R. H. Adamson, *Adv. Cancer Res.* **22,** 57 (1975).
2. J. M. Holt, A. H. T. Robb-Smith, S. T. Callender, and A. I. Spriggs, *Br. J. Haematol.* **22,** 633 (1972).
3. N. Marcovic, B.-G. Hansson, and J. Hallen, *Scand. J. Haematol.* **12,** 32 (1974).
4. C. Marsan, P. Henon, A. Quillard, A. Grimaldi, C. Cywiner-Golenzer, F. Adotti, A. Dryll, and J. Roujean, *Nouv. Presse Med.* **2,** 2958 (1973).
5. I. P. Law, H. S. Plovnick, and D. G. Beddow, *N. Engl. J. Med.* **294,** 164 (1976).
6. F. Gonzalez, J. M. Trujillo, and R. Alexanian, *Ann. Intern. Med.* **86,** 440 (1977).
7. D. Dubrovsky and P. Jacob, *Lancet* **1,** 1113 (1974).
8. F. Clement, *Schweiz. Med. Wochenschr.* **109,** 544 (1979).
9. J. C. Arseneau, R. W. Sponzo, D. L. Levin, L. E. Schnipper, H. Bonner, R. C. Young, G. P. Canellos, R. E. Johnson, and V. T. DeVita, *N. Engl. J. Med.* **287,** 1119 (1972).
10. P. L. Weiden, K. G. Lerner, A. Gerdes, J. D. Heywood, A. Fefer, and E. D. Thomas, *Blood* **42,** 571 (1971).
11. G. Bonadonna, M. De Lena, A. Banfi, and A. Lattuada, *N. Engl. J. Med.* **288,** 1242 (1973).
12. J. C. Arseneau, G. P. Canellos, V. T. DeVita, and R. J. Sherins, *Ann. N.Y. Acad. Sci.* **230,** 481 (1974).
13. C. N. Coleman, C. J. Williams, A. Flint, E. J. Glatstein, S. A. Rosenberg, and H. S. Kaplan, *N. Engl. J. Med.* **297,** 1249 (1977).
14. F. Rosner and H. Grünwald, *Am. J. Med.* **58,** 339 (1975).
15. F. Rosner, R. W. Carey, and M. H. Zarrabi, *Am. J. Hematol.* **4,** 151 (1978).
16. H. J. Lerner, *Cancer Treat. Rep.* **62,** 1135 (1978).
17. M. A. Portugal, H. C. Falkson, R. Stevens, and G. Falkson, *Cancer Treat. Rep.* **63,** 177 (1979).
18. M. R. Shetty and R. Freel, *Gynecol. Oncol.* **7,** 264 (1979).
19. R. R. Reimer, R. Hoover, J. F. Fraumeni, Jr., and R. C. Young, *N. Engl. J. Med.* **297,** 177 (1977).
20. K. Foucar, R. W. McKenna, C. D. Bloomfield, T. K. Bowers, and R. D. Brunning, *Cancer* **43,** 1295 (1979).
21. N. Einhorn, *Cancer* **41,** 444 (1978).

22. H. D. Preisler and G. H. Lyman, *Am. J. Hematol.* **3**, 209 (1977).
23. G. Sotrel, K. Jafari, A. F. Lash, and R. C. Stepto, *Obstet. Gynecol. (N.Y.)* **47**, Suppl., 675 (1976).
24. J. Morrison and J. L. Yon, *Gynecol. Oncol.* **6**, 115 (1978).
25. R. J. Cohen, P. H. Wiernik, and M. D. Walker, *Cancer Chemother. Rep.* **60**, 1257 (1976).
26. R. H. Adamson and S. M. Sieber, *Environ. Health Perspect.* **39**, 93 (1981).
27. P. Littman and C. C. Wang, *Cancer* **35**, 1412 (1975).
28. I. Penn, *Transplant Proc.* **9**, 1121 (1977).
29. J. G. Krikorian, J. L. Anderson, C. P. Bieber, I. Penn, and E. B. Stinson, *JAMA, J. Am. Med. Assoc.* **240**, 639 (1978).
30. S. M. Sieber, *Med. Pediatr. Oncol.* **3**, 123 (1977).
31. E. E. Pochin, *Br. Med. J.* **2**, 1545 (1960).
32. P. G. Smith and R. Doll, *Br. J. Radiol.* **49**, 224 (1976).
33. C. K. Wanebo, K. G. Johnson, K. Sato, and T. W. Thorslund, *N. Engl. J. Med.* **279**, 667 (1968).
34. J. McCann, E. Choi, E. Yamasaki, and B. N. Ames, *Proc. Natl. Acad. Sci. U.S.A.* **72**, 5135 (1975).
35. S. S. Epstein, E. Arnold, J. Andrea, W. Bass, and Y. Bishop, *Toxicol. Appl. Pharmacol.* **23**, 288 (1972).
36. J. H. Weisburger, D. P. Griswold, J. D. Prejean, A. E. Casey, H. B. Wood, and E. K. Weisburger, *Recent Results Cancer Res.* **52**, 1 (1975).
37. M. B. Shimkin, J. H. Weisburger, E. K. Weisburger, N. Gubareff, and V. Suntzeff, *JNCI, J. Natl. Cancer Inst.* **36**, 915 (1966).
38. T. P. Casey, *Clin. Exp. Immunol.* **3**, 305 (1968).
39. A. C. Griffin, E. L. Brandt, and E. L. Tatum, *JAMA, J. Am. Med. Assoc.* **144**, 571 (1949).
40. R. H. Adamson, *in* "Medical Primatology" (E. I. Goldsmith and J. Moor-Jankowski, eds.), Part III, p. 216. Karger, Basel, 1972.
41. M. G. Kelly, R. W. O'Gara, K. Gadekar, S. T. Yancey, and V. T. Oliverio, *Cancer Chemother. Rep.* **39**, 77 (1964).
42. M. G. Kelly, R. W. O'Gara, S. T. Yancey, and C. Botkin, *JNCI, J. Natl. Cancer Inst.* **40**, 1027 (1968).
43. S. M. Sieber, P. Correa, D. W. Dalgard, and R. H. Adamson, *Cancer Res.* **38**, 2125 (1978).
44. M. G. Kelly, R. W. O'Gara, S. T. Yancey, and C. Botkin, *JNCI, J. Natl. Cancer Inst.* **41**, 619 (1968).
45. H. Druckrey, S. Ivankovic, and R. Preussmann, *Naturwissenschaften* **51**, 144 (1964).
46. D. D. Leaver, P. F. Swann, and P. N. Magee, *Br. J. Cancer* **23**, 177 (1969).
47. J. V. Frei, *Chem.-Biol. Interact.* **3**, 117 (1971).
48. R. H. Adamson, F. J. Krowlikowski, P. Correa, S. M. Sieber, and D. W. Dalgard, *JNCI, J. Natl. Cancer Inst.* **59**, 415 (1977).
49. S. M. Sieber, P. Correa, D. M. Young, D. W. Dalgard, and R. H. Adamson, *Pharmacology* **20**, 9 (1980).
50. S. M. Sieber and R. H. Adamson, *Collect. Pap. Annu. Symp. Fundam. Cancer Res.* **27**, 401 (1975).
51. K. W. Chan, D. R. Miller, and C. T. C. Tan, *Med. Pediatr. Oncol.* **8**, 143 (1980).
52. N. M. Emanuel, E. M. Vermel, L. A. Ostrovskaya, and N. P. Korman, *Cancer Chemother. Rep.* **58**, 135 (1974).
53. C. Bertazzoli, T. Chieli, and E. Solcia, *Experientia* **27**, 1209 (1971).
54. R. R. Reimer and C. W. Groppe, *N. Engl. J. Med.* **90**, 989 (1979).
55. E. K. Weisburger, *Public Health Rep.* **81**, 772 (1966).
56. V. T. DeVita, T. H. Wasserman, R. C. Young, and S. K. Carter, *Cancer* **38**, 509 (1976).

16

Secondary Leukemia
and Non-Hodgkin's Lymphoma
in Patients Treated
for Hodgkin's Disease

C. NORMAN COLEMAN, JEROME S. BURKE, ANNA VARGHESE,
SAUL A. ROSENBERG, AND HENRY S. KAPLAN

I. Introduction

Leukemia and non-Hodgkin's lymphoma occurring in patients treated for, and often cured of, Hodgkin's disease have been the subject of recent reports from our institution (1–3) and from others (4–16). Leukemia appears to be a treatment-related complication, since it occurs predominantly in the subset of patients treated with both radiotherapy and chemotherapy (1, 5–9, 13–15). In our previous study on 680 patients no cases of leukemia occurred in patients treated with either chemotherapy or radiotherapy alone, whereas those given both modalities had a 3.9% actuarial risk of leukemia at 7 years (1). Similarly, in a group of 579 patients from our institution the 7-year actuarial risk of developing secondary non-Hodgkin's lymphoma was 2.3% in the subset of patients given combined treatment, with no cases occurring in patients given a single modality.

In July 1968, we began routinely to perform staging laparotomies and to incorporate chemotherapy consisting of mechlorethamine, vincristine, and procarbazine, with or without prednisone (MOPP) (17) into our treatment protocols. Since then almost 1100 previously untreated patients have received primary therapy for Hodgkin's disease at Stanford University Medical Center. This article will discuss the secondary leukemias and lymphomas occurring in these patients.

II. Materials and Methods

One thousand ninety-six previously untreated patients with all stages of Hodgkin's disease were evaluated and treated at Stanford University Medical Center in the period from July 1, 1968 to December 31, 1979. Details of staging and of radiotherapy technique have been described elsewhere (18). Adjuvant chemotherapy, consisting either of MOPP (17) or procarbazine, Alkeran, and vinblastine (PAVe) (19) is defined in this study as chemotherapy administered as part of the initial planned therapy. Radiotherapy usually preceded chemotherapy, but in some settings therapy was initiated with drug therapy or the chemotherapy and radiotherapy were alternated. Salvage chemotherapy was that given for relapse and consisted predominantly of MOPP, with adriamycin-containing combinations reserved for patients whose disease recurred after MOPP therapy.

Radiation therapy is usually given to one or more of three major anatomic regions—the mantle, the paraaortic nodes and splenic pedicle, and the pelvis. In certain clinical situations radiation therapy may also be delivered to the Waldeyer's field, the lungs, or the liver (18). Limited radiotherapy is defined as that given to lymphoid tissues on one side of the diaphragm only; subtotal lymphoid irradiation consists of treatment given to the mantle and to the paraaortic nodes and splenic pedicle but not the pelvis; total lymphoid radiotherapy treats all three anatomical regions. Some patients received liver irradiation in the form of intravenous injection of 25–40 mCi of colloidal gold (^{198}Au) in divided doses (18). This was in fact systemic therapy and often resulted in a transient lowering of the blood count.

For analysis patients have been divided into five major treatment groups: (1) radiotherapy alone; (2) radiotherapy and adjuvant chemotherapy (some patients later had further chemotherapy for relapse); (3) radiotherapy with chemotherapy for relapse (salvage chemotherapy); (4) radiotherapy and colloidal gold, with or without chemotherapy; and (5) chemotherapy alone. Acturial survival data are calculated by the method of Kaplan and Meier (20). Statistical analysis is performed by the method of Gehan (21).

III. Pathology

In 14 of the 19 patients with Hodgkin's disease who developed secondary leukemia, a preleukemic syndrome manifested primarily by peripheral cytopenia was observed. Thrombocytopenia represented the most consistent initial hematological abnormality and was often associated with giant platelets in the peripheral blood films. Normochromic, normocytic anemia was frequent, and nucleated red cells and macrocytes were common. Immature granulocytes averaging approximately 5% were present in the majority of the peripheral blood films and included both promyelocytes and myeloblasts.

Initial bone marrow studies generally revealed hypercellularity and dysplasia of all three main hematopoietic cell lines (Fig. 1). Dyserythropoiesis was the most prominent feature in the marrow, with numerous clusters of megaloblastoid erythroblasts replacing the normal hematopoietic elements (Fig. 2). Megakaryocytes were often increased in number and were atypical in appearance. There was usually increased reticulin. Although cells of the myeloid series were often less prominent than dysplastic erythroid and megakaryocytic cells in the initial marrow specimen, this series also showed altered maturation. Subsequent marrow examinations revealed increasing numbers of immature myeloid cells and a concomitant decrease in dysplastic erythrocytes and megakaryocytes. With the exception of three recently diagnosed patients, all patients eventually

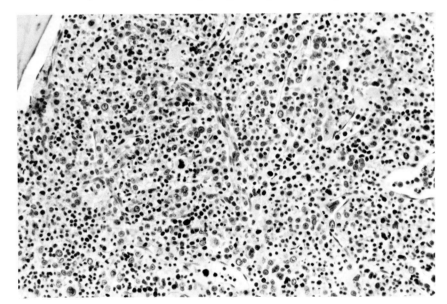

Fig. 1. Bone marrow biopsy demonstrating hypercellularity due to hematopoietic dysplasia. ×192.

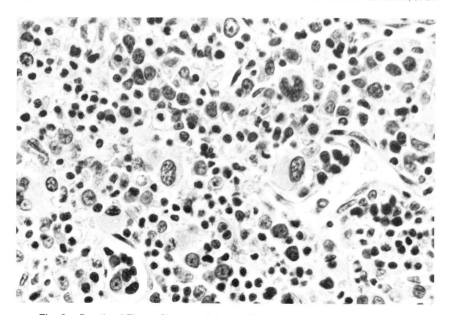

Fig. 2. Details of Fig. 1. Clusters of dysplastic erythrocytes predominate. ×480.

developed overt acute myeloid leukemia from 1 to 12 months following the onset of pancytopenia. In one patient the leukemia was not evident until a study of postmortem tissues. The remaining patients in the series presented with acute myeloid or undifferentiated blastic leukemia without a documented preleukemic phase.

Among the eight patients with Hodgkin's disease who developed secondary non-Hodgkin's lymphoma, five were classified as diffuse, small noncleaved (diffuse, undifferentiated) and three as large-cell (histiocytic) lymphoma (22, 23). In contrast to the polymorphous admixture of cells, including Reed–Sternberg cells, found in the initial biopsy diagnostic of Hodgkin's disease, the cell population of the secondary non-Hodgkin's lymphoma was relatively monomorphous (Figs. 3 and 4). The cells of the small noncleaved lymphomas were characterized by evenly dispersed nuclear chromatin, small but definite nucleoli, and well-defined amphophilic cytoplasm which stained intensely with methyl green–Pyronine stain. Three cases were associated with a "starry-sky" pattern and pronounced karyorrhexis; mitotic figures were frequent, with as many as four per high-power field. Three of the patients had small noncleaved lymphoma in the abdominal cavity, with involvement of the mesenteric or retroperitoneal soft tissues as well as the gastrointestinal tract; the diagnostic biopsies in the remaining two patients were obtained from lymph node and bone marrow.

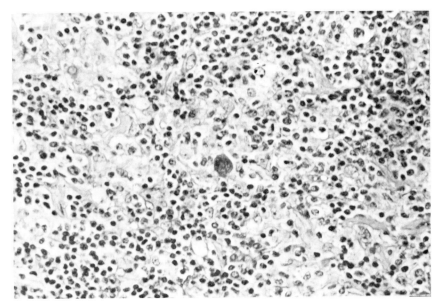

Fig. 3. Hodgkin's disease, mixed cellularity. The cell population is polymorphous. ×300.

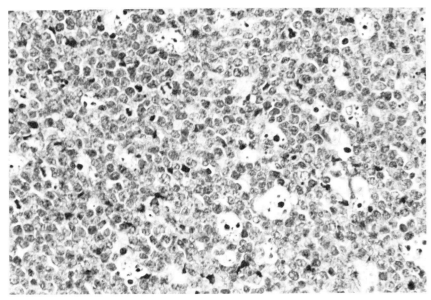

Fig. 4. Secondary small, noncleaved (undifferentiated) lymphoma. The cells are relatively monomorphous. Same case as in Fig. 3. ×300.

TABLE I

Patient Population (1096 Patients, 17 Leukemias)[a]

Extent of XRT	XRT alone	XRT adjuvant CX	XRT salvage CX	XRT plus gold	CX alone
Limited field	57	101 (3)	19	—	—
Subtotal nodal	171	68	39	1	—
Total nodal	189	284 (8)	66 (1)	64 (3)	—
None	—	—	—	—	37 (2)
Total	417	453 (11)	124 (1)	65 (3)	37 (2)

[a] The number of cases of leukemia is shown in parentheses. See text for treatment descriptions. XRT, Radiotherapy; CX, chemotherapy; gold, intravenous colloidal gold.

The gastrointestinal tract was also the initial site in two of the three patients with large-cell lymphomas. The diagnosis of secondary lymphoma was established at postmortem in one of these cases; the lymphoma was widespread, involving nodes, spleen, and other sites, in addition to the bowel. In the second patient the diagnosis was established at gastrectomy; although the pattern of the lymphoma in this patient was primarily diffuse, there was a focal follicular pattern. Diagnostic tissues from the third patient with large-cell lymphoma were obtained from lung and rib. All three patients with large-cell lymphoma were subclassified as the large, noncleaved type (22); double-nucleated or Reed–Sternberg-like cells were not found among these cases.

IV. Results

Table I shows the patient population. Each major subgroup is subdivided by the extent of radiotherapy administered. Table II demonstrates the major charac-

TABLE II

Characteristics of Treatment Groups

Group[a]	Mean age (years)	M/F ratio[b]	Median follow-up (years)	No. of cases of leukemia
XRT alone	30.0	1.35:1	4.7	0
Adjuvant CX	26.5	1.53:1	4.3	11
Salvage CX	30.3	1.64:1	5.3	1
XRT plus gold	30.8	2.09:1	7.2	3
CX alone	42.0	2.36:1	4.0	2

[a] XRT, Radiotherapy; CX, chemotherapy; gold, intravenous colloidal gold.
[b] M/F, Male/female.

teristics of the patients in those groups. The median follow-up is longer for the radiotherapy–gold group because that study was discontinued in 1975. It must be emphasized that the subset of patients given chemotherapy alone comprised only 3.4% of the total group; these patients had advanced disease and were older (mean age, 42 years).

Table III shows the clinical characteristics of the 17 patients who developed leukemia. Included also are data from two additional patients who developed secondary leukemia but whose treatment began prior to July 1968. Table IV summarizes the important clinical features. As noted above, most of the patients had a period of peripheral blood count depression prior to the diagnosis of leukemia. The leukemia itself was often an indolent leukemia, and the point of

TABLE III

Patients with Secondary Leukemia

Subgroup[a]	Age	Sex[b]	Stage[c]	Relapse	Duration of CX, years	Years from diagnosis to Cytopenia[d]	Leukemia	Death	HD status at last follow-up[e]
Adjuvant	19	F	IV$_{HS}$B	No		1.3	1.5[f]	1.5	NED
CX	47	M	III$_S$B	No		2.3	2.8	[g]	NED
	52	M	IV$_{HS}$A	No		2.6	2.7	[g]	NED
	24	M	III$_S$A	No		2.7	2.7[f]	3.4	NED
	32	M	IV$_{SB}$B	No		2.7	2.7[f]	3.1	NED
	51	M	IV$_{MS}$B	No		3.1	3.3	4.9	NED
	29	M	III$_S$B	No		3.3	4.0[f]	4.5	NED
	23	M (LF)	IIA	No		3.4	3.6	[g]	NED
	28	F	IIB	No		6.8	7.4	7.9	NED
	30	M (LF)	IV$_1$B	Yes		4.6	4.8	5.0	HD
	62	F	IIIB	Yes		7.3	7.3	7.5	NED
Salvage CX	40	M	IIA	Yes		4.6	5.6	5.9	NED
XRT plus	52	M	III$_S$A	Yes		?	4.1	4.8	NED
gold	25	M	III$_{ES}$A	Yes		6.1	6.2	6.4	HD
	32	M	III$_S$A	Yes		?	8.2	8.4	NED
CX alone	53	M	IV$_{HMS}$A		2.7	4.0	4.3	5.5	NED
	29	F	IV$_1$B		1.8	5.8	6.9	7.0	NED
Presented prior to	12	F	IIA	Yes		3.2	3.8	3.8	HD
study period	27	F	IIA	Yes		—	12.7	12.7	HD

[a] CX, Chemotherapy; XRT, radiotherapy; gold, intravenous collodial gold.
[b] LF, Limited-field radiotherapy.
[c] Ann Arbor (24).
[d] Cytopenia, peripheral blood count depression.
[e] NED, No evidence of disease; HD, Hodgkin's disease present.
[f] Aggressive treatment for AML.
[g] Alive.

TABLE IV

Characteristics of Secondary Leukemia (17 Patients)

Characteristic	Median time[a]	
Diagnosis to leukemia	4.1 Years	(1.3–8.1)
Duration of cytopenia	3 Months	(0–12)
Survival from diagnosis of leukemia	3 Months	(0–17)

[a] The range is shown in parentheses.

demarcation between cytopenia and leukemia was often not clearly definable. In fact, as the entity of therapy-related malignancy became well recognized, the diagnosis of leukemia was often made earlier. This accounts for the prolonged survivals of up to 17 months in some patients with leukemia.

Actuarial curves for the risk of leukemia for the entire group and the five subgroups are plotted in Figs. 5 and 6. The 17.6% risk at 7 years for patients treated with chemotherapy has a large standard error. The cumulative risks are in Table V; Table VI lists the results of a statistical comparison among groups. Compared to radiotherapy alone, there is a statistically significant increased risk

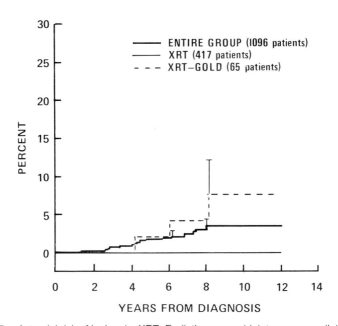

Fig. 5. Actuarial risk of leukemia. XRT, Radiotherapy; gold, intravenous colloidal gold.

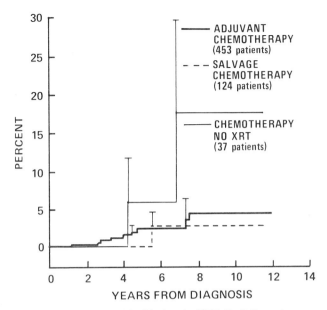

Fig. 6. Actuarial risk of leukemia. XRT, Radiotheraphy.

of leukemia in the three subgroups: adjuvant chemotherapy, chemotherapy alone, and radiotherapy plus gold. All other comparisons among major groups were not statistically significant. It must be emphasized that the 17.6% risk of the chemotherapy alone group is *not* statistically different from the 5.1% risk of the adjuvant group.

TABLE V

Actuarial Risk of Leukemia[a]

Group or subgroup[b]	5 Years from diagnosis	7 Years from diagnosis	9 Years from diagnosis
XRT alone	0	0	0
Adjuvant CX	3.0 (1.0)	3.0 (1.0)	5.1 (1.8)
Salvage CX	0	2.8 (1.8)	2.8 (1.8)
XRT plus gold	1.9 (1.8)	4.1 (2.9)	7.7 (4.5)
With CX			18
Without CX			0
CX alone	5.9 (5.7)	17.6 (12.1)	17.6 (12.1)
Entire group	1.5 (0.5)	2.3 (0.6)	3.4 (0.9)

[a] Percentage; SE is shown in parentheses.
[b] XRT, Radiotherapy; CX, chemotherapy; gold, intravenous colloidal gold.

TABLE VI

Statistical Significance of Leukemia Risk

Treatment[a]	*p* (Gehan) between actuarial curves[b]
Major groups compared	
Adjuvant CX versus XRT alone	.01
CX alone versus XRT alone	.016
XRT plus gold versus XRT alone	.034
Other comparisons	NS
Subgroups compared	
XRT plus gold plus CX versus XRT plus gold	.16
Adjuvant XRT by extent of XRT:	NS
LF, STLI, TLI	
Adjuvant CX versus adjuvant CX	NS
plus salvage CX	

[a] CX, Chemotherapy; XRT, radiotherapy; gold, intravenous colloidal gold; LF, limited field; STLI, subtotal lymphoid irradiation; TLI, total lymphoid irradiation. See text for description of treatment groups.

[b] NS, Not significant.

Three important points emerged from statistical comparison of the subsets of these major groups:

1. In the radiotherapy–gold group *all* leukemias occurred in patients who were also given chemotherapy (18 versus 0%), but the level of significance was $p = .16$.

2. In the adjuvant chemotherapy group the risk of leukemia was not affected by the extent of associated radiotherapy, i.e., involved-field, subtotal lymphoid, or total lymphoid irradiation.

3. The addition of salvage chemotherapy in the case of patients given adjuvant chemotherapy did not alter the risk of leukemia.

Three cases of leukemia occurred in patients given less than total lymphoid radiotherapy: One patient received hemiminimantle (involved-field) treatment with six cycles of MOPP; and second received treatment to the abdomen and liver with five cycles of MOPP; and the last patient received 800 rads to a mantle followed by MOPP and prolonged single-agent chemotherapy.

Secondary non-Hodgkin's lymphoma was diagnosed in eight patients, three of whom were included in this study population. The clinical characteristics of all eight cases are shown in Table VII; the actuarial risk data are in Table VIII. In the study group two patients received radiotherapy and chemotherapy, and one received radiotherapy alone. Similarly, among the pre-July 1968 patients, one received radiotherapy alone and four received combined-modality treatment.

TABLE VII

Patients with Non-Hodgkin's Lymphoma[a]

Age and sex	Stage[b]	XRT	CX	Years from diagnosis to		RX[c]	Last status of:	
				Lymphoma	Death		HD	Second Lymphoma
From a study population								
63 F	V$_{HS}$B	+	Salvage	3.8	3.9	CAT	NED[d]	Pos
28 M	IV$_L$B	+	Adjuvant	5.6	6.2	BACOP	NED	Pos
57 F	IA	+	0	6.6	[e]	C-MOPP	NED	NED
From a population prior to the study period								
13 F	IIB	+	Salvage	7.8	7.8	—	Pos	Pos
42 F	IIA	+	Salvage	9.3	11.0	CHOP, MTX	NED	NED
13 M	III$_S$B	+	Salvage	10.3	11.1	CHOP	NED	NED
51 M	IA	Plus gold	Salvage	10.7	10.8	—	Pos	Pos
38 F	IIIA	+	None	15.0	15.3	C-MOPP	NED	NED

[a] XRT, Radiotherapy; CX, chemotherapy; RX, treatment; HD, Hodgkin's disease.

[b] Ann Arbor (24).

[c] CAT, Cytosine arabinoside, adriamycin, 6-thioguanine; BACOP, bleomycin, adriamycin, cyclophosphamide, vincristine, prednisone (25); C-MOPP, cyclophosphamide, vincristine, procarbazine, prednisone (26); CHOP, cyclophosphamide, adriamycin, vincristine, prednisone (27); MTX, high-dose methotrexate.

[d] NED, No evidence of disease; Pos, positive.

[e] Alive 7.8 years after diagnosis.

TABLE VIII

Actuarial Risk of Secondary Non-Hodgkin's Lymphomas[a]

Group	5 Years from diagnosis	7 Years from diagnosis
Entire group	0.1 (0.1)	0.7 (0.4)
Adjuvant (three cases)	0.4 (0.4)	1.0 (0.8)

[a] Percentage; SD is shown in parentheses. Median time from diagnosis to second lymphoma, 6.3 years. Median survival from second lymphoma diagnosis, 6 months (2-15+).

The median time from diagnosis to secondary lymphoma was 6.3 years in the study group and 11.0 years in the prestudy group. This difference may be due in part to the fact that these pre-1968 patients had to survive long enough to receive MOPP chemotherapy. They were diagnosed, on average, 3 years before the routine use of MOPP. In the four pre-1968 cases who received combined treatment the median time from completion of MOPP to secondary lymphoma was 5 years (2.8–8.2 years). In the current study the median time of follow-up for the entire group from diagnosis is 5 years; therefore it is possible that additional non-Hodgkin's lymphomas may yet occur.

The actuarial risk of secondary lymphoma at 7 years is 0.8% for the entire population and 1.0% for patients given combined-modality treatment. Treatment of these lymphomas is slightly more successful than treatment of secondary acute leukemias. In the study group the one patient not previously treated with chemotherapy is still in complete remission 16 months after diagnosis of lymphoma, while the other patients died of lymphoma. In the group of patients treated before July 1968, three of three responded to therapy, and all were clinically free of lymphoma at the time of death, attributed to intercurrent disease.

V. Discussion

The occurrence of leukemia in patients treated for Hodgkin's disease is well established. In the treatment era prior to the advent of aggressive combined-modality treatment this complication was relatively rare, occurring in patients who received repetitive therapy with piecemeal radiotherapy and palliative single-drug chemotherapy (4, 28, 29). The data from this study on the modern treatment era corroborate our previous finding that combined-modality therapy is a significant risk factor in the development of leukemia (1). As before, we have no cases of leukemia in patients given radiotherapy alone; however, there are now two cases of leukemia in the chemotherapy alone group, both of whom received prolonged therapy. The risk of leukemia at 9 years in the chemotherapy group is 17.6% (SE 12.1%) which is *not* statistically different from the 5.1% (SE 1.7%) risk the group given adjuvant chemotherapy (Tables V and VI). That chemotherapy is a risk factor is further shown in the group of patients administered colloidal gold. All three cases of leukemia occurred in patients requiring chemotherapy in addition to external beam radiotherapy and intravenous gold (Table V).

Table IX lists the secondary leukemia data from other groups. As in the Stanford results, almost no cases of leukemia were seen following radiotherapy alone. Combined-modality therapy appears to be the major risk factor, although reports from two Italian groups yield a similar risk for chemotherapy alone and combined-modality treatment, as was seen in our study. The absence of leukemia in the small group of patients from Milan who received radiotherapy plus adriamycin, bleomycin, vinblastine, and dacarbazine (ABVD) (7) is of note in that

TABLE IX

Secondary Leukemia in Patients with Hodgkin's Disease

Author	Treatment group[a]	Risk of leukemia or number of cases[b]
Baccarani et al. (5)	XRT (117)	0% Actuarial, 7 years
	CX (152)	2.0% Actuarial, 7 years
	Combined (344)	2.04% Actuarial, 7 years
Valagussa et al. (7)	XRT (236)	0% Actuarial, 10 years
	CX (36)	5.5% Actuarial, 5 years
	Combined (492)	3.5% Actuarial, 10 years
	XRT-ABVD (55)	0% Actuarial, 10 years
Toland et al. (10)	XRT	0
	CX (intensive)	256 incidence density ratio
	Combined	253–1049 incidence density ratio
Canellos et al. (13,14)	XRT (149)	0 Cases
	CX (110)	0 Cases
	Combined (65)	4 Cases
Cadman et al. (8)	Combined (100)	1 Case
Wiernik et al. (9)	XRT (41)	1 Case
	Combined (33)	1 Case
Auclerc et al. (6)	XRT (450)	0
	CX (300)	4 Cases
	Combined (400)	17 Cases

[a] Number of patients is shown in parentheses. XRT, Radiotherapy; CX, chemotherapy; ABVD, adriamycin, bleomycin, vinblastine, dacarbazine; combined, radiation and chemotherapy.

[b] Incidence density ratio = observed/expected number of cases.

neither an alkylating agent nor procarbazine was in this drug combination, the latter being a potent carcinogen in animals (30).

Patients usually have a period of pancytopenia before the diagnosis of leukemia (5–7, 16, 31). It is often difficult to establish an exact date of onset of the leukemia, especially when it behaves in an indolent manner. The leukemia is usually an acute nonlymphocytic leukemia (5, 7), although erythroleukemia (5) and T-cell immunoblastic leukemia have been reported (32). Foucar *et al.* suggest that therapy-related leukemia is a panmyelosis (31). Cytogenetic studies were not done in our patients, but others describe abnormalities in most patients studied (5, 8, 31, 33). Rowley *et al.* (33) demonstrated that cells from eight of nine patients lacked a number 5 chromosome.

Aggressive treatment of therapy-related acute leukemia has been almost uniformly unsuccessful (5, 7, 8). The longest survivals in our group occurred in patients with indolent leukemia treated with supportive therapy. Schwartz *et al.* (34) recently analyzed the results of treatment at Stanford of acute myelogenous leukemia (AML) in 69 patients, 61 with primary AML and 8 with therapy-related AML. The complete response (CR) rates were equal in both groups, but the median duration of response was 12 months for primary AML versus only 2.8 months for patients with prior treatment ($p < .001$). Comparative mean survival times of CR patients were 21 months versus 8.6 months ($p < .01$) (34).

The data in this article and in Table IX strongly suggest that secondary leukemia is a consequence of therapy and not merely part of the natural history of the disease, unmasked by improved survival. Radiation and chemotherapy are both carcinogenic and immunosuppressive (35). Prolonged therapy with alkylating agents can lead to a substantial incidence of leukemia in patients treated for multiple myeloma (36), breast cancer (37, 38), ovarian cancer (39, 40), non-Hodgkin's lymphoma (41), and other conditions including nonmalignant diseases (29, 35) (Table X). Analysis of the adjuvant group in our study showed that the risk of leukemia was independent of the extent of irradiation and the amount of chemotherapy in that, once adjuvant therapy was given, the addition of further chemotherapy did not increase the risk.

Secondary non-Hodgkin's lymphoma was also seen predominantly in the combined-modality group, although two of eight patients had received radiotherapy alone. The different latency period in the study and prestudy groups may in part be artifactual, as discussed above. The lower actuarial risk of developing secondary lymphoma in this study compared that described in our previous published work (2) is probably due to slightly different study populations in that in the previous study only part of the population was at risk to receive MOPP (see above). Treatment of this complication is more successful than treatment of leukemia (see above).

Subsequent to our original report (2), there have been isolated case reports of non-Hodgkin's lymphoma developing after therapy for Hodgkin's disease (11,

TABLE X

Risk of Leukemia after Chemotherapy

Disease treated[a]	No. of cases of AML	Leukemia risk
Multiple myeloma (364) (36)	12	17.4% Actuarial, 4 years
Breast cancer (1460) (37)	4	—
Breast cancer, long-term chlorambucil (13) (38)	4	4/13
Ovarian cancer (5455) (39)	13	All patients receiving chemotherapy and living more than 2 years, 171-fold increase
Ovarian cancer >3 years of melphalan (48) (40)	4	All patients, 4/48; patients given >800 mg melphalan, 4/12

[a] Number of patients is shown in parentheses.

12, 42). These newly documented cases similarly were classified as diffuse, undifferentiated (small, noncleaved), or histiocytic (large-cell) lymphomas and displayed a propensity to involve the abdomen, as did five of our eight cases. Ultrastructural examination in one of the reports revealed features of transformed lymphocytes (42); the tumor cells in another expressed monoclonal surface immunoglobulin indicative of B-lymphocyte origin (11). In our initial report, immunofluorescent studies demonstrated IgM and monoclonal kappa light chains in the one patient studied (2). The combination of light microscopy, ultrastructure, and immunological studies suggests that the newly developed lymphomas likely derive from a different clone than the original Hodgkin's disease and represent disparate neoplasms.

It is beyond the scope of this report to discuss treatment options for the various stages of Hodgkin's disease. The 9-year actuarial risk of leukemia in our population was 0% for radiotherapy alone, 5.1% for radiotherapy and adjuvant chemotherapy, and 17.6% for a small subset of patients given chemotherapy (not statistically different from adjuvant chemotherapy). Thus secondary hematological neoplasms will occur in approximately 4.1% of patients treated for Hodgkin's disease. These can be called diseases of medical progress in that they would not occur if patients were not being cured of their Hodgkin's disease. Despite the fact that these diseases occur predominantly in the combined-modality group, the *overall survival* of patients given planned combined-modality therapy is at least as good as that of those given initial radiotherapy with chemotherapy reserved for patients who relapse (43). Clearly there are indications for primary treatment of certain stages of both modalities. However, this type of treatment should be discouraged if equivalent *survival* can be attained using primary radiotherapy, with chemotherapy reserved for treating patients who relapse.

VI. Summary

One thousand ninety-six patients have received primary treatment for Hodgkin's disease at Stanford since July 1968. The 9-year actuarial risk (and standard error) of developing leukemia is radiotherapy, 0%; adjuvant chemotherapy, 4.6% (1.7%); salvage chemotherapy, 2.8% (1.8%); chemotherapy alone, 17.6% (12.1%); entire population, 3.4% (0.9%). The median time from diagnosis of Hodgkin's disease to the diagnosis of leukemia is 4.4 years (range 1.3–8.1 years). Most patients have a period of pancytopenia preceding the diagnosis of leukemia; the median survival after the diagnosis of leukemia is 3 months (range 0–17 months). Eleven cases occurred in the adjuvant chemotherapy group. The extent of radiotherapy of chemotherapy within this group did not affect the risk of leukemia. Three cases of non-Hodgkin's lymphoma occurred in this study population, yielding a 9-year actuarial risk of 0.7 (0.4%). It appears that secondary hematological neoplasms are a complication of both combined-modality therapy and prolonged chemotherapy.

Addendum

After the completion of this article an additional case of leukemia was diagnosed in a 23-year-old female with Stage III$_s$B Hodgkin's disease. She was treated with total lymphoid irradiation and adjuvant MOPP chemotherapy and developed peripheral cytopenia with a dysplastic bone marrow 8.8 years after diagnosis. This changes the actuarial risk of leukemia (percentage and standard error) at 9 years to 3.9% (1.0%) for the entire group and to 7.1% (2.6%) for the adjuvant chemotherapy subgroup.

Acknowledgments

The authors wish to thank Richard Cox for statistical assistance and Marge Keskin for secretarial assistance. We wish to acknowledge the many physicians who administered medical care to these patients.

References

1. C. N. Coleman, C. J. Williams, A. Flint, E. J. Glatstein, S. A. Rosenberg, and H. S. Kaplan, *N. Engl. J. Med.* **297**, 249 (1977).

2. J. G. Krikorian, J. S. Burke, S. A. Rosenberg, and H. S. Kaplan, *N. Engl. J. Med.* **300,** 452 (1979).

3. R. S. D'Agnostino, *N. Engl. J. Med.* **301,** 1289 (1979).

4. K. Borum, *Cancer (Philadelphia)* **46,** 1247 (1980).

5. M. Baccarani, A. Bosi, and G. Papa, *Cancer (Philadelphia)* **46,** 1735 (1980).

6. G. Auclerc, C. Jacquillat, M. F. Auclerc, M. Wiel, and J. Bernard, *Cancer (Philadelphia)* **44,** 2017 (1979).

7. P. Valagussa, A. Santoro, R. Kenda, F. F. Bellani, F. Franchi, A. Banfi, F. Rilke, and G. Bonadonna, *Br. Med. J.* p. 216 (1980).

8. E. C. Cadman, R. L. Capizzi, and J. R. Bertino, *Cancer (Philadelphia)* **40,** 1280 (1977).

9. P. H. Wiernik, J. Gustafson, S. C. Schimpff, and C. Diggs, *Am. J. Med.* **67,** 183 (1979).

10. D. M. Toland, C. A. Coltman, and T. E. Moon, *Ca—Clin. Trials* **1,** 27 (1978).

11. R. E. Scully, J. J. Galdabini, and B. U. McNeely, *N. Engl. J. Med.* **302,** 389 (1980).

12. M. B. Spaulding, H. Mogavero, and M. Montes, *N. Engl. J. Med.* **301,** 384 (1979).

13. G. P. Canellos, V. T. DeVita, J. C. Arseneau, J. Whang-Peng, and R. E. C. Johnson, *Lancet* **1,** 947 (1975).

14. G. P. Canellos, *Lancet* **1,** 1294 (1975).

15. R. S. Brody and D. Schottenfeld, *Semin. Oncol.* **7,** 187 (1980).

16. J. W. Vardiman, H. M. Golomb, J. D. Rowley, and D. Variakojis, *Cancer (Philadelphia)* **42,** 229 (1978).

17. V. T. DeVita, A. A. Serpic, and P. P. Carbone, *Ann. Intern. Med.* **73,** 881 (1970).

18. H. S. Kaplan, Harvard University Press, Cambridge, Massachusetts (1980).

19. J. R. Eltringham and H. S. Kaplan, *Natl. Cancer. Inst. Monogr.* **36,** 107 (1973).

20. E. S. Kaplan and P. Meier, *J. Am. Stat. Assoc.* **53,** 457 (1958).

21. E. A. Gehan, *Biometrika* **52,** 203 (1965).

22. R. F. Dorfman, J. S. Burke, and C. W. Berrard (in preparation). Academic Press, New York, 1981.

23. H. Rappaport, "Atlas of Tumor Pathology," Sect. 3, Fasc. 8, U.S. Armed Forces Inst. Pathol., Washington, D.C., 1966.

24. P. P. Carbone, H. S. Kaplan, and K. Musshoff, *Cancer Res.* **31,** 1860 (1971).

25. P. Schein, V. DeVita, S. Hubbard, B. Chabner, G. Canellos, C Berard, and R. Young, *Ann. Intern. Med.* **85,** 417 (1976).

26. V. DeVita, G. Canellos, B. Chabner, P. Schein, S. Hubbard, and R. Young, *Lancet* **1,** 248 (1975).

27. L. Elias, C. S. Portlock, and S. A. Rosenberg, *Cancer (Philadelphia)* **42,** 1705 (1978).

28. F. Rosner and H. Grunwald, *Am. J. Med.* **58,** 339 (1975).

29. D. A. Casciato and J. L. Scott, *Medicine (Baltimore)* **58,** 32 (1979).

30. S. M. Sieber, *Med. Pediatr. Oncol.* **3,** 123 (1977).

31. K. Foucar, R. W. McKenna, C. D. Bloomfield, T. K. Bowers, and R. D. Brunning, *Cancer (Philadelphia)* **43,** 1285 (1979).

32. F. R. Dick, R. D. Maca, and R. Hankenson, *Cancer (Philadelphia)* **42,** 1325 (1978).

33. J. D. Rowley, H. M. Golomb, and J. Vardiman, *Blood* **50,** 759 (1977).

34. R. Schwartz, J. Halpern, and P. Greenberg, *Proc. Am. Assoc. Cancer Res. Am. Soc. Clin. Oncol.* **21,** 435, Abstr. C-460 (1980).

35. C. N. Coleman, *Am. J. Pediatr. Hematol. Oncol.* **3** (in press).

36. D. E. Bergsagel, A. J. Bailey, G. R. Langley, R. N. MacDonald, D. F. White, and A. B. Miller, *N. Engl. J. Med.* **301,** 743 (1979).

37. M. A. Portugal, H. C. Falkson, K. Stevens, and G. Falkson, *Cancer Treat. Rep.* **63,** 177 (1979).

38. H. J. Lerner, *Cancer Treat. Rep.* **62,** 1135 (1978).

39. R. R. Reimer, R. Hoover, J. F. Fraumeni, and R. C. Young, *N. Engl. J. Med.* **297,** 177 (1977).
40. N. Einhorn, *Cancer (Philadelphia)* **41,** 444 (1978).
41. M. H. Zarrabi, F. Rosner, and J. M. Bennett, *Cancer (Philadelphia)* **44,** 1070 (1979).
42. J. Rubins, B. Sischy, and J. C. K. Lee, *Am. J. Clin. Pathol.* **74,** 696 (1980).
43. S. A. Rosenberg, H. S. Kaplan, and B. W. Brown, *in* ''Adjuvant Therapy of Cancer II'' (S. E. Jones and S. E. Salmon, eds.), p. 109. Grune & Stratton, New York, 1979.

17

A Dual Mechanism of ERFC Blocking in Hodgkin's Disease: The Possible Role of Ferritin

BRACHA RAMOT

I. Introduction

In this article I would like (1) to summarize the present state of knowledge on ferritin as a tumor-associated glycoprotein in Hodgkin's disease (HD) and other malignancies, and (2) to demonstrate, by the use of levamisole, indomethacin, and thymic hormone, a dual immunological defect in patients with HD involving both a subset of T cells and monocytes or macrophages. Finally, I shall link these two topics by discussing the possible role of ferritin in the genesis of certain immunological abnormalities.

II. Background

Ferritin is a major iron storage protein in the tissues. The protein shell, apoferritin, consists of various combinations of two different subunits of 18,000–

19,000 daltons, called H (heart), more acidic, and L (liver), more basic. The subunit combinations and the iron content determine the isoferritin pattern of the tissue (1–3). Small amounts of ferritin can be detected in the serum of normal individuals, while in iron overload, the serum ferritin level reflects the iron content of reticuloendothelial tissues (4). Contrary to observations in normals, patients with malignancies such as HD, acute nonlymphatic leukemia (ANLL), breast cancer, hepatoma, lung cancer, and neuroblastoma have markedly elevated serum ferritin levels (5–14). Furthermore, blast cells in ANLL, neuroblastoma cells, and lymphoblastoid cell lines synthesize ferritin independently of iron supplementation (14, 15). Recently, an acidic isoferritin was isolated from a patient with monocytic leukemia (16). Ferritin has also been extracted from tumor tissue such as breast, pancreas, colon, and liver; however, the significance of these findings has not been resolved.

What is the evidence that ferritin is a tumor-associated glycoprotein in HD? Is ferritin responsible for some of the immunological derangements in such patients? Bieber and Bieber (17) demonstrated ferritin in the macrophages of HD patients, and Eshhar et al. (18) extracted normal ferritin from noncultured spleens of HD patients and considered it a tumor-associated antigen. Subsequently the same investigators cast doubt on the specificity of this finding. Recently, Hancock et al. (19), using isoelectric focusing and quantitative immunological reactions, isolated an acidic ferritin band from the spleens of HD patients. These authors suggested that their results, which are not consistent with those of Eshhar et al., could be due to the abolition of cadmium sulfate crystalization in their own system (20). Since this phenomenon causes a reduction in the number of isoferritin molecules obtained by electrofocusing, it could account for the failure of the other investigators to demonstrate acidic ferritin bands. Since the iron content and the number of monocytes can determine the ferritin pattern of the tissue, it is hard to draw any conclusions when the tissue studied is the spleen.

III. The Nature of the Immunological Derangement in Hodgkin's Disease

This subject has been studied for the last two decades and lately extensively reviewed by Kaplan (21) and Twomey and Rice (22). Although the results are conflicting, in essence there are aberrations in T-cell functions, such as response to mitogens, decreased or impaired responsiveness to new and recall antigens (23–27), prolonged homograft survival (28), dysfunction in T-cell autoreactivity (23–31), T-cell redistribution (32), and an increase in suppressor monocytes (33–35). These abnormalities are not detected in all patients, and qualitative and quantitative differences in immunological function possibly depend upon the patient populations under study.

IV. E-Rosette-Forming Cells

The decreased number of E-rosette-forming cells (ERFCs) in the peripheral blood of HD patients is probably the most consistent *in vitro* finding (21, 36, 37), although even on this point the reports are conflicting (38). We found no correlation between the percentage of ERFCs and the clinical stage of the disease (Table I) (39). The ERFCs could be raised to normal levels *in vitro* by incubation with levamisole, a known immunomodulator, independently of the clinical stage (39–41), or by fetal calf serum (42). Finally, *in vivo* administration of levamisole had the same effect (41). These findings suggested to us that a subpopulation of ERFCs in the peripheral blood of HD patients was blocked.

Since ferritin had been implicated as a tumor-associated protein in HD, it was important to determine whether this might be the blocking substance.

Enzymatic radioiodination of surface proteins of HD peripheral blood mononuclear cells confirmed the presence of a surface protein. This protein was shed into the medium after incubation with levamisole, which resulted in the unmasking of surface proteins similar to those on normal mononuclear cells on acrylamide–sodium dodecyl sulfate electrophoresis. The blocking substance reacted with an antibody specific for normal human spleen ferritin. It contained no detectable iron and was dissociated into monomeric subunits of 18,000 daltons by reduction and alkylation. We concluded therefore that apoferritin rather than ferritin was the blocking protein (43).

Subsequently, Sarcione *et al.* (44) demonstrated increased ferritin synthesis by HD spleens and peripheral blood lymphocytes, and we demonstrated ferritin in the peripheral blood lymphocytes (PBLs) of HD patients by electron microscopy (45).

Is there any evidence that ferritin can inhibit the immune response of lymphocytes? The answer is yes. Ferritin suppresses the blastogenic response of normal mononuclear cells to phytohemagglutinin (PHA) and concanavalin A (ConA) at a concentration of 1 μg/ml of culture medium; the response to pokeweed mitogen

TABLE I

Percentage of ERFCs in Symptomatic and Asymptomatic Hodgkin's Disease Patients

Stage	Total patients			Asymptomatic			Symptomatic		
	No.	Mean	SD	No.	Mean	SD	No.	Mean	SD
I	9	52	16	8	50	16	1	65	—
II	36	45	16	28	44	16	8	48	15
III	11	47	14	5	42	9	6	51	17
IV	11	43	17	1	38	—	10	44	18
Total	67	46	15	42	45	15	25	47	16

(PWM) is not affected (46). Furthermore, it can markedly reduce the capacity for cap formation with ConA and slightly inhibits the mixed lymphocyte reaction (MLR) (46). A similar defect in capping has been described in peripheral blood lymphocytes obtained from patients with HD (47).

Contrary to our findings, Bieber *et al.* (48) isolated a low-molecular-weight E-rosette inhibitory substance, probably a glycolipid, from the serum of HD patients. Since glycolipids are known to be shed from the cell surface of normal and abnormal cells (49), this finding is not surprising. The question remains as to whether the deficiency in ERFCs is a result of cell surface modulation or is due to a blocking factor such as apoferritin bound to a specific receptor, possibly a glycolipid. This apoferritin–receptor complex could be the blocking agent that is shed from the T-cell subpopulation after incubation with levamisole.

V. Macrophages in Hodgkin's Disease

In addition to T-lymphocyte abnormalities, Goodwin *et al.* showed that monocytes in HD secreted fourfold greater quantities of prostaglandin E_2 (PGE_2) which is known to suppress various immune responses, in part by elevating the intracellular levels of cyclic adenosine $3',5'$-monophosphate in lymphocytes (33). By removing the monocytes (35) or inhibiting prostaglandin synthesis with indomethacin (33), a markedly increased response of HD lymphocytes to PHA was observed. We were able to confirm the effect of macrophage removal on PHA response, although it was more marked in patients in remission. We also compared the effect of monocyte removal, indomethacin, levamisole, and thymic humoral factor (THF) on ERFCs in HD in order to see whether the deblocking effect of levamisole on ERFC was direct or mediated via macrophages (50).

Sixty HD patients of all stages were studied prior to or at different periods after completion of therapy. Peripheral blood was collected in heparin, and the mononuclear cells were separated on a Ficoll–metrizoate gradient. The effect of levamisole was studied by incubating $2-3 \times 10^6$ mononuclear cells with levamisole 40 μg/ml phospahte-buffered saline (PBS). The final concentration of indomethacin was 1 μg/ml PBS. The concentration of THF (supplied by N. Trainin, Weitzman Institute) was 30 μg/ml, which was found to be the optimal concentration in our system. Control cells were incubated in PBS without additives. After a 30-minute incubation at 37°C the cells were washed three times with PBS, and E-rosette formation was determined. Then 0.25 ml of the mononuclear cell suspension containing 10^6 cells was mixed with 0.25 ml of fresh 1% sheep red cells and 0.05 ml of absorbed and inactivated fetal calf serum (FCS). After centrifugation for 2 minutes at 200 g, the mixture was incubated at 4°C for 1 hour and gently resuspended, and ERFCs were counted.

Two methods for the removal of monocytes were used: incubation with carbonyl iron followed by sedimentation or adherence to plastic petri dishes by the method of Kumagai (51). Both methods yielded lymphocyte preparations almost free of monocytes as determined by esterase staining.

We were able to confirm our previous results that HD patients had a significantly lower percentage of ERFCs than normals (46.4 ± 12.3 compared to 62.4 ± 12.5, $p < .0005$). Preincubation of HD cells with levamisole, indomethacin, or THF resulted in an increase in the percentage of ERFCs to the normal level (Table II). The removal of monocytes abolished the effect of indomethacin on ERFCs, while the effect of levamisole persisted (Table III). In four experiments with THF the results were similar to those obtained with levamisole.

These *in vitro* results suggest a dual immune aberration in HD: (1) a subpopulation of T cells whose impaired ability to form E rosettes can be normalized by levamisole, THF, or FCS, and (2) a monocyte population that suppresses ERFCs via PGE_2 secretion. This effect can be blocked by indomethacin. Recently, Passwell *et al.*, in our laboratory, found that blood monocytes of untreated HD patients and of patients in prolonged remission secreted three- to fourfold more PGE_2 than normal monocytes (Table IV) (52). Although the range is very wide and therefore not significant, these findings can explain the prolonged anergy in some HD patients in remission.

Since a similar, although less pronounced, blocked lymphocyte population that can be unblocked by levamisole is found not only in HD but also in active systemic lupus erythrymatosus (SLE) (53), breast cancer (54), and other cancer patients, and since the suppressive effect of macrophages and the effect of indomethacin have also been demonstrated in these conditions (54), it is tempting

TABLE II

The Effect of Levamisole, Indomethacin, and Thymic Hormone Factor on the E-Rosette Percentage in Hodgkin's Disease Patients and Normal Mononuclear Cells

	No. of experiments	E Rosettes (%)
HD patients		
Control	60	46.4 ± 12.3[a]
Levamisole	60	60.8 ± 10.4[b]
Indomethacin	60	59.9 ± 11.1[b]
THF	41	56.7 ± 12.5[b]
Normals		
Control	20	62.4 ± 12.5

[a] Significantly different ($p < .0005$) from normal control.
[b] Not significantly different from normal control.

TABLE III

The Effect of Levamisole and Indomethacin on ERFCs in Hodgkin's Disease Patients after Monocyte Depletion

Source	No. of experiments	ERFCs (% ± SD)
HD PBLs	8	44.6 ± 3.8
HD PBLs plus levamisole	8	60.3 ± 5.8
HD PBLs plus indomethacin	8	63.1 ± 5.2
Monocyte-depleted[a] PBLs plus indomethacin	8	37.2 ± 7.8[b]
Monocyte-depleted[a,b] PBLS plus levamisole	8	58.5 ± 6.7

[a] By carbonyl iron.
[b] $p < .0025$.

to suggest that a similar mechanism is responsible for these *in vitro* aberrations in malignancy.

I would like to propose the following working hypothesis, namely, that ferritin or possibly other blocking agents, such as immune complexes shed from lyphocytes, are taken up by monocytes which are activated and secrete prostaglandins. The latter suppress the lymphocyte response to lectins as well as modulate the lymphocyte membrane, including expression of the endoplasmic reticulum receptor. The suppressive effect of ferritin on lymphocyte response to CoA (46) could be the result of ferritin uptake by monocytes, followed by their activation, prostaglandin secretion, and secondary inhibitory effect on lymphocytes.

Preliminary indications in this direction were obtained recently in collaboration with Zvi Metzger. He had previously reported that the activation of macrophages was associated with a release of free radicals as shown by chemiluminescence. Human liver ferritin (provided by I. Listowsky, Albert

TABLE IV

Prostaglandin E$_2$ Secretion by Blood Monocytes of Normals and Hodgkin's Disease Patients[a]

Source	No. of experiments	PGE$_2$ ± SEM ($ng/ml/2 \times 10^6$ cells)
Controls	12	9.13 ± 2.17
HD, untreated	7	27.91 ± 9.05
HD, remission	16	33.93 ± 8.38

[a] Monocyte monolayers were cultured in complete medium supplemented with 2% AB serum. Supernatants were harvested after 48 hours, stored at $-20°C$, and assayed by radioimmunoassay.

Einstein Medical School) at concentrations of 0.5–1 μg/ml markedly enhanced the chemiluminescence of mouse peritoneal macrophages.

These observations suggest that skin anergy during remission in HD and possibly other malignancies is related to the presence of activated macrophages.

References

1. J. W. Drysdale and R. M. Singer, *Cancer Res.* **34,** 3352 (1974).
2. P. Arosio, M. Yokota, and J. W. Drysdale, *Cancer Res.* **36,** 1735 (1976).
3. D. J. Lavoie, K. Ishikawa, and I. Listowsky, *Biochemistry* **17,** 5448 (1978).
4. G. M. Addison, M. R. Beamish, C. N. Hales, M. Hodgkins, A. Jacobs, and P. Llewellin, *J. Clin. Pathol.* **25,** 326 (1972).
5. P. A. E. Jones, F. M. Miller, M. Worwood, and A. Jacobs, *Br. J. Cancer* **27,** 212 (1973).
6. M. Worwood, M. Summers, F. Miller, A. Jacobs, and J. A. Whittaker, *Br. J. Haematol.* **28,** 27 (1974).
7. A. Jacobs, A. Slater, J. A. Whittaker, G. Canellos, and P. H. Wiernik, *Br. J. Cancer* **34,** 162 (1976).
8. W. Mori, H. Asakawa, and T. Taguchi, *JNCI, J. Natl. Cancer Inst.* **55,** 513 (1975).
9. D. M. Marcus and N. Zinberg, *JNCI, J. Natl. Cancer Inst.* **55,** 791 (1975b).
10. J. T. Hazard and J. W. Drysdale, *Nature (London)* **265,** 755 (1977).
11. M. C. Kew, J. D. Torrance, D. Derman, M. Simon, G. M. Macnab, R. W. Charlton, and T. H. Bothwell, *Gut* **19,** 294 (1978).
12. Y. Niitsu, S. Ohtsuka, Y. Kohgo, N. Watanabe, J. Koseki, and I. Urushizaki, *Tumor Res.* **10,** 31 (1975).
13. C. Gropp, K. Havemann, and F.-G. Lehmann, *Cancer (Philadelphia)* **42,** 2802 (1978).
14. H-W. L. Hann, H. M. Levy, and A. E. Evans, *Cancer Res.* **40,** 1411 (1980).
15. M. Worwood, F. Summers, A. Jacobs, and J. A. Whittaker, *Br. J. Haematol.* **28,** 27 (1974).
16. Y. Yoda and T. Abe, *Cancer (Philadelphia)* **46,** 289 (1980).
17. C. P. Bieber and M. M. Bieber, *Natl. Cancer Inst. Monogr.* **36,** 147 (1973).
18. Z. Eshhar, S. E. Order, and D. H. Katz, *Proc. Natl. Acad. Sci. U.S.A.* **71,** 3956 (1974).
19. B. W. Hancock, L. Bruce, K. May, and J. Richmond, *Br. J. Haematol.* **43,** 223 (1979).
20. J. T. Hazard, P. Arosio, and J. W. Drysdale, *in* "Oncodevelopmental Gene Expression" (W. H. Fishman and S. Sell, eds.), Academic Press, New York, 1977.
21. H. S. Kaplan, *Cancer (Philadelphia)* **45,** 2439 (1980).
22. J. J. Twomey and L. Rice, *Semin. Oncol.* **7,** 114 (1980).
23. M. W. Chase, *Cancer Res.* **26,** 1097 (1966).
24. J. E. Sokal and M. Primikirios, *Cancer (Philadelphia)* **14,** 597 (1969).
25. A. C. Aisenberg, *J. Clin. Invest.* **41,** 1964 (1962).
26. R. C. Young, M. P. Corder, H. A. Haynes, and V. T. DeVita, *Am. J. Med.* **52,** 63 (1973).
27. J. R. Eltringham and H. S. Kaplan, *Natl. Cancer Inst. Monogr.* **36,** 107 (1973).
28. W. D. Kelly, D. L. Lamb, R. L. Varco, and R. A. Good, *Ann. N. Y. Acad. Sci.* **87,** 187 (1960).
29. M. Bjorkolm, G. Holm, H. Mellstedt, and D. Pettersson, *Clin. Exp. Immunol.* **22,** 373 (1976).
30. J. J. Twomey, A. H. Laughter, S. Farrow, and C. C. Douglass, *J. Clin. Invest.* **56,** 467 (1975).
31. E. G. Engleman, C. J. Benike, R. T. Hoppe, H. S. Kaplan, and F. R. Berberich, *J. Clin. Invest.* **66,** 149 (1980).
32. S. Gupta and C. Tan, *Clin. Immunol. Immunopathol.* **15,** 133 (1980).
33. J. S. Goodwin, R. P. Messner, A. D. Bankhurst, G. T. Peake, J. Saiki, and R. C. Williams, Jr., *N. Engl. J. Med.* **297,** 963 (1977).

34. S. M. Hillinger and G. P. Herzig, *J. Clin. Invest.* **61,** 1620 (1978).
35. G. P. Schechter and S. Frances, *Blood* **52,** 261 (1978).
36. J. Cohnen, W. Augener, J. Brittinger, and S. D. Douglas, *N. Engl. J. Med.* **289,** 863 (1973).
37. B. Ramot, M. Biniaminov, A. Many, and E. Aghai, *Isr. J. Med. Sci.* **9,** 657 (1973).
38. K. J. Gajl-Peczalska, C. D. Bloomfield, H. Sosin, and Kersey, J. H., *Clin. Exp. Immunol.* **23,** 47 (1976).
39. B. Ramot, *Proc. Congr. Int. Soc. Hematol., Plen. Sess., 17th, 1978* (1978).
40. Y. Levo, B. Ramot, and V. Rotter, *Biomedicine* **23,** 198 (1975).
41. B. Ramot, M. Biniaminov, C. Shoham, and E. Rosenthal, *N. Engl. J. Med.* **294,** 809 (1976).
42. Z. Fuks, S. Strober, and H. S. Kaplan, *N. Engl. J. Med.* **295,** 1273 (1976).
43. C. Moroz, N. Lahat, M. Biniaminov, and B. Ramot, *Clin. Exp. Immunol.* **29,** 30 (1977).
44. E. J. Sarcione, J. R. Smalley, M. J. Lema, and L. Stutzman, *Int. J. Cancer* **20,** 339 (1977).
45. I. Ben-Bassat, B. Ramot, E. Aghai, and M. Djaldetti, *Acta Haematol.* **62,** 267 (1979).
46. Y. Matzner, C. Hershko, A. Polliack, A. M. Konijn, and G. Izak, *Br. J. Haematol.* **42,** 345 (1979).
47. H. Ben-Bassat and N. Goldblum, *Proc. Natl. Acad. Sci. U.S.A.* **72,** 1046 (1975).
48. M. M. Bieber, D. P. King, S. Strober, and H. S. Kaplan, *Clin. Res.* **27,** 81A (abstr.) (1979).
49. P. H. Black, *Adv. Cancer Res.* **32,** 75 (1980).
50. B. Ramot, E. Rosenthal, M. Biniaminov, and I. Ben-Bassat, *Isr. J. Med. Sci.* **17,** 232 (1981).
51. K. Kumagai, K. Itoh, S. Hinvma, and M. Tada, *J. Immunol. Methods* **29,** 17 (1979).
52. J. Passwell, M. Levanon, and B. Ramot, submitted for publication.
53. R. Michalevicz, A. Many, B. Ramot, and N. Trainin, *Clin. Exp. Immunol.* **31,** 111 (1978).
54. Z. Ram and B. Ramot, submitted for publication.

18

Polar Lipid Inhibitor of Phytohemagglutinin Mitogenesis in the Sera of Untreated Patients with Hodgkin's Disease

MARCIA M. BIEBER, HENRY S. KAPLAN, AND SAMUEL STROBER

I. Introduction

Hodgkin's disease (HD) has been associated with a deficiency of cell-mediated immunity. Although antibody response appears unimpaired, patients with HD have diminished delayed hypersensitivity to new and recall antigens at all stages of disease (1, 2). Early experiments showed that the delayed hypersensitivity response could not be passively transferred with normal immune lymphocytes to patients with HD (3–5). This indicated that a circulating inhibitor might play a role in the suppression of this response. It has been well established that peripheral blood lymphocytes (PBLs) from patients with HD are deficient in their *in vitro* blastogenic response to mitogens (6–9) and antigens (10). There are conflicting reports on whether a serum factor plays a role in this response (11–13). The ability of HD T cells to form erythrocyte (E) rosettes is also impaired (13–15). E-Rosette formation is restored to normal values by *in vitro* incubation with fetal calf serum (FCS) (16) and levamisole (17). Levamisole given to HD patients reportedly increased their percentage of E-rosette-forming cells to normal (18). E-rosette formation by HD PBLs, after restoration to normal by *in vitro* FCS incubation, could be inhibited by incubation in 20% HD serum (13). E-rosette formation by normal PBLs could also be inhibited by incubation in 60% HD serum or with a low-density substance extracted from HD spleen (19), indicating that a circulating inhibitor might play a role in the immune abnormalities seen in HD. Further studies have shown that the inhibitor is not a low-density lipoprotein complex but an immunologically active polar lipid.

II. Methods

A. Preparation of Inhibitor

Serum was collected from untreated patients with HD and from normal young adult donors. The patient serum was either pooled in lots or processed individually. Serum was first fractionated on a 5-ml sucrose gradient with a density range of 1.01–1.15 gm/ml by bringing an aliquot (1.5 ml) of serum to a density of 1.15 gm/ml with sucrose, then overlaying with 1.5 ml phosphate-buffered saline (PBS)–sucrose adjusted to a density of 1.10 gm/ml, and finally filling the tube with 2 ml PBS. The gradient was centrifuged in a Spinco SW 50.1 rotor (Beckman Instruments, Palo Alto, California) for 18 hours at 189,000 g. Fractions were removed, and the density calculated. The serum fraction with a density >1.12 gm/ml was dialyzed against PBS. The sucrose gradient fraction was then separated on a KBr gradient with a density of 1.01–1.15 gm/ml by bringing a 1.5-ml aliquot to a density of 1.15 gm/ml with KBr, then overlaying with 1.5 ml of PBS–KBr, density 1.1 gm/ml, and filling the tube with 2.0 ml PBS. This gradient was then centrifuged as above (20). Fractions with a density of 1.02–1.06 gm/ml were pooled and dialyzed overnight in PBS or in RPMI-1640 medium using Spectra/Por 3 dialysis tubing (Spectrum Industries, Los Angeles, California) and yielded a fraction called SKL. With an initial serum volume of 1.5 ml, the volume of the SKL fraction was 3 ml.

B. Thin-Layer Chromatography

Silica G plates (Merck, Darmstadt, Germany) were used for chromatography. A variety of polar lipids and steroids (Sigma, St. Louis, Missouri) were used as standards. Plates were developed in several solvent systems (21), as described in Section III. Bands were detected with orcinol, ninhydrin, and molybdate sprays and with 50% H_2SO_4 spray and charring. For preparative thin-layer chromatography (TLC), 600 μl of the sucrose–KBr gradient fraction was streaked on the plates. After development, strips were cut from the side of the plate, and spots identified with H_2SO_4 spray. The unsprayed portion of the plate was then scraped in the appropriate area. The scraped silica was eluted with chloroform, methanol, and water (1:1:0.1) overnight. Silica was removed by filtration, and the extract dried by vacuum evaporation.

In early experiments, the extract was incorporated into liposomes by adding 1.0 μmole lecithin and 0.5 μmole cholesterol and drying under vacuum, followed by the addition of 600 μl RPMI-1640 medium, warming, and vortexing or sonication. Subsequently, the dried extract was redissolved by warming and vortexing in 600 μl RPMI-1640 medium supplemented with 10% normal human serum (NHS) as described by Wolf and Merler (22). No difference between the two methods of preparation was observed in assays of duplicate eluates from TLC.

C. Assay of Activity

Peripheral blood from normal donors or patients with HD was separated on a Ficoll–Hypaque gradient. Mononuclear cells were washed and suspended in RPMI-1640 medium containing 10% NHS. Occasionally, PBLs that had been stored in the frozen state were utilized. For each assay PBLs from a patient with HD and from a normal donor were cultured simultaneously using the same materials.

Two methods of phytohemagglutinin (PHA) cell stimulation were used to assay suppression. In the first method, mononuclear cells were suspended at a concentration of 5×10^5/ml in RPMI-1640 containing 10% NHS. A cell aliquot of 0.2 ml/well was stimulated with PHA (Burroughs Wellcome, Bechenham, England) at a final concentration of 1μg/ml. The material to be assayed was added to test wells in 10 to 40 μl volumes. Since the amounts of biologically active material in the SKL fractions and TLC eluates were too small to be determined chemically, the quantity of material assayed was expressed as the final concentration of the SKL fraction or TLC eluate tested; i.e., a 5% test concentration of HD-SKL was prepared by adding 10 μl to the cell suspension. Cells were incubated for 48 hours, pulsed with tritiated thymidine (1 μCi/well), and harvested onto filter disks at 72 hours.

The second PHA assay was based on that described by Wolf and Merler (22). The PBLs were suspended at 2×10^6 cells/ml in RPMI-1640 medium containing 10% NHS. An aliquot (0.3 ml) of this suspension was added to 0.6 ml of RPMI-1640 medium with 10% NHS containing the substance to be tested. A sample (0.2 ml) of this mixture was added to each well and stimulated with 1 μg/ml PHA. Cultures were pulsed with tritiated thymidine (1 μCi/well) at 30 hours and harvested at 48 hours. All cultures were prepared in quadruplicate. Cell viability was checked at the end of culture and was consistently greater than 85%.

D. Protein and Carbohydrate Determinations

Protein was assayed using the Bio Rad protein assay (Bio Rad Laboratories, Richmond, California). Human albumin (Sigma) and human beta lipoproteins from gradient flotation NHS were used as standards. With the microassay procedure these proteins could be reproducibly detected at 2 μg/ml. Hexose was measured by the phenol–H_2SO_4 method (23) using a galactose–glucose 1 : 1 mixture as a standard.

E. Radiolabeling

Radiolabeling of the terminal sialic acid or sugar residues with tritium was done using the method of Van Lenten and Ashwell (24). The SKL fraction in 0.1 M sodium acetate was activated by periodate oxidation and reduced using 5 mCi sodium borotritide (8 Ci/mmole, Amersham, Arlington Heights, Illinois).

F. Glycolipids

Bovine brain gangliosides (Sigma) were assayed for their capacity to suppress PBL responses to PHA. They were evaporated under vacuum and redissolved in complete medium or incorporated into lipsomes for assay.

III. Results

Previous experiments (13, 19) had shown that serum from patients with HD contained an inhibitor of lymphocyte proliferation and E-rosette formation. After KBr gradient fractionation this substance was found in the low-density fractions, but on sucrose gradients it was found in the serum protein with a density greater than 1.12 gm/ml. When HD or normal serum was fractionated sequentially on sucrose and then on KBr gradients, the final low-density fraction contained no detectable (<2 μg/ml) protein or lipoprotein. The hexose contents of the SKL fractions from three pools of HD serum were 25, 32, and 35 μg/ml. The hexose contents of the SKL fractions from two normal serum pools were 28 and 30 μg/ml.

The SKL gradient fraction was assayed for its capacity to inhibit PHA stimulation, using the 72- or 48-hour PHA assay (Table I). At a 5% concentration, the HD serum SKL fraction (HD-SKL) inhibited the PHA response of PBL from

TABLE I

Inhibition of [³H]Thymidine Incorporation into Phytohemagglutinin Stimulated Peripheral Blood Leukocytes by the HD-SKL Fraction from Hodgkin's Disease Serum

Source of PBLs	PHA alone, 1 µg/ml (mean cpm ± SD)[a]	PHA + N-SKL at 30% conc. (mean cpm ± SD)[a]	Normal serum pool	PHA + HD-SKL at 5% conc. (mean cpm ± SD)[b]	HD serum pool	PHA + HD-SKL at 30% conc. (mean cpm ± SD)[b]	Inhibition of PHA stimulation at 30% conc. of HD-SKL (%)
HD patients	69,979 ± 4504	68,102 ± 4255	A	39,369 ± 1173	5	27,521 ± 1385	60
	51,233 ± 1989	49,329 ± 2060	A	21,454 ± 1044	6	21,761 ± 2141	57
	57,607 ± 2036	—		28,258 ± 3530	6	20,231 ± 1892	64
	28,581 ± 1583	23,787 ± 1943	A	17,131 ± 1051	7	1,334 ± 140	95
	28,854 ± 2228	28,514 ± 2420	A	12,414 ± 864	8	9,091 ± 434	68
	26,320 ± 1415	—		7,509 ± 942	9	—	—
	34,301 ± 1698	29,138 ± 1275	B	13,006 ± 755	9	4,429 ± 925	87
	41,830 ± 4136	37,325 ± 3516	B	31,363 ± 2160	11	6,619 ± 752	84
	75,925 ± 1361	—		7,120 ± 887	12	—	—
	23,946 ± 272	19,981 ± 932	B	13,324 ± 743	12	6,232 ± 317	73
Mean	37,827	36,596		19,086		12,151	67
Normal donors	77,950 ± 5399	75,832 ± 5112	A	71,613 ± 3164	5	35,079 ± 1941	54
	79,946 ± 4752	76,477 ± 4815	A	75,509 ± 5375	5	37,925 ± 1580	52
	68,740 ± 2083	63,125 ± 3212	A	38,033 ± 3619	6	26,121 ± 912	62
	26,666 ± 2866	26,842 ± 2696	A	25,212 ± 2611	6	18,932 ± 863	29
	20,763 ± 921	21,720 ± 1047	A	22,328 ± 1232	7	8,894 ± 360	57
	52,833 ± 3329	49,315 ± 3923	A	49,634 ± 5532	7	18,883 ± 782	64
	51,230 ± 1744	48,947 ± 2668	A	50,636 ± 2483	8	24,636 ± 2178	51
	49,257 ± 3329	49,565 ± 3827	A	49,488 ± 4015	8	21,003 ± 1191	57
	68,947 ± 3243	60,423 ± 3942	B	55,536 ± 1874	9	7,070 ± 881	89
	39,820 ± 2686	35,289 ± 2320	B	33,269 ± 2431	9	10,709 ± 394	73
	74,815 ± 4062	—		—	11	33,422 ± 2075	55
	49,897 ± 1510	—			12	19,832 ± 969	60
	63,965 ± 2333	—		60,265 ± 2082	12	7,538 ± 1015	88
Mean	55,756	50,749		48,319		20,772	60

[a] From two pools of normal human serum.
[b] From eight pools of sera from patients with untreated Hodgkin's disease.

HD patients but not that of normal donor PBLs. However, at a 30% concentration, HD-SKL also inhibited the PHA response of normal PBLs. The SKL fraction similarly prepared from normal serum (N-SKL) was not suppressive for either HD or normal PBLs (Table I). The SKL fractions from two HD serum pools were also assayed at a 1% concentration on PBLs of three HD patients, using the 48-hour PHA assay. One of these HD-SKL fractions did not inhibit the PHA response at this concentration. The other HD-SKL fraction, tested at a 1% concentration, inhibited the PHA response by 22, 29, and 10% (10% inhibition is not significant). When the SKL fractions from the sera of six individual HD patients were assayed for their capacity to inhibit the PHA response of HD PBLs from four different patients, all caused 50–70% suppression at 30% concentration, and only one patient's serum SKL fraction failed to produce inhibition of the PHA response when assayed at 5% concentration.

Aliquots (600 μl) of the HD-SKL and N-SKL fractions were run on TLC using a solvent system of chloroform, methanol, and water (60:35:8). After H_2SO_4 spray and charring, three or four bands of variable intensity were seen on the HD-SKL chromatogram (Fig. 1). After preparative TLC, the silica was scraped from four regions on each plate corresponding to the bands on the HD-SKL

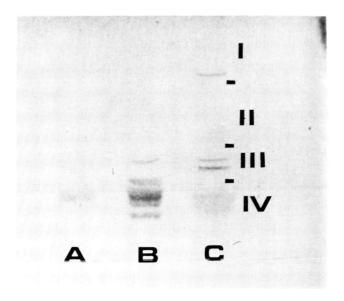

Fig. 1. Thin-layer chromatogram of SKL fractions on silica gel G. The solvent used was chloroform: methanol: water (60:38:8). Bands were identified by charring with 50% sulfuric acid. Lane A, SKL fraction from normal human serum. Lane B, bovine brain gangliosides. Lane C, SKL fraction from HD serum. Roman numerals indicate areas scraped and eluted (see text).

chromatogram and eluted (Fig. 1). After drying, each eluate was resuspended in 600 μl RPMI-1640 medium.

In the first set of experiments, eluates were incorporated into liposomes and tested at a 10% concentration in the PHA assay. Under these conditions, it was found that TLC eluate I from both normal and HD serum depressed the PHA response of both normal and HD PBLs by 25–35%. At a 60% concentration of eluate I dissolved in medium containing 10% NHS, depression of response was again 25–35% in the PHA assay. When eluate I was run on TLC with several standards in several solvent systems, it comigrated with one of two bands in a prednisolone standard (Sigma). Inhibition of PHA stimulation by glucocorticoids has been previously reported (25, 26). Eluates II and IV did not inhibit the PHA response, although eluate IV contained a band which was visible on TLC. Prostaglandins migrated near the solvent front in this solvent mixture.

When eluate III from the HD-SKL fraction was tested at a 10% concentration either in liposomes or dissolved in medium, it inhibited the PHA response of HD PBLs but not that of normal donor PBLs (Table II). However, at a 60% concentration in the 48-hour PHA assay, both normal and HD PBLs were inhibited by eluate III from the HD-SKL fraction (Table II). Eluate III from N-SKL fractions did not inhibit the PHA response of either normal or HD PBLs.

On TLC and SKL fractions from the sera of individual patients with HD were found to contain the eluate III band in 6 of 6 individuals. However, there was considerable variation from individual to individual in the amount of this material seen on TLC. In the SKL fraction of 6 individual normal donors and 10 individual patients with acute bacterial infections or carcinoma no band was seen in the eluate III region.

Bovine brain gangliosides at a final concentration of 100 μg/ml also inhibited the PHA stimulation responses of HD PBLs, but not those of normal PBLs. When these gangliosides were run on TLC, none had exactly the same R_f as eluate III from the HD-SKL fraction (Fig. 1). However, in several standard solvent systems HD-SKL eluate III migrates in the same region as gangliosides. In solvent systems more polar than that used for preparative TLC (chloroform, methanol, and water, 60:35:8), the HD-SKL eluate III material appeared to migrate as a double band. On the chromatogram, HD-SKL eluate III stained weakly purple with orcinol and was negative with ninhydrin and molybdate. The HD-SKL and N-SKL fractions had bands in the eluate IV region (Fig. 1), which also stained purple with orcinol.

The SKL fraction was radiolabeled by KIO_4 oxidation and reduction with tritiated NaB^3H_4. The labeled fraction was dialyzed, evaporated under vacuum, and extracted into chloroform–methanol (2:1). This was separated on TLC, and the bands identified with H_2SO_4–ethanol spray. Incorporated counts in bands and background areas of the plate were measured in a liquid scintillation counter. Background was 60 cpm, HD eluate III contained 1100 cpm, and HD and normal

TABLE II

Inhibition of Peripheral Blood Leukocyte Response to Phytohemagglutinin by Eluates from Thin-Layer-Chromatography Bands of HD-SKL and N-SKI Fractions[a]

Source of PBLs	HD-SKL eluate						N-SKL eluate						
	I		II	III		IV	I		II	III		IV	Gangliosides[b]
	10%	60%	60%	10%	60%	60%	10%	60%	60%	10%	60%	60%	
HD patients													
1[c]	22	—	—	60	—	—	24	—	—	1	—	—	—
2[c]	20	—	—	51	—	—	22	—	—	6	—	—	—
3[c]	25	—	—	59	—	—	27	—	—	11	—	—	—
4	26	29	3	48	55	8	27	27	5	3	9	6	53
5	26	30	-7	34	52	15	26	23	11	7	15	8	50
6	20	28	5	59	67	7	18	25	-1	6	10	1	49
7	—	26	1	—	62	6	—	28	2	—	12	3	42
8	—	29	8	—	57	8	—	26	2	—	7	4	62
9	—	24	—	—	54	—	—	28	—	—	4	—	—
Normal donors													
1[c]	25	—	—	14	—	—	19	—	—	8	—	—	—
2[c]	14	—	—	8	—	—	15	—	—	2	—	—	—
3	26	25	1	12	38	8	17	23	0	9	9	4	0
4	20	26	5	18	59	10	21	23	4	10	12	1	8
5	24	25	0	10	48	2	13	21	4	8	2	5	20
6	—	29	7	—	46	11	—	20	9	—	11	7	10
7	—	18	3	—	51	6	—	20	0	—	7	-1	16
8	—	22	-2	—	40	7	—	27	-1	—	8	3	—
9	—	—	—	8	49	—	—	—	—	-2	4	—	—
10	—	—	—	13	53	—	—	—	—	7	12	—	—

[a] Percentage inhibition of [³H]thymidine incorporation into PHA-stimulated PBLs by the indicated test concentration of each eluate. Numbers preceded by a minus symbo indicate slight stimulation rather than inhibition.

[b] Bovine brain gangliosides (Sigma), 100 µg/ml.

[c] 72-hour PHA assays with eluates prepared as liposomes; all other data refer to 48-hour PHA assays with eluates dissolved in medium.

eluate IV contained 6100 and 7500 cpm, respectively. The fast-migrating bands contained background counts.

IV. Discussion

We have previously reported an inhibitor of E-rosette formation and lymphocyte mitogenesis in the sera of patients with HD. Further pruification has shown this substance to be a glycolipid. A similar (or identical) glycolipid which inhibits the mitogen response of normal PBLs has been described by Wolf and Merler (22) and named SIF. This compound is produced after mitogen or antigen stimulation of normal PBLs *in vitro*. The glycolipid inhibitor we describe was consistently found in the sera of patients with HD but was not detected in normal serum at the concentrations tested. This glycolipid, when assayed *in vitro* at equivalent serum dilution of 1:3 to 1:20, inhibited the PHA mitogenic response of PBLs from patients with HD but failed to inhibit that of normal PBLs except at higher concentrations. The glycolipid inhibitor was found in all eight pools of HD serum and was present in the sera of all six individual patients tested, although its concentration varied. No attempt has yet been made to correlate this difference in concentration with clinical stage or histopathological type of disease.

The HD serum glycolipid was active as an inhibitor of lymphocyte proliferation after elution from a TLC plate. Staining of the TLC plates showed that one band or perhaps a double band was being eluted in a region which reveals no bands when normal serum is used. The substance migrated on TLC in the region of a small ganglioside or a large glycolipid. The band stained weakly purple with orcinol and could be radiolabeled with periodate, indicating the presence of a sugar, but the composition of the substance was otherwise unknown. However, gangliosides are known to have immunosuppressive effects. In this study, gangliosides from bovine brain at a concentration of 10 nmoles suppressed the PHA response of HD PBLs but not that of normal donor PBLs. Bovine gangliosides have also been reported to suppress mitogen responses of rat thymocytes (27). A specific ganglioside from mouse brain suppresses mouse B-cell differentiation (28). Human brain gangliosides have been reported to suppress human PBL mitogenic responses (29).

Preliminary results indicate that the HD-SKL fraction glycolipid, after elution from TLC plates, is also capable of depressing E-rosette formation by PBLs from patients with HD after they have been restored to normal levels by incubation with FCS (16). The depressed *in vitro* PHA response and E-rosette levels seen with PBLs from patients with untreated HD may be due to *in vivo* exposure of their lymphocytes to this circulating glycolipid inhibitor. The inhibitor may be produced by Hodgkin's cells. More likely it is a normal product for suppression of an immune response, which is uncontrolled in HD, or it may be a side effect of an increase in the number of suppressor cells, which has been reported in HD. Experiments are in progress to determine the chemical composition and structure of the glycolipid inhibitor, to study the source of its production in HD, and to assess its relevance to the immunological deficiency characteristic of untreated HD.

Acknowledgments

The authors would like to thank June Twelves, Nancy Ginzton, and Nicola Nanewicz for excellent technical assistance. This work was supported by research grants CA-05838 and CA-17004, and by research contract NO1-CP-91044 from the National Cancer Institute, NIH, DHEW.

References

1. J. R. Eltringham and H. S. Kaplan, *Natl. Cancer Inst. Monogr.* **36**, 107 (1973).
2. R. C. Young, M. P. Corder, H. Haynes, and V. DeVita, *Am. J. Med.* **52**, 63 (1972).
3. R. A. Good, W. D. Kelly, J. Rotstein, and R. L. Varco, *Prog. Allergy* **6**, 275 (1962).
4. A. U. Muftuoglu and S. Balkuv, *N. Engl. J. Med.* **277**, 126 (1967).
5. M. Fazio and A. Calciate, *Panminerva Med.* **4**, 164 (1962).
6. R. Levy and H. S. Kaplan, *N. Engl. J. Med.* **290**, 181 (1974).
7. E. M. Hersh and J. J. Oppenheim, *N. Engl. J. Med.* **273**, 1006 (1965).
8. R. S. Brown, H. A. Haynes, H. T. Foley, H. A. Godwin, C. W. Berard, and P. P. Carbone, *Ann. Intern. Med.* **67**, 291 (1967).
9. G. B. Faguet, *J. Clin. Invest.* **56**, 951 (1975).
10. J. M. Gaines, M. Gilmer, and J. S. Remington, *Natl. Cancer Inst. Monogr.* **36**, 117 (1973).
11. T. Han, *Cancer (Philadelphia)* **29**, 1626 (1972).
12. G. Holm, P. Perlmann, and B. Johansson, *Clin. Exp. Immunol.* **2**, 351 (1967).
13. Z. Fuks, S. Strober, and H. S. Kaplan, *N. Engl. J. Med.* **295**, 1273 (1976).
14. E. Ezdinli, K. L. Simonson, L. G. Simonson, and L. P. Wasser, *Cancer (Philadelphia)* **44**, 106 (1979).
15. A. M. Bobrove, Z. Fuks, S. Strober, and H. S. Kaplan, *Cancer (Philadelphia)* **36**, 169 (1975).
16. Z. Fuks, S. Strober, D. P. King, and H. S. Kaplan, *J. Immunol.* **117**, 1331 (1976).
17. C. Moroz, N. Lahat, M. Biniaminov, and B. Ramot, *Clin. Exp. Immunol.* **29**, 30 (1977).
18. B. Ramot, M. Biniaminov, C. Shoham, and E. Rosenthal, *N. Engl. J. Med.* **294**, 80–89 (1976).
19. M. M. Bieber, Z. Fuks, and H. S. Kaplan, *Clin. Exp. Immunol.* **29**, 369 (1977).
20. F. V. Chisari and T. S. Edgington, *J. Exp. Med.* **142**, 1092 (1975).
21. W. J. Esselman, R. A. Laine, and C. C. Sweeley, *in* "Methods in Enzymology" (V. Ginsburg, ed.), Vol. 28, Part B, p. 140. Academic Press, New York, 1973.
22. R. L. Wolf and E. Merler, *J. Immunol.* **123**, 1169 (1979).
23. M. Dubois, K. A. Gilles, J. K. Hamilton, P. A. Rebers, and F. Smith, *Anal. Chem.* **28**, 350 (1956).
24. L. Van Lenten and G. Ashwell, *in* "Methods in Enzymology" (V. Ginsburg, ed.), Vol. 28, Part B, p. 209. Academic Press, New York, 1973.
25. S. Gillis, G. R. Crabtree, and K. A. Smith, *J. Immunol.* **123**, 1624 (1979).
26. D. C. Tormey, H. H. Fudenberg, and R. M. Kamin, *Nature (London)* **210**, 282 (1967).
27. E. E. Lengle, R. Krishnaraj, and R. G. Kemp, *Cancer Res.* **39**, 817 (1979).
28. W. Esselman and H. C. Miller, *J. Immunol.* **119**, 1994 (1977).
29. R. L. Wihisler and A. J. Yates, *J. Immunol.* **125**, 2106 (1980).

19

Studies on Autologous and Allogeneic Mixed Leukocyte Reactions in Patients with Hodgkin's Disease

EDGAR G. ENGLEMAN

I. Introduction

The immunological status of patients with Hodgkin's disease has been a topic of intense investigation for the past two decades. Although antibody responses appear to be unimpaired (1, 2), patients frequently exhibit defects in T-cell-mediated immune functions manifested by diminished delayed hypersensitivity responses (3-7), impaired ability to reject skin allografts (8-10), and decreased resistance to certain types of infection (11, 12). Several *in vitro* functions of peripheral blood T cells have been shown to be defective, including the blastogenic response to soluble antigens (13-15), alloantigens (16-18), plant lectins (2, 19-29), and autoantigens (30). Although these abnormalities are of variable magnitude and are not diagnostic of Hodgkin's disease, their frequent occurrence in patients with this malignancy suggests that a defect of cell-mediated immunity may play a role in the pathogenesis of the disease.

In this report the status of allogeneic and autologous mixed leukocyte reactions (MLRs) is assessed in patients with Hodgkin's disease, untreated and treated. As shown, these reactions are often defective in Hodgkin's patients, but the explanation for the defects varies according to treatment status. Total lymphoid irradiation (TLI) in particular has profound effects on these T-lympocyte functions and results in the appearance of suppressor cells of the allogeneic MLR. On the other hand, untreated as well as treated patients frequently have impaired autologous MLRs, possibly suggesting a relationship between this immunologic defect and disease pathogenesis.

II. Materials and Methods

All patients with Hodgkin's disease underwent histological diagnosis as well as a staging lymphangiography and laparotomy at Stanford University Hospital. They were subsequently treated and followed at the Stanford University Radiation Therapy Clinic. Approximately 250 Hodgkin's patients were studied, of whom approximately 30 were untreated at the time of study. The remainder were studied 1-16 years following cessation of local, involved-field, or TLI with or without chemotherapy; these patients were in remission at the time of study. Although a variety of clinical stages and histological types of Hodgkin's disease were represented in our sample, the great majority of patients had stage II or III disease of the nodular sclerosing type.

Peripheral blood mononuclear leukocytes (PBMLs) were isolated by Ficoll-Hypaque gradient centrifugation (31) and suspended in RPMI-1640 medium supplemented with 25 mM HEPES buffer, 2 mM glutamine, and 10% heat-inactivated pooled human serum. Preparations enriched for T or non-T cells were obtained by a sheep erythrocyte (E)-rosetting technique described previously (30).

Allogeneic MLRs were carried out in round-bottom microtiter wells using 5 × 10^4 responder PBMLs and 5 × 10^4 X-irradiated (3000 rads) stimulator PBMLs in a volume of 0.2 ml. Triplicate cultures were incubated in air-10% CO_2 for 6 days at 37°C. At that time proliferation was measured by the addition of 1 μCi/well [^{3}H]thymidine, and the cells were harvested 18 hours later.

A screening test for the presence of PBMLs, which suppress the allogeneic MLR, is based on the observation that circulating suppressor cells of the MLR can be subjected to 1000 rads of X-irradiation without loss of suppressive activity (32–34). X-Irradiation of PBMLs abrogates the radiosensitive activities of other cell populations, leaving radio-resistant suppressor cells intact. In suppressor assays, 5×10^4 responder cells and 5×10^4 irradiated (6000 rads) allogeneic stimulator cells were cocultured with an additional 5×10^4 X-irradiated (1000 rads) responder cells in 0.2 ml. Each subject was tested against four unrelated stimulator cells, and the test was considered positive if the irradiated autologous cells inhibited at least two of four responses by a minimum of 40%.

Autologous MLRs were performed in a manner identical to allogeneic MLRs, except that 5×10^4 T lymphocytes were used as responders and 1×10^5 irradiated autologous non-T cells were used as stimulators.

III. Studies on Allogeneic Mixed Leukocyte Reactions

The allogeneic MLR is the proliferative response of one individual's (responder) lymphocytes cultured in the presence of another individual's (stimulator) lymphocytes. In humans, this reaction is elicited by cell surface antigens encoded by the *HLA-D* locus (35). This locus is among a cluster of genes located on the sixth chromosome which also includes genes coding for the major histocompatibility antigens HLA-A, -B, -C, and -DR. If the stimulator cell possesses D antigens not present on the responder, the lymphocytes of the latter undergo blast transformation resulting in DNA synthesis which can be measured (35). A vigorous response in the MLR to histoincompatible cells is the rule among healthy individuals.

A diminished allogeneic MLR is a characteristic feature of Hodgkin's disease, particularly in patients treated with TLI (36). The studies summarized below were an effort to determine if cells that suppress the MLR were responsible for the diminished alloreactivity of these patients.

A. Suppressor Cells in Untreated and Treated Patients

Normal volunteers as well as untreated and treated patients with Hodgkin's disease were tested for the presence of circulating MLR suppressor cells. An example of a positive suppressor test in a patient previously treated with TLI is shown in Fig. 1. As shown, this patient's responses to three of four stimulator cells were inhibited by the addition of his irradiated cells to the cultures. The results summarized in Table I indicate that detectable MLR suppressor cells are rare in healthy individuals but common in patients with Hodgkin's disease. The presence of MLR suppressor cells in patients showed no correlation with age,

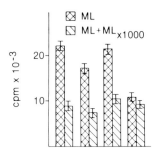

Fig. 1. Mixed leukocyte reaction suppressor activity in a patient with Hodgkin's disease. Cross-hatched columns represent a one-way MLR between cells from ML, a patient with Hodgkin's disease, and four different irradiated stimulator cells. Hatched columns represent the same MLRs in the presence of 5×10^4 ML cells exposed to 1000 rads. Each result represents the mean of triplicate cultures.

sex, duration of disease, histological classification, clinical stage, or HLA type (data not shown).

In an effort to determine the cell types responsible for MLR suppression in these patients, purified T and non-T lymphoid cells were tested for their capacity to suppress the MLR. The results summarized in Table II indicate that the majority of untreated and treated patients had detectable suppressor cells. However, in the majority of untreated patients suppression was in the non-T (monocyte and B-cell-enriched) fraction, whereas among treated patients E-rosette-forming (T) cells accounted for the majority of cases of observed suppression.

B. Induction of Suppressor Cells by Total Lymphoid Irradiation

The simplest interpretation of the above results was that treatment with, for example, TLI either induced suppressive lymphocytes or accentuated their detection.

TABLE I

Frequency of Mixed Leukocyte Reaction Suppressor Cells in Normal Subjects and Patients with Hodgkin's Disease

Subjects	Significant suppression	No significant suppression
Normal volunteers	1	51
Patients with untreated Hodgkin's disease	2	4
Patients with treated Hodgkin's disease	43	74

TABLE II

Mixed Leukocyte Reaction Suppressor Cell Types in Patients with Hodgkin's Disease

	Suppression of MLR by			
Patients	T cells alone	Non-T cells alone	Both T and non-T cells	No suppressor cells
Untreated ($n = 9$)	1	4	1	3
Treated ($n = 68$)	15	8	27	18

However, because untreated Hodgkin's patients frequently have immune defects and because the same patients were not available for study before and after treatment, additional studies were needed to test the hypothesis that TLI induces cells that suppress the MLR. Such studies were stimulated by the recent discoveries of Strober, Kaplan, and their colleagues at Stanford University that preparation of experimental animals with TLI allowed successful bone marrow transplantation across major histocompatibility barriers (37) and reversed autoimmune disease (38). Recently, these findings have led to clinical trials of TLI in organ transplantation and autoimmune diseases, the preliminary results of which are extremely encouraging.

The emergence of TLI as an immunosuppressive regimen for disorders other than Hodgkin's disease enabled us to examine its effects on non-Hodgkin's patients. Specifically, we sought to determine if MLR suppressor cells were induced in patients with advanced rheumatoid arthritis who underwent TLI at Stanford University Hospital. An initial report of the clinical results of this trial has appeared (39).

Six patients were studied before and after TLI. Five of six pretreatment patients responded normally in the MLR and had no detectable suppressor cells on the basis of comparing their responses in the absence and presence of irradiated autologous lymphocytes. To determine if suppressor cells were present 1 month after the completion of TLI, cryopreserved pretreatment lymphocytes were tested for the capacity to respond to allogeneic cells in the presence and absence of freshly obtained posttreatment lymphocytes. With this test, suppressor cells were detected in all six patients 1 month following TLI. Typical results in a TLI-treated patient who lacked detectable suppressor cells prior to treatment are shown in Table III.

Suppression appears to be mediated by a population of E-rosette-forming cells which lack most known T-lymphocyte differentiation markers. Kinetic studies revealed no early or delayed responses in cultures, consisting of 3 cell types, and cytotoxicity assays revealed no evidence of killing by suppressor cells. Suppression

TABLE III

Suppressor Cells of the Allogeneic Mixed Leukocyte Reaction in a Rheumatoid Arthritis Patient Treated with Total Lymphoid Irradiation[a]

Responder	Stimulator	Third-party cell	Response	Percentage of control response
Patient pre-TLI	Unrelated donor	None	25,230 ± 2,015	100
		Patient pre-TLI T	30,019 ± 2,394	119
		Patient pre-TLI non-T	27,606 ± 1,962	109
		Patient post-TLI T	10,556 ± 1,402	42
		Patient post-TLI non-T	13,990 ± 918	55
Healthy donor	Unrelated donor	None	43,512 ± 3,531	100
		Patient pre-TLI T	61,450 ± 5,419	141
		Patient pre-TLI non-T	56,683 ± 4,870	130
		Patient post-TLI T	30,894 ± 3,236	71
		Patient post-TLI non-T	20,757 ± 1,846	48

[a] PBMLs from a patient with rheumatoid arthritis were obtained 1 week prior to TLI. The cells were fractionated into T and non-T cells by E-rosetting and cryopreserved. One month after TLI, 5×10^4 thawed pre-TLI cells or 5×10^4 fresh PBMLs from a healthy donor were challenged with 5×10^4 irradiated (3000 rads) PEMLs from an unrelated donor in the presence or absence of the patient's pre- or post-TLI T or non-T cells. The results represent the mean of triplicate cultures ±SE.

was not antigen-specific in that the responses to all stimulator cells tested were usually inhibited, nor was suppression genetically restricted in that responder cells from healthy donors who had no HLA antigens in common with suppressor donors were inhibited (39). These observations are in agreement with those made for TLI-treated Hodgkin's patients. More importantly, the results clearly show that TLI plays a causal role in the appearance of suppressor cells, because patients were studied prospectively before and after treatment and because TLI was the only addition to an otherwise stable treatment regimen.

C. Discussion

On the basis of these findings, it is apparent that the presence of MLR suppressor cells in Hodgkin's patients who have undergone TLI may not be related to their primary disease. Moreover, the fact that this treatment has few long-term side effects suggests that suppressor cells of the type described are well tolerated. It is noteworthy that MLR suppressor cells have also been detected in the spleens of mice treated with TLI. Like the suppressor cells of TLI-treated humans, suppressor cells from TLI-treated mice consist of null lymphocytes, are radiation-resistant, are nonspecific with respect to stimulating antigen, and are not genetically restricted with respect to responder cell (40). The murine MLR suppressor cells not only inhibited alloreactivity *in vitro* but also prevented graft-versus-host disease when transferred to unirradiated syngeneic recipients. If, as the murine experiments suggest, TLI-induced MLR suppressor cells mediate immunological suppression *in vivo,* then by analogy the MLR suppressor cells described here may contribute to clinically significant immunosuppression in humans.

IV. Studies of the Autologous Mixed Leukocyte Reaction

The proliferative response of T lymphocytes cultured with autologous HLA-DR-positive non-T cells (B cells and monocytes) is known as the autologous MLR (41–48). The significance of this reaction *in vivo* is uncertain. Nonetheless it can be demonstrated reproducibly in healthy individuals, exhibits immunological memory and specificity, and has been shown to generate specific cytotoxic T cells as well as suppressor T cells. As described below, the autologous MLR is impaired in most patients with Hodgkin's disease regardless of their treatment status. The data provided in summary form here are presented in more detail elsewhere (30).

A. The Autologous Mixed Leukocyte Reaction in Untreated and Treated Patients

The T cells from normal volunteers or patients with Hodgkin's disease were cultured with either irradiated autologous non-T cells (the autologous MLR) or irradiated allogeneic PBMLs (the allogeneic MLR), and proliferation was measured after 1 week as described in Section II. As shown in Fig. 2, the mean autologous MLR of 29 normal subjects was 16,552 ± 6532 cpm. By comparison, the autologous MLR of 64 patients (untreated and treated) averaged only 3084 ± 1878 cpm. The response of T cells from the same patients to allogeneic lymphocytes was also diminished in patients (25,190 ± 9814) when compared to normals (37,218 ± 12,675). However, the reduction in the allogeneic MLR was modest as compared to the impairment of the autologous MLR, and many patients with vigorous responses to allogeneic lymphocytes failed to respond to autologous non-T cells.

There was no relationship between the level of autologous MLR and the histological classification or pathological stage (30). Treated patients in remis-

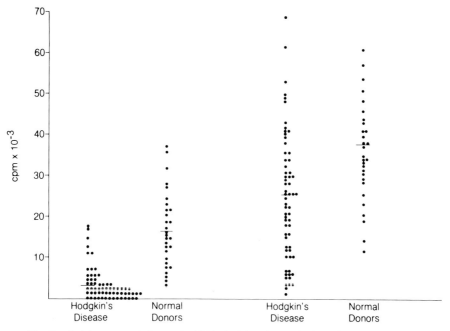

Fig. 2. Autologous and allogeneic MLRs in 64 patients with Hodgkin's disease and 29 healthy donors. The T cells (5 × 10⁴) were incubated with 1 × 10⁵ autologous non-T cells or 5 × 10⁴ allogeneic PBMLs from three different healthy donors. Results of the autologous MLR (left) are expressed as the mean of triplicate cultures. Results of the allogeneic MLR (right) are expressed as the mean response to three unrelated histoincompatible stimulator cells.

sion for 1–15 years, as well as untreated patients with active disease, had impaired autologous MLRs (30). However, the autologous MLR was more markedly depressed in recently treated patients than in patients who had been in remission for several years. For example, only 1 of 12 patients studied within 2 years of treatment had an autologous MLR greater than 2000 cpm compared to 14 of 23 patients tested 6 years or more after treatment, and 3 of 7 patients studied 10 or more years after treatment had autologous MLRs greater than 10,000 cpm.

B. Cellular Basis of Impaired Autoreactivity in Patients Treated with Total Lymphoid Irradiation

These findings could not be explained by abnormal kinetics or poor viability of stimulator or responder cells (30). Increasing the number of responder T cells in the culture or removing adherent cells from the stimulator population enhanced autoreactivity in some patients, indicating that the defect was not absolute (30). To determine whether the impaired autologous MLR was due to defective responder cells, defective stimulator cells, or both, two patients in remission following treatment with TLI and their healthy HLA-identical siblings were studied. In these studies, T lymphocytes from a patient, an HLA-A, -B, -DR-identical

TABLE IV

Cellular Basis of the Impaired Autologous Mixed Leukocyte Reaction in Two Patients with Hodgkin's Disease Treated with Total Lymphoid Irradiation

Responder	Response to stimulator non-T cells of		
	Patient A	Sibling of A	Unrelated donor 1
Patient A	1,611 ± 192	1,864 ± 1,341	22,823 ± 1,970
Sibling of A	29,915 ± 3,125	22,891 ± 2,450	47,510 ± 4,264
Unrelated donor 1	36,159 ± 4,029	39,670 ± 4,036	19,488 ± 2,090

Responder	Response to stimulator non-T cells of		
	Patient B	Sibling of B	Unrelated donor 2
Patient B	702 ± 95	1,140 ± 140	34,566 ± 2,822
Sibling of B	10,466 ± 907	8,572 ± 1,410	51,321 ± 4,398
Unrelated donor 2	18,595 ± 2,335	39,314 ± 3,589	13,286 ± 1,655

[a] Healthy siblings were HLA-A, -B, -C, and -DR-identical to Patient A (A2,Aw26/B8, Bw50/Cw6,-/DR3,DRw6) or B (A2,A24/B17,B35/Cw3,-/DR1,DR5). Patients A and B were unrelated and were in remission 4 and 7 years after TLI, respectively. Results represent the means ± SE of triplicate cultures.

TABLE V

Cellular Basis of the Defect in the Autologous Mixed Leukocyte Reaction Caused by Total Lymphoid Irradiation

Responder T cells	Autologous stimulator cells	Response
Pre-TLI	Pre-TLI non-T	14,611 ± 1156
	Post-TLI non-T	13,490 ± 1212
Post-TLI	Pre-TLI non-T	894 ± 150
	Post-TLI non-T	667 ± 95

" PBMLs from a Hodgkin's patient were obtained 1 week prior to TLI, fractionated into T and non-T populations, and cryopreserved. One month after completion of TLI, fresh T and non-T cells were obtained from the same patient and used in combination with either pre-TLI or post-TLI cells in the autologous MLR. Results represent the mean of triplicate cultures ±SE.

sibling, and an unrelated healthy volunteer were cultured with non-T cells from each of these three subjects. As shown in Table IV, autologous MLRs were diminished in patients but normal in their healthy siblings. The T cells from healthy siblings responded normally to the non-T cells of affected siblings, indicating that there was no defect in the capacity of the non-T cells of these patients to stimulate HLA-identical T cells. On the other hand, both patients failed to respond to their own non-T cells and to their siblings' non-T cells, indicating that a defective responder T-cell population was responsible for the failure of these patients to mount an autologous MLR.

Recently, Claudia Benike and Geoffrey Kansas of this laboratory have demonstrated in prospective studies that TLI virtually eliminates the autologous MLR in all patients so treated and that the defect is exclusively a responder T-cell defect (49). These data were obtained by utilizing pre-TLI cryopreserved T and non-T lymphocytes in combination with autologous lymphocytes obtained after TLI. As shown in an example in Table V, pre-TLI T cells proliferated normally in response to both pre-TLI and post-TLI stimulator non-T cells, whereas post-TLI T cells failed to respond either to pre- or posttreatment non-T cells.

This effect of TLI has been observed in patients with rheumatoid arthritis as well as in patients with Hodgkin's disease. Preliminary studies on these patients have not revealed cells that suppress the autologous MLR. Thus, in three patients studied to date, the addition of post TLI PBMLs to pre-TLI T cells did not inhibit the response of the latter cells in the autologous MLR (data not shown).

C. Cellular Basis of Impaired Autoreactivity in Untreated Patients

The previous studies did not clarify the nature of the defect in autoreactivity in untreated patients. The possibility existed, for example, that suppressor cells were responsible for this defect. Geoffrey Kansas has recently attempted to detect such suppressor cells by using a monoclonal antibody known to recognize T lymphocytes reactive in the autologous MLR (50) to separate these cells from the remaining T cells and test for autologous MLR activity. To date, suppressor cells of the autologous MLR have not been demonstrated in our patients. Furthermore, T cells of the responder phenotype were present in normal numbers, suggesting that autoreactive cells are present but dysfunctional in Hodgkin's disease (51).

D. Discussion

These data demonstrate that the T cells of patients with Hodgkin's disease respond poorly to autologous non-T cells. Although impairment of the autologous MLR precedes treatment, the explanations for defective autoreactivity in treated and untreated patients may or may not be the same. The nature of the defect in two patients who had been treated previously with TLI and were in remission was clarified by performing reciprocal mixing experiments involving patients and their HLA-identical healthy siblings. In each case, the T cells of the healthy siblings mounted vigorous proliferative responses to both autologous and affected siblings' non-T cells. Patients' T cells, however, failed to respond to both autologous and healthy siblings' non-T cells. Proof that TLI was responsible for this defect was obtained subsequently in prospective studies on patients with rheumatoid arthritis as well as Hodgkin's disease who underwent TLI. Thus T cells obtained after TLI failed to respond to autologous non-T cells obtained either before or after TLI, whereas post-TLI non-T cells stimulated pre-TLI T cells normally.

In both treated and untreated patients, impairment of the autologous MLR tends to be more common and more pronounced than impairment of the allogeneic MLR. Apparently, this difference is due to incompletely overlapping T-cell subpopulations, some responsive exclusively to allogeneic or autologous non-T cells and others responsive to both. In both untreated and TLI-treated patients, the autoreactive population is either dysfunctional or depleted. No evidence for active cellular suppression of the autologous MLR has been obtained.

It is conceivable that impairment of the autologous MLR and the pathogenesis of Hodgkin's disease are related. In this regard, the observations of Van de Stouwe et al. (46) are of particular interest. These investigators observed that the autologous reaction could serve as a proliferative stimulus for specific cytotoxic lymphocyte generation. Thus heat-treated allogeneic lymphocytes that alone did not stimulate proliferation or cytotoxic T-cell generation produced specific cytotoxic cells when added to the autologous system. Other investigators have found that lymphocytes from normal individuals sensitized to HLA-identical leukemic cells can, in the presence of an allogeneic proliferative stimulus, differentiate into cells specifically cytotoxic to leukemic cells (52). *In vivo*, the autologous MLR may provide the stimulus needed for the generation of cytotoxic lymphocytes against autologous neoplastic or virally infected cells. Conceivably, Hodgkin's disease might result from a failure of this protective mechanism.

Acknowledgments

This study was supported in part by grants CA 24607 and CA 05838 from the National Institutes of Health and grants from the Veterans Administration and the State of California.

References

1. M. W. Chase, *Cancer Res.* **26,** 1097 (1966).
2. R. S. Brown, B. A. Haynes, H. T. Foley, H. A. Godwin, C. W. Berard, and P. P. Carbone, *Ann. Intern. Med.* **67,** 291 (1967).
3. W. W. Schier, A. P. Roth, G. Ostroff, and M. H. Schrift, *Am. J. Med.* **20,** 94 (1956).
4. J. E. Sokal and M. Primikirios, *Cancer (Philadelphia)* **14,** 597 (1969).
5. A. C. Aisenberg, *J. Clin. Invest.* **41,** 1964 (1962).
6. R. C. Young, M. P. Corder, H. A. Haynes, and V. T. DeVita, *Am. J. Med.* **52,** 63 (1973).
7. J. R. Eltringham and H. S. Kaplan, *Natl. Cancer Inst. Monogr.* **36,** 107 (1973).
8. I. Green and P. F. Corso, *Blood* **14,** 235 (1959).
9. W. D. Kelly, D. L. Lamb, R. L. Varco, and R. A. Good, *Ann. N.Y. Acad. Sci.* **87,** 187 (1960).
10. D. G. Miller, J. G. Lizardo, and R. K. Snyderman, *JNCI, J. Natl. Cancer Inst.* **26,** 569 (1969).
11. A. R. Casazza, C. P. Duvall, and P. P. Carbone, *Cancer Res.* **26,** 1290 (1966).
12. D. R. Goffinet, E. J. Glatstein, and T. C. Merigan, *Ann. Intern. Med.* **76,** 235 (1972).
13. A. C. Aisenberg, *Nature (London)* **205,** 1233 (1967).
14. J. D. Gaines, A. Gilmer, and J. S. Remington, *Natl. Cancer Inst. Monogr.* **36,** 117 (1973).
15. G. C. DeGast and H. O. Nieweg, *Eur. J. Cancer* **11,** 217 (1975).
16. M. G. Bjorkolm, H. Holm, H. Mellstedt, and D. Pettersson, *Clin. Exp. Immunol.* **22,** 373 (1976).
17. J. J. Twomey, A. H. Laughter, S. Farrow, and C. C. Douglas, *J. Clin. Invest.* **56,** 467 (1975).
18. E. G. Engleman, C. Benike, R. T. Hoppe, and H. S. Kaplan, *Transplant. Proc.* p. 1827 (1979).
19. A. M. Bobrove, Z. Fuks, S. Strober, and H. S. Kaplan, *Cancer (Philadelphia)* **36,** 169 (1975).
20. E. M. Hersh and J. J. Oppenheim, *N. Engl. J. Med.* **273,** 1006 (1965).
21. S. Trubowitz, B. Masek, and A. Del Rosario, *Cancer (Philadelphia)* **19,** 2019 (1966).
22. T. Han and J. E. Sokal, *Am. J. Med.* **48,** 728 (1970).
23. M. P. Corder, R. C. Young, R. S. Brown, and V. T. DeVita, *Blood* **39,** 595 (1972).
24. K. M. Matchett, A. T. Huang, and W. B. Kremer, *J. Clin. Invest.* **52,** 1908 (1963).
25. K. J. Gajl-Peczalska, J. A. Hausen, C. D. Bloomfield, and R. A. Good, *J. Clin. Invest.* **52,** 3064 (1973).
26. R. Levy and H. S. Kaplan, *N. Engl. J. Med.* **290,** 181 (1974).
27. G. B. Faughet, *J. Clin. Invest.* **56,** 951 (1975).
28. J. B. Ziegler, P. Hausen, and R. Penny, *Clin. Immunol. Immunopathol.* **3,** 451 (1975).
29. J. S. Goodwin, R. P. Messner, A. D. Bankhurst, G. T. Peake, J. Saiki, and R. C. Williams, Jr., *N. Engl. J. Med.* **297,** 963 (1977).

30. E. G. Engleman, C. J. Benike, R. T. Hoppe, H. S. Kaplan, and F. R. Berberich, *J. Clin. Invest.* **66,** 149 (1980).
31. A. Boyum, *Scand. J. Clin. Lab. Invest.* **21,** 77 (1968).
32. E. G. Engleman and H. O. McDevitt, *J. Clin. Invest.* **61,** 828 (1978).
33. E. G. Engleman, A. J. McMichael, M. E. Batey, and H. O. McDevitt, *J. Exp. Med.* **147,** 137 (1978).
34. E. G. Engleman, *Transplant. Proc.* **10,** 901 (1978).
35. E. Thorsby and A. Piazzi, "Histocompatibility Testing 1975," (F. Kissmeyer-Nielson, ed.), p. 414. Munksgaard, Copenhagen, 1975.
36. Z. Fuks, S. Strober, A. M. Brobrove, T. Sasazuki, A. McMichael, and H. S. Kaplan, *J. Clin. Invest.* **58,** 803 (1976).
37. S. Strober, S. Slavin, M. Gottlieb, I. Zan-Bar, D. P. King, R. T. Hoppe, Z. Fuks, F. C. Grumet, and H. S. Kaplan, *Immunol. Rev.* **46,** 86 (1979).
38. B. Kotzin and S. Strober, *J. Exp. Med.* **50,** 371 (1979).
39. B. L. Kotzin, S. Strober, E. G. Engleman, A. Calin, R. T. Hoppe, G. S. Kansas, C. P. Terrell, and H. S. Kaplan, *N. Engl. J. Med.* **305,** 969 (1981).
40. D. P. King, S. Strober, and H. S. Kaplan, *J. Immunol.* (in press).
41. G. Opelz, K. Masahiro, M. Takasugi, and P. J. Terasaki, *J. Exp. Med.* **142,** 1327 (1975).
42. M. M. Kuntz, J. B. Innes, and M. E. Weksler, *J. Exp. Med.* **143,** 1942 (1976).
43. M. Takasugi, M. Kiuchi, and G. Opelz, *Transplant. Proc.* **9,** 789 (1977).
44. M. G. Beale, R. P. Macdermott, M. C. Stacey, G. S. Nash, B. H. Hahn, M. V. Seiden, S. L. Burkholder Jacobs, and L. S. Pletcher Lowenstein, *J. Immunol.* **124,** 227 (1979).
45. M. E. Weksler and R. Kozak, *J. Exp. Med.* **146,** 1833 (1977).
46. R. A. Van de Stouwe, H. G. Kunkel, J. P. Halper, and M. E. Weksler, *J. Exp. Med.* **48,** 1809 (1977).
47. J. B. Smith and K. P. Knowlton, *J. Immunol.* **123,** 419 (1979).
48. E. G. Engleman, D. J. Charron, C. J. Benike, and G. S. Stewart, *J. Exp. Med.* **152,** 99s (1980).
49. G. Kansas, C. Benike, B. Kotzin, H. S. Kaplan, and E. G. Engleman, unpublished observations.
50. E. G. Engleman, C. Benike, and E. L. Evans, *J. Immunol.* **127,** 2124 (1981).
51. G. Kansas, H. S. Kaplan, and E. G. Engleman, manuscript in preparation.
52. P. M. Sondel, C. O'Brien, L. Porter, S. F. Schlossman, and L. Chess, *J. Immunol.* **117,** 2197 (1976).

20

Immunological Surface Marker Studies in the Histopathological Diagnosis of Non-Hodgkin's Lymphomas Based on Multiparameter Studies of 790 Cases

ROBERT J. LUKES, CLIVE R. TAYLOR, AND JOHN W. PARKER

MALIGNANT LYMPHOMAS

I. Introduction

In 1972 at an international lymphoma conference in West Germany we proposed a functional classification of malignant lymphomas, accompanied by a multiparameter approach, for the study of malignant lymphomas (1). Our approach emphasized the importance of combining special morphology with a variety of techniques, including immunological surface marker studies, cytochemistry, heterologous antisera for T or B cells, and immunoperoxidase techniques, with a goal of redefining malignant lymphomas according to modern immunological concepts (2, 3). In the intervening years numerous investigators, including ourselves, using an ever-expanding armamentarium of techniques, have studied malignant lymphomas and related leukemias and established these disorders as immunological neoplasms that principally involved T- and B-cell types and rarely histiocytes (4–19). The nodular lymphomas of Rappaport have been established as lymphomatous follicles composed of follicular center cells (FCCs) (5), while diffuse lymphomas have been shown to be heterogeneous and composed of T- and B-cell subtypes (15, 17). The histiocytic type of Rappaport includes five of the cytological types of the Lukes–Collins classification (20), and evidence has been presented by Strauchen et al. (21) for their potential therapeutic significance. Acute lymphocytic leukemia (ALL) of childhood also is accepted as a heterogeneous disorder, accounting for the variability in the effectiveness of conventional therapy in the past and leading to new therapeutic approaches for the recently recognized specific cytological types. Attention has become focused on the need for precision in cytological identification for the diagnosis of malignant lymphomas and the potential role of immunological surface markers in these disorders.

The purpose of this article will be (1) to review the current effectiveness of the various technical parameters employed in cytological characterization and diagnosis of malignant lymphomas and related leukemias, and (2) to examine the potential and future roles of these techniques both in the diagnosis of malignant lymphomas and in investigation of the biology of these disorders. These views will be based on our experience with multiparameter studies in 790 cases of non-Hodgkin's lymphomas.

II. Background

Prior to the mid-1950s malignant lymphomas were commonly separated into three categories: lymphosarcoma, reticulum cell sarcoma, and giant follicle lymphoma. These groups have had little clinical significance because of the limited understanding of lymphopoiesis and the lack of technical precision for cytological identification. The approach of Rappaport focused on cytological identification of lymphoma cells and emphasized the distribution of each cytological type into both nodular and diffuse forms. Unfortunately, this proposal preceded the development of modern immunology and lacks biological relevance.

The functional or immunological approach of Lukes and Collins (1, 2, 3, 15, 17), initially presented in 1972, was based on two proposals: (1) Lymphomas involve the T- and B-cell systems and can be identified as being of either T- or B-lymphocytic origin by immunological surface marker techniques; and (2) malignant lymphomas develop as aberrations of lymphocyte transformation and represent either a blockage or a "switch-on" of the transformation process. From this basis a FCC concept was developed on the following principles: (1) The reactive follicular center is a site of normal B-cell transformation; (2) FCCs are plasma cell precursors; (3) FCC lymphomas occur in both follicular and diffuse histological patterns; and (4) FCC lymphomas are regarded as cytological types of lymphoma rather than as lymphomas of follicular structure as is implied by the term "follicular lymphoma."

A functional or immunological classification was proposed relating the various morphological types of lymphoma to the phases of transformation and development of the lymphocyte as shown in Table I.

The purpose of the classification was to redefine malignant lymphomas in modern immunological terms according to the T- and B-cell lymphocytic systems. Our approach from the beginning has been to establish initially the morphological diagnosis according to the proposed classification and then criti-

TABLE I

Immunologic Classification of Malignant Lymphomas

U Cell (undefined)
B-Cell types
  Small lymphocyte (B)
  Plasmacytoid lymphocyte
  Follicular center cell (FCC) types
    (Follicular, follicular and diffuse, and diffuse with or without sclerosis)
    Small cleaved FCC
    Large cleaved FCC
    Small noncleaved FCC
      Burkitt
      Non-Burkitt
    Large noncleaved FCC
  Immunoblastic sarcoma (B)
T-Cell types
  Small lymphocyte (T)
  Convoluted lymphocyte
  Cerebriform lymphocyte
    (Mycosis fungoides and Sézary's syndrome)
  Lymphoepithelioid lymphocyte
  Immunoblastic sarcoma (T)
Histiocytic Type

TABLE II

Multiparameter Techniques

Special morphology
Cytochemistry
Immunological surface markers
Monoclonal antibodies
Electron microscopy
Immunoperoxidase for cytoplasmic immunoglobulin and muramidase (lysozyme)
In vitro lymphocyte studies
Cell kinetics
HLA determinations

---

cally to relate the results of surface marker studies and cytochemical techniques to the morphological diagnosis. With a multiparameter approach, fresh biopsy tissue has been collected from a variety of sources, including lymph nodes, spleen, bone marrow, and peripheral blood, for over 6000 specimens, including over 800 cases of non-Hodgkin's lymphoma, from 30 hospitals in the Southern California Lymphoma Study Group, University of Southern California. The multiparameter approach is outlined in Table II. Through the use of this approach a wide variety of techniques have been evaluated continually for their potential usefulness. In addition, it permits a cross-check of the value of the various techniques in the definition of the cytological types of malignant lymphomas. Of major importance is the collection of tissue for special morphology, which emphasizes the importance of the manner of collecting and fixing tissue and preparing histological sections for ideal morphological evaluation and diagnosis. In subsequent sections the value of the various techniques applied in the study of non-Hodgkin's lymphomas will be evaluated, and the results for 790 cases of non-Hodgkin's lymphoma, evaluated as of June 1, 1980, will be summarized. The manner of collection of cells and tissue for these studies and the methodology have been summarized in previous reports (15, 17).

III. Multiparameter Approach

Characterization of non-Hodgkin's lymphomas as of B lymphocytic, T-lymphocytic, or histiocytic origin by immunological techniques is now widely accepted. Initially, rosetting techniques for the identification of cell receptors were relied upon for differentiating T and B cells and monocytes or macrophages (e.g., sheep erythrocyte receptors, Fc receptors, complement receptors). The development of specific antisera directed against the heavy and light chain classes of human immunoglobulin, and later against various B- and T-cell surface antigens, has provided methods that potentially are more specific and reliable. Recent reviews provide details of methodology, interpretation, and clinical application of these various procedures (22–25). The principal techniques employed are listed in Table III with the cell types identified and with critical comments on the multiparameter approach.

Histological evaluation is included here under the multiparameter technical

TABLE III

Markers for Distinguishing Human T and B Lymphocytes, Monocytes or Macrophages, and Third-Population Cells

Lymphocyte	Comments
T Lymphocytes	
Sheep erythrocyte receptors (E rosettes)	Also on other cells, but not B lymphocytes
T-Cell antigens	A variety of differentiation antigens identify T cells and subpopulations; monoclonal hybridoma antibodies particularly useful; antigen phenotypes associated with specific subset populations
Terminal deoxynucleotidyl transferase	In pre-T cells (prothymocytes, thymocytes); elevated in ALL and blast crisis of chronic granulyocytic leukemia; may recognize an early progenitor cell common for lymphocytes and granulocytes
IgG Fc receptors (Tγ), IgM Fc receptors (Tμ), IgA Fc receptors (Tα)	Also present on B cells and monocytes
β_2-Microglobulin	Associated with HL-A antigens; may also be on B cells
Acid phosphatase	Focally positive in T-cell ALL and convoluted T-cell lymphoma; diffuse cytoplasmic staining, resistant to tartrate, in hairy cell leukemia; diffuse staining of monocytes
Acid-naphthol acetic esterase	Focally positive cytoplasm
Proliferative response to PHA, Con A, alloantigens (in mixed lymphocyte culture), periodate, galactose oxidase, etc.	B Cells may also respond—possibly to secondary mitogenic factors produced by activated T cells
Peanut agglutinin receptors	Pre-T cells
B Lymphocytes	
Surface (membrane) and cytoplasmic immunoglobulin	Synthesized by B cells; T cells may synthesize small amounts of unique immunoglobulin, undetectable by standard techniques; monocytes adsorb immunoglobulin via Fc receptors and may endocytose immunoglobulin

(continued)

TABLE III (*Continued*)

Lymphocyte	Comments
Mouse erythrocyte receptors	Found on subset of mature B cells and possibly pre-T cells; commonly found in B-cell CLL
Epstein–Barr virus receptor	B cells only
Fc receptors for IgG, IgM, IgA	Also on T cells and monocytes
Complement receptors (C3b, C3d, C4b)	Also on subsets of T cells, erythrocytes, granulocytes, monocytes, eosinophils, and basophils; convoluted T-cell lymphoma and leukemia cells may possess C3 receptors
Tartrate-resistant acid phosphatase	Identifies hairy cell leukemia cells, but not restricted to them
Ia-like antigens (B-cell alloantigens)	Commonly used as a B-cell marker, but also on monocytes, some T cells, and third-population cells
B-Cell alloantigens	Stimulate T cells in the mixed lymphocyte reaction
Proliferative response to *Nocardia opaca,* insoluble protein A, pokeweed mitogen (PWM) (low dose)	PWM stimulates T and B cells at high concentrations; mitogens bound to solid state (polymer beads) may stimulate B cells preferentially, but soluble mitogens less specific
Monocytes	
Muramidase (lysozyme)	Immunocytochemistry
Phagocytosis	Functional test using erythrocytes, latex spheres, bacteria, etc. *in vitro*
Neutral red	"Vital" staining, measures endocytosis
α-Naphthyl butyrase (NSE)	Diffuse cytoplasmic staining; also seen in convoluted T-cell proliferations
Granulocyte or monocyte antigen(s)	Monoclonal hybridoma antibody detects common antigen (Ortho); reflects common progenitor cell
Third population	
IgG Fc receptors	This population has been called "null cells"
Complement receptors	because of lack of SRBC receptors and
Ia-like antigen	SIg, but does possess other markers;
ADCC	may be monocyte progenitors or T- or
Natural killer activity	B-cell progenitors or a mixed population

approach, since it is the basis of reference and requires special collection and processing of tissues and preparation of histological sections to achieve the required level of excellence for precise cytological identification and accurate morphological classification. As indicated earlier, biopsy material or tissue from resected masses is collected not only for cell suspensions but also to prepare tissue imprints for cytochemistry and to cut thin (3-mm) tissue blocks in order to achieve ideal fixation. Single-cell-thick sections, approximately 4 μm in thickness, are stained routinely by a variety of procedures, including hematoxylin-eosin, Giemsa, methyl green–Pyronine (MGP), and periodic acid–Schiff (PAS) methods. The histological material is evaluated and a morphological diagnosis made, and then this is related to the results of the range of other techniques employed.

A. Cytochemistry

A battery of cytochemical techniques is employed in the study of tissue imprints, smears of peripheral blood, and bone marrow and cytocentrifuge preparations (15, 17). They include the conventional stains mentioned above, stains for identifying peroxidase and chloracetate esterase activity and the Sudan black stain for lipid. The latter three are particularly helpful in making the diagnosis of poorly differentiated granulocytic leukemias. Others include stains for acid phosphatase activity with and without prior sodium fluoride exposure. Acid phosphatase activity that shows a single punctate globule in the Golgi region is present in a high proportion of convoluted T-cell lymphoma and leukemia cells. However, in our experience, its effectiveness and reproducibility depend upon the time interval between the preparation of imprints and fixation. In contrast, small T-cell proliferations show valuable acid phosphatase activity which is more diffuse and granular. In hairy cell leukemia acid phosphatase is usually tartrate-resistant, but in a small portion of cases the cells fail to stain for a reason that is not clear at the present time.

α-Naphthyl butyrase activity is seen diffusely in the cytoplasm of monocytes and histiocytes. Prior treatment of the slides with sodium fluoride blocks the staining of monocytes only. In our experience this nonspecific esterase (NSE) stain is an effective marker of these cells and correlates well with the immunoperoxidase staining of muramidase (lysozyme) on paraffin sections. However, T cells may also contain a single, intensely staining small globule with this method.

Other staining techniques are less specifically related to cell types but are useful. Methyl green–Pyronine stains RNA in nucleoli and cytoplasm and is particularly helpful in evaluating the small noncleaved FCC which includes Burkitt's lymphoma, large noncleaved FCC lymphoma, and immunoblastic sarcoma of the B-cell type. In general, immunoblastic sarcomas of the T-cell type and the rare, true histiocytic lymphomas stain with considerably less intensity with MGP, although individual cells may stain prominently. The PAS method identifies large blocklike cytoplasmic bodies in some cases of ALL and is particularly helpful in staining the intranuclear globules (Dutcher bodies) in plasmacytoid lymphocytes associated with IgM production. Chloroacetate esterase, MGP, and PAS may be applied to paraffin sections, but the remainder of the techniques are limited to tissue imprints and smears.

B. Sheep Erythrocyte Receptor

The observation that human T lymphocytes form rosettes with sheep or erythrocytes (26) is empirical, and the nature of the receptors remains unknown. However, until recently this was the only reliable marker of human T lymphocytes. With the development of antibodies directed against human T-lymphocyte surface antigens, it became possible to identify not only T lymphocytes but also T-cell subclasses. While the formation of E rosettes remains the standard against which the newer techniques are measured, it must be remembered that the E-rosette test is not specific for T cells since other human cell types, including fibroblasts and parenchymal cells from liver, lung, and prarthyroid, form E rosettes (27). This lack of specificity must be kept in mind when poorly differentiated neoplasms are studied.

The method for forming spontaneous sheep erythrocyte rosettes with lymphocytes is inherently simple, but technical modifications made by different laboratories have resulted in a range of normal values. Many factors may influence results, some technical, some physiological, and others interpretive; and a variety of experimental manipulations that effect E-rosette scores have been reported (25). Thus the first reports of spontaneous sheep erythrocytes rosetting with normal human lymphocytes indicated that as few as 5–15% of peripheral blood lymphocytes formed E rosettes, yet by 1975 laboratories were reporting scores of 50–80%, now regarded as the normal range. Much of this change has been due to modifications (improvements?) in technique.

These influencing factors make interpretation difficult in any individual case. In addition, with reference to cell suspensions derived from lymphomatous tissues or leukemic blood, it is important to remember that the population of rosetting cells is likely to be heterogeneous, consisting of residual T lymphocytes, activated T lymphocytes, and neoplastic E-rosette-forming cells. In such instances the usual E-rosette percentage score is not only valueless, it is misleading. Cytocentrifuge preparations must be examined to determine to what extent rosette formation is a feature of recognizable neoplastic cells.

Most investigators have reported E-rosette scores as percentages without reference to the total lymphocyte count of the peripheral blood. This may lead to serious errors in interpretation, because large fluctuations in absolute numbers of T lymphocytes may be masked. An example is seen in chronic lymphocytic leukemia (CLL) in which the percentage of E-rosette-forming T cells may be quite low as a result of the overwhelming number of neoplastic B lymphocytes, yet the absolute T-lymphocyte count is frequently markedly elevated; the absolute T-lymphocyte count in such situations may be of prognostic value (i.e., part of an immune response). Finally, there have been attempts, some successful, to adapt the E-rosette technique to tissue sections, but this approach has generally not proved reliable or clinically useful, for the attached red cells effectively obscure the underlying cells, hindering recognition by morphology.

C. Complement Receptors

Human B cells and a minor population of T cells bear receptors for the split products of activated C3 (C3b, C3d) and C4 (28, 29). The two major complement receptors CR1 and CR2 are detected by erythrocytes coated with C4b or C3b (CR1) and C3d (CR2). All lymphocytes with complement receptors have CR1, and about 50% also have CR2 (30); other cells (e.g., erythrocytes, granulocytes, monocytes, eosinophils, and basophils) also display complement receptor activity (31).

Most investigators have used sheep red cells (SRBCs) coated with sub-agglutinating amounts of rabbit antibody (IgM) to SRBCs and nonlytic complement (mouse or human) to detect complement receptor-bearing cells. This erythrocyte–antibody–complement (EAC) reagent is mixed with lymphocytes, and 5–25% of human peripheral blood lymphocytes (50% of B cells and a small number of T and null cells) form EAC rosettes. A problem presented by this method is that T lymphocytes may form rosettes with the E determinants on the sheep erythrocytes. This has been avoided by utilization of other species' red cells (32) and by incubation at 37°C, thereby inhibiting E-rosette formation. The former approach has proved to be useful in another way. Avian erythrocytes are nucleated and can be distinguished from sheep red cell E rosettes, giving a double label for lymphocytes which possess both sheep erythrocyte and complement receptors.

Another approach to identifying complement receptor-bearing cells has involved the use of zymosan beads (a polysaccharide extract of yeast cell wall) coated with C3b component of human complement (33). Zymosan activates the complement system by an alternate pathway, and thus antibody is not necessary. Any source of complement can be used since, unlike SRBCs, the zymosan particles are not lysed. This approach also provides a double-marking rosette method when combined with E or EA rosettes.

Shevach and colleagues (29) reported the adherence of EAC to frozen sections, demonstrating complement receptors on lymphoid cells and macrophages. Stein (22), also using this approach, found that binding was primarily by lymphoid cells and that C3d receptors could be detected on germinal center cells. C3d receptors were also present on cells at the periphery of the follicle and in the interfollicular areas, suggesting a means of distinguishing between follicular B cells and B cells differentiating into plasma cells. This approach may prove useful in distinguishing FCC lymphomas and plasmacytoid lymphocytic lymphomas but, as with the E-rosette method applied to sections, morphological details are obscured.

D. Null Cells

At this point it should be mentioned that a population of peripheral blood lymphocytes (10%) bearing neither sheep erythrocyte receptors nor surface membrane immunoglobulin (SIg) (a B-cell marker) has been designated "null cells." Since many of these cells may possess complement and Fc receptors and certain antigenic markers, it appears now that a more appropriate designation is third-population cells, not readily classified as either B or T; this third population appears to contain a variety of cells with different functions, including cells mediating antibody-dependent cellular cytotoxicity (ADCC), natural killer cells, early granulocytic forms, monocyte progenitors, and possibly B- and T-lymphocyte progenitors without SIg or E receptors. Whether certain non-T, non-B lymphomas arise from this third population is yet to be seen and will probably be determined by the demonstration of specific functions and/or the detection of identifying antigens with monoclonal antibodies.

E. Fc Receptors

Receptors for the Fc end of the IgG molecule are present on monocytes, macrophages, lymphocytes, and certain other cells. Sheep erythrocytes coated with anti-sheep erythrocyte antibodies (IgG) have commonly been used to form rosettes around Fc receptor-bearing cells. Another method involves the use of heat-aggregated IgG labeled with a fluorochrome or isotope.

Binding of IgG-EA to lymphocytes by using human erythrocytes sensitized with high-titer anti-D (rhesus) serum (34) or ox erythrocytes sensitized with IgG antibodies (35) avoids the problem of spontaneous E-rosette formation with SRBCs, but the presence of Fc receptors on nonlymphoid cells, including macrophages, granulocytes, cells from liver, kidney, breast, and various neoplastic cells (22), emphasizes the lack of specificity and limited value of the method as a means of positively identifying cells.

Approximately 60–90% of B lymphocytes possess Fc receptors, whereas most T cells lack them. A percentage of so-called null cells (third population) are also Fc receptor-positive (25–50%), and these cells appear to be involved in the mediation of ADCC. The Fc receptor on B cells is distinct from SIg and from the C3 receptor but appears to be associated (not identical) to the Ia determinants.

An interesting recent development is the observation that T cells expressing receptors for the Fc component of IgG (Tγ) express suppressor activity *in vitro*, whereas another population of T cells (Tμ) with IgM Fc receptors shows helper cell activity. These two populations have been isolated and to some extent characterized (36); since the cells bearing IgG receptors (Tγ) appear to be phagocytic and NSE-positive, the possibility of origin from a lymphocyte-like monocyte progenitor has remained. Quite recently it has been reported that the Tγ population is comprised of Ia-negative cells possessing a monocyte antigen and that Tμ cells make up the bulk of both suppressor and helper populations (37).

Because the Fc receptor exists on other hematological cell types and is capable of adsorbing aggregated IgG and antigen–antibody complexes, it has created problems in evaluating SIg results as discussed below. The issue has been further confused by reports of Fc receptors for immunoglobulin classes other than IgG and IgM (IgA, IgE, etc.) (38, 39).

F. Surface Immunoglobulin

Surface membrane immunoglobulin, by definition, refers to immunoglobulin manufactured by the lymphocyte and expressed at the cell membrane, as distinct from immunoglobulin adsorbed onto the surface. This synthesized membrane SIg acts as a specific receptor for antigenic determinants. It has proved to be a reliable marker for human B cells and can be detected using antiimmunoglobulin antibodies conjugated with fluorochromes, radioisotopes, peroxidase, red cells, or other particles. The methodology is straightforward but subject to error through a variety of mechanisms (Table IV). Of course, reliability is dependent on the sensitivity and specificity of the antisera used. The specificity of commer-

TABLE IV

Immunofluorescent Staining of Surface Immunoglobulin (B Cells) in Lymphocyte Suspensions: Problems in Interpretation

1. Inadequate washing leaves residual serum immunoglobulin nonspecifically bound to the cell surface, especially in hypergammaglobulinemia and hyperviscosity states (gives a false positive).
2. Fc receptors on non-SIg-synthesizing lymphocytes and other cells (granulocytes and monocytes) may adsorb IgG from serum *in vivo,* or may adsorb aggregates in reagent antisera. Existence of receptors for IgM, IgA, and IgE complicates the problem (gives a false positive or may risk a monoclonal pattern). Preincubation at 37°C and the use of F(ab)$_2$ fragments circumvents most of these problems.
3. Cell adsorption of antilymphoma or antilymphocyte antibodies in patient's serum gives false positivity or may mask a monoclonal population.
4. Neoplastic lymphocytes may rarely synthesize surface IgM with rheumatoid factor activity (anti-IgG). This anti-IgG activity on the surface of the cells may bind serum IgG *in vivo* and mask the monoclonality of the population as in item 2.
5. Any anti-Ig antibody in the serum may bind to SIg and mask the true pattern of synthesized SIg.

cial reagents is not always ensured, and each lot of antiserum obtained commercially must be subjected to a rigorous assessment of sensitivity and specificity with reference to positive and negative controls. Blocking studies and immunodiffusion against purified light and heavy chain components from sources other than those used in the production of antisera should also be used. The dilution of an antiserum should be determined by titration to the plateau end point, beyond which the percentage of SIg-positive cells falls progressively with dilution (15).

Precise cell identification in immunofluorescent preparations is generally difficult, and differentiation from monocytes may present a major problem. For this reason, the use of immunoperoxidase (40), immunomicrosphere methods (41), and direct antiglobulin rosettes (42) offers distinct advantages, permitting examination of the cytological features of stained cells in smears, touch imprints, frozen sections, or paraffin sections.

1. *Monoclonality*

Lymphomas and leukemias of B cells are commonly referred to as monoclonal because the cells which possess detectable surface or cytoplasmic immunoglobulin express only one or two heavy chains and one light chain (e.g., IgM κ chain), whereas a reactive or nonneoplastic lymphocyte population contains cells bearing a spectrum of heavy and light chains (polyclonal). Theoretically, monoclonality can be demonstrated by the use of antiidiotypic sera; in practice such antisera are rarely available, and a monoclonal pattern of surface or cytoplasmic immunoglobulin (exclusively one light and one heavy chain) is relied upon as an indicator of the neoplastic nature of the proliferative process.

Certain types of B-cell proliferations (e.g., CLL and hairy cell leukemia) not infrequently show a polyclonal SIg staining pattern upon testing with fluoresceinated antiimmunoglobulin sera. However, if the cells are incubated at 37°C and/or F(ab)$_2$ antisera are used, obviating some of the problems listed in Table IV, a monoclonal pattern emerges. Any residual polyclonality after incubation and utilization of F(ab)$_2$ antisera is presumably due to residual nonneoplastic B cells admixed with lymphoma or leukemia cells.

It is generally accepted that monoclonality reflects the proliferative expansion of a clone of B cells. The initial event may involve a single cell or several, but the end result is a dominant clone which expresses the immunoglobulin class of the parent cell. Observations that individual cells within a clonal proliferation may bear two heavy chains (e.g., CLL with both M and D expressed at the cell surface) are compatible with studies that have demonstrated a sequential switch in the production of heavy chains, controlled at the gene level (*C*-region genes). However, the antigen-combining site or idiotype (hypervariable sequence of the *V* region of the immunoglobulin molecule) is constant. It is this constancy of the idiotype expressed by neoplastic cells (43, 44) that holds great promise for the identification of neoplastic B cells which, because of a lack of morphological identity, are otherwise undetected within a mixed polyclonal population. For example, the identification of circulating B lymphocytes bearing idiotypes common to those produced by plasma cells in multiple myeloma supports the idea that multiple myeloma is a neoplasm of B cells with cells in different stages of differentiation (25, 44).

2. Rosetting Methods for Surface Immunoglobulin

The direct antiglobulin rosetting reaction (DARR) has been used to detect SIg on lymphocytes (42). The antiimmunoglobulin antibody is linked by chromic chloride to trypsin-treated ox erythrocytes. These antiimmunoglobulin-linked erythrocytes do not form E or EA rosettes with human lymphocytes but form rosettes with SIg-bearing lymphocytes. Comparisons between the DARR and direct immunofluorescence (42) have demonstrated that the DARR is the more sensitive of the two. The results obtained are quite comparable except that the DARR is more sensitive, is not influenced by various treatments of lymphocytes before testing, and offers the advantage that SIg-bearing cells can be viewed with conventional stains. In contrast to the direct immunofluorescence method, the DARR, according to Haegert et al. (42), gives essentially the same results whether the antiglobulin attached to red cells is IgG or F(ab)$_2$.

In addition to erythrocytes, a variety of other particles have been used to detect the SIg of B lymphocytes. The principle is essentially the same as for other indicators, e.g., fluorochromes, enzymes, and radioisotopes, but with added advantages. Rosettes can be stained for standard light microscopic examination; the lymphocytes forming rosettes can be isolated by gradient centrifugation methods; and by using particles of various size or appearance, multiple receptors can be identified in the same cell separations. The particle can be coated with antiimmunoglobulin antibodies so that it binds directly to the SIg-bearing lymphocytes, or it can be used in a "sandwich" technique.

Particles that have been used for these rosettes include polyacrylamide and other polymer beads (41, 45) and bacteria (46).

G. Specific Antisera and Identification of Lymphocyte Subsets

The increasing availability of antisera directed against T lymphocyte, B lymphocyte, and leukemic antigens offers the prospect of more precise cell identification (for reviews, see refs. 25, 47, 48). A variety of conventional heteroantisera have been prepared with specificity against T-cell antigen sources such as fetal thymus, separated peripheral blood lymphocytes, T lymphocytes from agammaglobulinemic patients, cultured T lymphoblasts, T-cell leukemia cells, and human brain (containing an antigen in common with some T cells); these antisera of course have differing specificities. B-Cell heteroantisera have been prepared against CLL cells, cultured B lymphoblasts, and spleen cell membrane digest. Alloantisera against B-cell antigens (Ia-like antigens) have also been utilized (sera from pregnant women).

More recently monoclonal antibodies, discussed by others in this volume, have been prepared against an increasing range of T- and B-cell antigens using a mouse hybridoma system (49). This approach involves the immunization of mice with human lymphocytes followed by *in vitro* fusion of the immunized mouse spleen cells with cells from a nonsecretory mouse myeloma cell line. The resulting antibody-producing hybrid cells are cloned, and the product of each antibody-producing clone is tested against a panel of target cells. Clones producing antibodies against a particular cell surface antigen are propagated *in vitro* or intraperitoneally in mice to produce large quantities of the desired antibody. Although such antibodies may react with related antigens, they are effectively monospecific, and extensive adsorption of antisera is unnecessary. The interest in these monoclonal antibodies is enormous because of the potential they offer

TABLE V

Commercially Available Anti-Human Monoclonal (Hybridoma) Antibodies[a]

Manufacturer	Code	Antigen or cell population identification[b]
Ortho Pharmaceutical	OKT-3	Peripheral T cells
	OKT-4	Inducer or helper T cells
	OKT-8	Suppressor or cytotoxic T cells
	OKT-6	Thymocytes
New England Nuclear	HU Lyt-1	Peripheral T cells, thymocytes, present on helper T cells and some killer T cells
	HU Lyt-2	Peripheral T cells, thymocytes, present in B-cell CLL
	HU Lyt-3	Peripheral T cells, thymocytes, receptor for SRBCs
	Ia	B Cells, monocytes, null lymphocytes, activated T cells
Becton-Dickinson	Anti-Leu-1	Peripheral T cells
	Anti-Leu-2	Suppressor or cytotoxic cells
	Anti-Leu-3	Helper inducer cells
	Anti-HLA-DR	Macrophage precursor, IgA, IgA2, β_2-microglobulin
Bethesda Research Lab	—	IgM (Fc), IgM (Fab), IgG (Fc), IgD (Fc), IgA-α_1, IgA-α_2, IgE (Fc), IgE (Fab), light chain κ, light chain λ, C3b but not C3c or C3d, HLA+ cells, T-cell ALL cells, null ALL cells, acute myelogenous leukemia cells

[a] Not intended as a complete list.
[b] According to manufacturer.

for identifying normal and neoplastic lymphocyte populations. A large number of monoclonal antibodies have already been produced, and some are available commercially (Table V).

1. B-Lymphocyte Alloantigens (Ia-Like Antigens)

A system of antigens resembling the Ia antigens of mice has been described in humans and designated the HL-B alloantigen system, the Ia-like antigen system, or the human B-lymphocyte alloantigen system (for an excellent review, see ref. 48). Recognition of this system came from utilization of pregnancy sera containing specific antibodies directed against paternal antigens. Absorption of these antisera with T cells and platelets to remove HL-A specificity reveals antibodies against B-cell-related cell surface antigens. As in the murine Ia system, the HL-B system antigens appear to have restricted cellular distribution, residing primarily on B lymphocytes but also on monocytes and some T-cell subsets. This system appears to be controlled by two loci located in the major histocompatibility complex, possibly between the HLA-B and HLA-D loci.

The study of lymphoproliferative disorders for expression of Ia antigens has provided some interesting information. B-Cell CLL lymphocytes possess Ia antigens, SIg, and receptors for complement of IgG Fc. In cases in which the SIg staining (by immunofluorescence) is weak or not detectable, Ia antigens usually stain more brightly. In T-cell CLL the cells form E rosettes and are Ia-negative, with rare exceptions (43).

The most common variety of ALL is characterized by the presence of Ia antigens and the absence of all other markers usually found on mature lymphocytes (so-called null cells). A second type of ALL (T-cell ALL) that possesses sheep erythrocyte receptors usually lacks Ia antigens. Cases of ALL with Ia antigens and intracellular or SIg are uncommon (B-cell ALL). Absolute null leukemia, lacking sheep erythrocyte receptors, Ia, and immunoglobulin, is rare. The Ia-positive, E-rosette-negative ALL cell is thought to represent an early stage of B-cell differentiation (50). So-called pre-B-cell ALL (cytoplasmic IgM, SIg-negative) and B-cell ALL (SIg-positive, Burkitt-like) are believed to be the neoplastic counterparts of later stages of this maturation process (51).

Plasma cells in multiple myeloma are negative for Ia antigens (52). On the other hand, plasmacytoid lymphocytes in Waldenström's macroglobulinemia may possess Ia antigens. It appears that Ia antigens represent differentiation antigens that are lost as the lymphocytes enter the terminal plasma cell phase.

There are, however, several technical problems which make it difficult to utilize anti-Ia antisera for routine studies (53). These include the small number of Ia-positive lymphocytes in peripheral blood, the varying quantity of Ia antigens from cell to cell, interfering substances in sera, and the presence of Ia-positive monocytes and other cells. Enrichment of B cells prior to staining with anti-Ia antisera helps, but introduces selection bias.

2. T-Lymphocyte Antigens

Several investigators have prepared heteroantisera (xenoantisera) with T-cell specificity; these are made against fetal brain, agammaglobulinemic lymphocytes, peripheral T cells, fetal thymus, T-cell lines, and leukemia cells and must be extensively absorbed with B cells, usually lymphoblastoid B-cell lines, to produce specificity. Approximately 80% of peripheral blood lymphocytes are identified by such antisera, along with over 90% of thymic cells, 50% of tonsil cells, and 20% of marrow lymphocytes. Some of these antisera show good correlation with E-rosette formation, but the T antigens identified are distinct from the E receptors. Because of the difficulty in preparing large numbers of purified T lymphocytes for immunization, alternate sources have been used, including brain tissue; in the mouse the Thy. 1 (θ) antigen is found in the brain, and analogous antigens appear to exist in humans.

By far the most exciting results have come with the utilization of monoclonal antibodies directed against a range of T-cell antigens. These have provided identification of subpopulations of human thymocytes and peripheral lymphocytes as well as corresponding or analogous populations in patients with ALL of the T-cell type (54). Such studies indicate that one can define the stages of human T-cell differentiation and relate them to T-cell lymphomas and leukemias.

Antibodies produced by the hybridomas are generally IgG, and standard procedures for indirect immunofluorescence, immunoperoxidase staining, or cytotoxicity of the cells can be employed, although cytotoxicity may not occur because the antibodies frequently do not fix complement. The cells can be examined by standard technology in live cell supensions with a fluorescent microscope or by cytofluorographic analysis (55). In addition, they can be viewed in fixed smears and frozen or paraffin sections with immunofluorescence or immunoperioxidase staining.

A potential problem relates to a possible surfeit of different monoclonal antibodies developed by many different groups and assigned different names. They may have common, closely related, or unrelated specificities and, as in the early days of HLA, confusion will reign until some means of comparing and standardizing these different reagents is devised.

3. Leukemia-Associated Antigens

A multiplicity of antigens are present on the different forms of leukemic cells; to date most studies have been on ALL. A major question that arises is whether such antigens are restricted to leukemic cells of a given type or are the expression of antigens present on normal analogous cells at different stages of differentiation. In some instances antigens designated leukemic antigens have been demonstrated to be normal differentiation antigens or oncofetal antigens. For instance, Stavem et al. (56) identified a leukemia-associated antigen in the serum of a small number of healthy blood donors, 12% of patients with CLL, and 41–75% of patients with acute or chronic myelogenous leukemia. The importance of the degree of specificity of these antisera for leukemic cells relates to immunotherapy and the clinical management of these diseases. Several groups have already used conventional antibodies to characterize leukemic cells, particularly those from patients with ALL, and have demonstrated different patterns of reactivity which have been associated with different clinical prognoses (25, 51). The use of monoclonal antibodies should permit a more critical analysis.

A related factor yet to be explored in any detail is whether such phenotyping of lymphocytes from patients with so-called preleukemic or prelymphomatous diseases (e.g., systemic lupus erythymatosus, rheumatoid arthritis, Sjogren's syndrome, Hashimoto's disease, etc.) will have any predictive value in identifying patients who have an even higher risk than others within their particular group.

H. Electron Microscopy

In general the ultrastructural characteristics of human lymphomas confirm light microscope impressions. However, additional information is obtained since subtle nuclear or cytoplasmic features are not always apparent with the light microscope. For example, minor degrees of nuclear irregularity in cleaved and convoluted cells are easily seen by electron microscopy but may be missed in paraffin sections. Cytoplasmic features indicating plasmacytoid differentiation, well-developed rough endoplasmic reticulum (RER), and the microvilli of hairy cells are also better appreciated with the electron microscope. Thus electron microscope examination of lymphomas may assist the pathologist in determining the cell type (57) and further may provide a means for studying the interrelationships between lymphoma cells and other cells of the lymphoid tissues, e.g., stromal elements.

In another sphere, the use of electron microscopy in the differential diagnosis of poorly differentiated neoplasms involving lymphoid tissues may be a significant clinical value. The presence of identifying features such as specific granules, melanosomes, desmosomes, and other organelles may be quite helpful.

A major problem in the use of electron microscopy by the pathologist relates to sample size. Specimens are by necessity quite small and are only representative of the lymphomatous process if there is diffuse and extensive involvement of the tissue studied or, if not, there is adequate sampling.

The use of immunocytochemical techniques (with a label such as ferritin or enzyme cytochemistry using electron-dense reaction products) and rosetting methods has increased the value of electron microscopy in lymphoma studies, particularly since the same techniques are used for light microscopy. Although there are some advantages and some forms of information are provided that cannot be obtained by light microscopy, most diagnoses are made by the pathologist on the basis of well-fixed 4- to 6-μm-thick paraffin sections or 1-2-μm sections of epoxy-embedded material, the former having the advantage of greater sample size.

For the pathologist the electron microscope is an extension of the light microscope. It provides information not made available by light microscopy, and, as with cytochemistry, it may assist in the diagnosis of difficult cases. The application of newer enzyme and immunological techniques to electron microscopy provides another dimension which may or may not be of significant value in diagnosis but surely promises to provide valuable information about the biology of lymphomas.

Lymphomas that have received special attention from electron microscopists are nodular or follicular lymphomas. Their cellular relationship to counterparts in reactive lymph node follicles or germinal centers has been described ultrastructurally by several workers (58–60). The observation of dendritic reticulum (stromal) cells and desmosomes in these FCC lymphomas has given rise to some controversy regarding their diagnostic value and biological meaning. Kojima *et al.* (59) regarded dendritic cells as lymphoid cell precursors and nodular lymphomas as dendritic cell neoplasms. Levine and Dorfman (60) found no desmosomes between lymphoid cells and determined that dendritic cells made up a very small portion of the total lymphoma population. They concluded that the cell was nothing more than a residual marker cell of a preexisting germinal center. Lennert and Niedorf (61) described dendritic cells with long cytoplasmic processes and prominent desmosomes in nodular lymphomas, whereas Glick *et al.* (58) observed similar cells, associated with collagen fibers, in lymphomas with both nodular and diffuse growth patterns. Lennert and his co-workers have more recently made the point that the stromal cells of lymphoid tissues are useful in differential diagnosis, with an association between dendritic reticulum cells and follicular lesions. Interdigitating reticulum cells are said to be associated with some T-zone lymphomas. Our own experience has been that the specificity of these associations is not sufficient to be more than supportive in diagnosis. Nevertheless, these relationships may become more readily apparent by combining morphology with enzyme and immunoelectron microscopy. Their importance lies in largely unexplored indications that stromal cells may play a role in immunoregulation. It is this type of electron microscope study which holds the most promise for providing meaningful answers about lymphomas.

I. Immunohistological Studies

In view of the empahsis given to immunological markers in the study of lymphoid neoplasms, it is important to remind ourselves that the diagnosis of these conditions continues to depend upon the use of cytological and histological criteria.

Rudolph Virchow and John Hughes Bennett were among the first to appreciate the importance of the microscope in the diagnosis of disease in general (Virchow, "Cellular Pathologie," 1850) (62) and diseases of the blood in particular (Bennett, "Leucocythemia," 1852) (63). Further advances in diagnostic hematopathology were dependent upon the development of cytological and histological criteria leading to the definition on a clinicopathological basis of an increasing number of entities within the general category of leukemia or lymphoma. Special stains and cytochemical methods were developed to aid the hematopathologist in the identification of normal and neoplastic lymphoid cells; however, many of these methods found only limited application because of requirements for fresh or specially processed tissues or because of limited specificity.

The advent of immunological surface marker techniques, and their application to the study of lymphoid neoplasms in humans, offered the prospect of a more specific means of cell identification. However, these methods, as described in the preceding sections of this article, were limited in their application to suspensions of viable cells and were of little direct help to the practicing hematopathologist faced with a tissue section and a diagnostic problem. It is in this area, the provision of a method for combining the specificity of immunological studies with traditional morphological criteria, that immunohistological methods have played a critical role in the evolution of the current concept that lymphomas are neoplasms of the immune system.

Although the potential for performing immunohistological studies had existed from the time that Coons and his collaborators first conjugated specific antibody with a fluorescence dye (64), pathologists were at first slow to adopt this method for diagnostic purposes. Initial difficulties centered upon the problems of obtaining specific antisera and upon the poor morphological resolution of immunofluorescence preparations. Application in diagnostic pathology was further hindered by the widely held belief that fresh or specially processed tissues were essential for studies using immunofluorescence.

Methods utilizing antibodies conjugated with enzymes (particularly horseradish peroxidase) as an alternative to fluorescent compounds were developed in response to these difficulties. Enzyme-labeled methods gave colored reaction products visible with light microscopy, but frozen sections were usually employed and morphological detail was poor. The final critical step in rendering the immunoperoxidase method more widely available for research, investigative, and diagnostic purposes was its application to routinely processed tissues (65, 66). For the first time a labeled antibody method was available for the demonstration of antigen in the types of processed tissues (fixed, paraffin-embedded tissue blocks) that abound in hospital and university pathology laboratories, and for the first time it was possible to achieve a standard of cellular detail that allowed pathologists to correlate immunological findings directly with traditional cytological and histological criteria (Fig. 1).

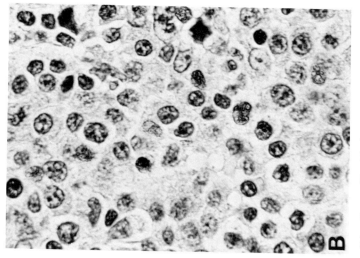

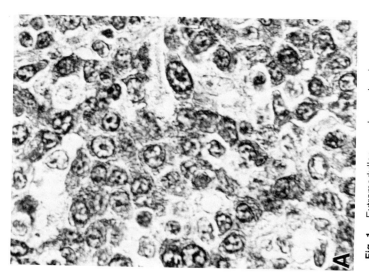

Fig. 1. Extramedullary myeloma showing monoclonal staining (A) anti-κ positive black staining in cytoplasm, (B) anti-λ negative, showing only nuclear staining with the hematoxylin counterstain. Morphological detail is good. Formalin paraffin section. ×200.

1. Immunofluorescence or Immunoperoxidase?

Immunofluorescence and immunoperoxidase methods should not be considered competitors, but rather techniques that complement one another. The immunofluorescence method is admirably suited to the study of surface markers (e.g., SIg) on viable cells in suspension as described in the previous section; it is relatively simple and quick and, when using some of the newer epiillumination fluorescence microscopes, is remarkably sensitive. Immunoperoxidase methods can similarly be employed for the demonstration of surface antigens (67, 68) but often are more time-consuming and are only to be preferred if detailed morphology is a requisite or if electron microscopic studies are contemplated.

With regard to immunohistological studies employing tissue sections, immunoperoxidase is generally the preferred method, this preference being based upon the requirement for good morphological detail. The immunoperoxidase method applied to fixed, paraffin-embedded tissues yields preparations in which the morphological detail is equivalent to orthodox hematoxylin–eosin-stained preparations (Fig. 1), thus permitting pathologists to correlate directly traditional morphological criteria with immunolabeling parameters. The principal limitation of the immunoperoxidase–paraffin section procedure relates to the possible destruction or denaturation of antigen by the processes of fixation, dehydration, paraffin embeddment, rehydration, etc.

That antigens survive this form of abuse at all is perhaps surprising; it has been established that without adequate fixation there is no survival, and thus the critical step in all these procedures is at the time of tissue fixation. In 1962 Ste. Marie (69) wrote: "Antigen and antibody acitivty is inactivated by conventional methods." This view effectively halted further work in the area until some 12 years later when it was shown that the immunoglobulin content of plasma cells could be immunostained using peroxidase-labeled conjugate on Formalin paraffin sections. The potential usefulness of such a method, demonstrating antigens within fixed, paraffin-embedded material, was clearly apparent and was soon to be explored by many groups of investigators (Table VI) (66, 70–107).

Within the field of hematopathology work concentrated upon the demonstration of immunoglobulin as a possible means of facilitating the diagnosis and classification of lymphomas of the B-lymphocyte series. As shown in Table VI, immunoperoxidase usually was the preferred procedure, whether by use of peroxidase-labeled conjugates or by use of the peroxidase–antiperoxidase (PAP) bridge procedure. Paraffin sections were employed to obtain good morphological detail, and a variety of fixatives were explored, including Formalin, Zenker's, B5, and Bouin's. Successful results were obtained with all these fixatives, though not all laboratories could emulate the standards of performance set by some investigators. On the basis of this last observation, some investigators tended to discredit the immunoperoxidase–paraffin section method; it now seems

TABLE VI

**Immunohistological Studies of Lymphoma—
Selected Key References**

Fixatives	(70–73)
Comparison of fluorescence and immunoperoxidase	(73–78)
Trypsinization studies	(79–83)
Findings in myeloma	(82, 84–87)
Findings in non-Hodgkin lymphomas	(66, 83, 88–93)
	(94, 95)
Central nervous system lymphoma	(66, 88, 90, 96–101)
Findings in Hodgkin's disease	
Cryostat sections"	(102) (IF); (103) (IF/IP); (104); (IF); (71) (IF/IP)
Comprehensive reviews of immunoperoxidase technology	(82, 105–107)

" If, Immunofluorescence; IP, immunoperoxidase.

clear that variations in the fixation and processing account for many of the observed discrepancies.

Immunofluorescence methods have been used less extensively in this period (Table VI) but sometimes have been employed as the standard against which to compare the immunoperoxidase technique. Most of the detailed comparisons that have been reported attest to a similar degree of specificity and sensitivity for the two methods. Again, discrepancies between the two methods appear to be related to differences in fixation and tissue processing and not to intrinsic differences between immunofluorescence and immunoperoxidase methods per se. Interestingly, these studies have revealed that the initial precept of Ste. Marie, that antigen and antibody activity is inactivated by conventional methods, does not hold true either for immunofluorescence or immunoperoxidase studies.

2. Fixation and Processing

Nonetheless, fixation and processing, whether by a method as simple as freezing and cryostat sectioning or by a technique more complex such as fixation in Formalin followed by dehydration and paraffin embeddment, have some effect upon tissue antigens. This effect varies among different fixatives and different antigens (70). In general terms some of the antigenicity is lost at the time of fixation, but that which remains following removal from fixative is preserved against the rigors of dehydration and paraffin embeddment and can be demonstrated in the deparaffinized sections by resorting to sensitive immunohistological methods. The PAP procedure is perhaps the most sensitive of the methods available, although under many circumstances peroxidase conjugates perform equally well, and the biotin–avidin–peroxidase system yields comparable results in our hands. Finally, immunofluorescence can give satisfactory results in paraffin sections, though hindered by the problems of tissue autofluorescence. A number of investigators recommend the use of partial predigestion of sections utilizing trypsin or pronase prior to immunostaining; it has been claimed that such digestion reduces nonspecific background staining (particularly in immunofluorescence preparations) and may actually enhance antigenicity, thus increasing the sensitivity of the procedure. The physiocochemical basis for this claim is unrealized, but advocates put forward the concept that antigen is unmasked or uncovered by the controlled protease digestion (Table VI). While predigestion may improve results for Formalin-fixed tissues, it has little or no effect on B5- or Zender-fixed tissues in which antigens are apparently better preserved *ab initio*.

Immunostaining of fixed paraffin sections for immunoglobulin reveals cytoplasmic, surface, and extracellular tissue immunoglobulin. Whereas plasma cells and related cells are readily demonstrated because of their relatively high concentration of intracellular immunoglobulin, staining of SIg is difficult to achieve, in part because of the denaturation of immunoglobulin in the fixation–embedding process and in part because of the difficulty in obtaining contrast between the small amounts of immunoglobulin on the cell surface and the immunoglobulin present in the extracellular fluids. Again trypsinization has its advocates as a means of facilitating demonstration of SIg, but results are inconsistent. There is a general consensus that SIg can reliably be demonstrated in frozen sections taken from quick-frozen blocks, cut by cryostat, and briefly fixed in acetone prior to immunostaining. Both immunofluorescence and immunoperoxidase techniques give comparable results, with equivalent sensitivity and specificity (71, 72, 78). With optimal conditions of freezing and sectioning, it is possible to achieve a useful degree of morphological definition such that, following counterstaining by hematoxylin, it is possible to recognize many cells types with some certainty. The quality is, of course, less than that obtainable by the use of fixed paraffin sections.

By these methods, or a combination of these methods, the pathologist can reliably demonstrate a variety of surface and cytoplasmic antigens in lymphoid tissues and with experience can use the pattern of immunostaining observed as a means of facilitating investigation and diagnosis of lymphoid neoplasms.

3. Cytoplasmic Antigens in Fixed Paraffin Sections

a. Cytoplasmic Immunoglobulin. The detection of cytoplasmic immunoglobulin within a cell has been taken as an indicator for the B-lymphocytic origin of that cell (the detection of SIg will be discussed later). In truth, such a statement must be subject to qualification, for immunoglobulin may be present within cells as a result of mechanisms other than synthesis; cells of the histocyte–monocyte series may contain immunoglobulin by virtue of phagocytosis of immune complexes; the same cells bear Fc receptors and are capable of adsorbing and internalizing immunoglobulin by this mechanism; other cells regardless of type might contain immunoglobulin as a result of an immune response directed against them or simply by virtue of passive absorption of serum immunoglobulin through membranes that have lost their integrity. In this respect the detection of a monoclonal (monotypic), as opposed to a polyclonal (polytypic), pattern of staining within a cell population is of great value in assessing the possible significance of the immunoglobulin staining. According to current concepts a monotypic pattern of staining (exclusively one light chain and one heavy chain) within a cell population is indicative of immunoglobulin synthesis and suggests that the population originated from a single clonal source. By the same token, the observation of a cell population in which some of the cells stain for κ chain and some for λ chain, with a similar distribution of staining among the different anti-heavy chain sera, is taken to indicate the origin of that population from many clonal precursors, a so-called polyclonal pattern. According to current concepts, neoplastic proliferations (malignant lymphomas and leukemias) can be expected to be monoclonal and reactive populations polyclonal (Fig. 1).

The detection of more than one light chain or more than one heavy chain within a single cell suggests that the cell contains immunoglobulin as a result of some mechanism other than synthesis, for individual B-lymphocytes are believed to synthesize only one light chain and one heavy chain (notwithstanding the known fact that changes in heavy chain do occur, the so-called heavy chain switch; the light chain type remains constant).

Application of the above principles is of value in the distinction of neoplastic B-cell proliferations from certain reactive processes (Table VII). For example, multiple myeloma may be distinguished from reactive plasmacytosis by its monoclonal staining pattern in sections or smears of bone marrow aspirates, even at a stage when the morphological criteria for multiple myeloma (108) are not fulfilled. Myeloma is characterized not only by the monoclonal nature of the proliferation but also by the marked lack of residual reactive B-cell clones in the biopsy material. It is this feature that is of most value in distinguishing early myeloma from benign monoclonal gammopathy, for in the latter condition immunoperoxidase staining of the marrow reveals the presence of a polyclonal proliferation that obscures the presence of the clone responsible for the serum monoclonal protein.

Recognition of a monotypic pattern is also of value in distinguishing certain lymphomas from proliferations of plasma cells and immunoblasts occurring in extramedullary tissues. In plasmacytoid lymphocytic lymphoma the monoclonal nature of the plasmacytoid lymphocytes is usually clearly apparent; Dutcher bodies when present also show the same pattern of staining. In immunoblastic

TABLE VII

Immunohistological Methods in Paraffin Sections and Frozen Sections[a]

Immunoglobulin:
  Paraffin sections (principally cytoplasmic immunoglobulin)
    Distinction of reactive B-cell proliferations from B-cell neoplasia; myeloma, plasmacytoid lymphocytic lymphoma, FCC lymphoma, immunoblastic sarcoma
    Subclassification of lymphomas; recognition and subclassification of B-cell tumors by immunoglobulin content
    Recognition of anaplastic tumor as B cell in origin according to content of monoclonal immunoglobulin (distinction of B-cell immunoblastic sarcoma from carcinoma, myeloma, etc.)
    Recognition of morphologically unusual tumors as B cell in origin, e.g., signet ring cell lymphoma
  Fixed cryostat sections (principally SIg)
    Identification of monoclonal SIg-bearing lymphomas—CLL and small lymphocytic, some FCC lymphomas
J Chain: Recognition of B-cell nature of normal or neoplastic cells (paraffin sections)
Lysozyme: Histiocytic or granulocytic marker in reactive and neoplastic proliferations; rapid identification of numbers of granulocytes in marrow (marrow granulocyte reserve); recognition of granulocytic sarcoma (paraffin sections)
α_1-Antitrypsin: Aid in recognizing reactive and neoplastic histiocytes (paraffin sections)
Lactoferrin: Aid in assessment of mature granulocytes in marrow (paraffin sections)
Hemoglobins A and F: Distinction of erythroid precursors from lymphoid cells; specific identification of marrow erythroid reserve; assessment of extent of hemoglobin F production in marrow in hemolytic diseases (paraffin sections)
Anti-T-cell sera: Identification of T cells in sections; recognition of T-cell lymphomas; distinction of T-cell subsets with specific antisera against subsets (including use of monoclonal hybridoma antibodies) (frozen sections)
Anti-B-cell sera (Ia-like): Identification of B cells in sections; recognition of B-cell lymphomas (monocytes also Ia-positive) (frozen sections)
Anti-terminal transferase: Recognition of terminal transferase-containing cells (T-cell precursors) in sections (frozen and paraffin)
Anti-common ALL antigen: Recognition of ALL subset in frozen sections
Research: Powerful investigative tool; widely applicable
Teaching: Morphological and functional correlations

---

[a] It is now apparent that both immunoperoxidase and immunofluorescence can be used in all these applications; with paraffin sections protease digestion is necessary prior to immunofluorescence; if good morphology is required, immunoperoxidase is preferred using fixed paraffin sections when possible, otherwise cryostat sections.

sarcoma of the B-cell type a monotypic staining pattern typically is seen within neoplastic immunoblasts and within plasmacytoid forms, including some apparently normal plasma cells present in the neoplastic population. Such a pattern of staining is of great value in identifying an immunoblastic proliferation as neoplastic (Fig. 1), in contrast to the polyclonal pattern seen in florid reactive immunoblastic responses which otherwise may be difficult to distinguish morphologically. With reference to FCC lymphoma, a smaller proportion of cases contain demonstrable cytoplasmic immunoglobulin within the tumor cells, but when present and monoclonal this finding is of great value in separating this process from reactive follicular hyperplasia.

The pattern of immunoglobulin staining is also of value in subclassifying B-cell tumors, facilitating the recognition of immunoblastic and plasmacytoid components, and enhancing the distinction of B-cell lymphomas from T-cell lymphomas. Anaplastic tumors, of uncertain cellular origin on the basis of morphological criteria, may also on occasion be assigned definitely to the B-cell series as a result of detection of monoclonal immunoglobulin within the neoplastic cells. Other morphologically ususual B-cell neoplasms, such as so-called signet ring cell lymphoma, have also been recognized with the aid of immunohistological methods (Table VII).

Staining for immunoglobulin is also of value in highlighting the presence of Reed-Sternberg cells and Hodgkin cells, the majority of which show an anomalous pattern of staining with individual cells staining both with anti-κ and anti-λ antisera. The significance of this observation has been warmly debated. Evidence continues to accumulate that the presence of immunoglobulin in these cells is indicative of synthesis, and thus a B-cell origin, in at least some cases, though probably not all (66, 75-77, 96, 109, 110; see also Table VI).

b. J Chain. J or junction chain serve to link together individual immunoglobulin molecules in the dimeric forms of IgA and in pentameric IgM. Assembly occurs within immunoglobulin-secreting cells, and such cells therefore synthesize J chain, which is demonstrable within the cytoplasm by the use of immunoperoxidase methods, thereby serving as an additional parameter for the identification of B cells (Table VII).

c. Lysozyme. Lysozyme, alternatively termed muramidase, is an enzyme present in certain human secretions such as tears, saliva, and milk, and in certain cells, most notably granulocytes and cells of the monocyte-histiocyte series. Among mononuclear cells, therefore, detection of cytoplasmic lysozyme is indicative of the histiocytic or monocytic nature of the cell, for lymphocytes are not known to contain this enzyme. In granulocytes lysozyme is present in both primary and secondary granules; staining for lysozyme can therefore be used to identify the granulocytic series from the stage of primary granule formation onward. This capability may be of particular value in the recognition of granulocytic sarcoma, in which a significant proportion of the otherwise anaplastic cells can be shown to contain lsyozyme by immunoperoxidase methods.

Detectable lysozyme is less consistently present in histiocytic proliferations. It appears that cells of the monocyte-histiocyte series immediately secrete the lysozyme they synthesize and thus contain only small amounts not readily detectable by light microscopy. So-called epithelioid histiocytes and giant cells, occurring under granulomatous conditions, contain much larger amounts of lysozyme and can readily be recognized by immunoperoxidase methods using antilysozyme antibody.

d. α_1 Antitrypsin. Some reports (e.g., ref. 93) have proposed the use of antiserum against α_1 antitrypsin as a possible additional parameter for identification of cells of the monocyte–histiocyte series. Clearly other parameters must also be considered in making this identification, for germ cells and liver cells, among others, are also capable of synthesizing α_1 antitrypsin.

e. Lactoferrin. Lactoferrin, like lysozyme, is present in many bodily secretions. Also, lactoferrin is present within granulocytes, specifically within the secondary granules of neutrophils, and thus can be used as an indicator of secondary granule formation in myelopoiesis and as a marker for mature neutrophils.

f. Hemoglobin A and Hemoglobin F. Hematologists and pathologists have almost a blind faith in their ability to distinguish nucleated red cell precursors from cells of the lymphoid series. The reliability of this distinction may be less than formerly supposed, as evidenced by the staining for hemoglobin F of nucleated cells within fetal thymic cortex (111); individual hemoglobin F-containing cells are indistinguishable from many cortical thymocytes on the basis of morphological criteria alone. Staining of cell populations for hemoglobin A and/or hemoglobin F facilitates rapid recognition of red cell precursors that have differentiated sufficiently to commence hemoglobin synthesis. This stain is of value in rapidly assessing erythropoietic reserve, particularly if significant numbers of small lymphocytes and so-called lymphoblasts are also present to confound the morphologist.

4. *Surface Antigens in Quick-Frozen Cryostat Sections*

The demonstration of patterns of staining of SIg in quick-frozen acetone-fixed cryostat sections, by either immunofluorescence or immunoperoxidase methods, offers an alternative to assessment of SIg by staining of viable cells in suspension. The usual method of staining lymphocytes in suspension (see previous sections), with counting of fluorescent cells, gives an impression of scientific accuracy; although it should not be forgotten that unknown selection bias may occur during the process of preparing a lymphocyte suspension from tissue, or in separating lymphocytes from other cells by density gradient centrifugation. In addition, SIg assay of viable cells counts only viable cells, and in many instances neoplastic populations show a very high rate of cell death, possibly leading to falsely low scores. For these reasons, our laboratory is moving toward analysis of SIg patterns on frozen sections using immunofluorescence, and particularly immunoperoxidase, techniques following methods modified from those of Burns *et al.* (73), Stein (112), Warnke and Levy (103), and Tubbs *et al.* (71). The pattern of staining with antisera specific for light chain types and heavy chain classes gives a reliable assessment of clonality, though the apparent precision of percent-age scores is not attainable. The method can be applied to all reactive and neoplastic tissues, particularly including large-cell lymphomas that are difficult to assess by cell suspension methods because of the high rate of cell death.

5. Other Antigens, Surface and Cytoplasmic

It is in this area that much of the current excitement lies.

Assays of terminal transferase have proven to be of value in distinguishing some of the acute T-cell leukemias (e.g., ref. 113). Preliminary evidence at hand indicates that immunostaining of cell populations using anti-terminal transferase antisera by immunofluorescence or immunoperoxidase methods provides a sensi-tive index of the T-cell nature of these proliferations and is simply and quickly performed.

There has also been much interest in the development of specific antisera for identifying and distinguishing B lymphocytes, T lymphocytes, and monocytes, corresponding to the use of analogous antisera in animal systems. The prospect of developing antisera for identifying subsets of T lymphocytes has proved particularly tantalizing. Such antisera have been developed, but have usually been applied to lymphocyte cell suspensions and only rarely to tissue sections, particularly cryostat sections. While these studies have excited a great deal of interest, their application has been of limited value diagnostically because of limited availability and inconsistent quality control of such antisera. Develop-ment of the monoclonal hybridoma antibody system promises to revolutionize this aspect of immunological recognition of lymphocytes, as described in the earlier part of this article.

Monoclonal antibodies that distinguish lymphocyte populations in suspension have been shown, in preliminary work, to identify reliably the same lymphocyte populations in cryostat tissue sections (104) and possibly also in fixed, paraffin-embedded sections (personal observation), although at present it is too early to determine if such staining patterns are entirely consistent and reliable.

The potential for identification of B cells, T cells, T-cell subsets, monocytes, and other cells in tissue sections offers the pathologist a further increment in refinement of cell identification. There arises a real possibility of still further extending immunological and morphological correlations, with a view toward defining and refining existing diagnostic criteria for lymphomas and leukemias. It is in this respect that immunoperoxidase and immunofluorescence methods are powerful investigative tools for hematopathologists, with a real prospect of more widespread application in diagnostic use.

The continuing application of methods such as those described in this chapter may provide much new information regarding the validity of current cytological and histological criteria for the diagnosis of lymphoma and leukemia and may prove of enormous value in teaching those who are prepared to learn.

IV. Results of Multiparameter Studies on Malignant Lymphomas

Our multiparameter studies, which began in early 1974, are based on the study of over 6000 specimens collected from 30 hospitals in our Southern California Lymphoma Group, of which 790 cases were interpreted morphologically within the non-Hodgkin's lymphoma group. Specimens evaluated principally were of lymph node, spleen, peripheral blood, and bone marrow and, in many cases, specimens from two or more sites were available for study prior to therapy. The multiparameter studies include special morphology, cytochemistry, immunological surface marker studies, including various rosette techniques, SIg, cytoplasmic immunoglobulin, electron microscopy and, in a significant portion of the cases, cell kinetics by flow cytofluorometry. The findings from the cell kinetic studies are the subject of a separate report (114). The results of all these studies demonstrate that the morphological findings of each of the cytological types are effective predictors of the manner in which the B- and T-cell subtypes mark. They also provide support for the proposal that the cytological types of the Lukes–Collins classification principally involve T- and B-cell subtypes and, rarely, the histiocytic type. It is acknowledged that there are problems in both technique and interpretation and that the cells in a limited proportion of the cases in each B-cell type have little or no detectable SIg and do not mark in a monoclonal fashion. Similarly, the T-cell types identified morphologically exhibit a wide range in the frequency of E rosettes and, at times, in low frequency, but lymphoma and leukemia cells were demonstrated to form E rosettes in cytocentrifuge preparations.

The distribution of the 790 cases of non-Hodgkin's lymphoma and related leukemias, according to major cytological types, is shown in Table VIII. The largest group is the B-cell type with 585 (74.1%) cases, while the histiocyte group is the least common with only 2 (0.2%) cases. There are 159 (20.1%)

TABLE VIII

Non-Hodgkin's Lymphomas: Distribution of Cases by Major Cytological Group[a]

Cell type	Number of cases	Percent
B Cell	585	74.1
T Cell	159	20.1
U Cell	44	5.6
Histiocyte	2	0.2
Total	790	100.0

[a] Study period: January 1974 through May 1980.

TABLE IX

Distribution of Malignant Lymphoma Cases by Lukes-Collins Cytological Types[a]

Cytological type	Number of cases	Percent
B Cell		
Small lymphocyte, B	90	11.4
Plasmacytoid or lymphocytic	52	6.6
Follicular center cell	(389)	(49.2)
Small cleaved	231	29.2
Large cleaved	39	4.9
Small noncleaved	59	7.5
Large noncleaved	60	7.6
Immunoblastic sarcoma, B	28	3.5
Hairy cell leukemia	26	3.3
T Cell		
Small lymphocyte, T	21	2.7
Convoluted T cell	73	9.2
Cerebriform lymphocyte (Sezary, mycosis fungoides)	24	3.0
Immunoblastic sarcoma, T	31	3.9
Lymphoepithelioid cell	10	1.3
Histiocytic	2	0.2
U-cell	44	5.6
Total	790	99.9

[a] Study period: January 1974 through May 1980.

cases in the T-cell group and 44 (5.6%) cases in the U-cell group which includes essentially only cases of ALL of the so-called non-B-, non-T-cell type.

In Table IX the cases in this study of non-Hodgkin's lymphoma are distributed according to the cytological types of the Lukes–Collins classification (1–3, 15, 17). Of the 585 cases in the B-cell group, 389 (49.2%) cases are of the FCC type. The small cleaved FCC is the most common cytological type with 231 (29.2%) cases. Of the 159 cases in the T-cell group, the convoluted T cell is the most common with 73 (9.2%) cases with the lymphoepithelioid cell, 10 (1.3%) cases, being the least common.

A. U-Cell Lymphomas

The U-cell type was created for primitive-appearing cytological types of lymphoma and leukemic processes that were not readily classifiable morphologically within the T-cell, B-cell, or histiocytic group, and multiparameter techniques failed to reveal specific characteristics. In this study there are 44 cases in the U-cell group that consists primarily of cases of ALL of childhood. The tumor cells in the U-cell group essentially failed to mark with any of the parameters, with the exception of 14 cases in which a low percentage of E rosettes was recorded (less than 20% and usually between 5 and 10%). In each of these cases a few tumor cells were shown to form E rosettes in cytocentrifuge preparations, but the tumor cells lacked the cytological features of the convoluted T cells. It is uncertain whether these cases represent a T-cell lymphoma or leukemia with low E-rosette formation or a non-B-, non-T-cell type. Clarification of this group must await a combined study of conventional immunological surface markers with monoclonal antisera for T cells.

B. B-Cell Lymphomas

Cases involving the B-cell type, as in each major group, were reviewed without knowledge of the results of the multiparameter studies and classified on the basis of morphological features according to the criteria of Lukes and Collins types (15, 17). The results of the SIg studies in the cases classified as B-cell types are recorded in Table X according to the cytological types of Lukes and Collins (17). Of the 585 cases within this group, 498 or 85.1% had sufficient cells for study. Lymphomas of the large cell, immunoblastic sarcoma, and large noncleaved FCC type exhibited a high rate of cell loss, with only approximately 67% of the cases having a sufficient number for study. In the cases identified as the small lymphocyte, plasmacytoid lymphocyte, and small cleaved FCC type, there was considerably less cell death. The large cleaved FCC cases, another large-cell type, also exhibited a high rate of cell death partially attributable to the prominent degrees of associated sclerosis encountered with this type.

Examination of the clonal character of the SIg in the B-cell group for the entire period of the study fails to reveal a strikingly high frequency of cases with monoclonal SIg in any of the cytological types. The frequency of monoclonality varies from a low in hairy cell leukemia of 26 (40%) cases to a high of 78% in the 70 cases with the small B lymphocyte usually associated with B-cell CLL. This limitation in the frequency of monoclonality is attributed to the technical problems encountered in the early period of our work in which monoclonality was often masked by absorption of immunoglobulins to the surface or Fc binding of immunoglobulin. This is reflected in the high frequency of polyclonality in the cytological types with low monoclonality, hairy cell leukemia, immunoblastic sarcoma, and the plasmacytoid lymphocytic types. There is also a significant degree of low marking where only a small proportion of the cells have immunoglobulin on the surface, and a few cases (23 or 5%) display little or no detectable SIg. Clearly, our results reflect a combination of the technical problems of the past and biological variations in the degree of immunoglobulin displayed on the surface by the cytological types of B-cell lymphoma.

A change in the technical approach to SIg studies in the past 3 years has tended to confirm the frequency of technical problems of immunoglobulin absorption and also that a significant proportion of cells exhibit only small amounts of

TABLE X

Surface Immunoglobulin Studies on B-Cell Lymphomas[a]

Cytological type	Total cases	Cases with sufficient cells	Pattern of SIg staining									
			Monoclonal		Bitypic		Polyclonal		Low marking		Unmarked	
			No.	%	No.	%	No.	%	No.	%	No.	%
Small lymphocyte, B	90	90	70	78	1	1	6	7	5	6	8	9
Plasmacytoid lymphocytic	52	41	20	49	1	2	10	24	9	22	1	2
Small cleaved	231	209	136	65	15	7	18	9	34	16	6	3
Large cleaved	39	24	12	50	0	0	3	12	8	33	1	4
Small noncleaved	59	49	33	67	1	2	7	14	4	8	4	8
Large noncleaved	60	41	20	49	0	0	6	15	14	35	1	2
Immunoblastic sarcoma B	28	19	8	42	2	11	5	26	2	11	2	11
Hairy cell leukemia	26	25	10	40	4	16	7	28	4	16	0	0
Total B	585	498	309	62	24	5	62	12	80	16	23	5

[a] Study period: January 1974 through May 1980.

immunoglobulin on their surface. Approximately 3 years ago we initiated the incubating of cell suspensions at 37°C for 45 minutes in an attempt to shed absorbed immunoglobulin or Fc-bound immunoglobulin. During the last 18 months of the study, Fab' reagents for the antisera study of SIg were employed. The results of our studies comparing the past 18 months with the earlier period of whole antisera study are demonstrated in Table XI. There is a striking difference in the frequency of monoclonality, with 125 (73%) of the 171 cases with sufficient cells interpreted morphologically as B-cell types exhibiting monoclonality as compared to 56% with whole antisera during the earlier period. By comparison, only four cases (2%) exhibited polyclonicity, while 32 cases (19%) exhibited low marking and 10 cases (6%) were essentially nonmarking cases by the SIg technique. The frequency of the low and nonmarking cases relates to the degree of established sensitivity of the antisera.

A similar comparison with the most common cytological type of lymphoma in our group, the small cleaved FCC type, is shown in Table XII. Of the 71 cases of this type with sufficient cells for evaluation with Fab' reagents, 55 (77%) cases exhibited monoclonality, while only one case showed a polyclonal SIg pattern. The frequency of low and nonmarking cases is very similar to the previous findings with whole antisera. The most dramatic change in the results for the B-cell types was observed in hairy cell leukemia in which all seven cases in the recent period marked in a monoclonal manner, in contrast to only three of the

TABLE XI

Comparison of Surface Marking Patterns Using Whole versus Fab' Antisera B-Cell Lymphomas[a]

	Antisera				Combined total	
	Whole[a]		Fab'[b]			
	No.	%	No.	%	No.	%
Total number cases	404	—	181	—	585	—
Cases with sufficient cells for marker studies	327	—	171	—	498	85
Surface immunoglobulin pattern						
Monoclonal	184	56	125	73	309	62
Anomalous patterns						
Bitypic	24	7	0	0	24	5
Polyclonal	58	18	4	2	62	12
Low marking	48	15	32	19	80	16
Nonmarking	13	4	10	6	23	5

[a] Study period: January 1974 through October 1978.
[b] Study period: November 15, 1978 through May 31, 1980.

TABLE XII

Comparison of Surface Marking Patterns Using Whole versus Fab' Antisera
Small Cleaved Follicular Center Cell Lymphomas

| | Antisera | | | | Combined total | |
| | Whole[a] | | Fab'[b] | | | |
	No.	%	No.	%	No.	%
Total number cases	160	—	71	—	231	—
Cases with sufficient cells for marker studies	138	—	71	—	209	90
Surface immunoglobulin pattern						
Monoclonal	81	59	55	77	136	65
Anomalous patterns						
Bitypic	15	11	0	0	15	7
Polyclonal	17	12	1	1	18	9
Low marking	22	16	12	17	34	16
Nonmarking	3	2	3	4	6	3

[a] Study period: January 1974 through October 1978.
[b] Study period: November 15, 1978 through May 31, 1980.

original 18 cases in this group. Hairy cell leukemia is confirmed as a B-cell process, accounting for its inclusion in the B-cell group, although admittedly it is not regarded as a lymphoma.

C. T-Cell Lymphomas

The identification of T-cell lymphomas was established on the basis of morphological features and then related to the results of multiparameter studies. In cases involving T-cell subtypes, lymphoma cells were demonstrated to form E rosettes in cytocentrifuge preparations, even though the frequency of E rosettes varied widely and was recorded at times as less than 20%. The frequency of demonstrated SIg was usually low in the T-cell subtypes, with the exception of a few cases in which all heavy and both light chains were observed in high frequency prior to the period of using Fab' reagents and incubation of cell suspensions at 37°C for 45 minutes. These findings were interpreted as indicating absorption of immunoglobulin or an autoantibody reaction.

The results of immunological surface marker studies on several T-cell subtypes will be commented upon briefly. In 73 cases of convoluted T-cell lymphoma there were sufficient cells for a complete study of 58 cases and enough for E-rosette studies of 69 of the 73 cases. There was a wide range of frequency of E rosettes, from 0 to 96%, with a median of 22%. In 17 cases the frequency exceeded 50%, and in 34 it was below 20%. In all the cases the lymphoma or leukemia cells were demonstrated to have acceptable E-rosette formation about the lymphoma or leukemia cell. The variation in the frequency of E-rosette formation undoubtedly reflects a degree of biological variation within this cell type that hopefully will be clarified further by future monoclonal antibody studies. The frequency of polyvalent SIg is usually low. In 46 cases it was below 10%, in 6 cases it exceeded 30%, and in no cases was monoclonal SIg encountered. The cases of immunoblastic sarcoma of the T-cell type, interpreted according to morphological criteria, also exhibited a wide range of E-rosette formation and failed to exhibit monoclonal immunoglobulin either on the surface or in the cytoplasm. Of the 31 cases, there were sufficient cells in 28 cases for E-rosette determinations. The frequency of E rosettes varied widely, from less than 5% to 87%, with a median of 53. Of the 24 with sufficient cells for polyvalent SIg determination, only 1 case exceeded 30% and 9 were less than 10%. Thirteen of the 17 cases with sufficient cells for the study of all heavy and light chains exhibited a low range of polyclonal SIg and none exhibited monoclonal SIg. Four cases failed to show any cells marking with SIg. The lymphoma cells, using immunoperoxidase techniques on paraffin sections, were not demonstrated to contain either immunoglobulin or muramidase (lysozyme) in their cytoplasm.

D. Histiocytic-Type Lymphomas

The cases interpreted as histiocytic lymphoma were strongly suspected on morphological features alone because they lacked the features of transformed lymphocytes. This interpretation was confirmed in imprints by positive staining of the lymphoma cell cytoplasm in the α-naphthyl butyrase stain and the presence of cytoplasmic muramidase in immunoperoxidase stains of paraffin sections. The cells failed to exhibit monoclonal SIg as well. None of the cells formed E rosettes in the cytocentrifuge preparations. In one case, a pretherapy bone marrow biopsy, leukemic involvement by primitive cellular proliferation was difficult to classify, partly because of technical factors, and possibly may have been of the monocytic leukemia type.

V. Significance

A. Current Role

The morphological features of the cytological types of the Lukes–Collins classification in this study are predictive of the T- and B-cell nature of lymphomas and can be effectively employed if the pathologist is experienced with this approach and the diagnostic material is properly collected, processed, and prepared for histological examination. It is acknowledged that in each B-cell subtype a small proportion of cases have little or no SIg, and in each of the T-cell subtypes the frequency of E-rosette formation varies widely even though the morphological features of the B- and T-cell subtypes are typical. It seems likely that this disparity between morphology and surface marking is a reflection of biological variability. This view of the high degree of reliability of the morphological features of the cytological types of the Lukes–Collins classification is based on our experience of evaluating the biopsy without knowledge of the results of the multiparameter studies. Unquestionably, cytochemical and ultrastructural studies contribute supportive information, and the immunological surface markers provide reassuring confirmatory results. The major problem pathologists encounter in morphological interpretation of these disorders, judging from our experience with large numbers of consultative cases received annually, results to a large extent from the less than optimal quality of the histological material available for study, which obscures the cytological details. To correct this deficiency, pathologists need to institute special handling of possible lymphomatous specimens by collecting biopsy specimens in the fresh state, in order to prepare tissue imprints for cytochemistry, and also to cut thin tissue blocks (3 mm) to ensure optimum penetration of the fixative. In our experience a mercurial type of fixative, either Zenker's solution or B-5 (115), is far superior to 10% Formalin in the preservation of cytological detail. The practice of immersing uncut specimens in a fixative which almost guarantees faulty fixation and obscuring of cytological details should be eliminated. Thus, there is need for the pathologist to provide special handling of specimens in order to portray the cytological details optimally and accomplish the maximum benefit of morphological evaluation.

Immunological investigative programs must continue the multiparameter studies, refining the definition of the character and function of B- and T-cell subtypes, with emphasis on morphological characterization as a base of reference. Morphological features, as indicated above, are effective predictors of B- and T-cell subtype, with lymphomatous follicles being essentially an absolute B-cell marker. Distinctive FCC types also accurately indicate the B-cell nature of the process. Undoubtedly, monoclonal antibody techniques will have an enormous impact on the degree of refinement of both cell characterization and function as new and more specific antigens are employed in their development. There are certain situations in which immunological surface marker studies and cytochemistry will ensure a high level of precision in diagnosis, classification, and reproducibility and, in addition, the necessary reassurance of diagnostic accuracy. Ideally, these techniques should be employed in all cases of ALL of both childhood and adults, the lymphomas of large cells, and three of the small cytological types, small T cell, plasmacytoid lymphocyte, and lymphoepithelioid cell lymphoma, formerly included in Lennert's lesion. With growing appreciation of the clinical entities represented by these subtypes the demand for precision will grow and will be essential in determining appropriate therapy. In community hospitals where the number of patients having malignant lymphomas and leukemias is relatively small, immunological surface marker studies will be desirable in the above selected problem areas. Thus, regional referral laboratories will be needed to characterize accurately these selected cytological types encountered for precise diagnosis and determination of therapy.

B. Future Role

Monoclonal antibodies produced by the hybridoma system seem likely to bring about a revolution in the understanding of the basic process and in the precision of cell characterization and the diagnosis of malignant lymphomas. Undoubtedly, these will be widely employed in the investigation and diagnosis of most neoplasms. The use of monoclonal antibodies in combination with morphology will bring cell characterization and identification to a new level of precision and reproducibility. Undoubtedly, it will promote the recognition of more homogeneous patient populations for each of the cytological types and, thus, permit more ideal comparison of case populations at medical centers around the world. Unquestionably, the comparative use of morphology and specific monoclonal antibodies will continue refinement of the morphological criteria and will enhance the accuracy of morphological diagnosis.

The availability of monoclonal antibodies will require the collection of fresh tissue and preparation of cell suspensions by pathologists and, as a result, will have a major impact on pathology departments in the handling of tumor tissue in general. The application of monoclonal antibody techniques on tissue sections, using fluorescent or immunoperoxidase techniques on frozen sections of tissue, will extend our understanding of the histological process, depending upon the specificity of the antibody available. In our view, the use of monoclonal antibodies in this manner will revolutionize pathology and transform it into a more dynamic field. Finally, the parallel use of monoclonal antibodies on histological sections and cell suspensions will eventually allow us to study cellular functional products and focus our attention on the important area of cellular interrelations which play a role in the development of lymphomas.

VI. Conclusions

Multiparameter studies employing a wide range of techniques by investigators throughout the world have yielded results that establish malignant lymphomas as neoplasms of the immune system that principally involve subtypes of the T- and B-cell systems and, rarely, histiocytes.

On the basis of the study of 790 cases of non-Hodgkin's disease and related leukemias, the morphological criteria for the recognition of the cytological types of the Lukes–Collins classification have proven to be reliable predictors of their immunological markers. Use of the criteria requires optimal fixation and technical preparation of sections and a pathologist experienced and knowledgeable of the criteria.

Morphological features of the T- and B-cell subtypes of the Lukes–Collins classification permit the identification of homogeneous clinical-morphological and immunological entities, many of which are new, i.e., the convoluted T-cell lymphoma or leukemia which interrelates with T-cell ALL, immunoblastic sarcoma of the T- and B-cell type, the small noncleaved FCC type which includes Burkitt's lymphoma, and the large cleaved FCC type which is often associated with sclerosis and disease of limited extent.

The multiparameter studies also demonstrated the heterogeneity of the cytological types of the past as well as childhood ALL. Undoubtedly, the diversity of clinical manifestations and therapeutic responsiveness of these disorders is attributable to their heterogeneity. The established heterogeneity of ALL has confirmed the clinical value of the immunological approach and has led to a change in the therapeutic approach to the ALL subtypes.

The role of multiparameter studies until the present time principally has involved redefinition of the T- and B-cell subtypes of malignant lymphoma and related leukemias, such as childhood ALL. These studies will continue and will be expanded as new techniques are developed, though monoclonal antibodies unquestionably will greatly enhance the precision of characterization and diagnosis of these disorders. Monoclonal antibodies have already demonstrated their value in the subclassification of ALL, and investigation is under way into the functional states of some T cells, particularly the characterization of helper and suppressor cells. Special investigative programs will continue to expand study of the biology of lymphomas. Clinical programs, on the other hand, will only require immunological surface marker studies for a limited portion of cases, such as childhood ALL, lymphomas of the large-cell subtypes, and the recently described small-cell subtypes, including the lymphoepithelioid T cell, the small T cell associated with T-cell CLL, and plasmacytoid lymphocytic B-cell lymphoma.

In the near future morphology combined with new generations of monoclonal antibodies will bring us to new levels of sophistication in the identification and characterization of cell types and cellular products of functional states. This approach will permit the study of cellular interrelationships in normal and defective immune states and provide information critical to the understanding of the development of lymphoma from prelymphomatous states.

Acknowledgments

The studies described are the results of a collaborative effort by the Lymphoma Group of the University of Southern California Cancer Center, Los Angeles, California, which includes A. D. Cramer, T. L. Lincoln, P. R. Meyer, P. K. Pattengale, S. Hill, and D. Dugas. Expert technical assistance has been provided by M. J. Cain, P. Lee, M. Clarke, J. Steiner, E. Runyan, R. Russell, D. Anderson, and R. Young. This work was supported in part by NIH grant 19449.

References

1. R. J. Lukes and R. D. Collins, *Recent Results Cancer Res.* **46**, 18 (1974).
2. R. J. Lukes and R. D. Collins, *Cancer* **34**, 1488 (1974).
3. R. J. Lukes and R. D. Collins, *Br. J. Cancer* **31**, Supl. 2 (1975).
4. J. H. Leech, A. D. Glick, J. A. Waldron, J. M. Flexner, R. G. Horn, and R. D. Collins, *JNCI, J. Natl. Cancer Inst.* **54**, 11 (1975).
5. E. S. Jaffe, E. M. Shevach, M. M. Frank, C. W. Berard, and I. Green, *N. Engl. J. Med.* **290**, 813 (1974).
6. A. C. Aisenberg and J. C. Long, *Am. J. Med.* **58**, 300 (1975).
7. I. Green, E. Jaffe, E. M. Shevach, R. L. Ederson, M. M. Frank, and C. W. Berard, *Monog. Pathol.* **16**, 282 (1975).
8. K. J. Gajl-Peczalska, C. D. Bloomfield, P. F. Coccia, H. Sosin, R. D. Brunning, and J. H. Kersey, *Am. J. Med.* **59**, 674 (1975).
9. R. C. Braylan, E. S. Jaffe, and C. W. Berard, *in* "Hematologic and Lymphoid Pathology Decennial 1966-1975" (S. C. Sommers, ed.), p. 213. Appleton, New York, 1975.
10. H. G. Kunkel, *Johns Hopkins Med. J.* **137**, 216 (1975).
11. F. R. Davey, J. Goldberg, J. Stockman, and A. J. Gottlieb, *Lab. Invest.* **35**, 430 (1976).
12. C. W. Berard, R. C. Gallo, E. Jaffe *et al.*, *Ann. Intern. Med.* **85**, 351 (1976).
13. C. R. Taylor, "Hodgkin's Disease and the Lymphomas. Annual Research Review," (D. F. Horrobin, ed.). Churchill-Livingstone, Edinburgh and London, Vol. 1, p. 11, 1977.
14. R. J. Lukes and R. D. Collins, *Cancer Treat. Rep.* **61**, 1 (1977).
15. R. J. Lukes, C. R. Taylor, J. W. Parker, T. L. Lincoln, P. K. Pattengale, and B. H. Tindle, *Am. J. Pathol.* **90**, 461 (1978).
16. K. Lennert, "Malignant Lymphomas Other than Hodgkin's Disease." Springer-Verlag, Berlin and New York, 1978.
17. R. J. Lukes, J. W. Parker, C. R. Taylor, B. H. Tindle, A. D. Cramer, and T. L. Lincoln, *Semin. Hematol.* **15**, 322 (1978).
18. R. J. Lukes, *Am. J. Clin. Pathol.* **72**, 657 (1979).
19. P. Van Heerde, *Cancer* **46**, 2210 (1980).
20. R. J. Lukes, *Recent Results Cancer Res.* **64**, 20 (1978).
21. J. A. Strauchen, R. C. Young, V. T. DeVita, Jr., T. Anderson, J. C. Fantone, and C. W. Berard, *N. Engl. J. Med.* **299**, 1382 (1978).
22. H. Stein, *in* "Malignant Lymphomas Other than Hodgkin's Disease" (K. Lennert ed.), p. 529. Springer-Verlag, Berlin and New York, 1978.
23. M. D. Cooper and A. R. Lawton, *in* "The Immunopathology of Lymphoreticular Neoplasms" (J. J. Twomey and R. A. Good, eds.), p. 1. Plenum, New York, 1978.
24. J. W. Parker *Am. J. Clin. Pathol.* **72**, Suppl., 670 (1979).
25. C. R. Taylor, "Hodgkin's Disease and the Lymphomas. Annual Research Review," (D. F. Horrobin, ed.). Churchill-Livingstone, Edinburgh and London, Vol. 1, p. 11, 1977; Vol. 2, 1978; Vol. 3, p. 15, 1979; Vol. 4, p. 49, 1980.

26. M. Jondal, E. Klein, and E. Yefenoff, *Scand. J. Immunol.* **4**, 259 (1975).
27. B. A. Woda, C. M. Fenaglio, E. G. Nette, and D. W. King, *Am. J. Pathol.* **88**, 69, (1977).
28. A. Eden, G. W. Miller, and V. Nussenzweig, *J. Clin. Invest.* **52**, 3239 (1973).
29. E. M. Shevach, E. S. Jaffe, and I. Green, *Transplant. Rev.* **16**, 3 (1973).
30. G. D. Ross, R. J. Winchester, E. M. Robellino, and T. Hoffman, *J. Clin. Invest.* **62**, 1086 (1978).
31. G. Brown and M. F. Greaves, *Scand. J. Immunol.* **3**, 161 (1974).
32. J. W. Chiao, V. S. Pantic, and R. A. Good, *Clin. Exp. Immunol.* **18**, 483 (1974).
33. N. F. Mendes, S. S. Mihi, and Z. F. Peixinho, *J. Immunol.* **113**, 531 (1974).
34. P. Brain and R. H. Marston, *Eur. J. Immunol.* **3**, 6 (1973).
35. M. Ferrarini, L. Moretta, R. Abrile, and M. L. Durante, *Eur. J. Immunol.* **5**, 70 (1975).
36. C. E. Grossi, S. R. Webb, A. Zicca, P. M. Lydyard, L. Moretta, C. Mingari, and M. D. Cooper, *J. Exp. Med.* **147**, 1405, (1978).
37. E. L. Reinherz, L. Moretta, M. Roper, J. M. Breard, M. G. Mingori, M. D. Cooper, and S. F. Schlossman, *J. Exp. Med.* **151**, 969, (1980).
38. S. Gupta, C. D. Platsoucas, and R. A. Good, *Proc. Natl. Acad. Sci. U.S.A.* **76**, 4025 (1979).
39. H. L. Spiegelberg and P. M. Dainer, *Clin. Exp. Immunol.* **35**, 286 (1979).
40. C. R. Taylor, *J. Histochem. Cytochem.* **28**, 777 (1980).
41. I. L. Gordon, C. R. Taylor, R. L. O'Brien, and J. W. Parker, *in* "Regulatory Mechanisms in Lymphocyte Activation" (D. O. Lucas, ed.), p. 349. Academic Press, New York, 1977.
42. D. G. Haegert, C. Hurd, and R. R. A. Coombs, *Immunology* **34**, 533 (1978).
43. S. M. Fu, N. Chiorazzi, C. Y. Wang, G. Montazeri, H. G. Kunkel, H. S. Ko, and A. B. Gottlieb, *J. Exp. Med.* **148**, 1423 (1978).
44. G. Holm, H. Mellstedt, D. Pettersson, and P. Biberfeld, *Immunol. Rev.* **34**, 139 (1977).
45. A. J. Ammann, D. Borg, L. Kondo, and P. W. Wara, *J. Immunol. Methods* **17**, 365 (1977).
46. M. Teodorescu, E. P. Mayer, and S. Dray, *Cell Immunol.* **24**, 90 (1976).
47. C. M. Balch and E. W. Ades, *RES, J. Reticuloendothel. Soc.* **25**, 635 (1979).
48. R. J. Winchester and H. G. Kunkel, *Adv. Immunol.* **28**, 221 (1979).
49. G. Koehler and G. Milstein, *Nature (London)* **256**, 495 (1975).
50. M. F. Greaves, G. Janossy, M. Roberts, W. T. Rapson, R. B. Ellis, J. Chessels, T. A. Lister, and D. Catovsky, *in* "Immunological Diagnosis of Leukemias and Lymphomas" (S. Theirfelder, H. Rodt, and E. Thiel, eds.), p. 61. Springer-Verlag, Berlin and New York, 1977.
51. J. H. Kersey, T. W. LeBien, R. Hurwitz, M. E. Nesbit, K. J. Gajl-Peczalska, D. Hammond, D. R. Miller, P. F. Coccia, and S. Leikin, *Am. J. Clin. Pathol.* **72**, Suppl., 746 (1979).
52. J. Halper, S. M. Fu., C. Y. Wang, R. Winchester, and H. G. Kunkel, *J. Immunol.* **120**, 1480 (1978).
53. S. Ferrone, J. P. Allison, and M. A. Pellegrino, *Contempo. Top. Mol. Immunol.* **7**, 239 (1978).
54. E. L. Reinherz, P. C. Kung, G. Goldstein, R. H. Levey, and S. F. Schlossman, *Proc. Natl. Acad. Sci. U.S.A.* **76**, 5061 (1979).
55. P. C. Kung, M. D. Talle, M. De Maria, M. Butler, M. Butler, J. Lifter, and G. Goldstein, *Transplant. Proc.* **12** (Suppl. I), 141 (1980).
56. P. Stavem, K. Berg, and G. Noer, *Scand. J. Haematol* **18**, 13 (1977).
57. J. W. Parker, *in* "Malignant Lymphoproliferative Diseases" (J. G. van den Tweel, C. R. Taylor and F. T. Bosman, eds.), Vol. 17, p. 149. Leiden Univ. Press, Leiden, The Netherlands, 1980.
58. A. D. Glick, J. H. Leech, J. A. Waldron *et al.*, *JNCI, J. Natl. Cancer Inst.* **54**, 23 (1975).
59. M. Kojima, Y. Imai, and N. Mori, *Gann Monog. Cancer Res.* **15**, 195 (1973).
60. G. D. Levine and R. F. Dorfman, *Cancer* **35**, 148 (1975).
61. K. Lennert and H. R. Niedorf, *Virchows Arch. B* **4**, 148 (1969).

62. R. Virchow, *Virchows Arch.* **8**, 3 (1855).
63. J. N. Bennett, "Leucocythemia, or White Cell Blood in Relation to the Physiology and Pathology of the Lymphatic Glandular System." Sutherland & Knox, Edinburgh, 1852.
64. A. H. Coons, H. J. Creech, and R. N. Jones, *Proc. Soc. Exp. Biol. Med.* **47**, 200 (1941).
65. C. R. Taylor, and J. Burns, *J. Clin. Pathol.* **27**, 14 (1974).
66. C. R. Taylor, *Lancet* **2**, 802 (1974).
67. F. Reyes, J. L. Lejonc, M. F. Gourdin, P. Mannoni, and B. Dreyfus, *Pathol. Biol.* **23**, 479 (1975).
68. O. Lees, *Eur. J. Cancer* **13**, 345 (1977).
69. G. Ste. Marie, *J. Histochem. Cytochem.* **10**, 250 (1962).
70. P. M. Banks, *J. Histochem. Cytochem.* **27**, 1192 (1979).
71. R. R. Tubbs, K. Sheibani, B. A. Sebek, and R. A. Weiss, *Am. J. Clin. Pathol.* **73**, 144 (1980).
72. R. Warnke, *J. Histochem. Cytochem.* **27**, 1195 (1979).
73. J. Burns, M. Hambridge, and C. R. Taylor, *J. Clin. Pathol.* **27**, 548 (1974).
74. D. M. Boorsma, J. G. Streefkerk, and N. Kors, *J. Histochem. Cytochem.* **24**, 1017 (1976).
75. S. Shu and B. Albini, *J. Immunol. Methods* **13**, 341 (1976).
76. D. M. Knowles, II, R. J. Winchester, and H. G. Kunkel, *Clin. Immunol. Immunopathol.* **7**, 410 (1977).
77. R. Warnke, M. Pederson, C. Williams, and R. Levy, *Am. J. Clin. Pathol.* **70**, 867 (1978).
78. R. C. Curran and J. Gregory, *J. Clin. Pathol.* **31**, 974 (1978).
79. H. Denk, T. Radaszkiewicz, and C. Witting, *Z. Krebsforsch.* **88**, 101 (1976).
80. H. Denk, T. Radaszkiewicz, and C. Witting, *Beitr. Pathol.* **159**, 219 (1976).
81. S. N. Huang, H. Minassian, and J. D. More, *Lab. Invest.* **35**, 383 (1976).
82. D. Y. Mason and P. Biberfeld, *J. Histochem. Cytochem.* **28**, 731 (1980).
83. P. Isaacson, *J. Histochem. Cytochem.* **28**, 761 (1980).
84. C. R. Taylor and D. Y. Mason, *Clin. Exp. Immunol.* **18**, 417 (1974).
85. G. S. Pinkus, and J. W. Said, *Am. J. Pathol.* **87**, 47 (1977).
86. C. R. Taylor, R. Russell, and S. B. Chandor, *Am. J. Clin. Pathol.* **70**, 612 (1978).
87. P. P. Clausen, M. Jacobsen, P. Johansen, and N. Thommesen, *Acta Pathol. Microbiol. Scand.*, **87C**, 307 (1979).
88. C. R. Taylor, *Eur. J. Cancer* **12**, 61 (1976).
89. C. R. Taylor, *J. Histochem. Cytochem.* **26**, 496 (1978).
90. C. R. Taylor, *J. Histochem. Cytochem.* **28**, 777 (1980).
91. C.-Y. Lee and E. G. Harrison, Jr., *Am. J. Clin. Pathol.* **70**, 721 (1978).
92. H. Stein, G. Tolksdorf, M. Burkert, and K. Lennert, *Adv. Med. Oncol., Res. Educ., Proc. Int. Cancer Congr., 12th, 1978*, Vol. 7, p. 141 (1979).
93. P. Isaacson and D. H. Wright, *J. Histochem. Cytochem.* **27**, 1197 (1979).
94. H. J. Houthoff, S. Poppema, E. J. Ebels, and J. D. Elema, *Acta Neuropathol.* **44**, 203 (1978).
95. C. R. Taylor, R. Russell, R. J. Lukes, and R. L. Davis, *Cancer* **41**, 2197 (1978).
96. C. R. Taylor, *Recent Results Cancer Res.* **64**, 214 (1978).
97. A. J. Garvin, S. S. Spicer, R. T. Parmley, and A. M. Munster, *J. Exp. Med.* **139**, 1077 (1974).
98. A. J. Garvin, S. S. Spicer, and P. E. McKeever, *Am. J. Pathol.* **82**, 457 (1976).
99. S. Poppema, J. D. Elema, and M. R. Halie, *Cancer* **42**, 1793 (1978).
100. S. Poppema, *J. Histochem. Cytochem.* **28**, 788 (1980).
101. M. Reynès, V. Paczynski, M. Galtier, and J. Diebold, *Int. J. Cancer* **23**, 474 (1979).
102. R. Levy, R. Warnke, R. F. Dorfman, and J. Haimovich, *J. Exp. Med.* **145**, 1014 (1977).
103. R. Warnke and R. Levy, *J. Histochem. Cytochem.* **28**, 771 (1980).
104. G. Janossy, A. Thomas, and J. A. Habeshaw, *J. Histochem. Cytochem.* **28**, 1207 (1980).

105. C. R. Taylor, *Arch. Pathol. Lab. Med.* **102,** 113 (1978).
106. K. Mukai and J. Rosai *in* "Progress in Surgical Pathology" Vol. 1. (C. M. Fenoglio and M. Wolff, eds.), p. 15. Masson, Paris and New York, 1980.
107. C. R. Taylor and S. B. Chandor, *in* "Monographs in Diagnostic Pathology" (S. S. Sternberg, ed.). Masson, Paris and New York, 1981.
108. D. D. Canale and R. D. Collins, *Am. J. Clin. Pathol.* **61,** 382 (1974).
109. C. R. Taylor, *in* "Malignant Lymphoproliferative Diseases" (J. G. van den Tweel, C. R. Taylor, and F. T. Bosman, eds.), p. 399. Leiden Univ. Press, Leiden, The Netherlands, 1980.
110. S. Poppema, E. Kaiserling, and K. Lennert, *Virchows Arch. B* **31,** 211 (1979).
111. C. R. Taylor and J. Skinner, *Blood* **47,** 305 (1976).
112. H. Stein, *J. Histochem. Cytochem.* **28,** 746 (1980).
113. J. H. Kersey, T. W. LeBien, R. Hurwitz, M. E. Nesbit, K. J. Gajl-Peczalska, D. Hammond, D. R. Miller, P. F. Coccia, and S. Leikin, *Am. J. Clin. Pathol.* **72,** Suppl., 746 (1979).
114. S. E. Shackney, K. S. Skramstad, R. E. Cunningham, D. Dugas, T. Lincoln, and R. J. Lukes, *J. Clin. Invest.* **66,** 28 (1980).
115. M. C. Bowling, "Histopathology Laboratory Procedures of the Pathological Anatomy Branch of the National Cancer Institute." U.S. Dept. of Health, Education, and Welfare, Washington, D.C., 1967.

21

A Working Formulation of Non-Hodgkin's Lymphomas: Background, Recommendations, Histological Criteria, and Relationship to Other Classifications

RONALD F. DORFMAN, JEROME S. BURKE, AND
COSTAN W. BERARD

I. Introduction

In 1968 one of us (R.F.D.) was responsible for the adoption by the Pathology Department at Stanford University Medical Center of Rappaport's classification of non-Hodgkin's lymphomas (1, 2). This was accepted by the clinicians at

Stanford under the direction of Henry Kaplan, chairman of the Department of Radiology, and Saul Rosenberg, head of the Division of Oncology. Subsequent reports emanating from Stanford (3), the National Cancer Institute (4, 5), and other institutions (6, 7) demonstrated the utility of this classification when applied to clinicopathological investigations. This consensus enabled clinicians from many medical centers in the United States and abroad to compare the results of various modes of therapy. Rappaport's classification was adopted by the Pathology Panel for Lymphoma Clinical Studies (8), which serves cancer chemotherapy groups throughout the United States.

The recognition that malignant lymphomas represent neoplasms of the immune system resulted in attempts to correlate morphology with function and the introduction of new classifications encompassing these concepts (9–11). This was followed by the publication of additional classifications of malignant lymphomas (12–18) purporting to represent more scientifically accurate alternatives to the Rappaport classification. This lack of unanimity among pathologists dismayed clinicians and statisticians faced with attempts to evaluate comparative clinical trials.

In an effort to resolve this controversy Vincent DeVita, Jr., at that time director of the Division of Cancer Treatment, United States National Cancer Institute, invited two of us (R.F.D. and C.W.B.) to convene a conference of pathologists and clinicians at Airlie House, Warrenton, Virginia, in September 1975. The Airlie Conference unfortunately failed to accomplish the desired aims of its organizers, but it enabled the clinicians to air their concerns and voice their objections to the pathologists responsible for the newly proposed classifications. All participants urged an early resolution of the current confusion and called for a universally acceptable classification.

II. Design and Implementation of Study

The Division of Cancer Treatment of the United States National Cancer Institute offered to support a large-scale study of six classifications of non-Hodgkin's lymphomas at four major institutions, the Milan Tumor Institute, the University of Minnesota, Stanford University, and Tufts University. Saul Rosenberg of Stanford University succeeded Eli Glatstein as principal investigator of this study, following Dr. Glatstein's move to the National Cancer Institute. One of us (C.W.B.) was selected as project director.

Complete clinical records and histopathological sections of initial diagnostic biopsies were collected for 1175 patients. Detailed forms of clinical data for analysis by computer were prepared for all cases by clinical principal investigators at each of the participating institutions. All histological sections were reviewed and classified independently by a panel of six expert pathologists and a counterpart group of six control pathologists. Each of the cases was classified according to six systems, i.e., those of Rappaport, Dorfman, Kiel, the British National Lymphoma Investigation, the World Health Organization, and Lukes–Collins. The expert pathologists, each of whom was required to classify the cases according to his or her own system, were Henry Rappaport, Duarte, California; Ronald F. Dorfman, Stanford, California; Karl Lennert, Kiel, West Germany; Kristin Henry, London, England; Gregory O'Conor, Bethesda, Maryland; and Robert Lukes, Los Angeles, California. The control pathologists, each of whom was required to classify the cases according to all six systems, were Costan W. Berard, Bethesda, Maryland; Robert Hartsock, Pittsburgh, Pennsylvania; Gerhard Krueger, Cologne, West Germany; Koji Nanba, Hiroshima, Japan; A. H. T. Robb-Smith, Woodstock, England; and Martin Sacks, Beer-Sheba, Israel.

To assess reproducibility as well as comparability of the various systems, 20% of the cases were selected at random and reviewed and classified a second time by each of the 12 pathologists.

Detailed statistical analyses of the results have been completed and discussed by all participating clinicians and pathologists. Although each of the systems has merit, as applied by either the expert pathologists or the control pathologists, none is clearly superior to the others. The control pathologists were able to use all six systems with comparable facility and there were no important differences in reproducibility among the various systems.

Based on this remarkable international effort the investigators reached a consensus on a working formulation of non-Hodgkin's lymphomas for clinical usage (Table I). A preliminary report incorporating the design and implementation of this study, results of clinicopathological analyses, and the histological criteria for the formulation is in preparation (19) and very likely will have appeared in the literature prior to the publication of this article.

III. Histological Criteria

Rigorous statistical analysis of the clinical and pathological data generated by this study delineated three major prognostic groups designated "favorable," "intermediate," and "unfavorable," respectively. It was proposed that the terms "low grade," "intermediate grade," and "high grade" be substituted as major headings in the working formulation (Tables I and II). The decision was made to use the term "follicular" in preference to "nodular" to indicate the architectural pattern. Provision has been made for the inclusion of additional observations under each major heading (Table I), e.g., plasmacytoid differentiation, diffuse areas, sclerosis, an epithelioid cell component, and follicular areas in lymphomas that are predominantly diffuse.

It must be emphasized that this formulation is based on morphological criteria applied to histological sections stained with hematoxylin and eosin or with Giemsa stains, depending upon the preference of the pathologists involved.

TABLE I

**A Working Formulation of Non-Hodgkin's Lymphomas for Clinical Usage:
Recommendations of an Expert International Panel**

Low grade
Malignant lymphoma
Small lymphocytic
    consistent with chronic lymphocytic leukemia; plasmacytoid
Malignant lymphoma, *follicular*
Predominantly small cleaved cell
    diffuse areas; sclerosis
Malignant lymphoma, *follicular*
Mixed, small cleaved and large cell
    diffuse areas; sclerosis

Intermediate grade
Malignant lymphoma, *follicular*
Predominantly large cell
    diffuse areas; sclerosis
Malignant lymphoma, *diffuse*
Small cleaved cell
    sclerosis
Malignant lymphoma, *diffuse*
Mixed, small and large cell
    sclerosis; epithelioid cell component
Malignant lymphoma, *diffuse*
Large cell
    cleaved cell; noncleaved cell; sclerosis

High grade
Malignant lymphoma
Large cell, immunoblastic
    plasmacytoid; clear cell; polymorphous; epithelioid cell component
Malignant lymphoma
Lymphoblastic
    convoluted cell; nonconvoluted cell
Malignant lymphoma
Small non-cleaved cell
    Burkitt's; follicular areas

Miscellaneous
Composite
Mycosis funqoides
Histiocytic
Extramedullary plasmacytoma
Unclassifiable
Other

TABLE II

Working Formulation	Rappaport Classification
Low grade	Related Terms
Small lymphocytic	Lymphocytic, well-differentiated
Follicular; predominantly small cleaved cell	Nodular, poorly differentiated lymphocytic
Follicular mixed, small cleaved and large cell	Nodular mixed lymphocytic–histiocytic
Intermediate grade	
Follicular, predominantly large cell	Nodular, histiocytic
Diffuse, small cleaved cell	Diffuse, poorly differentiated lymphocytic
Diffuse, mixed, small and large cell	Diffuse, mixed lymphocytic–histiocytic
Diffuse, large cell (cleaved/noncleaved)	Diffuse, histiocytic
High grade	
Diffuse large cell, immunoblastic	Diffuse, histiocytic
Lymphoblastic (convoluted/nonconvoluted)	Lymphoblastic (convoluted/nonconvoluted)
Small noncleaved cell (Burkitt's/non-Burkitt's)	Diffuse undifferentiated (Burkitt's/non-Burkitt's)

Cytoplasmic pyroninophilia naturally applies only to sections stained with the methyl green–Pyronine method. No immunological studies were employed in the development of this formulation, and it is not expected that they will be needed in its future application. Nonetheless it would be of interest and probable import if such studies could be performed prospectively in an endeavor to correlate structure with function.

Related terms in accordance with each of the classifications tested in this study are provided with each of the newly proposed terms using the following abbreviations: British National Lymphoma Investigation classification (BNLI) (15, 16); Dorfman classification (DORFMAN) (12, 14); Kiel classification (KIEL) (10, 17); Lukes–Collins classification (LUKES–COLLINS) (9); Rappaport classification (RAPPAPORT) (2); World Health Organization (WHO) (18).

Recommended designations of types are italicized in the following descriptions.

A. Low Grade

1. *Malignant Lymphoma, Small Lymphocytic (SL)*

Related terms: BNLI—diffuse lymphocytic, well differentiated (small round lymphocyte); DORFMAN—small lymphocytic; KIEL—lymphocytic, CLL, and

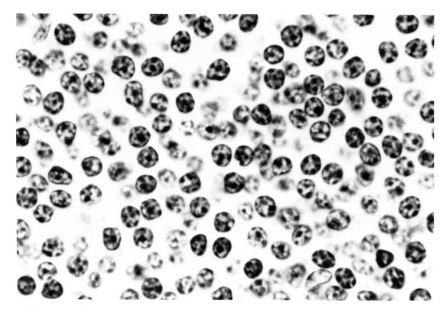

Fig. 1. Malignant lymphoma, small lymphocytic. The nuclei are round and indistinguishable from those of nonneoplastic lymphocytes. ×1200.

lymphoplasmacytic/lymphoplasmacytoid; LUKES–COLLINS—small lymphocytic and plasmacytoid lymphocytic; RAPPAPORT—lymphocytic, well differentiated; WHO—lymphocytic.

In principle, the pattern is diffuse, with effacement of architecture by small to medium-sized round lymphocytes exhibiting only slight variations in nuclear size and shape and, in most instances, an absence or paucity of mitotic figures (Fig. 1). A vague nodular pattern may be imparted by clusters of large cells with round vesicular nuclei and one or two prominent nucleoli (transformed lymphocytes, lymphoblasts, paraimmunoblasts). These clusters are referred to as proliferation centers (20). The above-described morphological features also apply to the tissue manifestations of *chronic lymphocytic leukemia*.

Plasmacytoid lymphocytes (lymphoid plasma cells) with the nuclei of lymphocytes, amphophilic or basophilic cytoplasm, and occasional intracytoplasmic and/or intranuclear inclusions of immunoglobin (so-called Russell or Dutcher bodies, respectively) may be prominent in patients with gammopathies and at times without detectable serum abnormalities. The terms plasma cell differentiation (BNLI), plasmacytoid differentiation (Rappaport), plasmacytoid lymphocytic lymphoma (Lukes–Collins), lymphoplasmacytic lymphoma, and lymphoplasmacytic/lymphoplasmacytoid lymphoma [LP immunocytoma (KIEL)] are variably employed in the respective classifications to describe these entities.

2. *Malignant Lymphoma, Follicular, Predominantly Small Cleaved Cell (FSC)*

Related terms: BNLI—follicular lymphoma, follicle cells, predominantly small; DORFMAN—follicular, small lymphoid; KIEL—centroblastic-centrocytic (small), follicular; LUKES-COLLINS—small cleaved follicular center cell (FCC), follicular, or follicular and diffuse; RAPPAPORT—nodular, poorly differentiated lymphocytic; WHO—nodular prolymphocytic.

The pattern is predominantly or partially follicular. *Diffuse* areas should be designated accordingly.

Follicles of relatively uniform size and shape, and lacking a prominent and well-defined lymphoid cuff, compress the intervening lymphoid regions which may or may not contain neoplastic cells. Tingible-body macrophages are usually absent, and there is no evidence of cellular polarization within the follicles, which are composed predominantly of small cells with scanty cytoplasm. These cells are usually slightly larger than normal lymphocytes and have irregular nuclei with prominent indentations and linear cleavage planes (Fig. 2). The chromatin pattern is fine, and nucleoli are small and inconspicuous. Cytoplasm can rarely be identified. Cells showing this morphology are called centrocytes in the Kiel classification. A small number of noncleaved cells is found, and there are always a few large cells with basophilic cytoplasm (centroblasts) scattered among the small cells. Mitotic figures are usually infrequent.

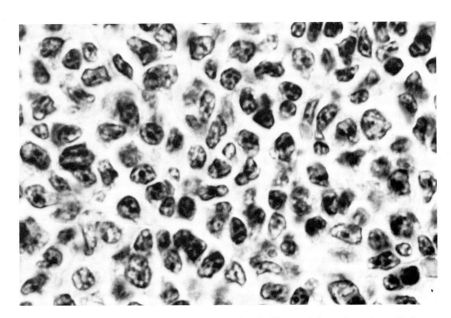

Fig. 2. Malignant lymphoma, small cleaved cell. The nuclei are irregular with linear cleavage planes. The pattern is predominantly follicular but may be diffuse. ×1200.

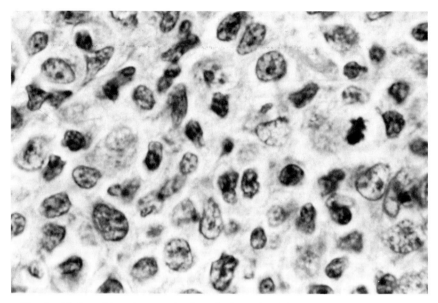

Fig. 3. Malignant lymphoma, mixed small cleaved and large cell. There is a relatively equal mixture of small cleaved and large cells. The pattern is predominantly follicular but may be diffuse. ×1200.

3. *Malignant Lymphoma, Follicular, Mixed Small Cleaved and Large-Cell (FM)*

Related terms: BNLI—follicular lymphoma, follicle cells, mixed small and large; DORFMAN—follicular, mixed small and large lymphoid; KIEL—centroblastic-centrocytic (small), follicular; LUKES–COLLINS—small cleaved FCC, follicular; also large cleaved FCC, follicular; RAPPAPORT—nodular, mixed lymphocytic-histiocytic; WHO-nodular, prolymphocytic-lymphoblastic.

A mixed cell category has been included to encompass cases of follicular lymphoma in which there is *no clear preponderance of one cell type* (small or large) over the other (Fig. 3). The large cells which may have cleaved or noncleaved nuclei are frequently two to three times the diameter of normal lymphocytes and have vesicular nuclei with one to three nucleoli. In the noncleaved type these nucleoli are often apposed to the nuclear membrane (9, 21) [centroblasts of the Kiel classification (20)].

B. Intermediate Grade

1. *Malignant Lymphoma, Follicular, Predominantly Large Cell (FL)*

Related terms: BNLI—follicular lymphoma, follicle cells, predominantly large; DORFMAN—follicular, large lymphoid; KIEL—centroblastic-centrocytic (large), follicular; LUKES-COLLINS—large cleaved and/or noncleaved FCC, follicular; RAPPAPORT—nodular histiocytic; WHO—nodular, prolymphocytic-lymphoblastic.

The majority of neoplastic cells within the follicles are large cleaved or noncleaved cells (Fig. 4) identical to those described in the follicular mixed type, although large noncleaved cells usually predominate. Moreover, mitotic figures are usually numerous. Partial follicularity, with diffuse effacement of architecture elsewhere, is more often encountered with this type than with other follicular lymphomas. Fine-banded *sclerosis* resulting in compartmentalization of cells may be a prominent feature, particularly in the *diffuse areas*.

2. Malignant Lymphoma, Diffuse Small Cleaved Cell (DSC)

Related terms: BNLI—diffuse lymphocytic, intermediate differentiation (small follicle lymphocyte); DORFMAN—diffuse atypical small lymphoid; KIEL—centrocytic, small; LUKES-COLLINS—small cleaved FCC, diffuse; RAPPAPORT—diffuse lymphocytic, poorly differentiated; WHO—diffuse pro-lymphocytic.

Based on criteria for the Lukes-Collins classification (9), this type represents the diffuse counterpart of the follicular lymphoma of corresponding cell type (small cleaved FCC) (Fig. 2). The frequency of mitotic figures varies but is often higher than that observed in the follicular type. As defined by Lukes and Collins

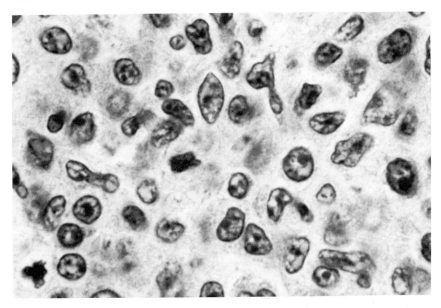

Fig. 4. Malignant lymphoma, large cell (cleaved and noncleaved). The nuclei are large and, in this lesion, are both cleaved and noncleaved. The pattern may be follicular but is predominantly diffuse. ×1200.

a small number of large noncleaved cells is invariably found; however, in the Kiel classification, the term centrocytic is applied only to lymphomas devoid of large noncleaved cells (20).

3. *Malignant Lymphoma, Diffuse, Mixed Small and Large Cell (DM)*

Related terms: BNLI—diffuse, mixed small lymphoid and large cell (mixed follicle cells); DORFMAN—diffuse mixed small and large lymphoid; KIEL—centroblastic-centrocytic, diffuse; also lymphoplasmacytoid, polymorphic; LUKES–COLLINS—small cleaved, large cleaved, or large noncleaved FCC, diffuse; RAPPAPORT—diffuse mixed lymphocytic-histiocytic; WHO—diffuse prolymphocytic-lymphoblastic.

This category represents a heterogeneous group of lymphomas of mixed cellular composition (Figs. 3 and 5). Some of these, in which the small lymphocytes are of the cleaved cell type, could represent the diffuse counterpart of category C, i.e., follicular lymphoma of mixed small cleaved and large cell type (Fig. 3) Others, in which large and small cells with irregular but noncleaved nuclear contours prevail (Fig. 5), may bear T-lymphocytic markers (22, 23). In the polymorphic lymphoplasmacytoid lymphomas of the Kiel classification a number of the neoplastic cells exhibit plasmacytoid features (20).

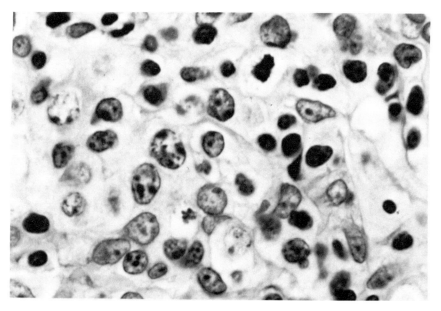

Fig. 5. Malignant lymphoma, small and large cell. The nuclei of the small cells are irregular but, in this instance, are not cleaved. ×1200.

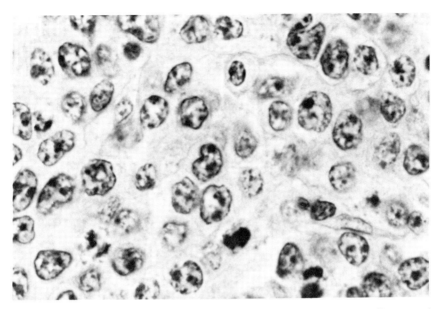

Fig. 6. Malignant lymphoma, large cell (noncleaved). The nucleoli are generally apposed to the nuclear membranes. ×1200.

4. *Malignant Lymphoma, Diffuse, Large Cell (DL)*

Related terms: BNLI—diffuse undifferentiated large cell (large lymphoid cell); DORFMAN—diffuse large lymphoid; KIEL—centroblastic-centrocytic (large), diffuse; centrocytic (large), and centroblastic, diffuse; LUKES-COLLINS—large cleaved or noncleaved FCC, diffuse; RAPPAPORT—diffuse histiocytic; WHO—diffuse lymphosarcoma, immunoblastic.

Lymphomas of this type may be composed of large cleaved and noncleaved cells (Fig. 4), or one of the two may be predominant (Fig. 6). Large-cell lymphomas may also contain small lymphocytes with cleaved or indented nuclei; however, the latter will clearly be in the minority. If the process is focally dominated by noncleaved cells, it is regarded as the noncleaved type (Fig. 6).

Cleaved and noncleaved cells differ not only in respect to the appearance of their nuclear membranes but also in the amount of cytoplasm and the prominence of nucleoli. Large cleaved cells have minimal cytoplasm and inconspicuous nucleoli. Large noncleaved cells usually possess a narrow rim of cytoplasm which may be amphophilic or basophilic and pyroninophilic. Their oval vesicular nuclei contain one or more prominent and distinctive nucleoli, typically situated at the nuclear membrane on the short axis of the oval nucleus (9) (Fig. 6).

Sclerosis, particularly of the fine trabecular type, may be prominent in association with large cleaved or noncleaved cell lymphomas, resulting in compartmentalization of cells simulating an epithelial neoplasm.

C. High Grade

1. *Malignant Lymphoma, Large-Cell, Immunoblastic (IBL)*

Related terms: BNLI—diffuse undifferentiated large cell (large lymphoid cell), plasma cell (extramedullary plasma cell); DORFMAN—diffuse large lymphoid; KIEL—immunoblastic and T-zone lymphoma; LUKES-COLLINS— immunoblastic sarcoma, T- or B-cell type; RAPPAPORT—diffuse histiocytic; WHO—diffuse lymphosarcoma, immunoblastic.

As defined by a number of authors (9, 10), immunoblasts have uniformly round to oval vesicular nuclei and one or more prominent centrally placed nucleoli which may be basophilic or eosinophilic. As defined in the BNLI classification (16) large-cell lymphomas showing prominent or predominant plasma cell differentiation are categorized as plasma cell types.

In this formulation immunoblastic lymphomas have been further subdivided into plasmacytoid and clear cell types based on their cytoplasmic characteristics. An additional category, polymorphous immunoblastic lymphoma, has been included to encompass the wide spectrum of T-cell lymphomas reported in Japan (22). It is likely that some of these are analogous to the malignant lymphomas of "peripheral T-lymphocytic" origin recorded in the United States by Waldron *et al.* (23), and T-zone lymphomas described by Lennert (20), and the T-cell immunoblastic sarcoma of Lukes and Collins (9, 21).

The plasmacytoid variant (Fig. 7) possesses an eccentrically placed nucleus with abundant amphophilic or basophilic and intensely pyroninophilic cytoplasm. Nuclei of the clear cell variant (Fig. 8) may be centrally placed and surrounded by abundant optically clear cytoplasm with little pyroninophilia. According to criteria defining the Lukes-Collins' T-cell immunoblastic sarcoma (21) nuclei of the clear cell variant have fine, evenly distributed chromatin and one or more small but distinct nucleoli. The polymorphous variant (Fig. 9) comprises an admixture of atypical small lymphoid cells with twisted nuclei and large clear cells similar to those described above. The latter may show considerable pleomorphism, and multinucleated or hyperlobated forms may resemble Reed-Sternberg cells. The stroma is vascular, and the vessels show an arborizing quality similar to that seen in the angioimmunoblastic lymphadenopathy of Frizzera *et al.* (24) and the immunoblastic lymphadenopathy of Lukes and Tindle (25). Plasma cells may occur in aggregates, and scattered epithelioid histiocytes may be evident. When the polymorphous immunoblastic variant is associated with a prominent epithelioid cell component, it may be indistinguishable from the lymphoepithelioid cell lymphoma of Lennert and associates (10, 20) and from the "Lennert's lymphoma" of other authors (26, 27).

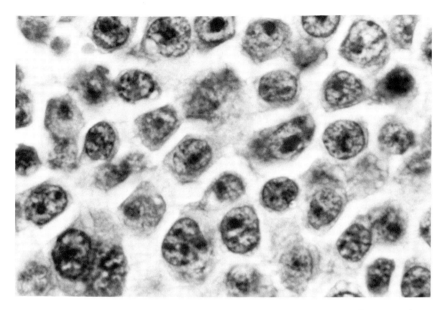

Fig. 7. Malignant lymphoma, large cell immunoblastic (plasmacytoid). The nucleoli are conspicuous and central, and the cytoplasm is abundant. Note the double-nucleated cell with plasmacytoid features (lower left). ×1200.

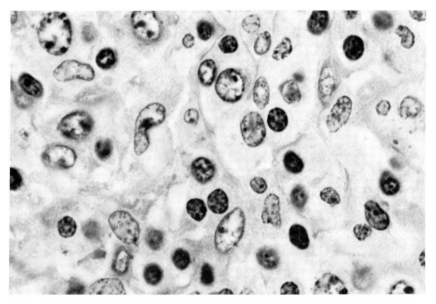

Fig. 8. Malignant lymphoma, large cell immunoblastic (clear cell). The cytoplasm of the large cells is optically clear, in contrast to the plasmacytoid variant. ×1200.

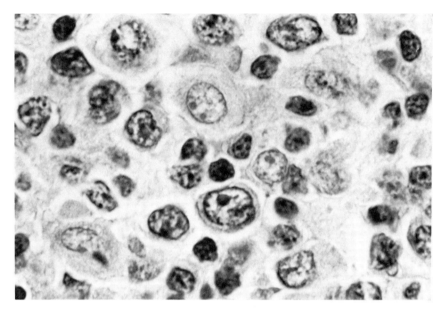

Fig. 9. Malignant lymphoma, large cell immunoblastic (polymorphous). The cells are heterogeneous and comprise a mixture of atypical small cells and large pleomorphic cells. ×1200.

2. *Malignant Lymphoma, Lymphoblastic (LBL)*

Related terms: BNLI—diffuse lymphocytic poorly differentiated (lymphoblast); convoluted cell mediastinal lymphoma; DORFMAN—lymphoblastic, convoluted/nonconvoluted; KIEL—lymphoblastic convoluted, or unclassified; LUKES–COLLINS—convoluted T-cell; RAPPAPORT—lymphoblastic convoluted/nonconvoluted; WHO—lymphoblastic.

Lymphoblastic lymphomas (28) are typically associated with diffuse effacement of architecture; however, the neoplastic cells appear to respect tissue planes in a manner similar to leukemic infiltrates and may impart a lobular (not follicular) appearance on occasion. A "starry-sky" pattern may be prominent, as a result of macrophages evenly dispersed among the lymphoblasts. The latter have lightly gray-stained nuclei with finely distributed chromatin and, as a rule, inconspicuous nucleoli. The nuclear membranes characteristically possess deep subdivisions of varying prominence, imparting a lobulated appearance or fine linear subdivisions in a round nucleus (29) (Fig. 10). The cytoplasm of both nuclear types is scanty or indistinct. Mitoses are invariably numerous (five to seven per high-power field). Lymphoblasts are usually of uniform size, with nuclei that are larger than those of small lymphocytes but smaller than those of immunoblasts or large cleaved or noncleaved follicular center cells.

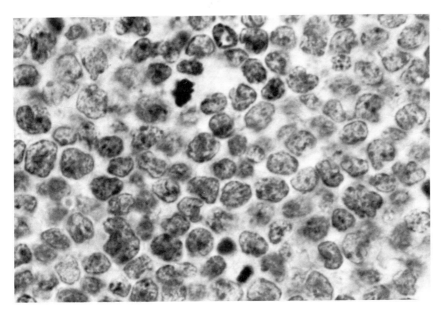

Fig. 10. Malignant lymphoma, lymphoblastic. Nuclear chromatin is evenly dispersed, nucleoli are inconspicuous, cytoplasm is indistinct, and mitoses are seen. Nuclear convolutions are evident in many cells. ×1200.

3. *Malignant Lymphoma, Small Noncleaved Cell (SNC)*

Related terms: BNLI—diffuse lymphocytic, poorly differentiated (lymphoblast) non-Burkitt's and Burkitt's tumor; DORFMAN—Burkitt's lymphoma; KIEL—lymphoblastic, Burkitt's type, and other B-lymphoblastic; LUKES-COLLINS—small noncleaved follicular center cell; RAPPAPORT—undifferentiated, Burkitt's and non-Burkitt's; WHO—Burkitt's tumor.

This category encompasses not only Burkitt's tumor but also lymphomas which heretofore have been designated undifferentiated non-Burkitt's type.

It must be emphasized that the term "small noncleaved" is relative to the size of large noncleaved cells. Clearly, the nuclei of small noncleaved cells are larger than those of small lymphocytes. As defined in the WHO bulletin (30), the nuclei of Burkitt's tumor are uniform in size and approximate those of macrophages (Fig. 11). They are usually round but may occasionally be ovoid and show a slight indentation. The nuclear membrane is prominent, and coarsely reticulated chromatin is irregularly distributed in a relatively clear parachromatin. Two to five prominent basophilic nucleoli are usually evident. The neoplastic cells may appear cohesive, but each cell possesses a distinct rim of amphophilic or basophilic and intensely pyroninophilic cytoplasm. A distinctive feature in well-fixed material is the manner in which the cytoplasm of individual cells "squares

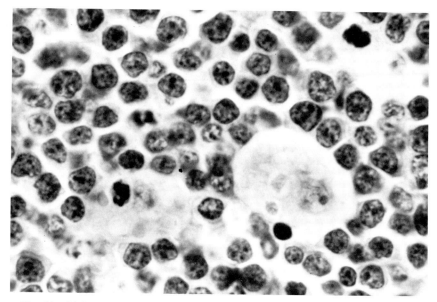

Fig. 11. Malignant lymphoma, small noncleaved cell. Cells are relatively homogeneous with round to ovoid nuclei containing coarse chromatin and one or more distinct nucleoli. In some, a thin rim of cytoplasm is evident, and mitotic figures are seen. Macrophages with abundant cytoplasm are present. ×1200.

off,'' forming acute angles where the cytoplasm of one cell abuts on that of another. Mitoses are numerous, and a "starry-sky" pattern is usually prominent (although not pathognomonic of Burkitt's lymphoma, as indicated in the discussion of lymphoblastic lymphomas). Although the growth pattern of Burkitt's tumor is classically diffuse, occasional lymphomatous follicles may be evident, implying a relationship to germinal centers (31).

Lymphomas which show a degree of nuclear variation and pleomorphism not considered acceptable for Burkitt's tumor and which were previously designated undifferentiated non-Burkitt's type (30, 32) should simply be termed "malignant lymphoma, small noncleaved cell type." They include cells varying from 15 to 35 nm with occasional bizarre or giant forms. Nuclear membranes are delicate, and chromatin is finely dispersed around a single inconspicuous nucleolus. The cytoplasm may be amphophilic and cohesive, but it is more commonly pale and scant. The cytological heterogeneity of these cases is striking to an observer conditioned to the cellular monotony of Burkitt's tumor (32).

IV. Miscellaneous

Although varying definitions of "composite lymphoma" have been proposed (2), in this formulation the term implies two distinctly demarcated types of non-Hodgkin's lymphoma, or the rare association of Hodgkin's disease with a form of non-Hodgkin's lymphoma, within a single organ or tissue. Recognition of a composite lymphoma is clearly important when the two components represent lymphomas of different grades, e.g., follicular, predominantly small cleaved cell type (low grade) and diffuse large-cell, immunoblastic type (high grade). According to a published report (33), prognosis is dependent on the high-grade component, even though disseminated lesions in the bone marrow may reflect the low-grade component. Thus both components of a composite lymphoma should be indicated in a pathology report.

The histological criteria for the identification of mycosis fungoides and extramedullary plasmacytoma have been described in numerous publications and will not be discussed in this article.

Whether or not malignant lymphomas composed of true histiocytes are morphologically identifiable is a matter of debate. Suffice it to say that the recognition of a true histiocytic lymphoma ideally requires both ultrastructural studies (34) and the identification of appropriate cell markers, similar to those associated with the cells of malignant histiocytosis (histiocytic medullary reticulosis) (35). The latter disorder is not included in classifications of malignant lymphomas.

V. Conclusions

It should be emphasized that this formulation was not devised to supplant any of the currently utilized classifications. By using the related terms which have been provided, pathologists and clinicians may continue to employ the systems with which they feel most comfortable. The formulation then provides a means for translation of terminology from one classification to another and for the comparison of clinical therapeutic trials, regardless of the classifications employed in such studies.

Acknowledgments

This work was supported in part by grants CA-05838 and CA-21555 from the National Cancer Institute, National Institutes of Health (R.F.D. and J.S.B.), and by contract grants NO1-CM-67072TQ and NO1-CM-67111TQ, awarded specifically for this study.

The histological criteria for this formulation were established by all pathologists involved in this project: C. W. Berard, R. F. Dorfman, R. Hartsock, K. Henry, G. Krueger, K. Lennert, R. Lukes, K. Nanba, G. O'Conor, H. Rappaport, A. Robb-Smith, M. Sacks, J. Burke, R. DeLellis, G. Frizzera, F. Rilke, J. Rosai, and R. Warnke. (19). We are especially grateful to Prof. K. Lennert and to Drs. Kristin Henry, Franco Rilke, Alistair Robb-Smith, Henry Rappaport, Robert Lukes, and Koji Nanba for their critical comments.

We take this opportunity to express our appreciation and admiration for the accomplishments of Dr. Saul Rosenberg, Dr. Richard Hoppe, Prof. Byron Brown and their associates at Stanford University Medical Center, in bringing this international project to its conclusion.

Mr. Philip Horne prepared the illustrations, and Ms. Gail Hicks typed the manuscript.

References

1. H. Rappaport, W. J. Winter, and E. B. Hicks, *Cancer (Philadelphia)* **9,** 792 (1956).
2. H. Rappaport, "Atlas of Tumor Pathology," Sect. 3, Fasc. 8. U.S. Armed Forces Inst. Pathol., Washington, D.C., 1966.
3. S. E. Jones, Z. Fuks, M. Bull, *et al., Cancer (Philadelphia)* **31,** 806 (1973).
4. R. E. Johnson, V. T. DeVita, L. E. Kun, *et al., Br. J. Cancer* **31,** Suppl. 2, 237 (1975).
5. G. P. Canellos, V. T. DeVita, R. C. Young, *et al., Br. J. Cancer* **31,** Suppl. 2, 474 (1975).
6. G. Bonadonna, M. DeLena, A. Lattuada, *et al., Br. J. Cancer* **31,** Suppl. 2, 481 (1975).
7. T. C. Brown, M. V. Peters, E. Bersagel, *et al., Br. J. Cancer* **31** Suppl. 2, 174 (1975).
8. V. T. DeVita, H. Rappaport, and E. Frei, *Cancer (Philadelphia)* **22,** 1087 (1968).
9. R. J. Lukes and R. D. Collins, *Cancer (Philadelphia)* **34,** 1488 (1974).
10. K. Lennert, N. Mohri, H. Stein, *et al., Br. J. Haematol.* **31,** Suppl., 193 (1975).
11. R. C. Braylan, E. S. Jaffe, and C. W. Berard, *Pathol. Annu.* **10,** 213 (1975).
12. R. F. Dorfman, *Lancet* **1,** 1295 (1974).
13. R. F. Dorfman, *Lancet* **2,** 961 (1974).
14. R. F. Dorfman, *Monogr. Int. Acad. Pathol.* **16,** 262–281 (1975).
15. M. H. Bennett, G. Farrer-Brown and K. Henry, *Lancet* **2,** 405 (1974).
16. K. Henry, M. H. Bennett, and G. Farrer-Brown, *Recent Results Cancer Res.* **64,** 38 (1978).
17. R. Gerard-Marchant, I. Hamlin, K. Lennert, *et al., Lancet* **2,** 406 (1974).
18. G. Mathe, H. Rappaport, G. T. O'Conor, and H. Torloni, "International Histological Classification of Tumours." No. 14. World Health Organ., Geneva, 1976.
19. S. A. Rosenberg, R. Hoppe, E. Glatstein, R. F. Dorfman, J. S. Burke, and C. W. Berard, *Cancer* (in press).
20. K. Lennert, *in* "Malignant Lymphomas Other than Hodgkin's Disease," p. 196. Springer-Verlag, Berlin and New York, 1978.
21. R. J. Lukes, J. W. Parker, C. R. Taylor, *et al., Semin. Hematol.* **15,** 322 (1978).
22. M. Shimoyama and S. Watanabe, eds., *Jpn. J. Clin. Oncol.* **9,** Suppl. I (1979).
23. J. A. Waldron, J. H. Glick, *et al., Cancer (Philadelphia)* **40,** 1604 (1977).
24. G. Frizzera, E. M. Moran, and H. Rappaport, *Am. J. Med.* **59,** 803 (1975).
25. R. J. Lukes and B. H. Tindle, *N. Engl. J. Med.* **292,** 1 (1975).
26. J. S. Burke and J. J. Butler, *Am. J. Clin. Pathol.* **66,** 1 (1976).
27. H. Kim, C. Jacobs, R. A. Warnke, and R. F. Dorfman, *Cancer (Philadelphia)* **41,** 620 (1978).
28. B. N. Nathwani, H. Kim, and H. Rappaport, *Cancer (Philadelphia)* **38,** 964 (1976).
29. M. P. Barcos, R. J. Lukes, *in* "Conflicts in Childhood Cancer. An Evaluation of Current Management" (L. F. Sinkes and J. O. Godden, eds.), Vol. 4, p. 147. Alan R. Liss, Inc., New York, 1975.
30. C. W. Berard, G. T. O'Conor, L. B. Thomas, *et al., Bull. W.H.O.* **40,** 601 (1969).
31. R. B. Mann, E. S. Jaffe, R. C. Braylan, *et al., N. Engl. J. Med.* **295,** 685 (1976).
32. C. W. Berard and R. F. Dorfman, *Clin. Haematol.* **3.** No. 1, 39 (1974).
33. H. Kim, M. R. Hendrickson, and R. F. Dorfman, *Cancer (Philadelphia)* **40,** 959 (1977).
34. K. Henry, *Br. J. Cancer* **31,** Suppl. 2, 73 (1975).
35. E. S. Jaffe, E. M. Shevach, E. H. Sussman, *et al., Br. J. Cancer* **31,** Suppl. 2, 107 (1975).

22

Radiation Therapy in the Management of Stage IIIA Hodgkin's Disease

RICHARD T. HOPPE, RICHARD S. COX, HENRY S. KAPLAN, AND SAUL A. ROSENBERG

I. Introduction

Only two decades ago, stage III Hodgkin's disease was considered incurable, and only palliative therapy was utilized in its management. In 1962, Dr. Henry S. Kaplan introduced the use of high-dose total lymphoid irradiation (TLI) in the treatment of these patients. At that time, the potential complications of this therapy were unknown, and its use was restricted to a clinical trial comparing

TLI with low-dose palliative irradiation restricted to involved sites. Within just a few years it was apparent that patient tolerance for TLI was acceptable and, moreover, that many patients were enjoying a continuous complete remission (1). Total lymphoid irradiation has now become the standard treatment for patients with stage IIIA Hodgkin's disease. Its success depends largely upon precise initial staging and fine attention to treatment details. Not only must all clinical sites of involvement be treated with adequate doses of irradiation, but sites at high risk of occult involvement must be treated as well. With adequate treatment, the majority of patients are cured. In this analysis we will discuss the radiation management of patients with stage IIIA Hodgkin's disease and review our results of treatment during the past 12 years.

II. Patients and Methods

At Stanford University Medical Center, 222 previously untreated patients with pathological stage (PS) IIIA Hodgkin's disease were evaluated and treated from July 1968 through December 1979. Twenty-one patients were excluded from this analysis: 13 pediatric patients who were treated with low-dose irradiation (1500–2500 rads) followed by mechlorethamine–vincristine–procarbazine–prednisone (MOPP) chemotherapy, 6 patients in whom there were contraindications to staging laparotomy and splenectomy, and 2 patients who had a diagnosis of composite lymphoma. The remaining 201 patients underwent complete staging studies including lymphography (with the exception of 1 patient) followed by staging laparotomy and splenectomy.

Sites of initial involvement were recorded according to the criteria defined at the Ann Arbor Conference (2). The extent of splenic involvement was scored according to its description in the laparotomy pathology report. Minimal splenic involvement was defined as microscopic disease only, or fewer than five nodules evident in the sectioned spleen. Extensive involvement was defined as five or more nodules evident in the sectioned spleen (3).

Delayed hypersensitivity was assessed in most patients by measuring their ability to become sensitized to and respond to a challenge of 2,4-dinitrochlorobenzene (DNCB) (4). The clinical stage of patients was scored by the Ann Arbor criteria (2), and the "anatomic substage" was determined using the criteria of Desser *et al.* (5).

Patients were treated with TLI with or without adjuvant chemotherapy. Treatment assignment was based in 109 cases on prospective randomized treatment protocols (6). In the remaining patients, usually because of protocol ineligibility, treatment was determined by general policies in effect at the time of their referral to Stanford.

The TLI program employed with these patients has been reviewed in detail (3, 7, 8). Usually patients were treated sequentially to the mantle and inverted-Y fields, however, occasional patients with extensive intraabdominal disease were treated first to the inverted Y. The dose to each field was 4000–4500 rads in 4–6 weeks. Important aspects of the mantle field treatment included the use of a "shrinking-field" technique in the presence of a large mediastinal mass, routine treatment of the pulmonary hilar lymph nodes in all cases, and low-dose irradiation of the lung (1650 rads) in the presence of ipsilateral hilar involvement (9). In addition, irradiation to the preauricular lymph nodes (3600 rads) was employed whenever high cervical lymphadenopathy was present. The inverted-Y field always included the splenic pedicle region and the pelvic lymph nodes. In the presence of splenic involvement the liver was irradiated, usually by means of a partial transmission liver block delivering a total dose of 2200 rads in 5–6 weeks (10). Some patients treated prior to 1972 also received fractionated doses of colloidal [198]Au as a component of their liver irradiation (11).

Patients scheduled to receive adjuvant chemotherapy generally did not receive irradiation to the lungs, preauricular region, or liver. In most cases the chemotherapy employed was the standard MOP(P) regimen (12). Several recently treated patients received procarbazine–alkeran–vinblastine (PAVe) chemotherapy (13).

Survival, freedom from relapse, and freedom from second relapse were calculated from the data first seen at Stanford using the actuarial technique of Kaplan and Meier (14). Survival and freedom from second relapse were also calculated from the date of first relapse in a separate analysis. The generalized Wilcoxon test of Gehan (15) and the actuarial test of Cox (16) were used to assess the significance of differences between treatment groups whenever appropriate. Selected groups, as noted, were compared using the multivariate regression technique of Cox (16).

One-hundred two patients were treated with TLI alone. Another 99 patients received adjuvant chemotherapy after completion of irradiation.

III. Results

A. Sites of Relapse

Table I summarizes the sites of initial relapse in the two different groups. One patient in each group failed to achieve a complete remission. Initial relapses were nodal in 76% (26/34) and 71% (10/14) of the patients in the two different treatment groups, respectively. The distribution of relapse sites was more generalized in the TLI group, 53% (18/34) of the patients having a component of

TABLE I

Initial Sites of Relapse in Patients with Pathological Stage IIIA Hodgkin's Disease

Relapse sites	Number of patients[a]	
	TLI	TLI + CHX
Nodal only	17	6
Extranodal only	8	4
Nodal plus extranodal	9	4
Supradiaphragmatic only	10	8
Subdiaphragmatic only	6	3
Generalized	18	3

[a] TLI, Total lymphoid irradiation; CHX, adjuvant chemotherapy. One patient in each group who failed to achieve an initial complete remission has been excluded.

relapse on both sides of the diaphragm, while only 21% (3/14) of the patients in the combined-modality group had a similar extent of relapsing disease. Overall, relapses limited to supradiaphragmatic sites were much more common than those at subdiaphragmatic sites (38 versus 19%).

B. Causes of Death

Table II summarizes the causes of death. The number of deaths due to Hodgkin's disease was quite small (9 and 6% in the two treatment groups). The

TABLE II

Causes of Death in Patients with Pathological Stage IIIA Hodgkin's Disease

Cause of Death	Number of Patients	
	TLI	TLI + CHX
Active Hodgkin's disease	9	6
Infection or sepsis	2[a]	2
Acute myelogenous leukemia	1[a]	1
Thrombocytopenia and hemorrhage	2[b]	—
Solid tumors	3[c]	—
Other	2[d]	—

[a] These patients received MOP(P) as salvage therapy.
[b] Both patients developed severe thrombocytopenia after treatment with colloidal [198]Au.
[c] Lung cancer (two cases) and colon cancer.
[d] Hypertension, automobile accident.

two patients who died from thrombocytopenia and hemorrhage had been treated with colloidal [198]Au as a component of their liver irradiation. They developed hematological complications shortly after [198]Au administration. This technique of liver irradiation was discontinued in 1972.

C. Prognostic Factors in the Group Treated with Total Lymphoid Irradiation Alone

A variety of possible prognostic factors including clinical stage, anatomic substage, extent of splenic involvement, DNCB reactivity, total number of sites of involvement, number of supradiaphragmatic sites of involvement, age, and sex were assessed in a univariate fashion to determine their influence on survival and freedom from relapse. Several factors had an adverse influence on freedom from relapse including the presence of extensive splenic involvement, negative DNCB reactivity, and a large number of initial sites of involvement, especially *supradiaphragmatic* sites. The relative importance of these prognostic factors was then assessed by a multivariate regression analysis (Table III). The most important covariate was the initial extent of splenic involvement. DNCB reactivity and the number of supradiaphragmatic sites involved also had a modest influence on prognosis. Other factors, including anatomic substage, clinical stage, age, and sex had no prognostic importance when incorporated into the multivariate analysis.

While the factors noted above adversely influenced freedom from relapse, survival differences were more difficult to demonstrate. The most important effect was related to the extent of splenic involvement. Ten-year survival rates after treatment with irradiation alone were 60 and 80% for patients with extensive versus minimal splenic involvement, respectively [p(Gehan) = .06].

TABLE III

Multivariate Analysis of Prognostic Factors and Their Influence on Relapse among 102 Patients Treated with Total Lymphoid Irradiation Alone for Pathological Stage IIIA Hodgkin's Disease

Covariate	Relative risk	p (Cox)[a]
Splenic involvement (extensive/minimal)	3.3	.0007
DNCB (negative/positive)	2.2	.01
Number of supradiaphragmatic sites (>3/≤3)	1.9	.08

[a] Relative risk represents the relapse risk for patients with condition X relative to the relapse risk for patients with condition Y (X/Y), and the p value is given for each variable after adjusting for all others.

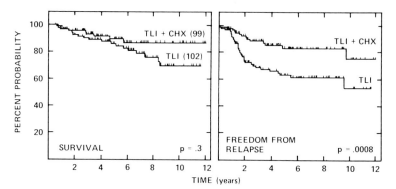

Fig. 1. Actuarial survival and freedom from relapse of 201 patients treated with either TLI alone (TLI) or TLI followed by adjuvant chemotherapy (TLI + CHX) for PS IIIA Hodgkin's disease at Stanford University. The *p* values noted were determined using a Gehan analysis. *p*(Cox) = .14 and .0002 for survival and freedom from relapse, respectively.

D. A Comparison of Total Lymphoid Irradiation Alone with Combined-Modality Therapy

Survival and freedom from relapse for the two different treatment groups are shown in Fig. 1. The survival difference is 4% at 5 years and 18% at 10 years. Tests of statistical significance reveal p(Gehan) = .3 and p(Cox) = .14. Differences in freedom from relapse achieve a greater degree of statistical significance [p(Gehan) = .0008 and p(Cox) = .0002], suggesting that there may be subgroups of patients at such high risk for relapse that initial management with

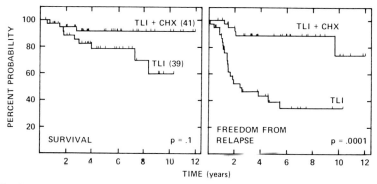

Fig. 2. Actuarial survival and freedom from relapse of patients with PS IIIA Hodgkin's disease and extensive splenic involvement who were treated either with TLI alone (TLI) or TLI followed by adjuvant chemotherapy (TLI + CHX). The *p* values noted were determined using the Gehan analysis. *p*(Cox) = .07 and 0.001 for survival and freedom from relapse, respectively.

combined-modality therapy may be justifiable. Therefore patients with specific unfavorable prognostic factors were analyzed further with respect to outcome after treatment with TLI alone or combined-modality therapy. Patients with extensive splenic involvement, negative DNCB reactivity, or a large number of initial sites of involvement had a significantly improved *freedom from relapse* when treated with combined-modality therapy. *Survival* differences, however, were less marked, the most important difference being in the group with extensive splenic involvement (Fig. 2). Freedom from relapse in the group with extensive spenic involvement treated with TLI alone was only 34% at 8 years, compared to 89% for patients treated with combined-modality therapy (p = .0001). Survivals at 8 years were 70 and 92%, respectively [p(Gehan) = .1, p(Cox) = .07].

E. Freedom from Second Relapse and Survival after First Relapse

In most instances, patients who relapsed after treatment with TLI alone were then treated with MOP(P) chemotherapy occasionally supplemented by low-dose adjuvant irradiation to involved sites. Patients who relapsed after initial treatment with combined-modality therapy were later treated with MOP(P) only if the interval from initial therapy was greater than 2 years—the others were treated with adriamycin–bleomycin–vinblastine–dacarbazine (ABVD) (17) or B-CAVe (18). Freedom from *second* relapse for the two different *initial* treatment groups calculated *from the date of presentation* is presented in Fig. 3. Treatment failure is scored in this analysis only if the patient fails to achieve an initial complete remission, fails to achieve a second complete remission after initial relapse, or relapses after achieving a second complete remission. The

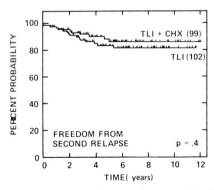

Fig. 3. Freedom from *second* relapse of 201 patients treated with either TLI alone (TLI) or TLI followed by adjuvant chemotherapy (TLI + CHX) for PS IIIA Hodgkin's disease.

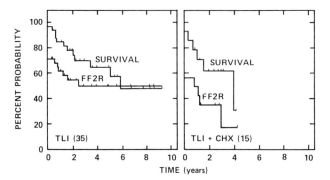

Fig. 4. Freedom from *second* relapse (FF2R) and survival after *first* relapse, calculated from the date of relapse, for patients with PS IIIA Hodgkin's disease treated initially either with TLI alone (left) or TLI followed by adjuvant chemotherapy (right).

long-term freedom from *second* relapse is excellent in both groups—82% for TLI alone and 87% for combined-modality therapy [p(Gehan) = .4].

The actual fate of patients after initial relapse is detailed more thoroughly in Fig. 4. In these curves, freedom from second relapse and survival are calculated *from the date of first relapse* rather than from the date of presentation. Among patients treated initially with TLI alone, 70% achieved a complete response to subsequent therapy. A second relapse occurred in 30% of these patients, yielding a long-term freedom from *second* relapse (or a salvage rate) of 50%. Second relapses in this group always occurred within the first 2 ½ years of retreatment. Ten patients have been in a second complete remission for 2 ½–10 years. Most of the patients who failed to achieve a second complete remission or suffered a second relapse have died, yielding a 48% long-term survival for this group.

Second remissions in patients treated initially with combined-modality therapy have been less durable. Although 65% of these patients have achieved a second complete response, the majority have subsequently relapsed—only 18% are still disease-free (salvaged) at 3 years, and only a single patient has been without evidence of disease more than 3 years after initial relapse.

IV. Discussion

Total lymphoid irradiation without adjuvant chemotherapy has proven to be effective management for most patients with stage IIIA Hodgkin's disease. Our 8-year survival is 70%, and freedom from relapse is 62% in this group of patients. Results reported from other centers have not been as good, and this may reflect differences in staging and treatment techniques. The subtle modifications of therapy which have evolved at Stanford in the past two decades are probably important in the management of these patients. Treatment of pulmonary hilar regions and pelvic lymph nodes in every case and treatment of the preauricular region, lungs, and liver in the presence of involvement of the upper cervical nodes, pulmonary hilar nodes, and spleen, respectively, all contribute to decreasing the likelihood of relapse. The use of combined-modality therapy in *all* patients with stage IIIA disease is not justified by our analysis. Despite the substantial differences in freedom from relapse, the ability to salvage patients with MOP(P) chemotherapy after failure of initial radiation management is good enough to yield similar overall survival rates in the two treatment groups. There is thus no valid reason to expose the entire population of Stage IIIA patients to the toxicities of combined-modality programs which include sterility in males (19), secondary acute myelogenous leukemia (20), and non-Hodgkin's lymphoma (21).

In confirmation of our previous study, this analysis fails to show any difference in either survival or freedom from relapse for anatomic substages III_1 and III_2 and no indication that *survival* is improved in either group by the addition of chemotherapy (3). There is disagreement in the literature regarding the significance of the anatomic substage, and this may again be a reflection of different treatment techniques (22). Policies involving routine treatment of the pulmonary hilar and pelvic lymph nodes and prophylactic treatment of the preauricular nodes, lungs, and liver under appropriate circumstances generally are not followed at centers where the anatomic substage has been found to be an important prognostic factor. It may be that our more aggressive and effective initial treatment program obscures the prognostic significance of the anatomic substage. The concept of anatomic substage also ignores the influence of disease above the diaphragm, where bulky mediastinal involvement is a well-documented adverse prognostic factor (23). Indeed, in our experience, relapse in *supradiaphragmatic* sites was more common than in *subdiaphragmatic* sites.

As in our previous analysis, the initial extent of splenic involvement continues to be an important prognostic factor (3). We hypothesize that this may be related to a greater likelihood of occult disseminated disease in patients with extensive splenic involvement. Freedom from relapse in this group of patients is markedly improved by the use of adjuvant chemotherapy. The survival difference is more modest because of successful salvage treatment in many patients treated initially with TLI alone, however, this is also approaching statistical significance.

In conclusion, TLI alone has proved to be appropriate treatment for most patients with stage IIIA Hodgkin's disease. In general the potential hazards of combined-modality programs should therefore be limited to patients who relapse. However, in view of the very high relapse rate among patients with extensive splenic involvement, and possible improvement in survival in these patients when they receive adjuvant chemotherapy, it is reasonable to employ systemic therapy in this unfavorable subgroup of patients with PS IIIA disease.

Acknowledgments

This work was supported in part by grant CA 05838 from the National Cancer Institute, National Institutes of Health. The authors thank Marge Keskin for secretarial assistance in the preparation of the manuscript.

References

1. H. S. Kaplan and S. A. Rosenberg, *Cancer Res.* **26,** 1268–1276 (1966).
2. P. P. Carbone, H. S. Kaplan, K. Mushoff, D. W. Smithers, and M. Tubiana, *Cancer Res.* **31,** 1860–1861 (1971).
3. R. T. Hoppe, S. A. Rosenberg, H. S. Kaplan, and R. S. Cox, *Cancer* 46, 1240–1246 (1980).
4. J. R. Eltringham and H. S. Kaplan, *Natl. Cancer Inst. Monogr.* **36,** 107–115 (1973).
5. R. K. Desser, H. M. Golomb, J. E. Ultmann, D. J. Ferguson, E. M. Moran, M. L. Griem, J. Vardiman, B. Miller, N. Oetzel, D. Sweet, E. P. Lester, J. J. Kinzie, and R. Blough, *Blood* **49,** 883–893 (1977).
6. S. A. Rosenberg, H. S. Kaplan, and B. W. Brown, *in* "Adjuvant Therapy of Cancer II" (S. E. Jones and S. E. Salmon, eds.), pp. 109–117. Grune & Stratton, New York, 1979.
7. H. S. Kaplan, "Hodgkin's Disease," 2nd ed. Harvard Univ. Press, Cambridge, Massachusetts, 1980.
8. R. T. Hoppe, *Semin. Oncol.* **7,** 144–154 (1980).
9. B. Palos, H. S. Kaplan, and C. J. Karzmark, *Radiology* **101,** 441–442 (1971).
10. H. P. Schultz, E. Glatstein, and H. S. Kaplan, *Int. J. Radiat. Oncol.* **1,** 1–8 (1975).
11. J. W. Kraut, H. S. Kaplan, and M. A. Bagshaw, *Cancer* **30,** 39–46 (1972).
12. V. T. DeVita, A. A. Serpick, and P. P. Carbone, *Ann. Intern. Med.* **73,** 881–895 (1970).
13. E. M. Wolin, S. A. Rosenberg, and H. S. Kaplan, *in* "Adjuvant Therapy of Cancer II" (S. E. Jones and S. E. Salmon, eds.), pp. 119–127. Grune & Stratton, New York, 1979.
14. E. S. Kaplan and P. Meier, *J. Am. Stat. Assoc.* **53,** 457–480 (1958).
15. E. A. Gehan, *Biometrika* **52,** 203–233 (1965).
16. D. R. Cox, *J. R. Stat. Soc. Ser. B* **34,** 187–220 (1972).
17. G. Bonadonna, R. Zucali, S. Monfardini, M. DeLena, and C. Uslenghi, *Cancer (Philadelphia)* **36,** 252–259 (1975).
18. K. J. Porzig, C. S. Portlock, A. Robertson, and S. A. Rosenberg, *Cancer (Philadelphia)* **41,** 1670–1675 (1975).
19. R. Chapman, S. B. Stucliffe, L. Reis, and J. S. Malpas, *Proc. Am. Assoc. Cancer Res.* **20,** 321 (1979).
20. C. N. Coleman, C. J. Williams, A. Flint, E. Glatstein, S. A. Rosenberg, and H. S. Kaplan, *N. Engl. J. Med.* **297,** 1249–1252 (1977).
21. J. G. Krikorian, J. S. Burke, S. A. Rosenberg, and H. S. Kaplan *N. Engl. J. Med.* **300,** 452–458 (1979).
22. R. S. Stein, R. M. Hilborn, J. M. Flexner, M. Bolin, S. Stroup, V. Reynolds, and S. Krantz, *Cancer* **42,** 429–436 (1978).
23. P. Mauch, R. Goodman, and S. Hellman, *Cancer* **42,** 1039–1045 (1978).

23

The Curative Potential of Chemotherapy in the Treatment of Hodgkin's Disease and Non-Hodgkin's Lymphomas

VINCENT T. DEVITA, JR., AND SUSAN MOLLOY HUBBARD

Lymphomas and leukemias have been models of the curability of cancer by drugs. We hope the data presented in this article and elsewhere in this volume will satisfactorily convey this point for lymphomas. In a previous publication lymphomas were used as an example of how, after a certain point in the evolution of the treatment of a disease, the human model takes over in directing research (1). The utility of the human model can be readily seen when we later discuss how prognostic factors impact on therapeutic results and alter the direction of new clinical trials. If lymphomas are curable by chemotherapy and other cancers are not, we need to ask ourselves why when we are examining the data on the treatment of Hodgkin's disease and non-Hodgkin's lymphomas, especially in light of certain new theories on factors that may influence the success of chemotherapy (2).

I. Primary Therapy of Advanced Hodgkin's Disease

The development and application of effective drug combinations in the treatment of advanced Hodgkin's disease have revolutionized the management of patients with this disease. Single-agent chemotherapy in patients with advanced disease is clearly less effective than drug combinations. Single agents, at best,

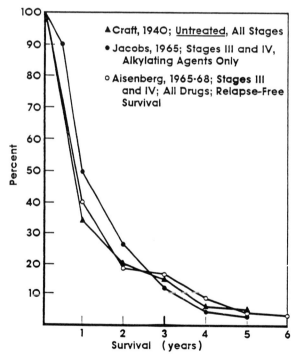

Fig. 1. Hodgkin's disease: survival in untreated patients and those treated with single agents (14).

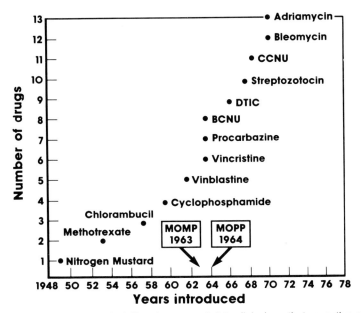

Fig. 2. Diagram depicting the influx of new agents into clinical use that are active against Hodgkin's disease (14).

produced overall response rates of 13–37% and complete remissions in approximately 20% of patients. The duration of response with single-agent therapy ranged from 3 to 6 months, and almost all patients with advanced disease were dead within 2 years of diagnosis. Fewer than 10% of patients with advanced disease survived 5 years, and virtually no patients were free of disease 5 years after diagnosis. The sequential use of alkylating agents, vinca alkaloids, and even procarbazine in the 1960s produced relapse-free survival that was not significantly better than the crude survival reported by Jacobs and associates utilizing alkylating agents alone (3). In fact, median survival of treated patients was not significantly better than the survival for untreated patients reported by Craft in the 1940s (4) (Fig. 1). Prior to 1963, the only class of drugs with clinical activity in Hodgkin's disease was the alkylating agents, although methotrexate appeared to have some activity. However, by 1963 a number of new drugs with activity in Hodgkin's disease were identified, making the development of an effective drug combination possible (Fig. 2).

The development of the MOPP program in 1964 represented an attempt to cure the disease using effective drugs in combination. The MOPP program, which followed a pilot study of a four-drug combination using methotrexate instead of procarbazine, embodied six principles which have remained important in the development of current therapeutic programs in all of the lymphomas: the use of multiple drugs, each with independent antitumor activity, and no known cross-resistance; the use of these drugs in full therapeutic doses in their optimal schedule of administration; the selection of an agent from each drug class based on nonoverlapping organ toxicity; cyclic drug administration to allow recovery of host tissue between cycles; a fixed schedule of administration within cycles, and a sliding scale for adjustment of doses of each subsequent cycle based on marrow toxicity; and discontinuation of treatment after clinical complete remission, followed by post-treatment restaging to determine the quality of complete remission.

From 1964 until February 1976, 198 patients with Hodgkin's disease were treated with the MOPP program as their primary treatment at the National Cancer Institute (NCI). Major characteristics of this patient population are shown in Table I. The staging and treatment policies and criteria for determining remission status have been reported in detail elsewhere (5). Eighty percent of patients (159 of 198) achieved complete remission, a fourfold increase over that achieved with

TABLE I

Major Characteristics of 198 Patients Treated with MOPP (5)

	Number	Complete remission (%)
Total	198	80.3
Male	130	77
Female	68	87
Major histology		
MC (mixed cellularity)	75	81
NS (nodular sclerosis)	74	84
LD (lymphocyte depleted)	43	70
LP (lymphocyte predominant)	4	100
U	2	100
Minor histology (for NS)		
MC	38	87
LD	16	63
None	20	95
Clinical stage		
II	14	93
III	70	84
IV	114	76
Pathological Stage		
II	11	100
III	78	82
IV	109	77
B Symptoms		
No	23	100
Yes	175	78

single agents. Sixty-eight percent of patients who attained complete remission, at risk for 5 years or longer, are continuously relapse-free 5 years after the end of all treatment, a 10-fold increase in duration of complete response as compared to that achieved with single-agent therapy. Only four relapses have occurred beyond 42 months after the cessation of therapy. Thus, the relapse-free survival of patients who achieved complete remission is, at 10 years, 63.4% (Fig. 3).

Survival of patients who attained complete remission is compared to that of patients who failed to achieve complete remission in Fig. 4. The median survival for the 39 patients who failed to achieve complete remission was 11 months. As shown in Fig. 4, no patient who failed to attain complete remission survived beyond 5 years. Only 44% of those in whom induction failed survived the first year, 26% survived the second year, and 10% survived the third year. In contrast, for patients who achieve complete remission, the probability of surviving beyond 5 years is 82%, and for 10 years it is 73%.

Confirmation of cure is substantiated by available autopsy data. Of the 98 recorded deaths, 23 (24%) represented patients who died without evidence of recurrent Hodgkin's disease. Autopsies were done in 15 of these patients, and no Hodgkin's disease was detected in 14 patients. In 1 patient who died of cerebral toxoplasmosis 18 months after attaining complete clinical remission, equivocal evidence of Hodgkin's disease was found in retroperitoneal lymph nodes. These data provide the evidence that has made us confident that the majority of patients who achieve complete remission are cured of their disease.

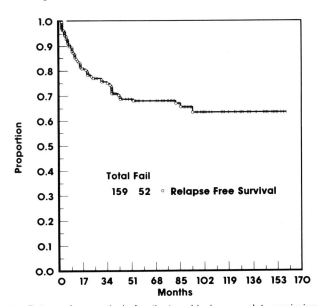

Fig. 3. Relapse-free survival of patients achieving complete remission (5).

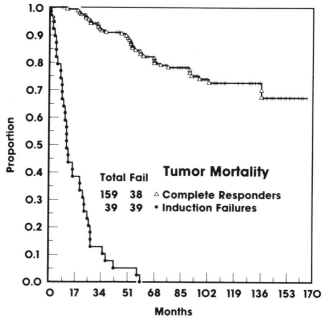

Fig. 4. Survival of patients who achieved complete remission and patients who failed to respond to MOPP (5).

A. Prognostic Factors Affecting the Curability with MOPP

Long-term follow-up in these MOPP-treated patients has allowed us to examine variables that influence the ability to achieve a complete response. We found that prior exposure to chemotherapy had a negative impact on the ability to achieve a complete and durable remission with MOPP, a fact that has been confirmed by others. In contrast, prior administration of radiotherapy did not compromise a patient's ability to be cured with MOPP chemotherapy, in fact, it may have helped. All but 2 of the 32 patients who received prior radiotherapy attained complete remission compared to a complete remission rate of 78% in previously untreated patients ($p = .065$). The fact that prior chemotherapy compromises the capacity to achieve complete remission with MOPP and radiotherapy does not has had a major impact on the design of current treatment protocols for patients with localized disease. This observation is consistent with all chemotherapy studies on malignant lymphomas.

The most important single factor influencing the ability to attain complete remission in patients with advanced Hodgkin's disease who had not received prior drug treatment was B symptoms. All 23 patients who were asymptomatic attained complete remission, while 78% of the patients with B symptoms achieved a complete response ($p = .025$). Sex, age, histological subclassification, and stage of disease did not exert a significant influence on the probability of achieving complete remission.

When we examined the variables that influenced the durability of complete remissions attainable with MOPP, we found that B symptoms also influenced the probability of remaining disease-free. All 23 asymptomatic patients achieved complete remission, and only 1 patient relapsed and died. Ninety-five percent of asymptomatic patients have remained disease-free compared to 58% of those with B symptoms, a highly significant difference ($p < .002$) (Fig. 5). With only one relapse in asymptomatic patients, the highly significant difference in tumor mortality was again noted between asymptomatic and symptomatic patients ($p < .002$).

The major histological subtype is also a significant factor in the durability of complete remissions attained with MOPP. Although patients with nodular sclerosing Hodgkin's disease had complete remission rates which were not significantly different than those of other histological subtypes, they had significantly shorter remission durations than patients with mixed cellularity ($p < .02$) or lymphocyte-depleted histology ($p < .02$), as shown in Fig. 6.

Further subclassification of nodular sclerosing Hodgkin's disease into minor categories of mixed cellularity or lymphocyte depletion has shown that progressive deterioration of histological characteristics has a negative effect on remission

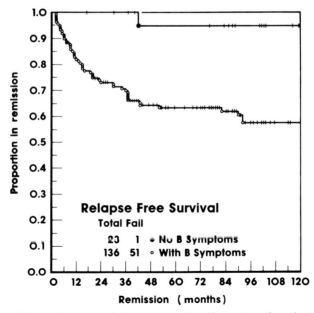

Fig. 5.   Relapse-free survival of asymptomatic and symptomatic patients (5).

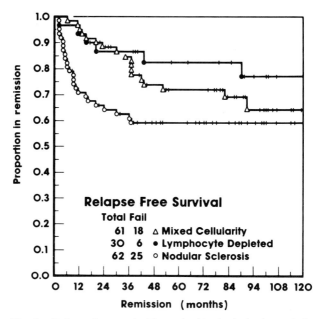

Fig. 6. Relapse-free survival by major histological subtype (14).

duration. Patients with nodular sclerosing Hodgkin's disease and a minor histological subtype of lymphocyte depletion had significantly shorter remissions than those with a minor histological subtype of mixed cellularity ($p < .05$). Furthermore, patients with nodular sclerosing Hodgkin's disease with a minor subtype of lymphocyte depletion experienced significantly shorter remissions than patients who had lymphocyte depletion ($p < .005$) or mixed cellularity as their major histological classification. Patients with nodular sclerosis who did not have a minor histology subtype recorded also had significantly shorter remission durations than patients with a major histological classification of mixed cellularity ($p < .005$) or lymphocyte depletion ($p < .005$) (Fig. 7).

The influence of a minor histological category (within the major classification of nodular sclerosis) on tumor mortality has not yet been noted. However, patients with nodular sclerosis and a minor classification of lymphocyte depletion did have a significantly greater tumor mortality than those with a minor histological subtype of mixed cellularity ($p < .005$) or those without a minor histological subtype recorded ($p < .025$). The same impact of minor histological classifications was noted on the survival of patients who failed to achieve complete remission. Only one patient with nodular sclerosing Hodgkin's disease who failed to achieve complete remission was not subclassified. The five patients with nodular sclerosing Hodgkin's disease with a subtype of mixed cellularity had a median survival of 25 months, compared to 7 months for the six patients with nodular sclerosing lymphocyte-depleted disease ($p < .02$) (Fig. 8).

When the data were analyzed by clinical stage, only patients with clinical stage IV (CS IV) experienced shorter remission durations than patients with CS II or III. Analysis of data by pathological stage revealed that patients with pathological stage II (PS II) had somewhat longer remissions than those with PS III or IV. However, the latter two groups had almost identical disease-free survivals. Only clinical evidence of pleural involvement conferred a significantly shorter disease-free survival when sites of visceral disease were analyzed.

The influence of clinical stage on tumor mortality was greater than that of pathological stage. Clinical stage II and III patients had similar tumor mortality, but CS IV patients had a higher tumor mortality than CS II patients ($p < .002$). Patients with clinical evidence of liver involvement had a significantly greater tumor mortality than those without clinical evidence of liver involvement ($p < .004$). Again, patients with clinical evidence of pleural involvement had a significantly higher tumor mortality than patients without pleural involvement ($p < .05$).

Stepwise regression analysis based on an additive proportional hazards model was used to evaluate the relative importance of the above factors on disease-free survival and tumor mortality and to evaluate whether the influences of these

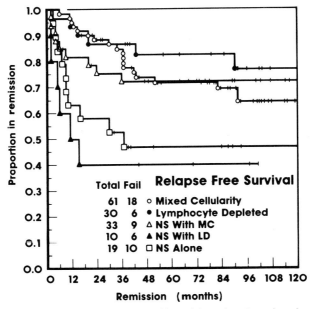

Fig. 7. Relapse-free survival of patients with nodular sclerosis and a minor histological subtype in relation to other major histological types.

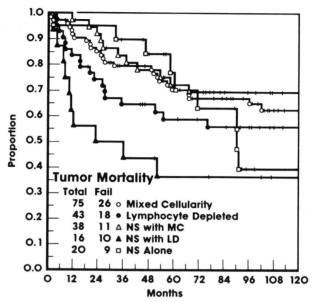

Fig. 8. Tumor mortality of patients with nodular sclerosis and a minor histological sub-type in relation to other major histological types.

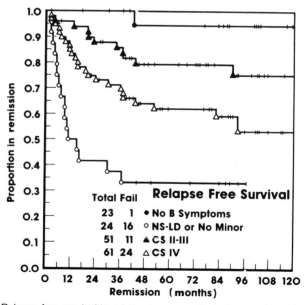

Fig. 9. Relapse-free survival in relation to prognostic factors as determined regression analysis.

factors were independent. The most important factor affecting remission duration was clearly the presence of B symptoms, and the second most important was histological subtype. After accounting for the influence of these two factors, clinical stage and clinical evidence of pleural involvement exerted a statistically significant influence on remission duration, while pathological stage did not (Fig. 9).

A stepwise regression analysis showed that the most important single factor influencing tumor mortality was again the presence of B symptoms. After adjustment for the effect of B symptoms, however, histological subtype and clinical stage were equally important influences on tumor mortality. After accounting for the effects of the three most important variables, B symptoms, histological subtype, and clinical stage, neither clinical evidence of liver involvement nor pleural involvement had a statistically significant effect on disease mortality. However, if one included B symptoms, histological subtype, and clinical evidence of either liver or pleural involvement in the regression, clinical stage no longer had prognostic importance.

B. Recurrence and Resistance: Implications for the Design of New Trials

While the durability of complete remissions attainable with MOPP demonstrates that a significant number of all patients with advanced disease can be cured with MOPP, a significant fraction of complete responders relapse at some point after achieving complete remission. Therefore, we investigated the effect of maintenance therapy to determine if it exerted a significant impact on tumor recurrence and found that relapse-free survival was not prolonged (6). Recent reanalysis of these data confirm that drug maintenance exerts no influence on remission duration or overall survival (Fig. 10). While other studies reported a beneficial effect for maintenance, it is now clear that maintenance therapy delays rather than prevents relapse (5). This conclusion has now been confirmed by others (7–12). This can be viewed as a further sign that cure has been achieved in many patients who attain complete remission. Cured patients should not need further treatment.

Faced with the fact that relapses after MOPP therapy occurred in approximately one-third of patients who achieved complete remission, we attempted to determine whether MOPP had value as a reinduction regimen. Fifty-nine percent of 32 patients who relapsed achieved a second complete remission when retreated with MOPP and intermittent maintenance with two cycles every 3 months for 2 years (13). As with primary MOPP therapy, no disease variable seemed to affect the second response rate. However, only 5 out of 17 patients whose initial complete remission was less than 1 year in duration achieved a second complete remission (29%) compared to 14 out of 15 patients whose initial complete remis-

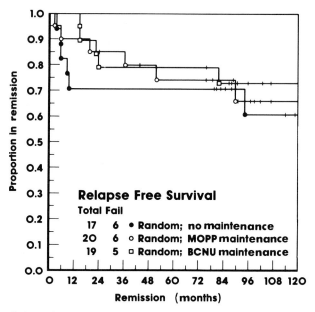

Fig. 10. Relapse-free survival of patients randomized to no further therapy or maintenance (14).

sion was a year or longer (93%), a statistically significant difference ($p < .001$). The duration of the second remission was longer in patients whose initial complete remission exceeded 1 year than in those whose initial remission was less than 1 year (Fig. 11). Overall survival is significantly improved in those who achieve second remissions over those who do not achieve a second remission ($p < .005$) (Fig. 12). Thus, the duration of an initial complete remission attained with MOPP represents an important variable that must be taken into consideration in the management of patients who relapse. In fact, the duration of the first complete remission represents an important variable that should influence the interpretation of any new treatment program evaluated in patients with Hodgkin's disease who relapse after combination chemotherapy.

Data on the importance of the initial remission duration and data demonstrating that maintenance therapy in complete responders does not improve relapse-free survival have led us to form several hypotheses (14). Patients who are truly cured during remission induction cannot experience beneficial effects from maintenance therapy. Long initial remissions and retained sensitivity to MOPP in patients who stay in remission in excess of 1 year probably indicate that they were almost cured by the intensive induction program. This is suggested by the fact that 14 out of 15 patients who relapsed 1 year or more after the end of therapy achieved a durable second remission. These data suggest that remission

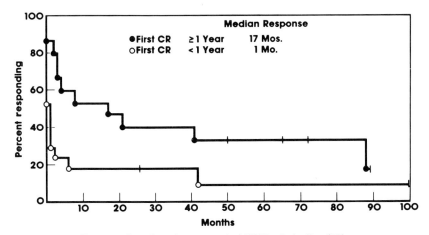

Fig. 11. Duration of response to MOPP reinduction (13).

induction was not continued long enough. The failure of maintenance programs to prevent relapse is therefore probably related to dose reduction and less intensive schedules of administration that are ineffective in eradicating occult residual tumor. The relative insensitivity of patients who experience short remissions (<12 months) suggests that the primary cause of treatment failure is the development of drug resistance.

Reasoning that drug resistance is the primary cause of induction failure and early recurrence following combination chemotherapy in Hodgkin's disease, Bonadonna and his associates initiated a randomized clinical trial evaluating MOPP alone as an induction regimen against MOPP alternating with adriamycin–bleomycin–vinblastine–dacarbazine (ABVD), a combination that is not cross-resistant with MOPP (15). Complete remissions were seen in 87% of

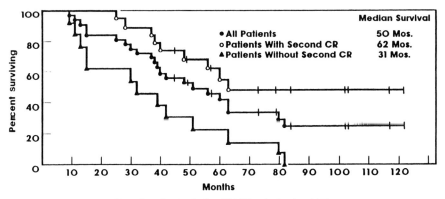

Fig. 12. Survival after MOPP reinduction (13).

patients given the alternating sequence as compared to 63% treated with MOPP alone in a series of 77 patients. All patients received 12 cycles of chemotherapy. With a median follow-up of 30 months 96% of patients achieving complete remission with MOPP-ABVD have remained disease-free as opposed to 65% of patients treated with MOPP alone.

Steady improvements in both disease-free and overall survival have been observed following the development and use of combinations that are not cross-resistant to MOPP in patients who fail to achieve complete remission with MOPP or in whom disease recurs rapidly following the cessation of therapy. These advances have stimulated a number of additional clinical trials evaluating the sequential use of other non-cross-resistant drug programs with MOPP in patients with advanced disease in an attempt to improve complete remission rates and prevent recurrence following primary treatment. At our institution MOPP alone is being compared to MOPP alternating with a non-cross-resistant combination containing streptozoticin, CeeNU, doxorubicin, and bleomycin as an induction regimen in patients with III_2A, IIIB, IVA, and IVB disease (Fig. 13).

Successful use of MOPP in advanced disease has led to clinical trials evaluating MOPP as an adjuvant to radiotherapy. Current data indicate that this approach may improve disease-free and/or overall survival in patients with PS, IA, IIA, IIIA, and IIIB Hodgkin's disease (16). Studies at the NCI randomizing patients between radiotherapy alone and radiotherapy plus MOPP indicate that disease-free survival has been improved by using MOPP in combination with radiotherapy in patients with PS I and II disease who have large mediastinal masses and widespread involvement of abdominal nodes (17). To answer questions about the ability of MOPP to cure patients with localized disease we have currently embarked on a protocol evaluating MOPP, and stage-tailored radiotherapy in early stages of disease (1) (Fig. 14).

HODGKIN'S DISEASE
MEDICINE BRANCH DCT AND CLINICAL
ONCOLOGY BRANCH BCRP

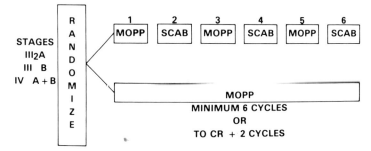

Fig. 13.   Current NCI protocol for advanced Hodgkin's disease (1). CR, complete remission.

HODGKIN'S DISEASE PROTOCOL
MEDICINE BRANCH AND CLINICAL
ONCOLOGY BRANCH, BCRP, DCT, NCI

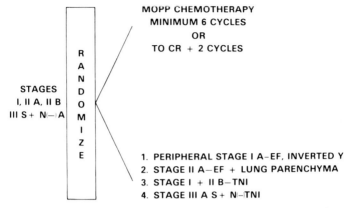

Fig. 14.   Current NCI protocol in early stages of Hodgkin's disease (1).

II. Primary Therapy of Advanced Diffuse Lymphoma

Diffuse histiocytic lymphoma (DHL), as designated by the Rappaport his-topathological classification, is a common, virulent lymphoma that when diag-nosed in advanced stages had a median survival in the range of 3 months prior to the advent of effective combination chemotherapy. Single-agent chemotherapy has consistently been shown to be ineffective. We have reported data on the use of three programs in the treatment of patients with advanced disease clearly indicating that a significant fraction of patients with DHL can be cured. We presented our evidence for cure at the Blood Club meeting in the spring of 1974, based on data dating back to 1964 (18). We reported a 41% complete remission rate achievable with MOPP and C-MOPP in untreated patients with advanced disease. Thirty-seven percent of all patients treated had experienced prolonged disease-free survival (Fig. 15). These data led us to examine prospectively new therapeutic programs to increase complete remission rates and to perform several retrospective analyses to identify important prognostic factors affecting the ability of chemotherapy to cure these patients.

Experience with DHL taught us several important points. While most patients demonstrated excellent responses to chemotherapy, with many rapidly achieving a complete or near-complete resolution of all clinically detectable disease, pa-tients often relapsed between cycles and only those who truly attained complete remission had a significant improvement in survival. To address the problem of recurrence between cycles, we evaluated a second program that substituted doxorubicin on days 1 and 8 for procarbazine and included two nonmyelosup-

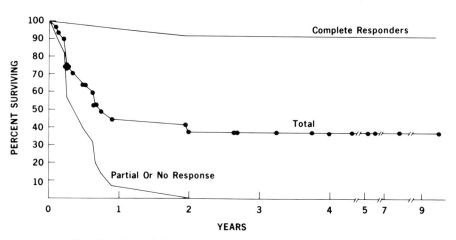

Fig. 15. Survival of patients with DHL treated with C-MOPP (18).

pressive agents that were administered during the period of bone marrow recovery. This program, known as BACOP, produced a slightly better complete remission rate (48%) in previously untreated patients with advanced disease (19). Again, only those achieving complete remission experienced prolonged disease-free and overall survival.

Because we noted that patients with DHL almost always responded to treatment but that the rate of regression tended to decrease over time, we attempted to design our current trial to address this problem. This protocol for patients with

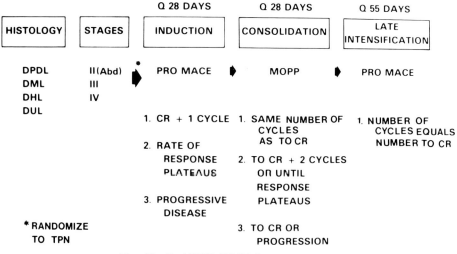

Fig. 16. ProMACE, MOPP flexitherapy (1).

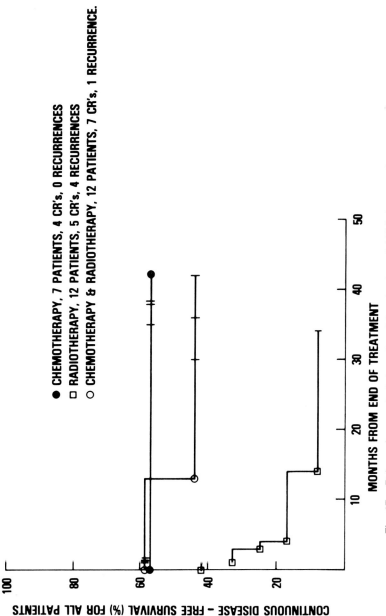

● CHEMOTHERAPY, 7 PATIENTS, 4 CR's, 0 RECURRENCES

□ RADIOTHERAPY, 12 PATIENTS, 5 CR's, 4 RECURRENCES

○ CHEMOTHERAPY & RADIOTHERAPY, 12 PATIENTS, 7 CR's, 1 RECURRENCE.

Fig. 17. Relapse-free survival stage II nodal and extranodal DHL by type of treatment (21).

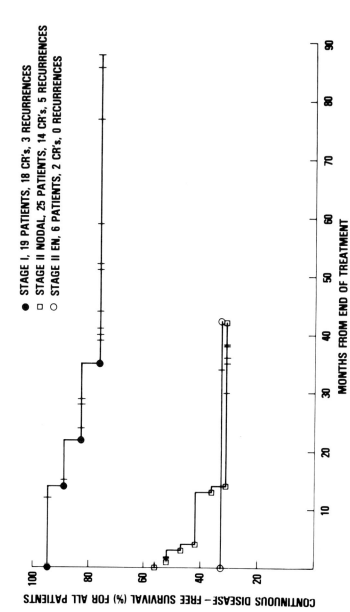

Fig. 18. Relapse-free survival of DS I DHL and PS II DHL by site organ (21).

diffuse lymphoma employs two non-cross-resistant combinations and incorporates a concept we refer to as "flexi-therapy" (1). The first combination consists of prednisone, cyclophosphamide high-dose methotrexate with leuvovorin rescue, adriamycin, and etoposide, VP-16. This regimen is administered as long as the rate of tumor regression remains constant, complete remission is achieved, or progressive disease occurs. When the rate of response decreases or all clinically detectable disease disappears, therapy is changed to the second regimen, the MOPP combination for consolidation (Fig. 16). Treatment is continued for the same number of cycles that were required to achieve complete remission plus one cycle, or until the rate of tumor regression plateaus. Finally, late intensification is administered using the ProMACE combination. The rate of response, therefore, determines the intensity and duration of the treatment. Early results using this approach in 33 patients with diffuse lymphomas have revealed a 67% complete remission rate (20).

In stage II DHL, data from a randomized trial of combination chemotherapy alone (C-MOPP), radiotherapy alone, or a combination of both treatments at our institution show that remission rates with chemotherapy are comparable to those achieved in patients with advanced disease (21) (Fig. 17). Only patients who remained stage I at the end of a thorough staging protocol that included laparotomy achieved a high complete remission rate (95% in 19 patients) (Fig. 18). Prognosis was excellent in stage I patients whether the tumor originated in nodal or extranodal sites. The apparent lack of influence of stage on survival in patients whose disease was not truly localized to a single site led us to look for clinical parameters that have prognostic significance in diffuse lymphoma and influence the ability to achieve durable complete remissions.

Prognostic Factors Affecting the Curability of Diffuse Non-Hodgkin's Lymphomas

A recent retrospective analysis of all patients with diffuse histologies at diagnosis who were treated at the NCI between 1964 and 1977 has shown that several prognostic factors can be identified as influencing response to therapy and survival (22). The major characteristics of this population of 151 patients are shown in Table II. Staging was originally performed according to the conventions of the time, but all staging data were reinterpreted according to our current criteria for staging, as defined by Chabner et al. in 1976 (23). If an inadequate evaluation of a given organ site was performed, the site was considered unevaluable for purposes of this study. As defined by the Ann Arbor Conference, 13% of patients were stage I, 23% stage II, 14% stage III, and 50% stage IV.

Initial therapy consisted of localized radiotherapy (involved or extended fields) in 29 patients (19%). More extensive fields were employed in an additional 8 patients (6%). Combination chemotherapy was the initial treatment in 91 patients

TABLE II

Clinical and Histological Characteristics of Patients with Diffuse Lymphomas

Characteristics	Number	Percent
Total patients	151	100
Sex		
Males	93	62
Females	58	38
Age (years)		
Less than 20	13	9
20–40	40	26
40–60	70	46
Over 60	28	19
Constitutional symptoms[a]		
A	83	55
B	68	45
Histological diagnosis[b]		
Diffuse mixed	31	20
Diffuse histiocytic	91	60
Diffuse undifferentiated non-		
Burkitt's	19	13
Unclassifiable	10	7
Stage		
I	20	13
II	34	23
III	21	14
IV	76	50
Initial therapy		
Radiation	37	25
Combination chemotherapy	91	61
Combined modality	16	11
Other	5	3

[a] Fever, night sweats, or loss of 10% of total body weight.
[b] According to the Rappaport classification (22).

(60%)—14 receiving CVP, 37 receiving MOPP or C-MOPP, and 40 receiving BACOP. The remaining patients received a combination of radiotherapy and combination chemotherapy (7%), or single agents (8%).

Actuarial survival for all 151 patients is shown in Fig. 19. With a median follow-up that exceeds 6 years, median survival is 34 months, with 43% of patients alive longer than 70 months. Only patients achieving complete remission have experienced prolonged disease-free survival. Fifty-four percent of patients achieved complete remission, and their median survival has not been reached with 76% of complete responders alive at 70 months. Median survival of the 37% of patients who achieved partial responses and the 9% who did not respond was 6 and 7 months, respectively.

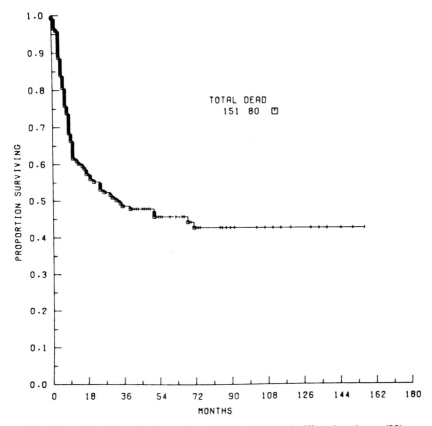

Fig. 19. Actuarial survival curve for all 151 patients with diffuse lymphoma (22).

Eight factors determined prior to the initiation of therapy affected the survival of this patient population. All save one tend to reflect a large volume of tumor cells. The only exception is a characteristic (sex) that significantly affected survival without influencing the complete remission rate (Fig. 20). Male survival was significantly poorer than the survival of females ($p = .05$). Factors that affected both response rate and survival are discussed below.

The complete response rate for patients with constitutional symptoms (fever, night sweats, or weight loss greater than 10% of total body weight) is 38% compared to 67% for asymptomatic patients ($p = .002$). Likewise, median survival for patients with B symptoms is 10 months, while the median for asymptomatic patients has not been reached ($p = .002$).

A patient's initial stage is inversely correlated with the complete response rate and also survival as shown in Fig. 21 ($p < .002$) except for patients with stage II disease who had a lower complete response rate and survival than patients with

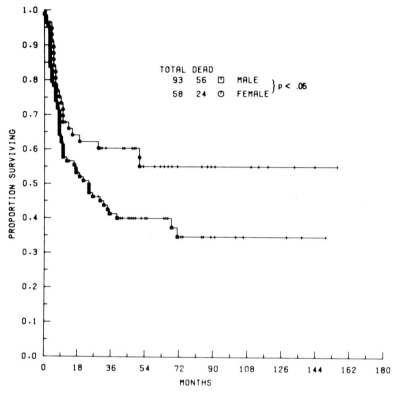

Fig. 20. Survival of all patients according to sex (22).

stage III lymphoma. This is related to the fact that patients with stage II disease and huge (>10 cm in diameter) gastrointestinal masses are included in this category.

Fifteen percent of evaluable patients had bone marrow infiltration, and their prognosis was extremely poor. The complete response rate was only 9% in these patients as compared to 62% in patients without marrow lymphoma ($p < .002$). As shown in Fig. 22, median survival drops from 51 months for patients without marrow involvement to 6 months for patients with marrow lymphoma ($p < .002$).

The prognosis of patients with a huge (>10 cm) abdominal mass and/or gastrointestinal involvement is shown in Fig. 23. Although only 10% of all evaluable patients had a huge mass and gastrointestinal lymphoma, their complete response rate of 7% and median survival of 6 months were significantly shorter than for all other patients (complete response rate of 60% and median survival of 51 months, respectively, $p < .002$). We could not demonstrate that gastrointestinal involvement without a huge mass or huge masses at other sites had prognostic significance.

Involvement of the liver also adversely affects the prognosis; 12% of evaluable patients had documented parenchymal liver disease. Of these, 25% had a complete response and median survival was only 6 months. This is significantly worse ($p < .002$) than survival in patients without liver involvement (complete response rate of 59% and median survival of 51 months, $p = .01$). No other site of extranodal involvement significantly affected survival.

Of the routine laboratory parameters analyzed, the patient's initial hemoglobin determination and serum lactate dehydrogenase (LDH) affected prognosis. Patients whose hemoglobin was less than 12 gm% had a 41% complete response rate and a 10-month median survival compared to 63% and 71 months for patients whose hemoglobin was equal to or greater than 12 gm% ($p < .002$). Patients with an LDH greater than 250 units had a 39% complete response rate

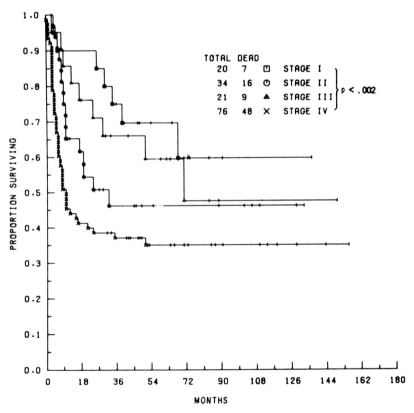

Fig. 21. Survival of all patients according to stage (22).

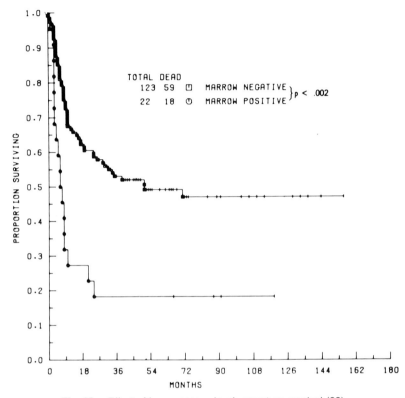

Fig. 22. Effect of bone marrow involvement on survival (22).

and a median survival of 13 months. In contrast, patients with an LDH of less than 250 units, had a 74% complete response rate and a median survival which has not been reached with 57% of the patients alive at 70 months ($p = .003$).

When histopathological subclassification was considered for prognostic influence in this patient population according to the Rappaport criteria, prognosis worsened from diffuse mixed to diffuse histiocytic to diffuse undifferentiated lymphoma, but there is no significant difference among the categories ($p = .27$) (Fig. 24).

When a multifactoral analysis was performed using a Cox regression model to delineate the relative importance of each prognostic factor, it was not possible to define the order of importance of these factors. In part, this is related to the fact that each factor was highly predictive of survival and that several prognostic factors were present in only a small number of patients. However, a patient's course could best be predicted by using a set of four variables that defined the patient's status in regard to bone marrow, huge abdominal masses with gastrointestinal involvement, constitutional symptoms, and sex. It is most important, however, to note that these clinical factors affected survival because fewer patients achieved complete remissions; survival of patients with poor prognostic factors was *not* compromised if complete remission was attained.

Knowledge of these prognostic factors should assist investigators in interpreting the results of clinical trials of drug regimens under evaluation in patients with diffuse lymphomas, since the distribution of these factors will vary from one study to another. Another reason for identifying prognostic factors is to permit the development of therapeutic approaches designed to take poor prognostic factors into consideration. At our institution, patients with advanced diffuse lymphoma who have bone marrow or bone involvement at diagnosis or at some time during the course of disease have a 25% chance of developing central nervous system involvement (24). Therefore, our current protocol for patients with these characteristics who achieve a complete response to ProMACE induction includes prophylactic treatment of the central nervous system in hopes of

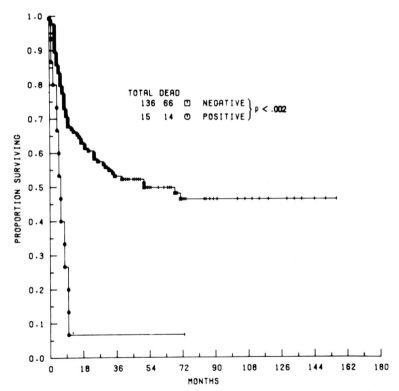

Fig. 23. Effect of huge (>10 cm) abdominal mass involving the gastrointestinal tract on survival (22).

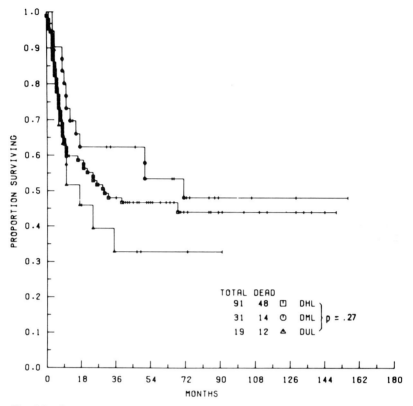

Fig. 24. Survival of 151 patients with diffuse lymphoma according to the Rappaport classification (22).

improving long-term disease-free survival in this subgroup of patients. Our interpretation of published literature suggests that differences in prognostic factors account for all differences in response rates with various drug combination programs utilized in the treatment of diffuse lymphoma.

III. Primary Therapy of Nodular Lymphomas

Nodular lymphomas represent a heterogenous class of diseases originating from B cells with differing natural histories and differing susceptibilities to currently available treatment modalities. It is valuable to consider response to treatment, disease-free survival, and overall survival in relation to specific histopathological subclassifications.

A. Nodular Mixed Lymphoma

Nodular mixed lymphoma (NML) comprises approximately 15–20% of all non-Hodgkin's lymphomas. Virtually all patients with this histological pattern have disseminated disease at the time of diagnosis. Results with combination chemotherapy in this population indicate that high complete remission rates (77%) and prolonged disease-free survivals can be achieved with aggressive therapy (25) (Figs. 25 and 26). The shape of the survival curve is different than that for nodular poorly differentiated lymphoma (NPDL), with a plateau indicating that the pressure of relapse is different and less when evolution toward large, undifferentiated cells occurs (Fig. 25). These data demonstrate that a significant difference in overall survival exists between patients who achieve a documented complete remission and those who fail to respond or respond partially to combination chemotherapy. This improvement in survival in complete responders has

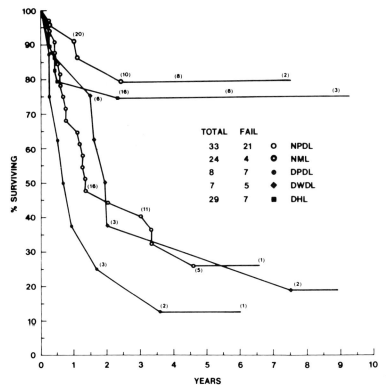

TOTAL	FAIL		
33	21	○	NPDL
24	4	◉	NML
8	7	●	DPDL
7	5	◆	DWDL
29	7	■	DHL

Fig. 25. Duration of complete remission in non-Hodgkin's lymphoma according to the Rappaport classification (25).

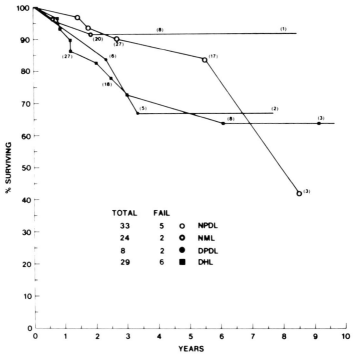

Fig. 26. Survival of complete responders—non-Hodgkin's lymphoma according to the Rappaport classification (25).

been confirmed by Ezdinli in 80 patients (26). Since the diagnosis of nodular mixed (instead of NPDL) is made with as few as 5% of large, undifferentiated lymphocytes, the success of chemotherapy cannot be due just to the successful eradication of this group of cells. More likely, the appearance of this small fraction of cells probably represents a change in the population kinetics of the entire group of cells that renders them more vulnerable to drug treatment. It should be noted that, in contrast to the treatment of NPDL (see below), drug combinations are more effective than single agents.

B. Nodular Histiocytic Lymphoma

Nodular histiocytic lymphoma (NHL) is an uncommon histological pattern with a poorly defined natural history. Of 473 patients seen at the NIH between 1953 and 1975, 16 patients (3.4%) were identified as having NHL (27). Thirteen of 16 patients had PS III or IV disease. Of the 9 who were PS IV, 3 had bone marrow involvement and 7 had liver involvement. Four patients received radiotherapy as their initial treatment; 11 patients received combination chemotherapy, and one received extended-field radiotherapy and C-MOPP. Eight of 11 patients who received combination chemotherapy attained complete remission, and two patients given radiotherapy achieved complete remission. The duration of complete remission and overall survival were better in patients who received chemotherapy despite the fact that 10 of these patients had advanced (PS III or IV) disease as compared to 2 who received radiotherapy. Both patients achieving complete remission with radiotherapy relapsed rapidly. Only 1 of 8 patients achieving complete remission with chemotherapy has relapsed. Seven are long-term disease-free survivors, and median survival of this group is in excess of 5 years (27) (Fig. 27).

Nine of the 16 patients had a repeat biopsy of a lymph node because of disease progression, or a review of lymph node histopathology at autopsy. In 7 of 9 patients, histopathological examination of nodal tissue revealed diffuse lymphoma (4 at the second biopsy, 3 at autopsy). One patient was free of disease at autopsy, and one patient who had had NML at rebiopsy did not have an autopsy. The majority of patients who originally presented with NHL eventually converted to a diffuse histology unless combination chemotherapy induced a durable complete remission.

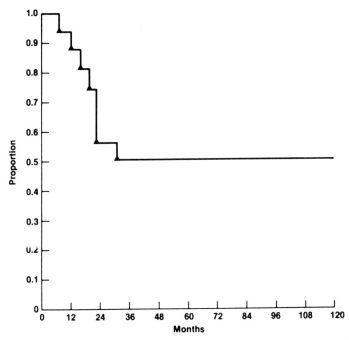

Fig. 27. Median survival of patients with nodular histiocytic lymphoma (27).

This report suggests that NHL also does not fit into the classification of indolent lymphomas. This histological subgroup exhibits certain characteristics that are commonly attributed to diffuse lymphoma: advanced stage at diagnosis and poor survival in partial or nonresponding patients. Treatment with combination chemotherapy rather than single agents is required to produce durable remissions and prolonged disease-free survivals similar to those achieved with patients with DHL. The fact that neither patient with PS I or II disease achieved a durable remission with radiotherapy alone as compared to seven out of eight treated with C-MOPP suggests that combination chemotherapy should be considered in all patients with NHL.

IV. Nodular Poorly Differentiated Lymphoma

Patients with NPDL often have with progressive nontender peripheral lymphadenopathy that slowly increases and sometimes waxes and wanes without treatment. The vast majority (85%) of patients are found to have advanced disease at the staging evaluation (23). Pathological evidence of disease is often easily documented by percutaneous liver and/or bone marrow biopsy.

This group of patients responds well to treatment with both radiotherapy and chemotherapy. Complete response rates on the order of 60–80% and median survivals of 6–7 years in responding patients are not unusual (Fig. 26). This has led to the commonly held belief that this population represents a good prognostic group. However, remissions are not durable, as evidenced by the continuous rate of relapse over time. This constant pressure of relapse has not been decreased by including new drugs such as adriamycin and bleomycin with (CVP) or alkylating agents, or by administering immunotherapy. This very drug-sensitive neoplasm provides one of the few striking examples where combination chemotherapy appears to be no better than single-agents treatment, an observation that requires further examination.

The best results in Stage III NPDL have been reported by Glatstein with radiotherapy. Of 51 patients with PS III who were treated with total lymphoid irradiation at doses between 3500 and 4000 rads (28), one-third remained in complete remission 10 years from diagnosis, with 90% of the relapses occurring in the first 5 years. Relapses mainly occurred in previously unirradiated nodes.

Total body irradiation in the range 100–150 rads can produce complete remissions in up to 85% of patients (29). Unfortunately, the pattern of relapse is continuous, resulting in median durations of complete remission ranging from 24 to 30 months.

Combination chemotherapy has also been utilized in an attempt to cure patients with NPDL. Our institution has reported a complete remission rate of 67% in 33 previously untreated patients with CVP (25). The median duration of remission was 16 months (Fig. 25). These results are comparable to others reported in the literature that range from 37 to 83% for complete remission and 16–36 months for median duration of response. Unlike the patients reported by Glatstein, virtually all the patients relapsed in previously involved lymph nodes.

Treatment with a single alkylating agent can produce complete remission on the order of 60–65% (30). The major difference between combinations such as CVP and single agents such as chlorambucil is the length of time required to induce complete remission. Patients receiving chlorambucil may require continuous therapy up to 20 months as compared to 3–6 months with CVP.

A. Histological Progression in Nodular Lymphoma: Implications for Treatment

There is a considerable amount of data, both old and new, supporting the hypothesis that the disease of patients with nodular lymphomas tends to evolve, albeit at varying rates of speed, from a nodular pattern to a diffuse pattern with effacement of lymph nodes by increasingly dedifferentiated tumor cells. This hypothesis is consistent with the finding that the tumor cells of most patients with DHL are cells of B-lymphocyte origin by surface marker studies. The true rate and frequency of this evolution are not known, nor has it been established whether the change in histology is accelerated by or related to therapy.

Current information suggests that normal cells in lymphoid follicles are motile and circulate through the lymphatic system with ease. Lymphomas of follicular center cells also appear to be motile as long as the lymphocytes retain the capacity to form nodules. This may explain why patients with nodular lymphomas usually have easily detectable disseminated disease. As the malignant lymphocytes dedifferentiate, the architecture of the lymph nodes changes from nodular to diffuse. These cells, like transformed lymphocytes, become less motile but more sensitive to eradication by drugs than cells found in nodular lymphomas. This lack of motility may account for the difficulty encountered in the identification of disseminated disease in patients designated, *per primum*, as having DHL. If the assumptions above are correct, there could indeed be a therapeutic advantage in allowing patients with advanced NPDL to evolve to a NML, NHL, or DHL histological subtype before treatment, since these histological subtypes are more sensitive to drug therapy, but treatment with combination chemotherapy is required

We, therefore, have retrospectively reviewed and analyzed the clinical course and serial biopsy specimens from 515 non-Hodgkin's lymphoma patients to determine the clinical importance of changes in histology over time (31). When initial diagnostic biopsies were subdivided according to the Rappaport classification, 39.8% of patients had nodular histologies, while 60.2% had diffuse types. The most common histological patterns were NPDL (20.2%) and DHL (18.6%).

Two hundred sixty-six patients had additional diagnostic biopsies at some time during their clinical course. One hundred fifty-two patients (29.5%) had another biopsy at a different site within 3 months of diagnosis. Thirty nine of the repeat biopsies demonstrated a histological pattern different from that seen in the original diagnostic specimen.

Prompted by the findings in these patients, we retrospectively reviewed the clinical course of 205 patients who had nodular lymphoma. Sixty-three patients had undergone a repeat biopsy more than 3 months after diagnosis (31). Thirty percent of these repeat biopsies revealed a changed histology, with histologic progression from a nodular pattern to diffuse histiocytic, mixed, or undifferentiated lymphoma, according to Rappaport's classification. When we compared the clinical characteristics of nodular patients showing histological progression with those who had not changed histology, no significant differences were found in the initial stage, duration and type of initial treatment, or reasons for repeat biopsy. Patients with nodular lymphoma whose histology was unchanged and patients whose histology revealed progression were rebiopsied at a time of relapse from complete remission or at the conclusion of an unsuccessful attempt to induce complete remission. The time that elapsed from initial diagnosis to repeat biopsy was approximately the same for patients showing histological progression (25 months) as compared to those whose histology was unchanged (27 months).

The impact of histological progression on overall survival was also examined. Patients with nodular lymphoma who converted to a diffuse lymphoma had a significantly shorter overall survival, 48 months. Those with unchanged repeat biopsies had a median survival of 92 months. ($p < .001$). This difference in survival was not due to a difference in the time from diagnosis to repeat biopsy but resulted from a markedly shorter survival after the repeat biopsy in those who demonstrated histological progression.

The reason for histological progression is unclear. One explanation is that progression represents an integral feature of the evolution of disease, similar to the blastic transformation of chronic granulocytic leukemia. A second factor influencing histological progression may be therapy. Alkylating agents and other anticancer drugs, but not necessarily ionizing irradiation, are known to be mutagenic for bacterial and mammalian cells and may hasten the appearance of a more transformed cell type. The early use of chemotherapy in patients with nodular lymphomas may increase the risk of selection of drug-resistant clones and may compromise later therapy. These considerations lend support to a conservative therapeutic approach to nodular lymphoma in its indolent phase.

In the present series, the survival of patients following histological progression was largely determined by response to intensive therapy. A complete response was achieved in 8 of 14 patients treated with combination chemotherapy, a response rate similar to that observed in previously untreated patients with DHL.

The median duration of survival in these patients after repeat biopsy was 40.5 months as compared to 4 months in those who did not achieve complete remission. This finding raises the intriguing possibility that a more successful strategy for treatment of nodular lymphoma might be to delay the use of any chemotherapy (especially low-dose continuous alkylating agents which might easily promote resistance) until the manifestation of histological progression, at which time long-term, disease-free survival may be attainable by using current drug combinations effective for diffuse lymphomas.

It is clear that new therapeutic strategies for the nodular phase of disease must be designed with the likelihood of eventual transformation to clinically more aggressive, but potentially curable, diffuse histology. Patients who have clinically progressed or relapsed but remain nodular on rebiopsy may anticipate prolonged survival with conservative therapy. However, progression from a nodular to a diffuse histology confers a prognosis similar to that usually associated with diffuse histologies diagnosed *de novo*. Histological progression should be suspected in all patients with nodular lymphoma who respond poorly to therapy, relapse, or develop disease at new extranodal sites. In these settings, a biopsy should be obtained whenever possible. Detection of histological progression is of considerable importance, since attainment of complete remission following this change can yield prolonged disease-free survival. Failure to attain complete remission is associated with a median survival (following rebiopsy) of 4 months (31a).

Studies comparing chemotherapy to radiotherapy and/or radiotherapy plus chemotherapy in NPDL have failed to show the clear superiority of any treatment approach. The failure of treatment administered with curative intent to render a significant fraction of patients disease-free for prolonged periods has led us to develop a protocol that prospectively compares aggressive chemotherapy to conservative radiotherapy administered only when patients become symptomatic from tumor masses in order to determine what fraction of patients with NPDL can be managed without initial therapy. Patients with NPDL will be randomly allocated either to receive aggressive treatment with chemotherapy combination at the outset of their disease, or to the alternative of no treatment if possible, or treatment with localized radiotherapy only (Fig. 28). We hope to derive several important pieces of information from this prospective study, such as the true rate at which an unselected population of patients with NPDL convert from an indolent to a progressive disease that requires treatment. By biopsying all growing tumors or new lesions, we should also be able to derive the true rate and frequency of conversion from a nodular to a diffuse pattern in aggressively and conservatively treated patients (31a).

At Stanford University the results of conservative watchful waiting followed by palliative intervention when necessary are comparable in a selected group of patients with indolent NPDL to results obtained with combination chemotherapy

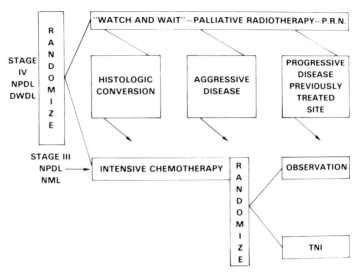

Fig. 28. Schema of watch-and-wait protocol for nodular lymphoma (1). TNI, Total nodal irradiation.

(32). The median actuarial survival for 21 selected patients followed until symptoms demanded treatment was 10 years. The median time between diagnosis and treatment was 32 months, and the 4-year actuarial survival was not significantly different from that of patients who had been entered on more aggressive treatment protocols at diagnosis.

The potential advantages of withholding drug treatment until aggressive therapy is required are considerable. The uncomfortable side effects of chemotherapy can be avoided at a time when patients otherwise are asymptomatic. Drug-related myelosuppression with its attendant risk of infection is also avoided. Pharmacological considerations also support the withholding of therapy until absolutely essential. Exposure to chemotherapy during indolent phases of the disease's natural history is known to compromise the ability of patients' to respond to drug treatment at a later time. Withholding chemotherapy, especially chlorambucil, until the disease becomes more aggressive, may place untreated or radiotherapy-treated patients whose tumor evolves to NML or DHL at a distinct advantage, since the tumor cells are more vulnerable to eradication by drug combinations. Avoidance of chlorambucil is critical because we know that prolonged exposure to low-dose alkylating agents increases the risk of a second malignancy in addition to fostering the development of resistance.

However, the safety and well-being of patients depend largely on careful observation by an experienced oncologist who will make appropriate and prudent decisions about therapeutic intervention.

In summary, the findings on the treatment of NPDL at Stanford University have an important influence on the choice of treatment of asymptomatic patients with NPDL. For these patients, the withholding of initial therapy must be considered a reasonable alternative to aggressive intervention. However, it will be increasingly important to attract these patients to centers where this conservative approach can be adequately tested before being utilized in general oncological practice.

B. General Comments on the Curability of Neoplasms by Chemotherapy with Lymphomas in Mind

How do the results of the treatment of lymphomas with chemotherapy fit with the critical elements thought to have a favorable influence on response to treatment? There are three important influences on the curability of cancer with drugs that were called to our attention by the remarkable work of Skipper and his colleagues in the early 1960s (33, 34) and more recently by a highly provocative piece of work described in an article by Goldie and Coldman (2): cell number at the time of treatment, growth characteristics of the tumor population, and sensitivity to chemotherapy (35–37).

Drugs kill a constant fraction and not a constant number of cancer cells in a population of uniform composition (first-order kinetics). There is an invariable inverse relationship between cell number at the time of treatment and curability by drugs. Growth characteristics influence the outcome because tumors with high growth fractions (such as Burkitt's lymphoma and DHL) are more vulnerable to chemotherapy. Experimental evidence indicates that growth fraction increases as population size decreases (and vice versa), again emphasizing the importance of cell number. For some time sensitivity to chemotherapy has been considered the major block to successful cancer chemotherapy. Cancer cells were thought to be inherently resistant or to develop resistance as a consequence of exposure to chemotherapy. Goldie and Coldman have reemphasized work reported by Luria and Delbruck in 1943 (with bacteria and phage) showing that mutation toward resistance does not require preexposure to the agent in question (38). This is now known to be true for resistance of tuberculosis to chemotherapy (39), and expansion of the resistant line may not require selective pressures. The Goldie and Coldman mathematical expression says that, for a population of tumor cells with an inherent tendency to mutate, the existence of at least one resistant cell will go from a condition of low to high probability over a very short interval in the biological history of the tumor. In fact, this may occur over an increase in size of approximately 2 logs or only six doubling times. The percentage and absolute number of resistant cells in tumor colonies of the same size will vary depending on whether the mutations occur as an early or a late event. If mutations occur as an early event, then the proportion and absolute number of resistant cells may already be high at the time of diagnosis of a 1-cm tumor mass, because the cell population has already doubled about 30 times to reach this size (40).

The basic assumption of this hypothesis is that spontaneous, stable, genetically based phenotypic drug resistance occurs in all exponentially growing populations of cells. After Goldie and Coldman wrote their paper, Skipper (41) analyzed the implications of their work for animal data and drug-curable human tumors, particularly lymphomas. The data suggest that the somatic mutation hypothesis goes a long way in explaining resistance to chemotherapy. Skipper points out that the inverse relationship between neoplastic cell burden and curability of murine lymphomas is observed over a range of 10^3–10^8 tumor cells where the growth fraction is known to be essentially constant. Therefore, growth fraction differences should not account for the superiority of combinations of drugs over the maximally tolerated doses of single drugs for these tumors. He also reemphasizes something that has bothered clinicians for many years. The cells of the bone marrow and gastrointestinal tract seem never to become resistant to the toxic effects of chemotherapy. These normal cells do not have an inherent tendency to mutate toward resistance to the available chemotherapy, while this clearly occurs in tumor cells.

Some lymphoma treatment data are interesting in this respect. One of the reasons for success in the treatment of Hodgkin's disease with drugs may involve an inherently low mutation rate related to the low number of malignant cells in any given tumor mass, even when this disease is advanced. The risk of mutation to a condition of high probability of resistance may be delayed relative to, say, lung cancer.

Clinical observations from chemotherapy studies on lymphomas are also compatible with the inferences of the somatic mutation theory. It is extraordinarily interesting that patients with NPDL, whose tumor is morphologically closest to the nomal tissue counterparts, are not curable by chemotherapy, but as they evolve to NML, NHL, and DHL they are. This observation is enhanced by the fact that, for NPDL, single agents are quite as good as drug combinations, and the same drug may be used effectively and repeatedly; but it is only possible to cure NML, NHL, and DHL with drug combinations. This suggests that in NPDL there is no tendency toward spontaneous or selective development of phenotypic drug resistance. The failure to cure NPDL is more likely related to the indolent growth characteristics of the tumor. The fact that prior treatment with radiotherapy does not compromise the later ability of patients who relapse to be cured by MOPP (in fact, it may help them) suggests that radiotherapy may narrow the number of resistant cell lines effectively.

When NPDL cells dedifferentiate, growth accelerates. The follicular pattern is effaced, and a diffuse lymphoma is the product. Now the high growth makes the disease more vulnerable to cure with drugs, but drug combinations are a requisite for cure. Treatment with drugs prior to dedifferentiation makes the likelihood of subsequent cure less likely, since chemotherapy can be expected to increase the mutation pressure on the malignant cell. Other observations consistent with this theory are:

1. There is a marked advantage of combinations of drugs over single drugs in achieving durable complete remissions, compatible with a cure, in both Hodgkin's disease and DHL, even though for the B-cell parent, NPDL, this is not true (5, 18).

2. Four drug combinations, however, have failed to achieve 100% complete remission rates. Approximately 40% of patients with Hodgkin's disease who achieve complete remission eventually relapse even though the groups of patients are uniformly classified and staged.

3. Some Hodgkin's patients treated with MOPP relapse after complete remission and achieve a second complete remission when retreated with MOPP, while others do not. The fact that the duration of initial remission has prognostic value suggests that there may be an inherently different somatic mutation rate in early and late relapsing patients which could account for their difference in response to retreatment with MOPP. Diffuse histiocytic lymphoma patients who relapse soon after achieving a clinical complete remission are also rarely ever successfully retreated with any combination of drugs, suggesting that the resistant cell lines have overgrown rapidly.

4. All prognostic indicators that influence complete remission rates implicate volume of tumor as the main reason for treatment failure in previously untreated patients.

5. The theory explains why the intuitive movement toward the current protocols, in which two non-cross-resistant combinations of drugs are delivered in alternating manners, offers promise (MOPP cycled with ABVD, and ProMACE cycled with MOPP).

These observations lead us to conclude that alternating cycles of combinations or alternating dosing of single drugs needs to be explored further for remission induction. They also raise the question as to whether the use of drugs thought to be ineffective against patients with advanced DHL (6-mercaptopurine, 5-flurouracil, and methotrexate), based on clinical studies in patients with advanced disease, should be reexamined in early stage disease or in treating patients further after they appear to be in remission. Incorporation of antimetabolite chemotherapy into the treatment of early stages of the disease or its use after other drugs have reduced the tumor mass (as in the COMLA and ProMACE studies) might prove to be effective (20, 42).

The hypothesis proposed by Goldie and Coldman offers an explanation for the invariable inverse relationship between tumor cell burden and curability by drugs independent of the growth characteristics of the tumor but dependent on growth rate and mutation rate.

References

1. V. T. DeVita, Human models of human disease: Breast cancer and the lymphomas. *Int. J. Radiat. Oncol. Biol. Phys.* **5**, 1855-1867 (1979).
2. J. H. Goldie and A. J. Coldman, A mathematic model for relating the drug sensitivity of tumors to their spontaneous mutation rate. *Cancer Treat. Rep.* **63**, 1727-1733 (1979).
3. E. M. Jacobs, F. C. Peters, J. K. Luce, C. Zippin, and D. A. Wood, Mechlorethamine HCl and cyclophosphamide in the treatment of Hodgkin's disease and the lymphomas. *JAMA, J. Am. Med. Assoc.* **203**, 104-110 (1968).
4. C. B. Craft, Results with roentgen ray therapy in Hodgkin's disease. *Bull. Staff Hosp. Univ. Minn.* **11**, 391-409 (1940).
5. V. T. DeVita, R. M. Simon, S. M. Hubbard, R. C. Young, C. W. Berard, J. H. Moxley, III, E. Frei, III, P. P. Carbone, and G. P. Canellos, On the curability of advanced Hodgkin's disease with chemotherapy: Long-term follow-up of MOPP treated patients at NCI and the influence of disease variables on prognosis. *Ann. Intern. Med.* **92**, 587-595 (1980).
6. R. C. Young, B. A. Chabner, G. P. Canellos, P. S. Schein, and V. T. DeVita, Maintenance chemotherapy for advanced Hodgkin's disease in remission. *Lancet* **1**, 1339-1343 (1973).
7. C. A. Coltman, E. Frei, III, and T. E. Moon, MOPP maintenance versus unmaintained remission of advanced Hodgkin's disease: 7.2 year follow-up. *Proc. Am. Soc. Clin. Oncol.* Abstr. C-211, p. 289 (1976).
8. J. R. Durant, R. A. Gams, E. Velez-Garcia, A. Bartolucci, D. Wirtschafter, and R. Dorfman, BCNU, Velban, cyclophosphamide, procarbazine, and prednisone (BCVPP) in advanced Hodgkin's disease. *Cancer* **42**, 2101-2110 (1978).
9. R. F. Bakemeier, V. T. DeVita, and J. Horton, Chemotherapy and immunotherapy of Hodgkin's disease. *Proc. Am. Soc. Clin. Oncol.* Abstr. C-225, p. 293 (1976).
10. J. R. Durant, A. Bartolucci, R. A. Gams *et al.*, Southeastern Cancer Study Group trials with nitrosoureas in Hodgkin's disease. *Cancer Treat. Rep.* **60**, 781-787 (1976).
11. C. H. Diggs, P. H. Wiernik, J. S. Levi, and L. K. Klovs, Cyclophosphamide, vinblastine, procarbazine, and prednisone with CCNU and vinblastine maintenance for advanced Hodgkin's disease. *Cancer* **39**, 1949-1954 (1977).
12. S. B. Sutcliffe, P. F. M. Wrigley, J. Peto, T. A. Lister, A. G. Stanfeld, J. M. A. Whitehouse, D. Crowther, and J. S. Malpas, MVPP chemotherapy regimen for advanced Hodgkin's disease. *Br. Med. J.* **1**, 679-683 (1978).
13. R. I. Fisher, V. T. DeVita, S. P. Hubbard, R. Simon, and R. C. Young, Prolonged disease-free survival in Hodgkin's disease with MOPP reintroduction after first relapse. *Ann. Intern. Med.* **90**, 761-763 (1979).
14. V. T. DeVita, The consequence of the chemotherapy of Hodgkin's disease. The 10th David A. Karnofsky Lecture. *Cancer* **47**, 1-13 (1981).
15. A. Santoro, G. Bonadonna, V. Bonfante, and P. Valagussa, Non-cross-resistant regimens (MOPP and ABVD) versus MOPP alone in stage IV Hodgkin's disease. *Proc. Am. Soc. Clin. Oncol.* **16**, 470 (1980).
16. R. T. Hoppe, S. A. Rosenberg, H. S. Kaplan, and E. Glatstein, The treatment of Hodgkin's disease stage I-IIA—Subtotal lymphoid irradiation versus involved field irradiation plus adjuvant MOPP. *In* "Adjuvant Therapy of Cancer" (S. E. Jones and S. E. Salmon, eds.), pp. 137-144. Grune & Stratton, New York, 1979.

17. P. H. Wiernik and J. L. Lichtenfeld, Combined modality therapy for localized Hodgkin's disease: A seven year up-date of an early study. *Oncology* **32**, 208 (1975).
18. V. T. DeVita, G. P. Canellos, B. Chabner, P. Schein, R. C. Young, and S. P. Hubbard, Advanced diffuse histiocytic lymphoma, a potentially curable disease: Results with combination chemotherapy. *Lancet* **1**, 248–280 (1975).
19. P. S. Schein, V. T. DeVita, S. P. Hubbard, B. A. Chabner, G. P. Canellos, C. W. Berard, and R. C. Young, Bleomycin, adriamycin, cyclophosphamide, vincristine, and prednisone (BACOP): Combination chemotherapy in the treatment of advanced diffuse histiocytic lymphoma. *Ann. Intern. Med.* **85**, 417–422 (1976).
20. R. I. Fisher, V. T. DeVita, S. M. Hubbard, M. F. Brennan, B. A. Chabner, R. Simon, and R. C. Young, ProMACE-MOPP combination chemotherapy: Treatment of diffuse lymphomas. *Proc. Am. Soc. Clin. Oncol.* **16**, 468 (1980).
21. V. T. DeVita, E. J. Glatstein, R. C. Young, S. P. Hubbard, R. M. Simon, J. L. Ziegler, and P. H. Wiernik, Changing concepts: The lymphomas. *In* "Adjuvant Therapy of Cancer" (S. E. Jones and S. E. Salmon, eds), pp. 173–190. Grune & Stratton, New York, 1972.
22. R. I. Fisher, S. M. Hubbard, V. T. DeVita, C. W. Berard, R. Wesley, J. Cossman, and R. C. Young, Factors predicting long-term survival in diffuse mixed, histiocytic and undifferentiated lymphoma. *Blood* **58**, 45–51 (1981).
23. B. A. Chabner, R. E. Johnson, R. C. Young, G. P. Canellos, S. P. Hubbard, S. K. Johnson, and V. T. DeVita, Sequential nonsurgical staging in non-Hodgkin's lymphoma. *Ann. Intern. Med.* **85**, 149–154 (1976).
24. R. C. Young, D. M. Howser, T. Anderson, R. I. Fisher, E. Jaffe, and V. T. DeVita, Central nervous system complications of non-Hodgkin's lymphoma: The potential role of prophylactic therapy. *Am. J. Med.* **66**, 435–443 (1979).
25. T. Anderson, R. A. Bender, R. I. Fisher, V. T. DeVita, B. A. Chabner, C. Berard, L. Norton, and R. C. Young, Combination chemotherapy in non-Hodgkin's lymphoma: Results of long-term follow-up. *Cancer Treat. Rep.* **61**, 1057–1066 (1977).
26. E. Z. Ezdinli, W. G. Costello, I. Fikri, R. E. Lenhard, G. J. Johnson, M. Silverstein, C. W. Berard, J. M. Bennett, and P. P. Carbone, Nodular mixed lymphocytic, histiocytic lymphoma: Response and survival. *Cancer* **45**, 261–267 (1980).
27. C. K. Osborne, L. Norton, R. C. Young, A. J. Garvin, R. M. Simon, C. W. Berard, S. M. Hubbard, and V. T. DeVita, Nodular histiocytic lymphoma: An aggressive nodular lymphoma with potential for prolonged disease-free survival. *Blood* **56**, 98–103 (1980).
28. E. Glatstein, Z. Fuks, D. R. Goffinett *et al.*, Non-Hodgkin's lymphoma of stage III extent: Is total lymphoid irradiation appropriate treatment? *Cancer* **37**, 2806–2809 (1976).
29. R. C. Young, R. E. Johnson, G. P. Canellos, B. A. Chabner, H. D. Brereton, C. W. Berard, and V. T. DeVita, Advanced lymphocytic lymphoma: Randomized comparisons of chemotherapy and radiotherapy, alone or in combination. *Cancer Treat. Rep.* **61**, 1153–1159 (1977).
30. S. E. Jones, S. A. Rosenberg, H. S. Kaplan *et al.*, Non-Hodgkin's lymphoma. II. Single agent chemotherapy. *Cancer* **30**, 31–38 (1972).
31. R. Jones, S. M. Hubbard, C. Osborne, G. J. Merrill, R. Young, and V. T. DeVita, Histologic conversion in non-Hodgkin's lymphoma: Evolution of nodular lymphomas to diffuse lymphomas. *Clin. Res.* **26**, 437A (1978).
31a. Hubbard, S. M., Chabner, B. A., DeVita, V. T., Simon, R., Berard, C. W., Jones, R. B., Garvin, A. J., Canellos, G. P., Osborne, C. K., and Young, R. C., Histologic progression in non-Hodgkin's lymphoma. *Blood,* February, 1982 (in press).
32. C. S. Portlock and S. A. Rosenberg, No initial therapy for stage III and IV non-Hodgkin's lymphomas of favorable histologic types. *Ann. Intern. Med.* **90**, 10–13 (1979).
33. H. E. Skipper, F. M. Shabel, and W. S. Wilcox, Experimental evaluation of potential anti-

cancer agents. XIII. On the criteria and kinetics associated with "curability" of experimental leukemia. *Cancer Chemother. Rep.* **35**, 1–111.

34. H. E. Skipper, Reasons for success and failure in treatment of murine leukemia with the drugs now employed in treating human leukemias. Cancer Chemotherapy, Vol. 1. University Microfilms International, Ann Arbor, Michigan, 1978.

35. R. W. Brockman, Mechanisms of resistance. *In* "Antineoplastic and Immunosuppressive Agents" (A. C. Sartorelli and D. G. John, eds.), pp. 352–410. Springer-Verlag, Berlin and New York, 1974.

36. M. Harris, Mutation rates in cells at different ploidy levels. *J. Cell. Physiol.* **78**, 177–184 (1971).

37. L. H. Thompson and R. M. Baker, Isolation of mutants of cultured mammalian cells. *In* "Methods in Cell Biology" (D. M. Prescott, ed.), p. 209. Academic Press, New York, 1972.

38. S. E. Luria and M. Delbruck, Mutations of bacteria from virus sensitivity to virus resistance. *Genetics* **28**, 491–498 (1943).

39. H. L. David, Probability distribution of drug resistant mutants in an unselected population of *Mycobacterium tuberculosis*. *Appl. Microbiol.* **20**, 810–814 (1970).

40. V. T. DeVita, R. C. Young, and G. P. Canellos, Combination versus single agent chemotherapy. *Cancer* **35**, 98–110 (1975).

41. H. E. Skipper, personal communication.

42. D. L. Sweet, H. M. Golomb, J. E. Ultmann, B. Miller, R. S. Stein, E. P. Lester, U. Mintz, J. D. Bitran, R. A. Streuli, K. Daly, and N. O. Roth, Cyclophosphamide, vincristine, methotrexate with leucovorin rescue and cytarabine (COMLA) combination sequential chemotherapy for advanced diffuse histiocytic lymphoma. *Ann. Intern. Med.* **92**, 785–790 (1980).

24

Primary Chemotherapy for Hodgkin's Disease and Non-Hodgkin's Lymphoma

JOHN M. GOLDMAN

I. Introduction

In 1970 a group of radiation and medical oncologists gathered in an effort to standardize the treatment of Hodgkin's disease (HD) in the United Kingdom. Studies were designed to compare different treatment approachs for patients with

Copyright © 1982 by Academic Press,Inc.
All rights of reproduction in any form reserved.
ISBN 0-12-597120-6

specific histological subtypes and clinical stages of HD. Thereafter the number of participants in this collaborative group, which came to be known as the British National Lymphoma Investigation (BNLI), increased annually. In 1974 the group established criteria for the histological grading and clinical staging of non-Hodgkin's lymphoma (NHL), and comparisons of different treatment regimens for NHL were initiated. As of November 1980 the BNLI represented collaborating clinicians from 26 medical centers in the United Kingdom. The BNLI pathology panel has examined material from 4380 patients considered by the referring clinician to have lymphoma. Of these, 1550 patients with HD and 960 patients with NHL have been entered in one or another of the treatment studies.

In this article I will review briefly selected results obtained in comparisons of different treatment approaches for patients with advanced HD entered in BNLI studies since 1970 and for patients with advanced NHL entered since 1974. I will refer also to a pilot study designed to prolong the duration of complete remission (CR) and perhaps to increase the chance of cure for patients with NHL.

II. Methods and Results

A. Criteria for Diagnosis and Assessment of Response

Histological material from all patients entered in BNLI studies was reviewed by members of the central pathology panel. Biopsy material from patients with HD was classified according to the criteria of Lukes and Butler (1), and patients were thereby divided into one of two grades (grade I—lymphocytic predominance or nodular sclerosis, or grade II—mixed cellularity or lymphocytic depletion). Biopsy material from patients with NHL was classified in accordance with criteria established by the BNLI pathology panel in 1973 (2) and divided also into one of two prognostic grades: grade I was the "good prognosis" category, and grade II the "poor prognosis" category.

For staging patients with HD the BNLI used the Rye classification as modified at Ann Arbor (3), with certain additional minor changes intended to facilitate the administration of radiotherapy to convenient single fields. A number of investigations including bipedal lymphography were mandatory for staging patients with HD; laparotomy, however, was performed at the option of the clinician. Criteria similar to those established for HD were used for the staging of NHL, but the presence or absence of constitutional symptoms (A or B) was not considered relevant in NHL.

When staging procedures were completed, patients were randomized according to stage and histological grade by the central secretariat. Complete remission was defined as the disappearance of all known disease as demonstrated originally during pretreatment investigation of the patient. Confirmation of CR was ob-

TABLE IA

Clinical Details of All Patients Entered in BNLI Studies up to February 1980[a]

	Patients		Histology[b]		Stage						
Disease	Males	Age <46 years	Grade I	Grade II	I	II	III	IV	A	B	Total
Hodgkin's disease	923 (66)	1023 (73)	LP 112 (8) NS 993 (71)	MC 240 (17) LD 50 (4) H 12 (1)	335 (24)	368 (26)	412 (29)	294 (21)	943 (67)	463 (33)	1410 (100)
Non-Hodgkin's lymphoma	430 (61)	169 (24)	414 (60)	275 (40)	124 (18)	106 (15)	196 (28)	282 (40)	—	—	708 (100)

[a] Some data on a small number of patients summarized in this table are still being evaluated; individual rows do not therefore always add up to the correct total number of patients. Percentages are shown in parentheses.

[b] LS, Lymphocytic predominance; NS, nodular sclerosis; MC, mixed cellularity; LD, lymphocytic depletion; H, histiocytic.

tained by repeating all investigations (other than laparotomy) that were originally abnormal. For subsequent analyses such patients were only regarded as having achieved CR if it persisted for at least 3 months. Partial remission (PR) was defined as 50% or greater reduction in measurable tumor masses. A response of less than 50% was classified as no response (NR).

TABLE IB

Results of Treatment for All Patients Entered in BNLI Studies up to February 1980[a]

	Response[b]				Survival		
Disease	CR, no recurrence	CR, recurrence	PR	NR	Alive	Dead	Total
Hodgkin's disease	785 (56)	351 (25)	204 (17)	40 (3)	1074 (76)	336 (24)	1410 (100)
Non-Hodgkin's lymphoma	309 (44)	98 (14)	235 (33)	66 (9)	487 (69)	221 (31)	708 (100)

[a] Data analysis, October 1980. Percentages are shown in parentheses.

[b] CR, Complete remission; PR, partial remission; NR, no response.

TABLE II

MOPP versus MOP (BNLI Regimens)[a]

Either MOPP:
    Mustine hydrochloride, 6 mg/m^2 (max. 15 mg), days 1 and 8
    Vincristine, 1.4 mg/m^2 (max. 2.0 mg), days 1 and 8
    Procarbazine, 100 mg/m^2 (max. 200 mg), daily, po, days 1–10
    Prednisone 25 mg/m^2 (max. 60 mg), daily, po, days 1–14
Or MOP:
    As above, with the omission of steroids

---

[a] Patients in this study were planned to receive six courses of MOPP or MOP. (Subsequently provision was made to increase the total number of courses if necessary; see Table IV.) po, Orally.

Clinical details, including histological subtype and stage, and the results of treatment are summarized in Tables IA and IB for all patients with HD or NHL entered in BNLI studies up to February 1980.

B. MOPP versus MOP for Stage IV Hodgkin's Disease

The four-drug combination of cytotoxic drugs [nitrogen mustard, vincristine, procarbazine, and prednisone (MOPP)] designed originally by De Vita included prednisone in cycles 1 and 4 of the six-cycle regimen (4). In 1970, however, the evidence supporting the use of corticosteroids as single agents in the treatment of HD was equivocal (5, 6), and we therefore elected to compare results of treating patients with advanced (stage IV) HD either with corticosteroids in each of six courses (MOPP) or without corticosteroids in any course (MOP) (Table II). The initial results of this study were published in 1975 (7). Forty-nine patients had

TABLE III

Results of Treating Patients with Stage IV Hodgkin's Disease by MOPP or MOP over the Period 1970–1975[a]

Treatment	Response[b]				Survival		Total
	CR, no recurrence	CR, recurrence	PR	NR	Alive	Dead	
MOPP	25	9	12	3	25	24	49
	(51)	(18)	(25)	(6)	(51)	(49)	(100)
MOP	5	10	21	6	10	32	42
	(12)	(24)	(50)	(14)	(24)	(76)	(100)

[a] Data analysis, September 1980. Percentages are given in parentheses.
[b] CR, Complete remission; PR, partial remission; NR, no response.

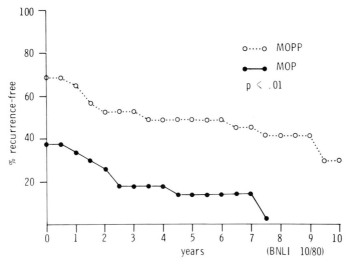

Fig. 1. Probability of recurrence-free survival for patients with stage IV HD treated by MOPP ($n = 34$) or MOP ($n = 15$).

received MOPP and 41 patients MOP. The rates of CR were 80 and 44%, respectively. At the time of the publication, 13 (27%) of the MOPP-treated patients and 17 (41%) of the MOP patients were dead. Both these results were significantly in favor of MOPP. The patients in this trial were followed up to September 1980 (Table III). The differences between patients in the two treat-

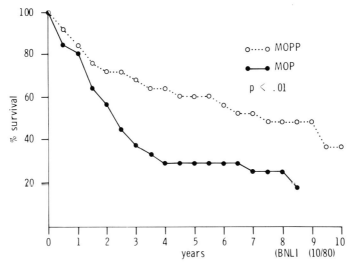

Fig. 2. Probability of overall survival for patients with stage IV HD treated by MOPP ($n = 49$) or MOP ($n = 42$).

ment groups with respect to age, sex, histological type, and stage of disease (IVA or IVB) were not significant. More rigorous application of criteria for accepting individual patients in CR led to reassessment of the proportion of patients reported in 1975 to have achieved CR; moreover, one additional patient treated by MOP was included in the recent analysis. The revised incidence of CR for MOPP-treated patients was 69%; the corresponding value for MOP-treated patients was 36%. Of the 34 MOPP-treated patients who achieved CR, 9 (26%) subsequently had recurrent disease; the corresponding figure for the 15 MOP-treated patients who achieved CR was 10 (67%). Actuarial curves for recurrence-free survival (Fig. 1) and overall survival (Fig. 2) confirmed that MOPP was significantly superior to MOP as primary treatment for stage IV HD in this group of patients.

C. MOPP versus B-MOPP for Stage IV Hodgkin's Disease

In 1973 Coltman and his colleagues from the Southwest Oncology Group reported preliminary data which suggested that the addition of bleomycin to MOPP for treatment of HD significantly improved the CR rate (8). As a result of this report [the data for which were not subsequently confirmed (9)], the BNLI terminated the comparison of MOPP versus MOP and initiated a study of MOPP versus bleomycin combined with MOPP (B-MOPP) (Table IV) for patients with stage IV HD.

This study ended in 1978, and the results were analyzed in September 1980. Sixty-eight patients had been randomized for treatment with MOPP, and 71 patients had received treatment with B-MOPP. A comparison of the two groups of patients with respect to age, sex, histological type, and presence or absence of symptoms showed no significant differences. The overall incidences of CR were 52 and 65% for patients treated with MOPP and B-MOPP, respectively (Table V). The actuarial curve for recurrence-free survival is shown in Fig. 3. There was no significant difference between treatment with MOPP and with B-MOPP. Twenty-one patients in the MOPP arm and 25 patients in the B-MOPP group died. Actuarial survival curves for the two treatment arms are shown in Fig. 4.

TABLE IV

MOPP versus B-MOPP (BNLI Regimens)[a]

Either MOPP:
  Drugs as in Table II
Or MOPP plus:
  Bleomycin, 2 mg/m^2 (max. 4 mg), days 1 and 8

---

[a] Bleomycin may be given intravenously or intramuscularly. The intention was to give at least three courses after CR had been achieved, with a minimum total number of six courses.

TABLE V

Results of Treating Patients with Stage IV Hodgkin's Disease by MOPP or B-MOPP over the Period 1976–1979[a]

| Treatment | Response[b] | | | | Survival | | |
	CR, no recurrence	CR, recurrence	PR	NR	Alive	Dead	Total
MOPP	27	8	26	7	47	21	68
	(40)	(12)	(38)	(10)	(69)	(31)	(100)
B-MOPP	41	5	18	7	46	25	71
	(58)	(7)	(25)	(10)	(65)	(35)	(100)

[a] Data analysis, September 1980. Percentages are shown in parentheses.
[b] CR, Complete remission; PR, partial remission; NR, no response.

Again there was no significant difference. The total scheduled dose of bleomycin for patients in the B-MOPP arm of the study was low (24 mg/m² for six courses). No patients randomized to receive B-MOPP failed to complete treatment with bleomycin. No pulmonary or other major toxicity attributable to bleomycin was seen.

The two combinations, MOPP and B-MOPP, were also compared in another group of patients. Patients with Stage IIIB HD for whom laparotomy was deemed

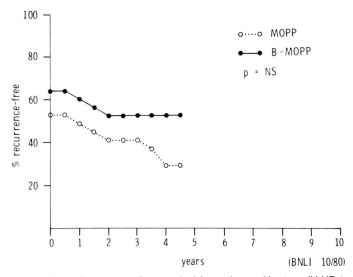

Fig. 3. Probability of recurrence-free survival for patients with stage IV HD treated by MOPP (*n* = 35) or B-MOPP (*n* = 46).

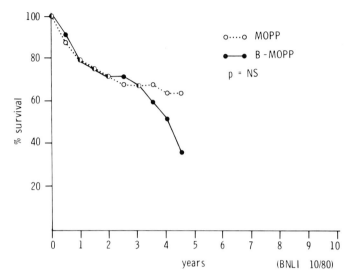

Fig. 4. Probability of overall survival for patients with stage IV HD treated by MOPP (*n* = 68) or B-MOPP (*n* = 71).

inadvisable were randomized as if they had had stage IV disease. Ten such patients were treated with MOPP, and 12 received B-MOPP. The incidences of CR were 70 and 60%, respectively. Actuarial survival curves show no significant difference between the two treatment arms.

D. Maintenance with CVB for Patients with Stage IV Hodgkin's Disease in Complete Remission

The question of how best to manage patients with advanced HD who achieve CR after treatment with combination chemotherapy remains unresolved. Because we knew that the combination of 1-(2-chloroethyl)-3-cyclohexyl-1-nitrosourea (CCNU), vinblastine, and bleomycin [CVB (10)] could be valuable for treatment of patients with advanced resistant HD, we chose to randomize patients with

TABLE VI

CVB for Maintenance in Stage IV Hodgkin's Disease Patients in Complete Remission[a]

CCNU, 100 mg/m², po, day 1 only
Vinblastine, 6 mg/m², iv, days 1 and 8
Bleomycin, 4 mg/m², iv or im, days 1 and 8

---

[a] The intention was to give six courses. The interval between the beginning of each course was 6 weeks. po, Orally; iv, intravenously; im, intramuscularly

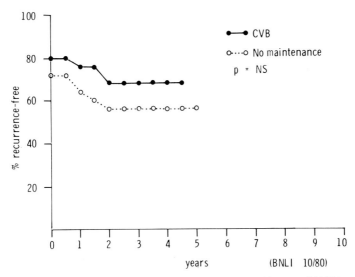

Fig. 5. Probability of recurrence-free survival for patients with stage IV HD treated with CVB (*n* = 16) or receiving no maintenance (*n* = 29) after achieving CR. (Data are calculated from date of completion of CVB maintenance or equivalent date for patients not receiving maintenance. A proportion of patients in each group relapsed before this date).

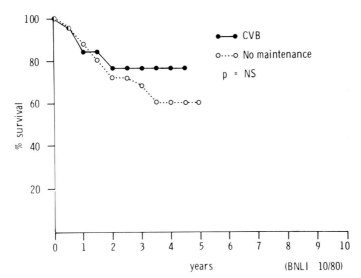

Fig. 6. Probability of overall survival for patients with stage IV HD treated with CVB (*n* = 20) or receiving no maintenance (*n* = 36) after achieving CR.

stage IV disease who had achieved CR after treatment with MOPP or B-MOPP to receive (or not to receive) a further six courses of treatment with CVB (Table VI). By September 1980, 20 patients had completed treatment with six courses of CVB (10 had achieved CR with MOPP and 10 with B-MOPP) and 36 patients who had received no maintenance (15 treated initially with MOPP and 21 with B-MOPP) served as controls. The actuarial survival curves for patients maintained with CVB and control patients are shown in Figs. 5 and 6.

E. MOPP versus LOPP for Stage IV Hodgkin's Disease

The trial of MOPP versus B-MOPP described above was finished at the end of 1978. During the year results reported from the Royal Marsden Hospital in London suggested that the use of chlorambucil in place of mustine in the mustine–vinblastine–procarbazine–prednisone (MVPP) combination gave equally good initial CR rates (11). The BNLI therefore decided to compare MOPP with chlorambucil-OPP (designated LOPP, Table VII) for treating patients with stage IV HD. It was thought necessary to design the study so that patients who failed to obtain progressive benefit with either combination would be reassessed and, if necessary, assigned to other treatment at the latest by the end of the third course of therapy. In view of the possibility that LOPP might prove inferior to MOPP, either because chlorambucil was intrinsically less valuable for advanced HD than mustine or because of relatively poorer patient compliance, it was decided that patients failing on LOPP should be changed over to MOPP; the reverse changeover, using LOPP for patients failing on MOPP, was not deemed necessary. For patients who failed on MOPP, radiotherapy was recommended. This could be administered either to localized resistant disease or as total body irradiation or hemicorporeal irradiation. The study is summarized in Fig. 7.

In October 1980, 26 patients had been randomized to receive treatment with MOPP, and 23 patients had completed treatment with LOPP. Further patients will be entered in this study, but as yet there is no significant difference between the incidence of CR in the two treatment arms. Hitherto no patient who failed to achieve CR with LOPP has subsequently benefited from treatment with MOPP.

TABLE VII

LOPP Regimen (BNLI Version)[a]

Chlorambucil (Leukeran), 10 mg daily, po, days 1–10
Vincristine, 1.4 mg/m² (max. 2.0 mg), iv, days 1 and 8
Procarbazine, 100 mg/m² (max. 200 mg), daily, po, days 1–10
Prednisone, 25 mg/m² (max. 60 mg), daily, po, days 1–14

[a] The same number of courses was given as with MOPP; i.e., three courses were given after CR was achieved with a minimum total number of six. po, Orally; iv, intravenously.

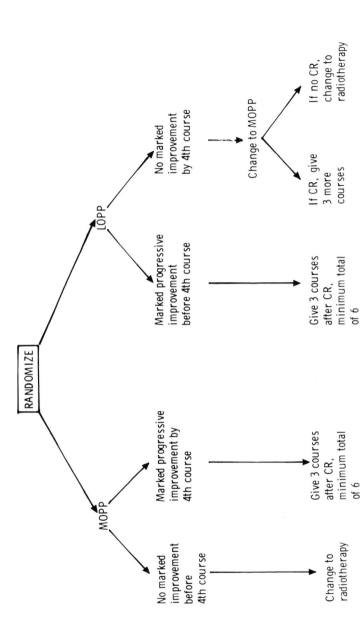

Fig. 7. Scheme of treatment for patients with stage IV HD randomized to receive either MOPP or LOPP as primary treatment.

This is important, because it implies that any patient who proves resistant to LOPP would also probably have been resistant to primary therapy with the MOPP combination.

Patients who achieve CR with MOPP or LOPP are subsequently randomized to receive or not to receive maintenance with the two drugs CCNU and vinblastine. It is too early to comment on the possible value of such maintenance.

F. CHOP versus Total Body Irradiation for Stage III and IV Non-Hodgkin's Lymphoma

In 1975 available data suggested that the best combinations of cytotoxic drugs for the treatment of patients with advanced stage NHL of poor prognosis histology were those that incorporated cyclophosphamide, adriamycin, vincristine, and prednisone (CHOP) (12). It was also known that whole-body irradiation (TBI) could induce CR in a significant proportion of patients with NHL so treated (13). A BNLI study was therefore begun to compare the results of using these two different modalities of therapy in the treatment of patients with Stage III or IV NHL with grade II histology. The TBI was administered by daily radiotherapy from a linear accelerator or a ^{60}Co source at a midline dose of 10 cGy/day to a total dose of 150 cGy over a 3-week period. The technique was modified from that described by Johnson *et al.* (13). CHOP dosage is given in Table VIII.

This study ended in 1979, and the results were analyzed most recently in October 1980. Differences between the patients in the two groups with respect to age and sex were not significant. The respective proportion of patients with stage III or IV disease differed, however—22 (45%) patients in the TBI group but only 21 (31%) patients in the CHOP group were stage III. The incidences of CR for patients treated by CHOP and TBI were 40 and 22%, respectively (Table IX). Actuarial curves for recurrence-free survival and for overall survival are shown

TABLE VIII

CHOP Regimen (BNLI Version)[a]

Cyclophosphamide, 750 mg/m^2 iv, days 1 and 8
Hydroxydaunorubicin (adriamycin), 25 mg/m^2, iv, days 1 and 8
Vincristine, 1.4 mg/m^2 (max. 2.0 mg), iv, days 1 and 8
Prednisone, 50 mg/m^2, daily, po, days 1–8

---

[a] Courses were repeated every 4–6 weeks. Three courses were given as "consolidation" after CR was achieved; the minimum total number of courses was six. Adriamycin was omitted from the schedule after a total of 550 mg/m^2 was reached, i.e., after 11 courses. A small proportion of patients at the beginning of this study was treated with an earlier version of CHOP—this consisted of cyclophosphamide (750 mg/m^2, day 1 only), adriamycin (50 mg/m^2, day 1 only), and vincristine and prednisone as above. po, Orally; iv, intravenously.

TABLE IX

Results of Treating Patients with Advanced-Stage Poor Histology Non-Hodgkin's Lymphomy by CHOP or Total Body Irradiation

Treatment	Response				Survival		
	CR, no recurrence	CR, recurrence	PR	NR	Alive	Dead	Total
CHOP	17	10	26	14	28	39	67
	(25)	(15)	(39)	(21)	(42)	(58)	(100)
TBI	8	3	17	21	12	37	49
	(16)	(6)	(35)	(43)	(24)	(76)	(100)

" Data analysis, October 1980. Percentages are shown in parentheses.
^{b} CR, Complete remission; PR, partial remission; NR, no response.

in Figs. 8 and 9. It is apparent that treatment with CHOP gave remission rates and survival values somewhat, but not significantly, better than those achieved by TBI. When, however, CHOP and TBI are compared with stratification for the patients' stage of disease, the overall survival for patients treated by CHOP was significantly better than that of patients treated by TBI ($\chi^2 = 4.125$, $p < .05$).

The plateau on the CHOP curve (Fig. 8) that appears after $2\frac{1}{2}$ years suggests that approximately half the patients who achieve CR with combination chemotherapy may anticipate prolonged disease-free survival.

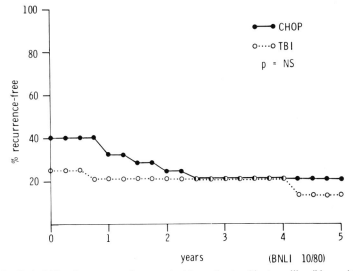

Fig. 8. Probability of recurrence-free survival for patients with stage III or IV poor histology NHL treated with CHOP ($n = 27$) or TBI ($n = 11$).

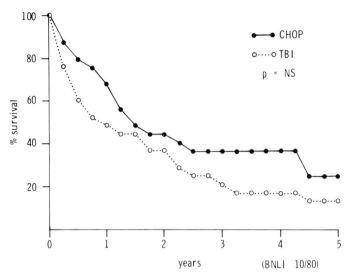

Fig. 9. Probability of overall survival for patients with stage III or IV poor prognosis histology NHL treated by CHOP (n = 67) or TBI (n = 49). (A number of patients treated by CHOP after the end of this study were nonetheless included in the analysis; the numbers of patients in the two arms are therefore not equal.)

G. LOAP Maintenance for Patients with Advanced-Stage Grade II Non-Hodgkin's Lymphoma

In 1978 a small pilot study was initiated to test the hypothesis that the rate of relapse in patients who achieved CR after treatment with CHOP could be reduced by continuation of chemotherapy for a further year. Therefore patients with stage III or IV grade II NHL who had been treated with six or more courses of CHOP (including three courses after they achieved CR) were treated with LOAP (Table X) for a further 12 months. Ten patients at the Hammersmith and North Middlesex Hospitals in London were treated by this approach. One patient had stage III and nine patients had stage IV disease. Three patients relapsed while

TABLE X

LOAP Regimen[a]

Chlorambucil (Leukeran), 12 mg/m² (max. 20 mg), daily, po, days 1–5
Vincristine, 1.4 mg/m² (max. 2.0 mg), iv, day 1
Cytosine arabinoside, 100 mg/m², sc, daily, days 1–5
Prednisone, 40 mg/m², daily, po, days 1–5

[a] Courses were given every 4 weeks, and the total number of courses was 12. Prednisone was given only in odd-numbered courses, i.e., in alternate courses. po, Orally; iv, intravenously; sc, subcutaneously.

TABLE XI

Results of Treating Patients with Stage III or IV Non-Hodgkin's Lymphoma in Complete Remission with LOAP[a]

Patients treated	Patients relapsed	Mean time to relapse (months)[b] ($n=5$)	Mean overall survival in CR (months)[c] ($n=5$)
10	5	10.8 (3–23)	26.6 (17–34)

[a] Data analysis, November 1980. Ranges are given in parentheses.
[b] Measured from the time when the patient achieved CR.
[c] Measured from the initial diagnosis.

still receiving LOAP, and two relapsed thereafter (Table XI). Five patients remained in continuing CR. Some patients complained of nausea while receiving cytosine arabinoside, but in general the combination was well tolerated. No other toxicity was seen. It is too early to comment on the possible long-term benefits of this additional chemotherapy.

III. Discussion

If it is fair to assume that the 2118 patients with lymphoma entered in BNLI studies up to February 1980 are representative of all patients with lymphoma, the accumulated data provide a unique picture of the pattern of disease at presentation and of the response to initial treatment for lymphoma patients diagnosed in England and Wales in the 1970s. Of patients with HD two-thirds were male and nearly three-quarters were relatively young (<46 years). No one stage was especially probable at presentation; one-third of patients had B symptoms. As a result of treatment 81% of all patients at all stages achieved CR, but at least one-third of these subsequently relapsed. Of patients with NHL again the majority were males, but three-quarters were older than 45 years. Of all NHL patients 68% had advanced (stage III or IV) disease at diagnosis; 58% of all patients achieved CR after treatment, and of these at least one-quarter relapsed.

This article deals only with results of chemotherapy trials designed for the treatment of patients with stage IV HD or advanced-stage NHL with a poor prognosis histology.

A. Hodgkin's Disease

The role of corticosteroids either as single agents or in combination with other drugs in treating advanced HD remains ill-defined. The study reported here seems to show that steroids are an essential component of the MOPP combination. However, the incidence of CR in the MOP-treated patients was so low as to cast some doubt on the validity of the comparison—it could, for example, be a result produced indirectly if the omission of steroids from the first course led frequently to a delay or reduction in drug dosage in the second (and subsequent) courses. In a retrospective comparison of response to chemotherapy of advanced-stage HD patients treated with or without prednisone at Stanford University, Jacobs and his colleagues were unable to detect any adverse effects of omitting steroids (14). Moreover, it should be noted that the incidence of CR in the BNLI studies in which steroids were included in all courses was comparable but not greater to that in other studies employing steroids only in courses 1 and 4 (4). One may for the present conclude that the use of steroids as originally recommended by De Vita need not be modified.

Various efforts have been made to improve the incidence of CR or to prolong recurrence-free survival for patients with advanced HD by modifying the MOPP combination (15). In the BNLI study the addition to MOPP of bleomycin gave an incidence of CR slightly higher than that for patients treated by MOPP alone, but this difference and analysis of actuarial survival curves lack statistical significance. Coltman and his colleagues have reported remission rates ranging between 54 and 84% for patients treated with MOPP plus bleomycin, but the results of the treatment regimen that proved to be best in the earlier study, MOPP plus low-dose bleomycin (8), were not reproduced in the subsequent study (9). The case for adding bleomycin to the MOPP combination has not been established. At present the most encouraging approach reported to have improved the results of MOPP treatment remains the addition to MOPP of adriamycin, bleomycin, vinblastine, and imidazole carboxamide (ABVD) or of ABVD plus radiotherapy (16, 17). For the present the BNLI has chosen to study the possibility that results comparable to those obtained with MOPP may be achieved with less overt toxicity by substituting chlorambucil for mustine.

Because about 40% of patients with advanced HD who achieve remission with combination chemotherapy will relapse, attempts have been directed toward improving the duration of recurrence-free remission. In general, such attempts have consisted either of continuing the original induction regimen for an additional arbitrary number of courses after CR has been achieved or of administering a maintenance regimen consisting of drugs to which the patient has not previously been exposed; such maintenance regimens may be comprised of single agents or combinations of cytotoxic drugs. Because no form of maintenance has clearly been shown to benefit patients with HD whose disease is truly in CR (15), it is important that regimens being tested confer on the patient no major toxicity. The CVB combination appears to satisfy this criterion. Patients who received CVB maintenance showed a disease-free survival slightly but not significantly superior to that for untreated control patients. The patients in this study must be followed for a longer period before any firm conclusions can be drawn.

B. Non-Hodgkin's Lymphoma

The results of the BNLI study on treatment of patients with advanced-stage poor histology NHL cannot be compared directly with those of other studies in which histological classification was based on that of Rappaport. It is clear, however, from the BNLI study that TBI is not an appropriate primary treatment for these patients. McKelvey *et al.* reported remission rates of 68% in patients with diffuse poorly differentiated lymphocytic lymphoma and in patients with diffuse histiocytic lymphoma using a CHOP regimen similar to that of the BNLI (12). By these standards the 40% CR rate obtained in this study is not impressive and emphasizes the need for a fundamentally new approach to the initial management of these patients.

The observation that the recurrence-free survival curve for patients with advanced-stage poor histology NHL shows a plateau has been made previously (18, 19). Previous reports have, however, stressed that cure is more probable for patients with diffuse histiocytic or diffuse undifferentiated disease than for patients with other poor prognosis histologies. In the BNLI study no one histological subtype predominated in those who remained free of recurrence at 4 years. It seems therefore that all patients with poor histology who achieve CR should receive further treatment aimed at cure. Whether such additional treatment should consist of further courses of the drugs that induced CR, of intensive courses of other drugs for a further defined period, or of low-dose maintenance for a further 12 months (such as LOAP) remains to be determined.

IV. Summary

Multicenter studies on the treatment of patients with advanced HD and NHL were carried out under the auspices of the BNLI. In HD the omission of prednisone from the MOPP combination gave initial CR rates and overall survival inferior to that of MOPP (36 versus 69%) The addition of bleomycin to the MOPP combination (i.e., B-MOPP) gave an incidence of CR slightly but not significantly greater to that of MOPP (65 versus 52%). Differences in recurrence-free survival were not significant. The use of the CVB combination as maintenance resulted in slightly improved recurrence-free survival for patients with HD in CR as compared with patients not so maintained; this trend too lacked statistical significance. For patients with advanced-stage poor histology NHL a comparison of CHOP with TBI showed that the former could produce somewhat better rates of CR (40 versus 22%) and better long-term survival, though these differences fell short of statistical significance.

Acknowledgments

We gratefully acknowledge the collaboration of many clinicians, pathologists, and other specialists throughout the United Kingdom who have contributed to the study of patients in the BNLI.

Financial support for these investigations was provided by the Cancer Research Campaign, the Cooperative Clinical Cancer Therapy Trust Fund, the Middlesex Hospital Trustees, and many patients, relatives, and other benefactors.

The following centers and clinicians participated in this study. Barking: R. Storring and Joy Edelman. Belfast: J. H. Robertson. Birmingham: G. A. Newsholme and M. J. Leyland. Cambridge: E. Kingsley-Pillers, F. G. J. Hayhoe, D'A. Kok, N. M. Bleehen, and T. K. Wheeler. Canterbury: Shirley R. Drake, A. D. O'Connor, M. O. Rake, H. Sterndale, C. I. Roberts, Y. F. Williams, D. G. Wells, and D. A. Lillicrap. Cardiff: I. Howell Evans. Cheltenham: D. J. Mahy. Coventry: T. W. Backhouse, R. N. Das, and L. A. Birchall. Guildford: A. Folkes. Ipswich: C. R. Wiltshire and T. J. Mott. Yorks: T. S. Worthy, J. Stone, S. Cartwright, A. V. Simmons, and D. A. Ashe. Liverpool: W. B. Dawson, M. J. Garrett, J. E. S. Brock, J. Bradley, J. Martin, and J. E. Dalby. London: Greenwich, B. J. Cuddigan and P. J. Black; Kings College: D. Brinkley and K. W. Pettingale; London Hospital: H. Hope-Stone and B. S. Mantell; Middlesex: A. M. Jelliffe, M. F. Spittle, R. J. Berry, and C. Coulter; Hammersmith: D. A. G. Galton, J. M. Goldman, A. W. G. Goolden, C. G. McKenzie, and J. Lambert; Northwood: P. Strickland, A. M. Jelliffe, S. Dische, R. Dickson, L. Grosch, and A. J. Moon. Newcastle: W. M. Ross, A. L. Hovenden, and O. M. Koriech. Norwich: A. W. Jackson, A. J. Black, and J. M. Hughes. Nottingham: P. J. Toghill and M. Benton. Plymouth: A. F. Broad and C. J. Tyrrell. Stevenage: S. Watkins. Stoke-on-Trent: J. H. Friend, R. Lindup, and E. R. Monypenny. Southampton: R. Buchanan, H. McDonald, P. E. Bodkin, V. L. Hall, and R. H. Ryall. Southend: D. L. Phillips. Exeter: C. R. H. Penn.

We also acknowledge the contributions of M. H. Bennett, G. Farrer-Brown, K. Henry, and J. Newman, members of the pathology panel; G. Vaughan Hudson, research associate; and J. L. Haybittle and B. Vaughan Hudson who provided statistics and the computer analysis.

Acknowledgment

The LOAP pilot study was conducted in conjunction with G. W. Marsh and T. O. Kumaran at the North Middlesex Hospital (London).

References

1. R. J. Lukes and J. J. Butler, *Cancer Res.* **26**, 1063 (1966).
2. K. Henry, M. H. Bennett, and G. Farrer-Brown, *Recent Results Cancer Res.* **63**, 38–56 (1978).
3. P. P. Carbone, H. S. Kaplan, K. Musshoff, D. W. Smithers, and M. Tubiana, *Cancer Res.* **31**, 1860 (1971).
4. V. T. DeVita, A. A. Serpick, and P. P. Carbone, *Ann. Intern. Med.* **73**, 881 (1970).
5. S. Kofman, C. P. Perlia, E. Boesen, R. Eisenstein, and S. G. Taylor, *Cancer* **15**, 338 (1962).
6. A. M. Jelliffe and J. D. N. Nabarro, *Br. J. Radiol.* **34**, 577 (1961).
7. British National Lymphoma Investigation, *Br Med. J.* **3**, 413 (1975).
8. C. A Coltman and F. C. Delaney, *Clin. Res.* **31**, 876 (1973).
9. C. A. Coltman, S. E. Jones, P. N. Grozea, E. De Persio, and T. E. Moon, *In* "Bleomycin: Current Status and New Developments" (S. K. Carter, S. T. Crooke, and H. Umezawa, eds.), p. 227. Academic Press, New York, 1978.
10. J. M. Goldman and A. A. Dawson, *Lancet* **2**, 1224 (1975).
11. T. J. McElwain, J. Toy, E. Smith, M. J. Peckham, and D. E. Austin, *Br. J. Cancer* **36**, 276 (1977).

12. E. M. McKelvey, J. A. Gottlieb, H. E. Wilson, A. Hant, R. W. Talley, R. Stephens, M. Lane, J. F. Gamble, S. E. Jones, P. N. Grozea, J. Gutterman, C. Coltman, and T. E. Moon, *Cancer* **38**, 1484 (1976).
13. R. E. Johnson, *Br. J. Cancer* **31**, Suppl. 2, 450 (1975).
14. C. Jacobs, C. S. Portlock, and S. A. Rosenberg, *Br. Med. J.* **2**, 1469 (1976).
15. R. C. Young and V. DeVita, *Clin. Haematol.* **8**, 625 (1979).
16. D. C. Case, C. W. Young, L. Nisce, B. L. Lee, III, and B. D. Clarkson, *Cancer Treat. Rep.* **60**, 1217 (1976).
17. G. Bonadonna, V. Fossati, and M. De Lena, *Proc. Am. Soc. Clin. Oncol.* **19**, 363 (C227) (1978).
18. V. T. DeVita, G. P. Canellos, B. Chabner, P. Schein, S. P. Hubbard, and R. C. Young, *Lancet* **1**, 248 (1975).
19. L. Elias, C. S. Portlock, and S. A. Rosenberg, *Cancer* **42**, 1705 (1978).

25

Chemotherapy of Malignant Lymphomas of Unfavorable Histology

STEPHEN E. JONES AND THOMAS P. MILLER

I. Introduction

Remarkable progress in the chemotherapy of malignant lymphoma (ML) has occurred in the last decade, and several histological types of ML are now considered potentially curable with chemotherapy. Table I lists the subtypes which have been reported either as curable (confirmed by at least two reports) or potentially curable (preliminary reports still require confirmation).

The definition of "cure" for an individual patient implies a durable complete remission (CR) free of signs of lymphoma, and for groups of patients implies survival and relapse-free survival curves which demonstrate a clear plateau. Follow-up in some series and with some programs is necessarily brief because of

TABLE I

Malignant Lymphomas Which May Be Cured with Chemotherapy

Histological type[a]	Rappaport abbreviation[b]	Relative frequency (%)
Diffuse large-cell ("histiocytic")	DH	30
Diffuse small noncleaved (undifferentiated, Burkitt's or non-Burkitt's)	DU	5
Follicular large cell (nodular "histiocytic")	NH	4
Follicular mixed small cleaved and large cell (nodular mixed)	NM	8
Lymphoblastic (same)	—?	4
Diffuse mixed small cleaved and large cell (diffuse mixed)	DM?	7

[a] Rappaport classification. Histological terms are consistent with the recently agreed upon working formulation for malignant lymphoma (see other articles in this volume). Rappaport classification equivalents and their abbreviations are also included where applicable.

[b] Question marks indicate lymphomas which may be curable, but confirmatory series are required.

the newness of the treatment. Nonetheless, for all the lymphomas without a question mark listed in Table I there has been convincing evidence of curability from one source and confirmation by at least one other report.

The first step in realizing a cure of lymphoma is the initial achievement of CR. This concept is well established (1, 2). Definitions of CR have changed over the last decade and are now generally based on careful reevaluation of the patient who has achieved a clinical complete response. Repetition of initially abnormal tests such as lymphangiography, computed tomographic (CT) scanning, bone marrow and liver biopsies, and even laparotomy have revealed that about 20% of those with ML still harbor occult disease and, therefore, will require additional treatment (1). Attainment of a carefully documented CR followed by no further therapy has provided the critical information about the potential curability of lymphoma.

It is not possible in this brief article to include or even mention all the chemotherapy programs which have been or currently are being tested, or to discuss all types of lymphoma. Instead, we have chosen to limit our discussion to relatively few programs which illustrate some of the progress and remaining challenges of chemotherapy of lymphoma, particularly of the unfavorable histological types [diffuse "histiocytic" (DH) and diffuse undifferentiated (DU)]. Since the other types listed in Table I are relatively rare, the results of treatment of DH serve as a model for all the potentially curable lymphoma subtypes.

II. Prognostic Factors in Diffuse Lymphoma

Besides the usual prognostic factors of stage and histology, recent information has revealed that other factors are also important in determining the likelihood of patients achieving CR or remaining in CR. Some of these are listed in Table II. Older patients who may have concurrent illnesses or impaired bone marrow reserves are less likely to achieve CR. Unfortunately, 40% of patients with diffuse lymphoma are over the age of 60 (3), so that this is a frequent adverse prognostic factor. As will be discussed later, the stage of the disease at presentation is also an extremely important factor. Several studies have determined that patients with involvement of particular sites (e.g., gastrointestinal tract, bone marrow) and those with bulky tumor have a much reduced chance of achieving CR with chemotherapy (4, 5). Although relatively little information is available about tumors kinetics in lymphoma, some cases of DH and DU have been shown to have extremely high-growth fractions, in instances similar or higher than those seen in acute leukemia (6). This undoubtedly accounts for the clinical observation in some patients of rapid regression after pulse chemotherapy followed by rapid regrowth before the next course of chemotherapy. Finally, we are just now beginning to appreciate the impact of the chemotherapy dose on the outcome of lymphoma (7). Low-dose regimens produce low CR rates and probably lead to the acquisition of tumor cell drug resistance (8).

All these factors must be taken into consideration when evaluating the outcome of new treatment programs. Exclusion of patients with adverse prognostic factors (e.g., older patients and those with bulky tumor or gastrointestinal tract involvement) would lead to spurious conclusions in comparison to clinical trials where adverse prognostic factors are substantially more frequent.

Even when patients with diffuse lymphoma (DH, DU) achieve CR, the problem of drug sanctuaries [e.g., the central nervous system (CNS)] may become an

TABLE II

Potential Prognostic Factors for Diffuse Lymphoma

Age
Stage
Sites of involvement
  Gastrointestinal tract
  Bone marrow
Tumor bulk (cell mass)
Tumor kinetics
Dose of chemotherapy
Emergence of drug-resistant stem cells

important factor. As many as 10–20% of patients with diffuse histologies develop CNS lymphoma (9, 10). Initial tumor bulk, advanced-stage, extranodal involvement (particularly of the bone marrow), and constitutional symptoms are all prognostic factors which indicate a higher likelihood of an individual patient developing CNS lymphoma (9, 10). Even so, relatively few programs have incorporated any form of CNS prophylaxis into the treatment of high-risk patients.

III. Treatment of Early-Stage Disease

The relatively common unfavorable histology lymphoma, diffuse large cell (DH), can be cured in 40–50% of patients with advanced stages (III and IV) of disease (11), and, in general, adriamycin-based regimens [e.g., cyclophosphamide, adriamycin, vincristine, and prednisone (CHOP)] have CR rates superior to those of non-adriamycin-based regimens (12). Historically, radiotherapy alone has been employed in treating patients with localized disease with disappointing results except in the most limited stages (I and I_E). The reasons for the failure of radiotherapy to eradicate disease in the majority of cases of localized disease have recently been summarized by us (3). Briefly, the reasons are as follows: (a) A small but definite percentage of patients have occult disease in the abdomen not detectable by noninvasive clinical means. The older age and general condition of many of these patients preclude a diagnostic laparotomy to find occult disease. (b) Unlike other lymphomas, there is no clear dose–response relationship for radiation therapy in these patients, so that even at high doses of radiation it may be impossible to achieve local control in a substantial fraction of patients (13). (c) Diffuse histiocytic lymphoma is a high-growth-fraction tumor (6) which has a marked propensity for rapid hematogenous and lymphatic spread. Clinically, this is manifest by 10–25% of patients developing new disease outside the radiation ports prior to the completion of local radiotherapy.

For these reasons there has been considerable interest in combining chemotherapy with radiotherapy for stage I and II disease. The results of three trials of adjuvant chemotherapy administered after completion of local irradiation have been reported. Both relapse-free survival and survival have been improved by this approach (14, 15). However, an appreciable number of failures still occur. The reasons for this appear to be as follows: (a) Since chemotherapy is delayed until radiotherapy is completed, new disease still develops before the completion of radiotherapy (3, 14). (b) The chemotherapy employed in these series did not contain adriamycin and was less than optimal (12). (c) Kinetic resistance or drug-resistant stem cells could account for failure even when the chemotherapy was administered promptly.

For these reasons we chose to study the effects of primary chemotherapy for stage I and II unfavorable histology lymphoma. The preliminary results have been reported previously (17) and recently compared to results of radiotherapy alone or with adjuvant chemotherapy (3). The use of initial immediate chemotherapy obviates the need for extensive staging (particularly surgical staging) and may prevent the rapid dissemination which may occur in DH lymphoma.

As of October 1980, 31 patients with clinical stage I or II disease have been treated with adriamycin-based combination chemotherapy (CHOP) as initial therapy at the time of diagnosis. Twelve patients received adjuvant radiotherapy as previously described (3, 17). The clinical and prognostic characteristics of the group of patients are summarized in Table III. Importantly, 15 of 31 patients had gastrointestinal tract involvement or bulky disease, factors known to influence prognosis adversely (4, 5). Eleven patients were older than 60 years of age. These patients might have been excluded from study if laparotomy staging had been necessary. Nineteen patients received chemotherapy alone, consisting of eight courses of CHOP every 3 weeks followed by careful restaging for residual disease (17). Complete remissions have been achieved in 18 of 19 (95%) patients treated with chemotherapy alone and in 12 (100%) patients treated with chemotherapy and adjuvant radiotherapy. Twenty-eight of 31 patients (90%) have remained continuously free of disease, and 3 have had recurrences (2 at initial sites of involvement and 1 at an initially uninvolved site). Relapse-free

TABLE III

**Clinical and Prognostic Features of Patients
(October 1980)**

Clinical features	Chemotherapy, 19 patients	Chemotherapy and XRT, 12 patients[a]
Median age[b]	55 (24–70)	59 (25–83)
Male/female ratio	10:9	7:5
Stage I	3	0
Stage I_E	1	3
Stage II	6	2
Stage II_E	9	7
B Symptoms	2	2
Extranodal disease	10	10
Gastrointestinal involvement	5	2
Bulky disease	4	6
>60 Years of age	5	6

[a] XRT, Involved-field radiation.

[b] The range is shown in parentheses.

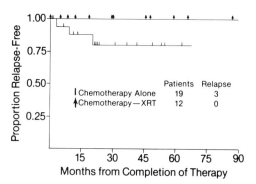

Fig. 1. Relapse-free survival from the completion of therapy as of November 1980 for 31 patients with stage I or II lymphoma who received chemotherapy alone (19 patients) or chemotherapy plus adjuvant radiotherapy (12 patients).

survival is shown in Fig. 1, and survival is shown in Fig. 2 (only a single patient has died from disease).

The approach of immediate chemotherapy followed by adjuvant radiotherapy seems particularly well suited to an older population who might not tolerate prolonged, high-dose chemotherapy (e.g., eight courses of full-dose CHOP) or to patients with initial bulky disease. For example, six patients in this series received minimal treatment: five received two courses of CHOP, and one received four courses of CHOP followed by local radiotherapy. All remain free of disease.

These results for the use of immediate systemic chemotherapy for localized lymphoma have been confirmed by the M. D. Anderson Hospital (Houston, Texas) group (18). In their series, 18 of 22 (82%) patients are currently free of disease (F. Cabanillas, personal communication).

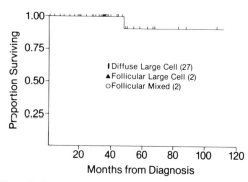

Fig. 2. Overall survival as of November 1980 for all 31 patients with localized disease treated at the University of Arizona.

The results of initial effective systemic chemotherapy have apparently improved the prognosis for patients with clinically staged localized lymphoma. Other, less common, histological subtypes (Table I) are expected to benefit similarly from this approach. The role of radiotherapy as an adjuvant or consolidative treatment in areas of initial bulky disease remains to be defined and should be further studied.

IV. Treatment of Advanced-Stage Disease

Stage of disease (see Section II) is a major determinant of outcome. In our trial of early-stage lymphoma, 95% of 19 patients treated with CHOP alone achieved CR, in contrast to 33 of 59 (56%) patients with advanced disease (stage III or IV). Thus, new approaches for improving the results in advanced disease are needed.

A. Chemoimmunotherapy

The rationale for the use of biological response modifiers in lymphoma has been recently reviewed (19). In the early 1970s we became interested in combining immunotherapy with bacillus Calmette Guérin (BCG) with chemotherapy. Accordingly, in 1974 the Southwest Oncology Group (SWOG) initiated a large-scale, prospective, controlled clinical trial of chemoimmunotherapy in advanced stages of ML. The protocol (SWOG 7426/7427) compared three remission induction treatment regimens: one consisting of combination chemotherapy (CHOP) plus Pasteur strain lyophilized BCG administered by scarification between courses of chemotherapy, and two other regimens consisting of combination chemotherapy alone (CHOP plus bleomycin or COP plus bleomycin). Patients achieving CR were then rerandomized to unmaintained remission or immunotherapeutic maintenance with monthly BCG scarifications. In this trial, major efforts were made to ensure quality control by incorporating routine submission of pathological material for expert histopathological review (20) and by using systematic restaging to define CR more accurately (1). The documentation of complete remission through restaging was considered an essential decision point prior to discontinuation of chemotherapy and allocation to either unmaintained remission or BCG maintenance immunotherapy. The early results of this trial have been reported previously (12, 21–23). Entry of patients into this study ceased in August 1977, and the results are now essentially final (23). In this study we were able to demonstrate that BCG exerted a favorable impact on the CR rate for large-cell lymphoma (Table IV) of both diffuse and follicular patterns. It failed to affect CR duration (Fig. 3), although both adriamycin-based programs (CHOP plus BCG and CHOP plus bleomycin) were superior to COP

TABLE IV

Complete Remission Rates by Treatment for Patients with Large-Cell ("Histiocytic") Lymphoma (October 1980)

		No. treated[a]			
Subtype	No.	CHOP + BCG	CHOP + bleomycin	COP + bleomycin	P Value
Diffuse (DH)	147	57 (65)	53 (49)	37 (41)	0.05
Nodular (NH)	24	8 (88)	8 (38)	8 (63)	0.12
All cases	171	65 (68)	61 (48)	45 (44)	<0.03

[a] Percentages of complete responses are shown in parentheses.

plus bleomycin. However, survival of patients treated with CHOP plus BCG was significantly longer than that observed with chemotherapy alone (Fig. IV). As previously reported, BCG had no effect on CR duration or survival when it was administered as maintenance, but only when it was given from the outset along with remission induction chemotherapy (23). The improved survival of patients

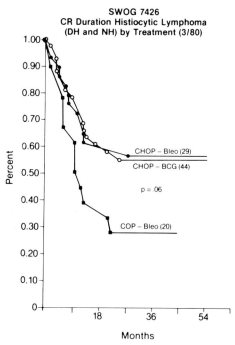

SWOG 7426
CR Duration Histiocytic Lymphoma
(DH and NH) by Treatment (3/80)

CHOP – Bleo (29)
CHOP – BCG (44)
p = .06
COP – Bleo (20)

Fig. 3. Complete remission duration for large-cell ("histiocytic") lymphoma according to initial remission induction treatment.

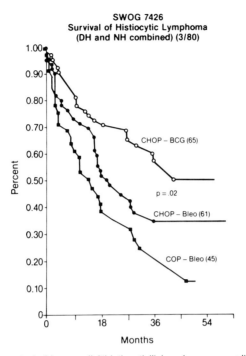

Fig. 4. Overall survival of large-cell ("histiocytic") lymphoma according to initial remission induction treatment.

treated with CHOP plus BCG presumably reflects the higher CR rate (Table IV), since CR duration (Fig. 3) was not affected by BCG. The mechanism whereby BCG affects the CR rate and survival of patients with large-cell lymphoma remains unclear.

Because of the results of this trial, we initiated a new SWOG study in 1977 which continues to accrue patients at the present time. With the same induction scheme, patients with all types of non-Hodgkin's lymphoma are randomized to one of three remission induction programs: chemotherapy alone (CHOP), chemotherapy (CHOP) plus levamisole, and chemotherapy (CHOP) plus levamisole plus BCG by scarification. We hope that such continued exploration of immunomodulation will define whether there will be a role for combination immunotherapy (e.g., levamisole and BCG) with additive or synergistic effects which can further augment the chemotherapeutic effectiveness of the CHOP regimen in the management of ML.

B. New Chemotherapy Programs

Recently several new approaches to the drug treatment of DH lymphoma have been reported. For purposes of comparison we have analyzed our experience at the University of Arizona with the CHOP regimen in 74 previously untreated patients (15 with stage II disease and 59 with stage III or IV disease) and used this as a basis for comparing five other programs: cyclophosphamide, vincristine, methotrexate with leucovorin rescue, and cytosine arabinoside (COMLA) (24); VP-16, cyclophosphamide, adriamycin, methotrexate with leucovorin rescue, and prednisone plus MOPP consolidation (ProMACE-MOPP) (25); high-dose methotrexate with rescue plus CHOP (M-BACOD) (26); alternating non-cross-resistant combinations (CVP/ABP) (27, 28); and escalated doses of CHOP in a protected environment (29). Although these series differ in some respects (e.g., prognostic factors in some and inclusion of stage II cases in others), their comparison provides some useful information (Table V).

The basic CHOP program used at Arizona (3, 12, 21–23) produced a CR rate of 93% in 15 patients with stage II disease and of 56% in 59 patients with stage III or IV disease, for an overall CR rate of 64%. The non-adriamycin-based COMLA regimen produced an equivalent 60% CR rate. The Milan group recently reported the results of alternating two combinations which they believe are non-cross-resistant: cyclophosphamide, vincristine, and prednisone (CVP) and adriamycin, bleomycin, and prednisone (ABP) (27). In their original studies on these two combinations, the ABP regimen produced a 40% CR rate in 14 patients with DH lymphoma compared to a 33% CR rate with CVP (27). Complete remission duration was longer with ABP. These facts are consistent with the later observations, supporting the view that adriamycin-based chemotherapy is superior to CVP in DH lymphoma (12) (also see Figs. 3 and 4). Subsequently, these investigators compared the results of alternating courses of CVP and ABP to their results with either regimen alone. This investigation showed a 49% CR rate (28) significantly superior to that of CVP. The Milan group did not include stage II patients, so that the 49% CR should be compared to the 56% CR rate we observed in comparably staged patients treated with CHOP.

Two new regimens were recently reported: ProMACE-MOPP and M-BACOD

TABLE V

Comparison of Selected Regimens Used for Diffuse Large-Cell Lymphoma

Regimen and institution	No. treated	CR (%)	Ref.
CHOP (Arizona)	74	04	—
COMLA (Chicago)	48	60	24
ProMACE-MOPP (NCI)	40	57	25
M-BACOD (Boston)	51	77	26
CVP-ABP (Milan)	37	49	28
CHOP + Bleo + PEPA (M. D. Anderson)	16	81	29

(25, 26). In the first study stage II patients were included. Five of 40 patients died of toxicity during induction (25). Thus, the overall CR rate of 57% does not seem superior to that of CHOP, COMLA, or CVP/ABP. In the M-BACOD program Skarin and associates added high-dose methotrexate with rescue to CHOP with excellent results: a 77% CR rate and only nine relapses to date (26). Furthermore, since methotrexate crosses the blood-brain barrier, only two patients have developed CNS lymphoma. This is a very promising regimen, but the difficulties and expense in using high-dose methotrexate will limit the general use of this program. Long-term follow-up of these programs will be needed to assess their relative importance compared to that of CHOP in the management of patients with DH lymphoma.

One other program deserves mention, although it requires special facilities (laminar flow isolation units) and special expertise in managing severely myelosuppressed patients. In this study a CR rate of 81% was reported in 16 patients with DH lymphoma treated with CHOP plus bleomycin plus a protected environment and prophylactic antibiotics (PEPA) (Table V) (29). This CR rate was not superior to that of patients treated without PEPA, but CR duration was superior for patients treated with escalated doses of drugs with PEPA (29).

V. Future Directions

Despite the advances in the chemotherapy of lymphoma, new approaches are required. Several investigational agents appear promising for use in new combinations: m-AMSA, vindesine (another vinca alkaloid), new anthracyclines, other new DNA binders (e.g., dihydroxyanthracenedione), gallium nitrate, platinum compounds, and methyl-GAG. The exploration of biological response modifiers (e.g., BCG and interferon) is also in its infancy and should have continued impact on the treatment of lymphoma.

Another area for potential study involves developing methods of modifying or limiting myelosuppression. Evidence exists suggesting a dose–response relationship in the treatment of lymphoma, and conceivably better results could be achieved with high-dose regimens. However, myelosuppression is the usual dose-limiting factor. Lithium, which stimulates granulopoiesis, has been reported to reduce treatment-induced myelosuppression in leukemia and oat cell lung cancer (6). Lithium needs to be evaluated in lymphoma. Isolation of patients (i.e., protected environments) and administration of prophylactic antibiotics has reduced the infectious complications of escalated dose treatment of lymphoma in one study and needs to be evaluated further, particularly since survival of patients treated at high-dose levels appeared to be superior to that achieved at lower doses (29). Myelosuppression may also be limited by autologous marrow infusion, and this approach will need to be investigated too.

VI. Summary

The past decade has seen marked progress in the chemotherapy of malignant lymphoma. Many types of malignant lymphoma are now potentially curable with drugs. Approximately 60% of patients with advanced stages of disease can achieve CR with prototype drug combinations (CHOP, COMLA, CVP/ABP). The addition of high-dose methotrexate with rescue or the addition of nonspecific immunotherapy with BCG has improved the CR rate and survival of patients with unfavorable large-cell ("histiocytic") lymphomas.

Favorable results in advanced stages have led to similar treatment in earlier stages with encouraging preliminary results. For example, we have obtained a 95% CR rate in 19 patients treated with chemotherapy (CHOP) and a 100% CR rate in 12 patients treated with CHOP plus adjuvant radiotherapy. In the future, development of new agents and new combinations, use of biological response modifiers, and development of methods to limit myelosuppression should result in continued progress in the treatment of lymphoma.

References

1. T. S. Herman and S. E. Jones, *Cancer Treat. Rep.* **61,** 1009 (1977).
2. P. S. Schein, V. T. DeVita, S. Hubbard *et al., Ann. Intern. Med.* **85,** 417 (1976).
3. T. P. Miller and S. E. Jones, *Cancer Chemother. Pharmacol.* **4,** 67 (1970).
4. R. I. Fisher, V. T. DeVita, B. L. Johnson, *et al., Am. J. Med.* **63,** 177 (1977).
5. F. Cabanillas, J. S. Burke, T. L. Smith *et al., Arch. Intern. Med.* **138,** 413 (1978).
6. H. Hansen, B. Koziner, and B. Clarkson, in press.
7. E. Frei and G. P. Canellos, *Am. J. Med.* **69,** 585 (1980).
8. S. E. Salmon, *in* "Cloning of Human Tumor Stem Cells" (S. E. Salmon, ed.), p. 223. Alan R. Liss, Inc., New York, 1980.
9. P. A. Bunn, Jr., P. S. Schein, P. M. Banks *et al., Blood* **41,** 3 (1976).
10. T. S. Herman, N. Hammond, S. E. Jones, *et al., Cancer* **43,** 390 (1979).
11. V. T. DeVita, G. P. Canellos, B. A. Chabner, *et al., Lancet* **1,** 248 (1975).
12. S. E. Jones, P. N. Grozea, E. N. Metz, *et al., Cancer* **43,** 417 (1979).
13. Z. Fuks and H. S. Kaplan, *Radiology* **108,** 675 (1973).
14. G. Bonadonna, A. Lattuada, S. Monfardini, *et al., in* "Adjuvant Therapy of Cancer II" (S. E. Jones and S. E. Salmon eds.), p. 145. Grune & Stratton, New York, 1979.
15. T. G. Landberg, L. G. Häkansson, T. R. Möller, *et al., Cancer* **44,** 831 (1979).
16. N. I. Nissen, J. Ersbøll, H. S. Hansen, *et al., Proc. Amer. Assoc. Cancer Res.* **21,** 194 (1980).
17. T. P. Miller and S. E. Jones, *Lancet* **1,** 358 (1979).
18. F. Cabanillas, G. P. Bodey, and E. J. Freireich, *Proc. Amer. Assoc. Cancer Res.* **20,** 19 (1979).
19. S. E. Jones, *in* "Clinical Immunotherapy" (A. LoBuglio, ed.), p. 201. Dekker, New York, 1980.
20. S. E. Jones, J. J. Butler, G. E. Byrne, Jr., *et al., Cancer* **39,** 1071 (1977).
21. S. E. Jones, S. E. Salmon, T. E. Moon, *et al., in* "Immunotherapy of Cancer: Present Status of Trials in Man" (W. D. Terry and D. Windhorst eds.), Vol. 6, p. 519. Raven, New York, 1978.
22. S. E. Jones, S. E. Salmon, and R. Fisher, *in* "Adjuvant Therapy of Cancer II" (S. E. Jones and S. E. Salmon, eds.), p. 163. Grune & Stratton, New York, 1979.

23. S. E. Jones, *in* "Immunotherapy of Cancer: Present Status of Trials in Man II" (W. Terry, ed.). Raven Press, New York (in press).

24. R. S. Stein, R. D. Collins, and J. E. Ultmann, *Proc. Amer. Soc. Clin. Oncology* **21,** 469 (1980).

25. R. I. Fisher, V. T. DeVita, S. M. Hubbard, *et al., Proc. Amer. Soc. Clin. Oncology* **21,** 468 (1980).

26. A. Skarin, G. Canellos, D. Rosenthal, *et al., Proc. Amer. Soc. Clin. Oncology* **21,** 463 (1980).

27. S. Monfardini, G. Tanini, M. DeLena, *et al., Med. Pediatr. Oncol.* **3,** 67 (1977).

28. R. Canetta, E. Villa, R. Musumeci, *et al., Proc. Amer. Assoc. Cancer Res.* **21,** 189 (1980).

29. G. P. Bodey, V. Rodriguez, F. Cabanillas, *et al., Am. J. Med.* **66,** 74 (1979).

30. T. Anderson, *Ariz. Med.* **36,** 762 (1979).

26

The Role of Radiation Therapy in the Treatment of Stage I and II Hodgkin's Disease

PETER MAUCH, ALAN LEWIN, AND SAMUEL HELLMAN

I. Introduction

The survival of patients with early-stage Hodgkin's disease has dramatically improved over the last 10–15 years (1). This has been in part due to the use of high-dose wide-field radiation therapy as initially proposed by Rene Gilbert, modified by Vera Peters, and systematically studied and elaborated upon by the group at Stanford University Medical Center (1–4). The routine use of staging laparotomies has allowed more precise localization of initial disease and more accurate use of localized therapy (5, 6). The development of effective chemotherapy has produced gratifying results in the treatment of more advanced Hodgkin's disease patients (7) and has provided a high percentage of salvage for patients who relapse following initial treatment with radiation therapy (8). One of the early studies reported 82% 3-year relapse-free survival and greater than 90% overall survival in pathologically staged IA and IIA Hodgkin's disease patients treated with total nodal irradiation (9). Similar relapse-free and overall survival

MALIGNANT LYMPHOMAS

rates were reported for a group of pathologically staged IA and IIA patients who received mantle and paraaortic irradiation with sparing of the pelvis (10). This approach avoided the high risk of sterility associated with pelvic irradiation in men and the necessity for oophoropexy in women (11, 12), while demonstrating that the untreated pelvis was at low risk for recurrence in patients with pathologically staged supradiaphragmatic Hodgkin's disease (10). Among these early-stage patients was a subgroup identified at higher risk for relapse (13, 14). These were patients with initial large mediastinal adenopathy. Characteristically, they had relapsed extranodally in the lung or pleura or at nodal sites above the diaphragm with the mediastinum at high risk for relapse. As a result of successful chemotherapy with nitrogen mustard, vincristine, procarbazine, and prednisone (MOPP) at the time of recurrence, similar survival rates have been reported for these patients regardless of whether initial combined-modality therapy or radiation therapy alone with MOPP reserved for treatment failure was used (14).

Pathologically staged IB and IIB Hodgkin's disease occurs less frequently than similarly staged IA and IIA disease. One report has randomized stage IB and IIB Hodgkin's disease patients to treatment with either initial total nodal irradiation (TNI) alone or to treatment with combined TNI and MOPP chemotherapy. Patients treated with TNI had an actuarial 89% survival at 8 years as compared to an 87% actuarial survival with TNI and MOPP (15).

This report summarizes the experience in treating early-stage I and II Hodgkin's disease patients at the Joint Center for Radiation Therapy. These patients have been primarily treated with radiation therapy alone, with pelvic irradiation omitted in most cases. We have evaluated adverse prognostic features in this group of early-stage patients, and alternative treatment recommendations are discussed.

II. Patients and Methods

At the Joint Center for Radiation Therapy, Harvard University, 257 patients with stage IA, IIA, or IIB Hodgkin's disease were treated between April 1969 and July 1978. Routine evaluation of these patients included chest radiography, whole-lung tomography (if hilar nodes were enlarged), bipedal lymphangiography, and biochemical evaluation. All patients underwent a staging laparotomy and splenectomy. Patients were staged using the Ann Arbor classification (16).

Two hundred and thirty-seven patients had supradiaphragmatic Hodgkin's disease. Pathological staging included 64 patients with stage IA, 128 patients with stage IIA, and 45 patients with stage IIB Hodgkin's disease (Table I). Thirteen of these patients were subclassified as ''E'' because of a single area of non-lymph node disease contiguous with an involved lymph node-bearing area. Patients had a median age of 23 years (range 6–68 years) and a median follow-up

TABLE I

**Supradiaphragmatic Hodgkin's Disease
(April 1969–July 1978) (237)**

Pathological stage (no. of patients)	
IA	64
IIA	128
IIB	45
Median age (years)	23
Median follow-up (months)	68

from initiation of treatment of 68 months (range 18–128 months). There were 130 men and 107 women with supradiaphragmatic disease. The histological subtypes included 131 patients with nodular sclerosis (55%), 79 patients with mixed cellularity (33%), 23 patients with lymphocyte predominance (10%), and 4 patients with lymphocyte depletion (2%) histology.

Patients were analyzed for the presence of mediastinal or hilar adenopathy. To determine the extent of mediastinal involvement the width of the mediastinal mass was divided by the thoracic cage diameter at its widest dimension as measured by PA chest radiography. Patients with a ratio of mediastinal adenopathy to thoracic cage diameter greater than 1:3 were considered to have large mediastinal involvement. The remaining patients had lesser or no mediastinal disease. Table II outlines the frequency of mediastinal adenopathy by stage. Large mediastinal adenopathy was present in only 3% of patients with stage IA Hodgkin's disease. In contrast, 19% of patients with stage IIA and 27% of patients with stage IIB Hodgkin's disease had mediastinal masses measuring greater than one-third the chest diameter. Of all patients with pathologically staged IA IIA, or IIB Hodgkin's disease 60% had mediastinal adenopathy at presentation and 40% had no evidence of mediastinal involvement. Although nodular sclerosing histology made up 55% of the patients in this study, 67% of

TABLE II

Mediastinal Adenopathy (237)

	Number of patients		
Mediastinal adenopathy	Stage IA	Stage IIA	Stage IIB
Greater than one-third (38)	2	24	12
One-third or less (105)	15	66	24
None (94)	47	38	9
Total	64	128	45

patients with mediastinal adenopathy were of this histological type while only 33% of patients without mediastinal involvement had nodular sclerosing histology ($p < 0.001$). There was a total of 23 patients with lymphocyte predominant histology, and out of this group only 2 had evidence of mediastinal involvement.

Twenty patients had infradiaphragmatic Hodgkin's disease. These patients had inguinal-femoral disease and were pathologically staged. Six patients had stage IA, eight had stage IIA, and six had stage IIB disease.

The treatment of patients with supradiaphragmatic stage IA IIA, or IIB Hodgkin's disease is outlined in Table III. Patients were treated with a 4- or 8-MeV linear accelerator at 100–130 cm FSD. A total dose of 3600–4000 rad was delivered to each field in 150- to 200-rad fractions at five fractions per week. In some patients areas of initial bulk disease were treated to an additional 400 rad. Thirteen patients with large mediastinal or hilar involvement received whole-lung irradiation for a total of 1500 rad delivered in 150-rad fractions. Blocks were then fashioned to reduce the volume of heart and lung treated without omitting known disease. Technical factors included simulation, individually contoured divergent blocks, thermoluminescent dosimetric monitoring, the arms-up position, and one to two fields per day. In general, patients with stage IA or IIA Hodgkin's disease received mantle irradiation followed by a 2- to 3-week rest period and then paraaortic and splenic pedicle treatment. Eleven patients with disease limited to the neck received lesser-field irradiation. Eighteen patients with stage IIB Hodgkin's disease were treated with radiation therapy alone. Twenty-seven stage IIB patients received initial combined-modality therapy with two to three cycles of MOPP followed by irradiation followed by the remainder of the MOPP chemotherapy. Radiation fields included mantle and paraaortic treatment in the majority of stage IIB patients. The choice of treatment for stage IIB patients appeared to be based on individual physician preference, as we were unable to detect differences in the extent of disease or

TABLE III

Treatment

| | Number of patients[a] | | | | |
Stage	Minimantle or mantle	M-PA	TNI	M-PA-MOPP	TNI-MOPP
IA	9	51	4	0	0
IIA	2	118	6	2	0
IIB	0	15	3	23	4

[a] M-PA, Mantle and paraaortic irradiation; TNI, total nodal irradiation; M-PA-MOPP and TNI-MOPP, combined-modality therapy.

symptoms in these patients. Actuarial survival curves were calculated using the Cutler modification of the Berkson Gage technique (17). Statistical comparisons were made using the chi square analysis with a Yates correction factor for small numbers. Patients dying from treatment-related complications were counted as relapsing and dying of Hodgkin's disease for statistical purposes.

III. Results

The survival of patients with supradiaphragmatic Hodgkin's disease is outlined in Table IV. Patients with stage IA disease have an actuarial 8-year freedom from relapse of 91% and an actuarial overall survival of 95% (Table IV). Stage IIA patients have an actuarial 79% relapse-free and a 92% overall survival at 8 years. The actuarial freedom from first relapse is 79%, and the overall survival rate is 89% for patients with stage IIB Hodgkin's disease at 8 years.

Patients were evaluated for size of initial mediastinal adenopathy. There were 26 patients with stage IA or IIA Hodgkin's disease who had mediastinal masses measuring greater than one-third of the chest diameter; 12 of these patients have relapsed. The freedom from first relapse at 8 years is 49%, and the probability of survival 88% (Fig. 1) for this group of patients with large mediastinal adenopathy. In contrast, there have been only 14 relapses in 166 patients with stage IA or IIA disease who had lesser or no mediastinal adenopathy. This group of patients has an actuarial freedom from first relapse at 8 years of 88% and a probability of survival of 95% (Fig. 2). Table V outlines the relapse patterns of these two groups of patients. Patients with initial large mediastinal adenopathy appear to relapse in the lung or pleura (4 patients) or at lymph node sites sbove the diaphragm (8 patients). The mediastinum was the most common site of relapse, and this occurred in 6 of the 8 patients with nodal relapses. Multiple sites of nodal relapse were noted in the majority of patients (13). None of the patients who initially had large mediastinal disease have relapsed below the diaphragm. In contrast, patients who had lesser or no mediastinal disease on initial presentation have relapsed at sites both above and below the diaphragm. These have

TABLE IV

Actuarial Survival by Stage at 8 Years

Stage	Number of patients	Percent relapse-free	Percent survival
IA	64	91	95
IIA	128	79	92
IIB	45	79	89

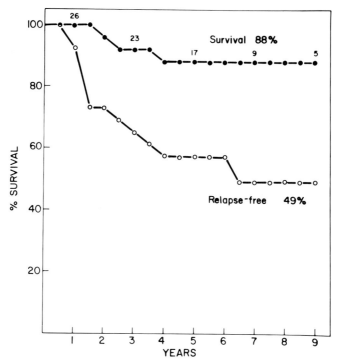

Fig. 1. Actuarial survival and relapse-free survival for pathologically staged IA and IIA Hodgkin's disease patients with large mediastinal adenopathy.

included 2 patients with liver relapse, 2 patients with pelvic nodal relapse, 2 patients with pelvic nodal plus pelvic bone relapse, and 1 patient with bone marrow relapse. None of the patients who received less than mantle and paraaortic irradiation have relapsed. There were no lung or pleura relapses in patients who received initial whole-lung irradiation.

The 45 patients with supradiaphragmatic stage IIB Hodgkin's disease were treated in a variety of ways based on individual physician preference. Eighteen patients were treated initially with radiation therapy alone, and 27 patients received combined-modality treatment. Six of the radiation therapy patients have relapsed. Three of 6 are disease-free following treatment with MOPP chemotherapy, and 1 patient is alive with disease. These patients have an actuarial freedom from first relapse at 8 years of 66% and an overall survival of 89% (Table VI). Out of 27 patients who were initially treated with combined-modality therapy there have been two relapses and one treatment-related death. Both the 8-year actuarial relapse-free and overall survival were 89%, as both patients treated with salvage chemotherapy have expired. Table VII outlines the sites of

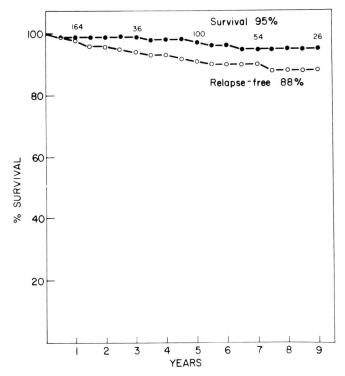

Fig. 2. Actuarial survival and relapse-free survival for pathologically staged IA and IIA Hodgkin's disease patients with lesser or no mediastinal adenopathy.

TABLE V

Stage IA and IIA Sites of Relapse

Large mediastinal adenopathy	(12)
Nodal (above diaphragm)	8
Lung or pleura	4
Lesser or no mediastinal disease	(14)
Liver	1
Liver plus retroperitoneum	1
Lung, chest wall, or pleura	4
Bone marrow	1
Pelvic nodal plus bone	2
Pelvic nodal	2
Nodal (above diaphragm)	3

TABLE VI

Stage IIB: Results of Treatment

Treatment[a]	Number of patients	8-year actuarial relapse-free (%)	8-year actuarial survival (%)
XRT	18	66	89
CMT	27	89	89

[a] XRT, Mantle and paraaortic or total nodal irradiation; CMT, combined-modality therapy.

relapse for stage IIB patients. There were 12 stage IIB patients with large medias-tinal adenopathy. Five were treated with radiation therapy alone; 7 received combined-modality therapy. With radiation therapy alone 3 out of 5 patients with large masses have relapsed, and 2 have died. Only 1 of the 7 patients receiving initial combined-modality therapy has relapsed.

The influence of histology upon relapse and subsequent survival was evaluated (Table VIII). Nodular sclerosis and lymphocyte predominance histology appeared to confer a more favorable prognosis in patients with stage IA or IIA Hodgkin's disease. Only 10 out of 102 patients with nodular sclerosing histology have relapsed, with 2 deaths. These patients have a significantly better relapse-free and overall survival than patients with mixed-cellularity disease in whom 15 of

TABLE VII

Stage IIB: Sites of Relapse

Initial treatment[a]	Size of mediastinal adenopathy	Relapse site	Time to relapse (months)	Status[b]
TNI	>One-third	Chest wall	4	Dead (pneumocystis)
M-PA	>One-third	Mediastinum	29	Dead (HD)
M-PA	>One-third	Preauricular node	25	NED (99 months)
M-PA	≤One-third	Lung	53	NED (72 months)
M-PA	≤One-third	Lung, pericardium	19	AcD (30 months)
M-PA	≤One-third	Right inguinal node	18	NED (106 months)
CMT	>One-third	Mediastinum	9	Dead (HD)
CMT		—	10	Dead (pneumocystis)
CMT	≤One-third	PA, inguinal nodes	20	Dead (HD)

[a] TNI, Total nodal irradiation; M-PA, mantle and paraaortic irradiation; CMT, combined-modality therapy.

[b] HD, Hodgkin's disease; NED, free of relapse; AcD, alive with active Hodgkin's disease; PA; paraaortic nodes.

TABLE VIII

Influence of Histology

Stage	Histology[a]	Number of patients	Number relapsed	Number dead
IA and IIA	NS	102	10	2
	MC	68	15	7
	LP	22	1	0
IIB	NS	11	6	2
	MC	5	0	0
	LP	1	0	0
	LD	1	0	0

[a] NS, Nodular sclerosis; MC, mixed cellularity; LP, lymphocyte predominance; LD, lymphocyte depletion.

68 have relapsed and 7 have died ($p < .05$). In contrast, patients with stage IIB Hodgkin's disease receiving radiation therapy alone appeared more likely to relapse with nodular sclerosis histology than with the other three histologies. Six of 11 patients with nodular sclerosis histology have relapsed, and there have been 2 deaths. Because of the conflicting results in the two groups and the small number of stage IIB patients it is difficult to know whether these results are meaningful. They require additional stage IIB patients and confirmation from other institutions. Nonetheless, the pattern of relapse in stage IA, IIA, and IIB patients appeared to relate to histology. Eight of 15 patients relapsing with mixed-cellularity disease relapsed extranodally in liver, lung, bone, or bone marrow. None of the 16 relapses among patients with nodular sclerosing histology were in the liver, bone, or bone marrow, and there was only 1 relapse below the diaphragm. Four patients relapsed in the lung or pleura, 2 patients developed chest wall recurrences, and the remaining 9 patients relapsed at nodal sites above the diaphragm.

Infradiaphragmatic Hodgkin's disease was an unusual presentation in this study. Out of 257 stage IA, IIA, and IIB patients only 20 (8%) had infradiaphragmatic presentations. This included 6 patients with stage IA, 8 patients with stage IIA, and 6 patients with stage IIB Hodgkin's disease. The treatment techniques and results are outlined in Table IX. All stage IA patients are free of disease. Two of the 8 patients with stage IIA disease have relapsed and are currently disease-free following retreatment with MOPP chemotherapy. All the patients with stage IIB disease received initial combined-modality treatment, and 5 of the 6 are alive without disease. All 20 patients had inguinal or femoral adenopathy, and all patients were pathologically staged.

Complications were recorded for stage IA, IIA, and IIB patients treated with radiation therapy alone. There was a 3.4% incidence of radiation pneumonitis

TABLE IX

Infradiaphragmatic Hodgkin's Disease (20)

Stage	Treatment[a]	Number of patients	Relapsed	Dead
IA	P, PA	6	0	0
IIA	P, PA	4	2	0
	TNI	2	0	0
	CMT	2	0	0
IIB	CMT	6	1	1

[a] P, Pelvic irradiation; PA, paraaortic irradiation; TNI, total nodal irradiation; CMT, combined-modality treatment.

and a 1.5% incidence of pericarditis largely in patients with significant mediastinal adenopathy (Table X). One patient died of pneumonitis following whole-lung irradiation—2000 rad in 10 fractions. Prednisone was prescribed for four of the patients with pneumonitis, and indomethocin for one patient with pericarditis. The acute pericarditis and pneumonitis resolved in all patients without sequelae, and there have been no cases of chronic dyspnea or constrictive pericarditis. Two second tumors were seen within the radiation therapy fields, a basal cell carcinoma in one patient and a pancreatic carcinoma in another. Of interest was the development of thyroiditis and exophthalmus in three patients. Two patients died

TABLE X

Complications of Mantle Irradiation (206)

Complication		Number
Pneumonitis		7 (3.4%)
Fatal	1	
Prednisone-treated	4	
No prednisone	2	
Pericarditis		3 (1.5%)
Hypothyroidism (clinical)		7 (3.4%)
Xerostomia		6 (2.9%)
(second tumors)		2
Hyperthyroidism		1
Thyroiditis, exophthalmus		3 (1.5%)
Brachial neuritis		1
Basilar artery thrombosis		1
Myocardial infarction		4 (1.9%)
Fatal	2	
Nonfatal	2	

of presumed myocardial infarctions, although autopsy or clinical confirmation could not be obtained. One was an 18-year-old male who expired while jogging; the other was a 45-year-old male who died in his sleep. Xerostomia of a mild to moderate nature was noted in six patients. Residual deficits were noted both in the patient with brachial neuritis and in the patient who developed a basilar artery thrombosis. As it is difficult to implicate the role of radiation therapy alone in the development of the myocardial infarctions or second tumors, the cases reported herein appear in parentheses in Table X.

Serious complications of staging laparotomy were unusual. Out of 257 staging laparotomies two patients developed a subdiaphragmatic abscess requiring surgical draining (0.8%), two patients developed small-bowel obstructions within 6 months of the initial laparotomy, requiring surgical intervention for lysis of adhesions (0.8%), and one patient died of complications from the staging laparotomy.

IV. Discussion

Patients with pathologically stage IA or IIA Hodgkin's disease have an excellent relapse-free and overall survival when treated with radiation therapy alone (13, 15). Treatment with mantle and paraaortic irradiation allows sparing of the pelvic bone marrow and potential preservation of fertility. From the results reported herein, patients with stage IA Hodgkin's disease have a 91% relapse-free and a 95% overall survival at 8 years. Stage IIA patients have a 79% relapse and a 92% overall survival. There have been only 4 pelvic nodal failures out of 169 patients who have received mantle and paraaortic irradiation (2.4%). In some patients there may be a role for lesser irradiation, especially when the initial disease is limited to high neck nodes. Very young or elderly patients with limited Hodgkin's disease might be the most likely candidates for lesser-field irradiation. Of 11 such patients treated with mantle or less than mantle irradiation in this study there have been no relapses.

There appears to be a subgroup of patients with large mediastinal adenopathy who are at high risk for relapse (13, 14). These relapses characteristically occur extranodally in the lung or pleura, as mediastinal recurrences within the treated volume, as recurrences at the margin of the treated field, and at other lymph node sites above the diaphragm (13, 14, 18–20). The judicious use of whole-lung irradiation and perhaps a higher total dose administered to the mediastinum may help prevent some of these recurrences, but this may significantly increase the risk of complications. In the current study the relapse-free survival of patients with large mediastinal adenopathy is only 49%, although the overall survival is 88% at 8 years. Several studies have reported no difference in overall survival of patients with large mediastinal adenopathy treated initially with combined-modality therapy as compared to radiation therapy alone with MOPP reserved for relapse (14, 21). However, at present only 5-year survival rates are available to evaluate the treatment of patients with MOPP chemotherapy following relapse, and a longer follow-up is needed before the potential for cure in these patients is known (8, 22, 23). There are other problems with patients having large mediastinal masses. Anesthesia, especially extubation, is more difficult with such masses, and thus the mass may require initial radiation to reduce its size (24). Further, the radiation fields required may be very large, increasing the risk of pneumonitis and pericarditis or causing extended treatment breaks which may increase the local failure possibility (25). Therefore the proper treatment of patients with large mediastinal masses is uncertain (26).

In patients with lesser or no mediastinal disease it is unlikely that the addition of MOPP chemotherapy can significantly improve the 88% actuarial freedom from first relapse reported herein for stage IA and IIA patients. When good technical radiation therapy is available, the acute morbidity (7, 27) and the substantial risk of sterility in both males and females (28, 29) with the administration of MOPP chemotherapy can be avoided in early-stage patients.

There is a paucity of information available on the treatment of stage IIB Hodgkin's disease, as the number of patients from any one center is small. In this study only 19% of patients with stage I or II Hodgkin's disease had symptoms of fever, weight loss, or night sweats. One of the early studies reported a 5-year 70% survival in clinically staged IIB patients who were treated with total nodal irradiation. Their treatment results with extended-field irradiation were not as satisfactory, presumably because of the presence of occult disease below the diaphragm (30). In a randomized study from Stanford, pathologically staged IIB Hodgkin's disease patients had similar relapse-free and overall survivals whether they were treated with total nodal irradiation alone or with initial combined-modality therapy. Patients had a freedom from relapse at 8 years of 79% with radiation therapy alone, and of 84% with combined treatment, however, the overall survivals were 89 and 87%, respectively (15). Patients with stage IIB Hodgkin's disease reported herein have an 89% survival at 8 years regardless of whether initial radiation therapy alone or combined-modality therapy was used. The majority of patients in this study, however, were treated with mantle and paraarotic irradiation with sparing of the pelvic lymph nodes.

The influence of histology upon the relapse-free and overall survival patients with early-stage Hodgkin's disease has been somewhat controversial. Several early studies reported a more favorable prognosis in patients with lymphocyte predominance or nodular sclerosing Hodgkin's disease as compared to the mixed-cellularity or lymphocyte-depleted type (30, 31). However, in both these studies a large proportion of patients were not surgically staged, and these results may simply reflect a lower probability that clinically staged I and II patients with nodular sclerosis of lymphocyte predominance histology have occult disease below the diaphragm. These differences have not been seen in studies in which surgical staging has been routinely performed (32, 33). Our results are unclear on this point. Nodular sclerosis has a better prognosis in stages IA and IIA but not in stage IIB. The patterns of relapse for the two histologies are quite different; patients with nodular sclerosing histology appear to fail at lung, pleura, or nodal sites above the diaphragm, and patients with mixed-cellularity histology have a much higher relapse rate in liver, bone, and bone marrow.

Infradiaphragmatic Hodgkin's disease with inguinal or femoral adenopathy has a prognosis similar to that for supradiaphragmatic disease. Patients with asymptomatic Hodgkin's disease were treated with radiation therapy alone, and patients with infradiaphragmatic stage IIB disease received combined-modality therapy. Out of 20 patients, 3 have relapsed, and there has been only 1 death. Similar results have previously been reported in another study (34).

The most frequent complications of radiation therapy are associated with mantle irradiation. It is unusual to see complications from the staging laparotomy or from paraaortic treatment. In the results reported herein the incidence of pericarditis was 1.5%, radiation pneumonitis 3.4%, clinical hypothyroidism 3.4%, and mild to moderate xerostomia 2.9%. Occasionally more serious complications were seen. A higher rate of radiation pericarditis and pneumonitis has been described in some studies, however, this appears to be related to volume irradiated, daily fractionation, total treatment time, and total dose (35, 36). When equally weighted anterior and posterior fields are used and when normal lung can be blocked after 1500 rad and heart after 2500–3000 rad, the complication rates are low (36, 37). The 3.4% incidence of clinical hypothyroidism reported herein appears somewhat lower than that reported previously (38). This may be due in part to our use of larynx block at 2000 rad and a posterior spine block at 3000 rad. In addition, many patients are now followed with routine thyroid-stimulating hormone determinations and, if elevated levels are noted, receive thyroid supplementation before potential clinical hypothyroidism develops.

This study described the results of treatment in patients with stage IA, IIA, and IIB Hodgkin's disease. Patients with large mediastinal adenopathy appear at higher risk for relapse; the implications of this for patient survival is not known at the present time. Treatment options include mantle and paraaortic irradiation with salvage MOPP therapy when indicated, no laparotomy, but MOPP initially, with radiation to sites of initial involvement, or this treatment following surgical staging proceeded by an initial small dose of irradiation to shrink the mediastinal mass. Treatment for the large majority of stage I and II patients who do not have large mediastinal masses is clear. Following surgical staging we recommend treating these patients with mantle and paraaortic irradiation alone. This approach has resulted in a low risk of relapse in the untreated pelvis and potentially preserves fertility in the majority of patients. The actuarial relapse-free and overall survival rates for these patients have been excellent.

References

1. H. S. Kaplan, *Radiology* **123**, 551 (1977).
2. R. Gilbert, *Am. J. Roentgenol. Radium. Ther.* **41**, 198 (1939).
3. R. Gilbert, *J. Radiol. Electrol.* **9**, 509 (1925).
4. M. V. Peters, *Am. J. Roentgenol. Radium Ther.* **63**, 299 (1970).
5. M. E. Kadin, E. Glatstein, and R. F. Dorfman, *Cancer (Philadelphia)* **27**, 1277 (1970).
6. A. J. Piro, S. Hellman, and W. Moloney, *Arch. Intern. Med.* **130**, 844 (1972).
7. V. DeVita, A. Serpick, and P. Carbone, *Ann. Intern. Med.* **73**, 881 (1970).
8. S. A. Weller, E. Glatstein, H. S. Kaplan, and S. A. Rosenberg, *Cancer (Philadelphia)* **37**, 2840 (1976).
9. H. S. Kaplan and S. Rosenberg, *Natl. Cancer Inst. Monogr.* **36**, 363 (1973).
10. R. L. Goodman, A. J. Piro, and S. Hellman, *Cancer (Philadelphia)* **37**, 2834 (1976).
11. J. Slanina, K. Musskoff, T. Rohner, and R. Staisny, *Int. J. Radiat. Oncol. Biol. Phys.* **2**, 1 (1977).
12. O. LeFloch, S. S. Donaldson, and H. S. Kaplan, *Cancer (Philadelphia)* **38**, 2263 (1976).
13. P. Mauch, R. Goodman, and S. Hellman, *Cancer (Philadelphia)* **42**, 1039 (1978).
14. R. T. Hoppe, C. N. Coleman, H. S. Kaplan, and S. A. Rosenberg, *Proc. Am. Soc. Clin. Oncol.* **21**, 471 (1980).
15. S. A. Rosenberg, H. S. Kaplan, E. J. Glatstein, and C. S. Portlock, *Cancer (Philadelphia)* **42**, 991 (1978).
16. P. Carbone, H. S. Kaplan, K. Musshoff, D. W. Smithers, and M. Tubiana, *Cancer Res.* **31**, 1860 (1971).
17. S. J. Cutler and F. Ederer, *J. Chronic. Dis.* **8**, 669 (1958).
18. T. L. Thar, R. R. Million, R. J. Hausner, and H. H. B. McKetty, *Cancer (Philadelphia)* **43**, 1101 (1979).
19. M. J. Peckham, *B.T.T.A. Rev.* **2**, 1 (1972).
20. J. A. Levi, P. H. Wiernik, and M. J. O'Connell, *Int. J. Radiat. Oncol., Biol. Phys.* **2**, 853 (1977).
21. C. A. Coltman and L. M. Fuller, *Blood* **50**, 188 (1977).
22. C. S. Portlock, S. A. Rosenberg, E. Glatstein, and H. S. Kaplan, *Blood* **5**, 825 (1978).
23. P. Mauch, M. E. Ryback, D. Rosenthal, R. Weichselbaum, and S. Hellman, *Blood* **56**, 892 (1980).
24. A. J. Piro, D. R. Weiss, and S. Hellman, *Int. J. Radiat. Oncol., Biol. Phys.* **1**, 415 (1976).
25. T. Landberg, K. Liden, and H. Forslo, *Acta Radiol.* **12**, 33 (1973).
26. P. Mauch and S. Hellman, *Int. J. Radiat. Oncol., Biol. Phys.* **6**, 947 (1980).
27. V. DeVita, J. C. Arseneau, R. J. Sherins, and G. P. Canellos, *Natl. Cancer Inst. Monogr.* **36**, 447 (1973).
28. R. Sherins, S. Winokur, V. T. DeVita, and J. Vaitukaitus, *Clin. Res.* **23**, 343A (1975).
29. R. J. Sherins and V. T. DeVita, *Ann. Intern. Med.* **79**, 216 (1973).
30. R. E. Johnson, L. B. Thomas, M. Schneiderman, D. W. Glenn, F. Faw, and M. D. Haferman, *Radiology* **96**, 603 (1970).
31. A. R. Patchefsky, H. Brodovsky, M. Southard, H. Menduke, S. Gray, and W. S. Hoch, *Cancer (Philadelphia)* **32**, 150 (1973).
32. F. M. Torti, R. F. Dorfman, S. A. Rosenberg, *et al.*, *Proc. Am. Assoc. Cancer Res. Am. Soc. Clin. Oncol.* **20**, 401 (1979).
33. L. M. Fuller, H. Madoc-Jones, J. F. Gamble *et al.*, *Cancer (Philadelphia)* **39**, 2174 (1977).
34. J. G. Krikorian, C. S. Portlock, S. A. Rosenberg, and H. S. Kaplan, *Cancer (Philadelphia)* **43**, 1866 (1979).
35. J. R. Stewart, K. E, Cohen, L. F. Fajardo *et al.*, *Radiology* **89**, 302 (1967).

36. R. J. Carmel and H. S. Kaplan, *Cancer* (*Philadelphia*) **37,** 2813 (1976).
37. S. Hellman, P. Mauch, R. L. Goodman, D. S. Rosenthal, and W. C. Moloney, *Cancer* (*Philadelphia*) **42,** 971 (1978).
38. E. Glatstein, S. McHardy-Young, N. Brast, J. R. Eltringham, and J. P. Kriss, *J. Clin. Endocrinol. Metab.* **32,** 833 (1971).

27

A Working Formulation of Non-Hodgkin's Lymphomas for Clinical Usage: Clinicopathological and Prognostic Correlations

RICHARD T. HOPPE

I. Introduction

The background for this study and the histopathological criteria for the entities defined in the working formulation of non-Hodgkin's lymphomas for clinical usage are outlined elsewhere in this volume by Dorfman *et al.* (1). Intrinsic to the design of this study was the idea that the working formulation be founded not only upon histopathological differences, but also upon important differences in the natural history, clinical course, and outcome of these diseases (2). Clinicopathological correlation was available from detailed abstracts completed by clinicians at four institutions—Istituto Nazionale Tumori (G. Bonadonna), University of Minnesota Hospitals (C. Bloomfield), New England Medical Center (R. Rudders), and Stanford University (R. Hoppe). The data available included baseline demographic information, symptoms at presentation, sites of initial diagnostic biopsies, results of initial staging procedures, a summary of sites of involvement, final pathological stage, type and duration of initial therapy, extent of initial treatment evaluation, relapse data, and follow-up information for each patient. An analysis of the important clinical characteristics of each disease entity in the six classification systems was facilitated by computer entry of these data. The survival data for the six classification systems utilizing the diagnoses of the expert for each system (3–11) are summarized in Fig. 1. It is evident from examination of these curves that each system is effective in predicting prognosis. In each case there is a spectrum of patient survival ranging from good to poor. The similar appearance of these survival curves suggests that the six systems share some important features.

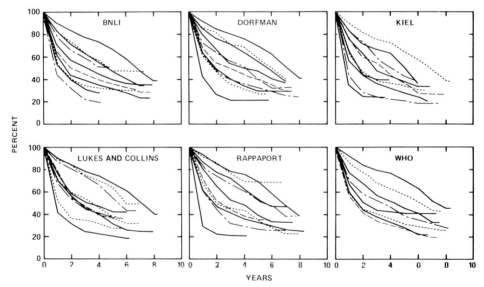

Fig. 1.   Actuarial survival of patients with non-Hodgkin's lymphoma utilizing the experts' diagnosis in each of the six major classification systems. Only categories with 20 or more patients are included. BNLI, British National Lymphoma Investigation Classification; WHO, World Health Organization.

II. The Clinicopathological Entities of the Working Formulation of Non-Hodgkin's Lymphomas for Clinical Usage

A. Small Lymphocytic Lymphoma

Despite the differences in concept and terminology employed in the six major classification schemes, there are some entities which bear substantial similarity in each system. One such example is summarized in Table I. Histologically, this type of lymphoma is marked by diffuse effacement of the lymph node architecture by small to medium-sized lymphocytes with only slight variations in nuclear size or shape and little evidence of mitotic activity. A true nodular or follicular pattern is never present. The lymphocytes may occasionally have plasmacytoid features. The terms used to describe this lymphoma in each system are listed in Table I. Important characteristics of the patients in this study with each diagnosis also are summarized in Table I. In each system this lymphoma accounts for approximately 5% of the patients. The median age is 55–60 years, and cases in patients less than 40 years old are extremely rare. Pathological stage (PS) IV disease can be documented in 70–80% of patients and is usually due to bone marrow involvement. The prognosis for these patients is good, with a median survival of nearly 5 years.

In the working formulation, this type of lymphoma is termed *small lymphocytic*. The clinical characteristics of these patients, which closely parallel those in each of the classification systems, are summarized at the bottom of Table I. A detailed clinical printout for small lymphocytic lymphomas is displayed in Fig. 2. This computer printout includes histograms of the age and stage distribution, sites of initial involvement, response rates, survival, and relapse-free survival curves.

B. Diffuse Large-Cell Lymphomas

Several clinicopathological entities *do not* have clear equivalents in each system. An important example is the group of lymphomas called diffuse histiocytic in the Rappaport system (11).

Despite the terminology of the Rappaport system, very few of these lymphomas are truly of histiocytic origin. Other systems, including those of Lukes and Collins (9) and Lennert (7, 8) more accurately consider the majority of these lymphomas to be derived from transformed lymphocytes. Furthermore, included in this group are lymphomas with rather diverse morphological characteristics which can be subclassified into several *different* groups in the Lukes–Collins and Kiel systems. In this study, cases identified as diffuse histiocytic by Rappaport

TABLE I

The Equivalents of Small Lymphocytic Lymphoma in Six Classification Systems

System and diagnosis[a]	Number of cases	Median age (years)	PS IV (%)	Marrow positive (%)	Sex ratio, M/F	5-Year survival (%)
BNLI: Diffuse lymphoma, lymphocytic, well differentiated (small round ymphocyte), with or without plasmacytoid differentiation	65	58.2	82	60	1.4	47
Dorfman: Diffuse small lymphocytic, with or without plasmacytoid differentiation	57	61.7	86	63	1.0	56
Kiel: Lymphocyic or lymphoplasmacytoid	49	58.8	67	45	.9	43
Lukes-Collins: B-Cell type, small lymphocytic, or B-cell type, plasmacytoid lymphocytic	39	55.7	83	62	1.2	55
Rappaport: Diffuse lymphocytic, well differentiated, with or without plasmacytoid features	47	60.7	86	66	.9	53
WHO: Diffuse lymphosarcoma, lymphocytic or lymphoplasmacytic	62	58.5	76	53	1.1	45
Working formulation: Small lymphocytic	41	60.5	81	66	1.2	59

[a] BNLI, British National Lymphoma Investigation; WHO, World Health Organization.

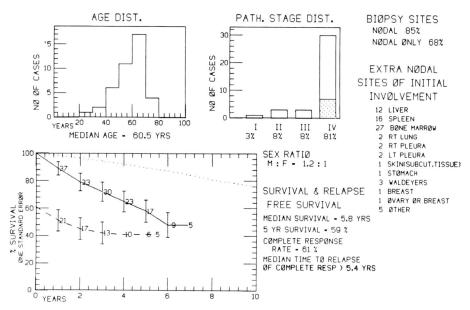

Fig. 2. A clinical printout showing the characteristics of the working formulation group of lymphomas identified as small lymphocytic. These 41 cases represented 3.6% of the total patient population in this study. The stippled area in the histogram of stage distribution indicates the proportion of patients with systemic (B) symptoms. "Extranodal sites of initial involvement" includes sites involved by *either* clinical or pathological criteria. On the survival curve, the solid line represents actuarial survival, the broken line shows freedom from relapse, and the dotted line represents predicted survival for an age, sex, and geographically matched population.

TABLE II

Interclassification Analysis of Diffuse Histiocytic Lymphomas (Rappaport) According to Cell Types within the Lukes–Collins System (Lukes) and Kiel System (Lennert)

Lukes–Collins system	Number of cases	Kiel system	Number of cases
Large noncleaved FCC	74	Immunoblastic	93
Small noncleaved FCC	35	Centroblastic—centrocytic	63
Large cleaved FCC	25	Centroblastic	36
Immunoblastic sarcoma (B-cell type)	22	High grade, unclassified	25
Small cleaved FCC	21	Composite lymphoma	19
Immunoblastic sarcoma (T-cell type)	20		
Composite lymphoma	17		

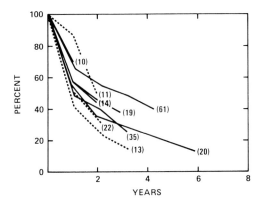

Fig. 3. An interclassification analysis of cases called diffuse histiocytic by Rappaport subclassified according to the diagnosis of Lukes utilizing the Lukes–Collins system. The actuarial survivals of patients with the various subtypes are shown.

were subclassified according to the diagnosis recorded by Lukes using the Lukes–Collins system, and by Lennert using the Kiel system. A summary of the distribution of diagnoses obtained in these two systems is provided in Table II. Survival curves can be calculated for each of these subtypes. For example, Fig. 3 shows the survival of the various groups as classified by Lukes (Lukes–Collins system). Although a spectrum of survival curves is produced, the large number of categories and relatively few patients in each prevent the demonstration of statistically significant differences. Conceptually and histologically there appear to be two major subtypes of histiocytic lymphomas—lymphomas of follicular center cell (FCC) origin and non-FCC origin (immunoblastic sarcomas of the B- or T-cell type). Figure 4 summarizes the survival of these two major subgroups. In the working formulation, lymphomas considered diffuse histiocytic in the Rappaport system but which have histological features consistent with the

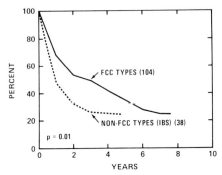

Fig. 4. Actuarial survival of patients with diffuse large-cell lymphomas and immunoblastic lymphomas utilizing a consensus diagnosis of pathologists.

TABLE III

Comparison of Diffuse Large-Cell and Immunoblastic Lymphomas

Working formulation group	Number of cases	Median age (years)	Sex ratio, M/F	PS I (%)	PS IV (%)
Diffuse large cell	227	56.8	1.0	16	44
Large cell immunoblastic	91	51.3	1.5	23	33

Working formulation group	5-Year survival (%)	Median survival (years)	Complete response rate (%)	Median time to relapse (years)
Diffuse large cell	35	1.5	59	>8.4
Large cell immunoblastic	32	1.3	53	3.5

Lukes–Collins FCC type have been termed *diffuse large-cell* lymphomas. The remaining large-cell lymphomas are termed *immunoblastic*. As shown in Fig. 4, in which a consensus diagnosis of pathologists was employed, the survival difference between these two subtypes of large-cell lymphoma is statistically significant. Other clinical series have supported a similar subclassification (12, 13).

Table III summarizes the clinical characteristics of these two types of large-cell lymphoma. The features of immunoblastic lymphoma were identified in 29% of the cases. The immunoblastic type affected slightly younger individuals, was more common in males, and presented more often with early-stage disease than diffuse large-cell lymphoma. The response-to-treatment and survival curves were not greatly different in the two groups, but the duration of remission was longer in the diffuse large-cell type.

The ability of pathologists to differentiate between these two entities is good.

TABLE IV

Reproducibility of Diagnosis of Types of Large-Cell Lymphomas[a]

Second call	First call	
	FCC type	Non-FCC type, immunoblastic
FCC type	41	0
Non-FCC type, immunoblastic	10	16

[a] Analysis based on panelist A. Sixty-seven cases of large cell lymphoma were examined on two separate occasions. At the time of the second review the initial diagnosis was not known to the panelist. Overall reproducibility 85.1%.

TABLE V

Correlation of Architectural Patterns and Cell Types in Six Classification Systems

BNLI	Dorfman	Kiel	Lukes–Collins	Rappaport	WHO
Cell types					
Small follicle lymphocyte	(Atypical) small lymphoid	Centroblastic—centrocytic	Small cleaved FCC	Lymphocytic, well differentiated	Prolymphocytic
Mixed follicle cell	Mixed, small and large lymphoid	—	Large cleaved FCC	Lymphocytic, poorly differentiated	Prolympho-cytic-lympho-blastic
Large lymphoid	Large lymphoid	—	Small noncleaved FCC	Mixed lympho-cytic and histiocytic	
			Large noncleaved FCC	Histiocytic	
Architectural patterns					
Follicular	Follicular (or follicular and diffuse)	Follicular	Follicular	Nodular	Nodular
		Follicular and diffuse	Follicular and diffuse		
Diffuse	Diffuse	Diffuse	Diffuse	Diffuse	Diffuse

This was tested easily in this study, since a random 20% of cases were examined twice by each pathologist. Table IV shows the first and second diagnoses in 67 cases of large-cell lymphoma examined by one of the panelist pathologists. Overall reproducibility was 85.1%.

C. Lymphomas with Follicular or Diffuse Patterns

Each of the six major classification systems of non-Hodgkin's lymphomas includes a description of the architectural pattern of lymph node involvement. Most systems specify either a follicular (nodular) or a diffuse pattern, while the Kiel and Lukes–Collins systems also specify a mixed architectural pattern (follicular and diffuse). In some systems, the importance of the architectural pattern is considered secondary to that of the cell type, in others the two characteristics are thought to be of equal importance, and in some the architectural pattern takes precedence over the cell type.

A summary of the terminology employed for specifying architectural pattern in each system and a description of the possible cell types present in these patterns are provided in Table V. The number of cytological types with a variable architectural pattern ranges from a single group in the Kiel system (centroblastic— centrocytic) to four types in the Lukes–Collins and Rappaport systems. In each of the six systems, the reproducibility of pathologists in assigning architectural patterns was excellent (2).

The impact of architectural pattern (neglecting cell type) is displayed in the survival curves in Fig. 5. Based upon Table V, patients with follicular (nodular)

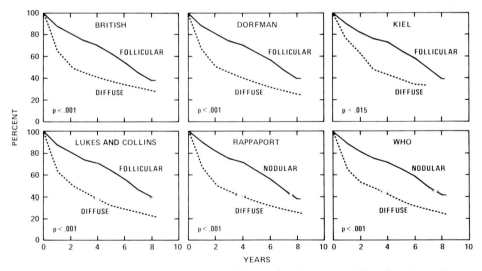

Fig. 5. Actuarial survival of patients with follicular (nodular) versus diffuse lymphomas in each of the six major classification systems.

lymphomas of all cytological types were combined and compared to the group of patients with diffuse lymphoma of the same cytological types. In each system, patients with follicular (nodular) lymphomas had a significantly more favorable prognosis than patients with diffuse lymphomas. This suggests an important prognostic effect for the architectural pattern, however, architectural pattern and cell type are correlated in systems which have more than one cytological type. Cell types with more favorable prognoses are more often present in the follicular pattern. This figure should therefore be interpreted with caution. Figure 6 shows the effects on survival of both architectural pattern *and* cell type using the FCC lymphomas of the Lukes–Collins system. Figure 6A shows the survival of cases with a follicular pattern, and Fig. 6B the survival of cases with a diffuse pattern. It is clear, especially within follicular lymphomas, that the cell type is also an important variable. A multivariate analysis which included architectural pattern, cell type, stage, age, sex, and symptoms confirmed that both architectural pattern and cell type were important covariates in predicting survival (2).

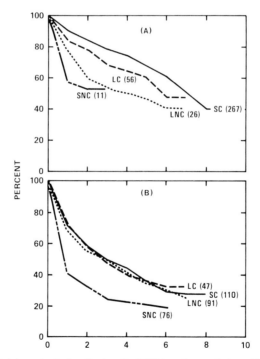

Fig. 6. Actuarial survival of patients with FCC lymphoma (Lukes–Collins system). (A) Actuarial survival of patient with follicular lymphomas of the four different FCC subtypes. (B) Actuarial survival of patients with diffuse lymphomas of the four different FCC types. SC, Small cleaved; LC, large cleaved; SNC, small noncleaved; LNC, large noncleaved.

TABLE VI

Comparison of Follicular and Diffuse Lymphomas—Clinical Factors at Presentation

Working formulation group	Number of cases	Median age (years)	Sex ratio, M/F	PS I and II (%)[a]	Marrow positive (%)
Follicular					
Small cleaved	259	54.3	1.3	18	51
Mixed	89	56.1	0.8	27	30
Large	44	55.4	1.8	27	34
Diffuse					
Small cleaved	79	57.9	2.0	28	32
Mixed	77	58.0	1.1	45	14
Large	227	56.8	1.0	46	9.5

[a] PS, Pathological stage (12).

In the working formulation, three cytological types were identified which could show either a follicular or a diffuse pattern: small cleaved cell, large cell, and mixed small (cleaved) and large cell. The clinical characteristics of these groups are summarized in Table VI, and the outcome of therapy in Table VII. The small cleaved cell type is usually follicular (77%) and is the most common follicular subtype (67%), while the large-cell type is less frequently follicular (16%) and is the least common follicular subtype (11%). An opposite distribution of cell types is noted among diffuse lymphomas, where the large-cell type accounts for 60% of cases.

Patients with follicular lymphomas less often present with early-stage (PS I and II) disease—21% of cases. In contrast, 42% of patients with diffuse lymphomas

TABLE VII

Comparison of Follicular and Diffuse Lymphomas—Treatment Response and Outcome

Working formulation group	5-Year survival (%)	Median survival (years)	Complete response rate (%)	Median time to relapse (years)
Follicular				
Small cleaved	70	7.2	73	5.0
Mixed	50	5.1	65	5.2
Large	45	3.0	61	>8.0
Diffuse				
Small cleaved	33	3.4	56	2.1
Mixed	38	2.7	69	4.3
Large	35	1.5	59	>8.4

have early-stage disease at presentation. The advanced stage of patients with
follicular lymphoma is due primarily to a high frequency of bone marrow
involvement—in 41% of cases. Only 11% of patients with diffuse lymphomas of
these cell types have documented bone marrow involvement at presentation.

Complete remission rates are slightly higher among patients with follicular
lymphoma, and 5-year survivals and median survivals are significantly better in
follicular than in diffuse lymphomas of similar cell type. The majority of patients
with small cleaved or mixed-cell lymphomas of either architectural pattern will
ultimately relapse, despite achieving initial complete remission. However, the
time to relapse is much shorter for patients with the diffuse than with the follicular pattern. Finally, the median time to relapse for patients with large-cell lymphomas, whether follicular or diffuse, has not yet been reached, suggesting that a
significant proportion of patients who achieve complete remission may be cured.

D. Malignant Lymphoma, Lymphoblastic

Malignant lymphoma, lymphoblastic is another entity with an approximate
equivalent in each classification system (14, 15). In the working formulation,
cases with nuclei of either a convoluted or nonconvoluted appearance are included together. A detailed clinical printout showing the characteristics of these
patients is provided in Fig. 7. The majority of cases occur in young males, but

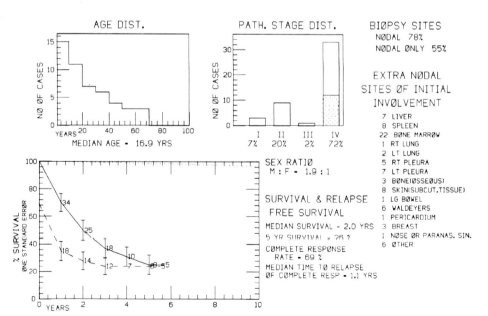

Fig. 7. A clinical printout for the 49 patients with lymphoblastic lymphoma.

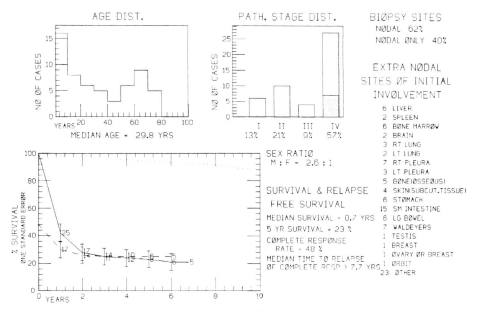

Fig. 8. A clinical printout for the 58 patients with small noncleaved cell lymphoma.

occasional patients are elderly. Most patients have PS IV disease, usually because of bone marrow infiltration. Survival and freedom from relapse are poor in this series.

E. Malignant Lymphoma, Small Noncleaved Cell Type

This group actually includes two different clinicopathological entities—*small noncleaved cell* lymphomas of *Burkitt's* or *non-Burkitt's* type. The clinical characteristics of these patients are summarized in Fig. 8. Patients with a diagnosis of Burkitt's lymphoma are younger than those with the non-Burkitt's type, thereby producing a bimodal age distribution. The majority of patients have PS IV disease, often because of gastrointestinal tract involvement or unusual extranodal sites of disease. Bone marrow involvement is not common. The survival and freedom from relapse for this type of lymphoma are the poorest observed in all the groups in the working formulation.

III. Discussion

The entities included in the working formulation of non-Hodgkin's lymphomas for clinical usage can be identified histologically and have characteristic clinical features. Based on these diagnoses, Fig. 9 shows the spectrum of survival curves that results. This closely resembles the distribution of survival when any of the six major classification systems is employed (Fig. 1).

Only 10 major groups are identified in the working formulation, however, within each group are subgroups with microscopic characteristics that a pathologist may wish to include in a description of the diagnosis (1, 2). These characteristics, such as the plasmacytoid features noted in some cases of small lymphocytic lymphoma, have no specific clinical features identifiable from this analysis. However, there may be important and interesting clinical characteristics, such as associated serum immunoglobulin abnormalities, which were not examined in this study.

The groups of the working formulation are divided into low-grade, intermediate-grade, and high-grade lymphomas based purely upon survival characteristics (1, 2). As shown in Fig. 9, however, there is a spectrum of survival, and the definition of three grades of malignancy is somewhat arbitrary. In addition, as more effective treatments are identified for high-grade lymphomas, the survival of these lymphomas may become better than that which can be achieved in low- or intermediate-grade lymphomas.

The working formulation of non-Hodgkin's lymphomas for clinical usage is proposed to define distinct clinicopathological entities within non-Hodgkin's lymphomas. It is not intended to supplant any of the classification systems currently employed but rather to permit translation of terminology from one classification system to another for the purpose of comparing the results of clinical trials.

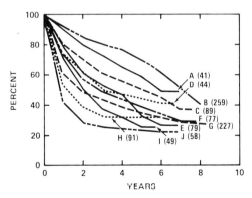

Fig. 9. Actuarial survival for the 10 groups of the working formulation. (A) Small lymphocytic; (B) follicular, small cleaved cell; (C) follicular, mixed cell; (D) follicular, large cell; (E) diffuse, small cleaved cell; (F) diffuse, mixed cell; (G) diffuse, large cell; (H) immunoblastic; (I) lymphoblastic; and (J) small noncleaved cell. Numbers in parentheses indicate the frequency of the various types.

Acknowledgments

The data reported herein are a result of the efforts of many investigators, including A. Banfi, C. W. Berard, C. Bloomfield, G. Bonadonna, B. W. Brown, J. S. Burke, R. DeLellis, V. T. DeVita, R. Dorfman, G. Frizzera, E. J. Glatstein, R. Hartsock, K. Henry, M. S. Hu, H. S. Kaplan, G. Krueger, K. Lennert, R. J. Lukes, K. Nanba, G. T. O'Conor, H. Rappaport, F. Rilke, A. H. T. Robb-Smith, J. Rosai, S. A. Rosenberg, R. A. Rudders, M. Sacks, R. Simon, R. A. Warnke, R. L. Ziegler; however, the opinions expressed are primarily those of the author and not of the other collaborators, many of whom did not have an opportunity to review this manuscript.

This work was supported in part by grant CA 05838 from the National Cancer Institute, National Institutes of Health, and contract grants NO1-CM67072TQ and NO1-CM-6711TQ awarded specifically for this study. The author acknowledges the efforts of Margie Koslow for statistical analysis, Marge Keskin for secretarial assistance, and Janet Morgan for research assistance.

References

1. R. F. Dorfman, J. S. Burke, and C. W. Berard, this volume, Chapter 21.
2. National Cancer Institute Sponsored Study of Classifications of Non-Hodgkin's Lymphomas: Summary and Description of a Working Formulation for Clinical Usage, *Cancer* (in press).
3. R. F. Dorfman, *Lancet* **1**, 1295 (1974).
4. R. F. Dorfman, *Monogr. Pathol.* **16**, 262 (1975).
5. M. H. Bennett, G. Farrer-Brown, K. Henry, *et al.*, *Lancet* **2**, 405 (1974).
6. K. Henry, M. H. Bennett, and G. Farrer-Brown, *Recent Results Cancer Res.* **64**, 38 (1978).
7. K. Lennert, N. Mohri, H. Stein, *et al.*, *Br. J. Haematol.* **31**, Suppl. 193 (1975).
8. R. Gerard-Marchant, I. Hamlin, K. Lennert, *et al.*, *Lancet* **2**, 406 (1974).
9. R. J. Lukes and R. D. Collins, *Cancer* **34**, 1488 (1974).
10. G. Mathe, H. Rappaport, G. T. O'Conor, *et al.*, *in* "International Histological Classification of Tumours," No. 14. World Health Organ. Geneva, 1976.
11. H. Rappaport, "Atlas of Tumor Pathology," Sect. 3, Fasc. 8. U.S. Armed Forces Inst. Pathol., Washington, D.C., 1966.
12. J. A. Strauchen, R. C. Young, V. T. DeVita, *et al.*, *N. Engl. J. Med.* **299**, 1382 (1978).
13. R. Warnke, J. Strauchen, J. Burke, *et al.*, *Cancer* (accepted for publication).
14. M. P. Barcos and R. J. Lukes, *in* "Conflicts in Childhood Cancer. An Evaluation of Current Management" (L. F. Sinkes and J. O. Godden, eds.), Vol. 4, p. 147. Alan R. Liss, Inc., New York, 1975.
15. B. N. Nathwani, H. Kim, and H. Rappaport, *Cancer* **38**, 964 (1976).

28

The Place of Radiation Therapy in the Management of Patients with Localized Non-Hodgkin's Lymphoma

R. S. BUSH AND M. GOSPODAROWICZ

I. Introduction

There are many reasons which prevent a physician from confidently being able to base management decisions on published data from studies on patients with non-Hodgkin's lymphoma. Great stress has been placed on the pathological type of lymphoma, at a time when different pathological classifications are being proposed, all of which differ from each other significantly. Reports of improved survival for subgroups of patients with non-Hodgkin's lymphoma, often based on short follow-up periods, frequently do not give any consideration to the separate effect of staging procedures on the results being reported, nor any mention of any change in the survival of the total patient population. This discussion will try to distinguish the major factors we believe should influence management decisions at this time, particularly as they affect the use of radiation therapy for patients with non-Hodgkin's lymphoma. The significant factors, and their interactions, which will be emphasized are (a) extent of disease (stage), (b) pathological subtype, (c) bulk of disease, (d) age of the patient, and (e) radiation dose.

Data will be presented to support the following conclusions:

1. A significant fraction of patients with "nodular" pathologies have truly localized disease presentations.

2. "Diffuse" pathology identifies the subgroup of patients with a high risk of early death.

3. The use of the simple clinical parameters of age and bulk allows the accurate identification of patients in stage IA or IIA with a high likelihood of cure by irradiation alone.

4. A radiation dose–response curve is clearly evident for patients with diffuse histiocytic (DH) lymphoma.

II. Patients and Methods

Nine hundred and seventy-six (976) patients older than 16 years of age have been seen at the Princess Margaret Hospital (PMH), Toronto, between January 1, 1967 and December 31, 1975 for primary evaluation and management of non-Hodgkin's lymphoma. Staging has been carried out retrospectively, using the criteria and recommendations for the staging of Hodgkin's disease derived from the Ann Arbor Conference (1971).

The original biopsy material for each patient was reviewed by T. C. Brown, chief of pathology at the PMH. Classification was by the criteria of Rappaport (1).

Relapse was determined on the basis of both clinical and pathological findings. The date of relapse was taken as the day recorded on the chart of the clinical opinion of relapse, or the date of any biopsy demonstrating lymphoma. The site of relapse was recorded, and in particular whether relapse occurred within an irradiated volume.

Actuarial survival curves were determined from the date of diagnosis of lymphoma. The Wilcoxon–Gehan test for significance was used for comparisons between survival curves and logrank analysis for variables having multiple levels, or when there was a need to adjust for confounding or interaction. One standard error is shown in the figures.

III. Results

The overall actuarial survival of this group of 976 patients is shown in Fig. 1. The percentage of survival is plotted on a logarithmic scale, and time linearly, so

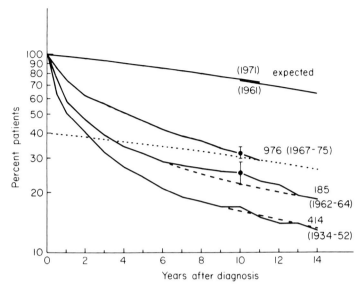

Fig. 1. The long-term survival (actuarial) for new patients with non-Hodgkin's lymphoma seen at the PMH between 1934 and 1975. The dotted line running from 40% of patients is drawn parallel to the expected survival for a 1971 Ontario population of the same age and sex as the patient population seen between 1967 and 1975.

that curves with similar rates of change will be parallel. Out to 10 years, the survival of the treated population always decreases at a more rapid rate than that of the general population with the same age and sex distribution. Thus cure is not demonstrated in the total population, although, as has been reported (2) and will be discussed below, evidence of cure has been obtained for some specific subpopulations. The 5- and 10-year survival is improved over that of our previous experience, and to illustrate this, also plotted in Fig. 1, is the survival of patients seen between 1934–1952, and 1962–1964 (3, 4).

In order to determine which patients may be cured with the use of radiation therapy, it is necessary to examine a number of patient and treatment attributes likely to be important prognostic factors for radiation therapy. These were listed in Section I, and the following analysis will deal with them in that order. First, the significance of the extent of disease will be discussed. As there appears to be a relationship between the Rappaport nodular or diffuse classification and the risk of generalized disease (5, 6), extent of disease and pathology will be discussed together.

The evidence for the "generalized" nature of nodular disease has come from the data generated from pathological staging. Nevertheless, how these findings correlate with long-term survival following local regional radiation to the primary site following less extensive pretreatment evaluation needs to be examined. The survival experience of patients with nodular non-Hodgkin's lymphoma at the PMH is quite different from what would be expected on the basis of published sequential staging data (5). Approximately the same proportion of patients at the PMH (41%) have been classified as having nodular disease as at the National Cancer Institute (NCI) (48%). After full pathological staging, only 6% of the NCI patients remained classified as stage IA or IIA. This result suggests that not just the majority but probably all nodular lymphoma patients have generalized disease, and that current evaluative tests are not sensitive enough to obtain the appropriate information. However, at the PMH, 46% (181/397) of the nodular lymphoma patients were clinically staged as stage IA or IIA (lymphography done in 65%). Only 130 were treated with local regional radiation with the objective of cure. The actuarial 10-year relapse-free rate for these 130 patients is 53% (Fig. 2). This leads to an estimate of 0.17 (130/397 × 0.53) as the fraction of nodular patients with "localized" disease, defined in terms of efficacy of local regional treatment. This is approximately three times higher than that determined by the staging procedures at the NCI (17 versus 6%). That the definition of localized disease is a problem is supported by Stein *et al.* (7) who found that bone marrow interpreted as being involved by lymphoma did not affect prognosis in follicular center cell lymphomas. This was in contrast to involvement of other viscera such as lung. Most nodular patients in Chabner's report from the NCI were upstaged on the basis of bone marrow being interpreted as being involved by disease. If no

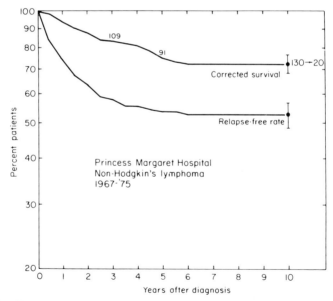

Fig. 2. The relapse-free rate and corrected survival (actuarial) for patients with nodular non-Hodgkin's lymphoma, stage IA or IIA, treated by local regional irradiation with the objective of cure.

treatment, or treatment with modalities other than radiation, for patients with localized disease yields the same outcome in terms of quality, quantity, and efficiency, then there would be no concern. However, no data exist showing that other methods achieve cure in all patients with nodular lymphoma, particularly nodular lymphocytic poorly differentiated (NLPD). Thus it becomes important not to classify falsely patients with localized nodular lymphomas as stage III or IV. In order to ensure that all patients with localized nodular lymphomas (as defined above) receive radiation therapy, the criteria for evaluation must be such that some patients with advanced disease run the chance of being falsely classified as localized, rather than vice versa. The policy followed then would be one in which it is preferable to treat patients with generalized disease using local regional radiation rather than the reverse. Then all, or the great majority, of those with localized disease will be treated with the objective of cure utilizing local regional radiation.

In contradistinction to nodular non-Hodgkin's lymphomas, patients with diffuse lymphomas are more frequently classified as having localized disease on the basis of pathological staging if their clinical presentation is with localized disease (5). However, the ability of current staging procedures, or the criteria being used, to determine accurately distant spread of disease is poor. Monfardini *et al.* have reported the preliminary results of a randomized trial comparing local regional radiation versus chemotherapy plus local regional radiation for patients with pathologically staged IA or IIA non-Hodgkin's lymphoma (8). In the diffuse group, the actuarial estimate is that approximately 55% of those treated with local regional radiation have relapsed. The fraction who relapsed outside the treatment field formed the majority of failures. Thus, in one series, even when aggressive staging techniques were followed, the information obtained did not correlate well with the survival data, nor the failure analysis. In the PMH past experience, without laparotomy, multiple bone marrow, or liver biopsies, 47% of those with diffuse lymphomas were classified as stage IA or IIA. Seventy-five percent (75%) were treated with radiation therapy with the objective of cure. The actuarial relapse-free rate and overall survival for these patients is illustrated in Fig. 3. Thirty-nine percent (39%) are relapse-free 10 years after initial treatment with radiation therapy alone. This 61% relapse rate in clinically staged patients is similar to the 55% reported for surgically staged patients. Because the application of surgical staging has yet to be shown to influence cure rates, its value must be questioned if it fails to predict distant relapse. A further point to be made from Fig. 3 is that diffuse histologies of Rappaport clearly include the majority of patients who die very rapidly. As other factors are examined, any association between them and the subpopulation which dies quickly will be identified, as it has potential importance for medical decision making.

After radiation therapy, the patient may be relapse-free, or suffer relapse within and/or outside the treatment volume (local and/or distant relapse). Patients who develop only distant relapse must have had unrecognized disease beyond the

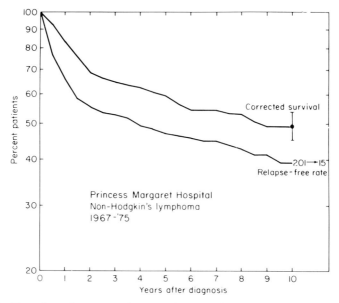

Fig. 3. The relapse-free rate and corrected survival (actuarial) for patients with diffuse non-Hodgkin's lymphoma, stage IA or IIA, treated by local regional irradiation with the objective of cure.

treatment volume at the time of treatment, discounting the possibility of reinduction of the malignancy at another site. In Fig. 4 the actuarial estimates for patients with stage IA or IIA DH pathology have been made for those with no relapse and those with local and/or distant relapse at 10 years and with the assumption that the risk of relapse from initial unrecognized distant spread of disease is the same for those with or without local relapse.

From Fig. 4, the actuarial estimate was that 31.7% of patients surviving would be relapse-free at 10 years and 12.6% would develop local relapse only. It is these first two groups that have demonstrated localized disease from the viewpoint of management of disease. The fraction of patients who could develop distant relapse can be calculated by actuarial methods to be 55%. The management problem is one of identifying those with a high risk of unrecognized distant disease, as well as determining factors influencing local control. It is at this point that one has to return to the question of whether current staging techniques are entirely appropriate for doing this or whether clinical findings may yield this information more reliably. On the basis of our previous arguments, the criteria used for staging are suspect if long-term relapse-free survival after local regional radiation is used to define localized disease, and thus examining clinical findings in more detail is justified. Consequently, we will analyze all the pathological

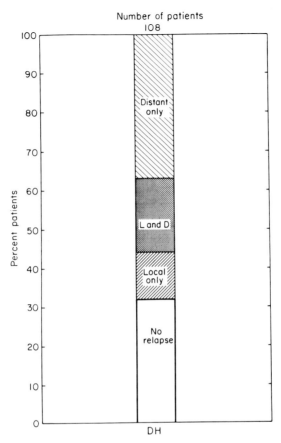

Fig. 4. Actuarial estimates of patients with no evidence of disease (no relapse), with local relapse only (local only), with local and distant relapse (L and D), and with distant relapse only (distant only). All patients were stage IA or IIA, had DH lymphoma, and were treated by radiation for cure.

subgroups in the same manner as we have for DH and then investigate the effect of bulk.

Figure 5 illustrates by means of block diagrams the estimates of the 10-year relapse rates of the different categories by individual Rappaport subgroups. Three groupings can be recognized. First is the numerically small group 1, made up of those classified as diffuse lymphocytic well-differentiated and intermediately differentiated (DLWD and DLID) lymphomas. Seventy percent (70%) of patients are cured by the initial radiation therapy, and the only failures are due to distant relapses. Group 2 is the group comprised of nodular and diffuse lymphocytic poorly differentiated (NLPD and DLPD), mixed cell (MC), and

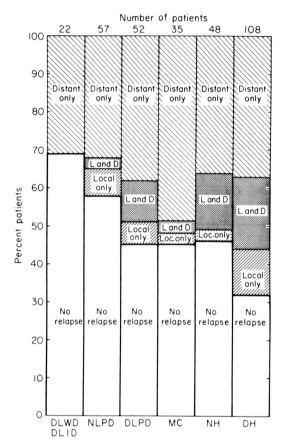

Fig. 5. Actuarial estimates of the relapse pattern for all patients, stage IA or IIA, following radiation therapy for cure by pathological subtype.

nodular histiocytic (NH), where approximately 50% of the patients are estimated actuarially to be relapse-free at 10 years, and 5–10% will develop a local relapse. Group 3 is made up only of patients classified as DH. This analysis indicates that three main groups of pathological subgroups can be identified with different patterns of relapse after local regional radiation. These three groups are illustrated in Fig. 6, and further comparisons will be by these groups rather than individual pathological subgroups.

As would be expected, the majority of patients cured by initial radiotherapeutic treatment were those classified as Ann Arbor stage IA or IIA (2). However, bulk of disease within stages IA and IIA at the time of radiation therapy also appears to play a significant part in determining the probability of long-term survival for patients. Small (S) disease is defined as any lymph node enlargement 2.5 cm or less, or extranodal disease 2.5 cm or less. The number of S nodes influenced only the stage, not the classification by bulk. Medium (M) is defined as nodal disease 2.5–5 cm in each node, extranodal disease 2.5–5 cm, or clearly positive evidence of involvement by lymphography. Large (L) disease is nodal or extranodal disease larger than 5 cm. Survival appears to be related to the bulk of the disease at the time of treatment. As bulk of disease is likely to have a major effect on the radiation dose required for control, its interaction with the various pathological subgroups will be examined next, in particular how the results of any interaction may affect the decision to use radiation therapy.

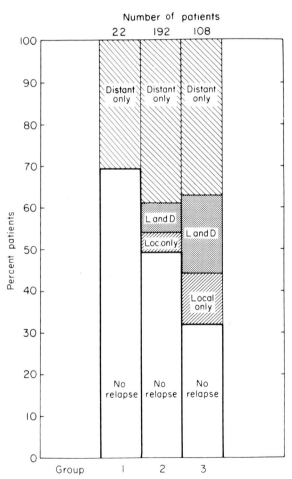

Fig. 6. Patterns of relapse for the patients included in Fig. 5, but assembled into three groups. Group 1: DLWD, DLID. Group 2: NLPD, DLPD, MC, NH. Group 3: DH.

In Fig. 7 the estimates of the frequency of both local and distant relapse are seen to increase with bulk. With S bulk disease, group 2 shows 65% of patients relapse-free, and 48% for group 3. However, when the bulk is classified as M or L, only 20% of patients at risk with DH are expected to be relapse-free 10 years following diagnosis and initial treatment with local regional radiation in the doses we have used. Thirty-five percent (35%) of those in group 2 will be relapse-free and cured. Thus patterns of relapse after local regional therapy also depend strongly on the bulk of disease at the time of treatment.

The age of the patient is important to the physician having to recommend management. Not only does age dictate what treatment may be tolerated, but the lethality of the disease may correlate with increasing age. Logrank analysis of

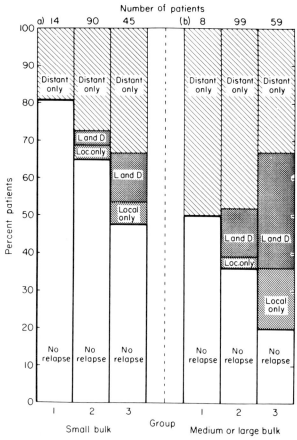

Fig. 7. Patterns of relapse for the groups in Fig. 5, but divided into those with S and M or L bulk. See text for the definition of bulk.

survival data adjusted for bulk of disease and age demonstrates an interaction between these two factors for DH (group 3). This interaction is demonstrated in Table I. The survival data used are corrected for deaths unrelated to disease or treatment, but there is no change in the conclusions even when all deaths are utilized. Clearly, those in group 3 less than 60 years of age with S bulk have fewer disease-related deaths than those in the other subgroups ($p < .0005$). Conversely, those 60 or older with L bulk have nearly twice the expected deaths from disease. These patients, because of their age, are often not included in prospective studies, yet are a major factor in lowering the results of treatment, particularly as reported by radiation therapy centers. The relapse-free rates for each of these subgroups are illustrated in Fig. 8. These data demonstrate that patients younger than 60 with S bulk have a relapse-free survival consistent with 77% being cured as a result of primary treatment by local regional radiation therapy. This appears then to be adequate primary treatment. The remaining three subgroups have relapse-free rates similar to each other. The data demonstrate that relapses still occur out to 8 years following diagnosis when only 21–35% are still relapse-free. Management methods which might improve this relapse-free rate and be tolerated by these patients, who are mostly older than 60 years, need to be studied.

The interaction of age and bulk of disease is not as strong in group 2 (NLPD, DLPD, MC, NH), although interaction is still present. Figure 9 illustrates the relapse-free rates for the same age and bulk classifications as in group 3. As in that group, those younger than 60 with S bulk have a high relapse-free rate (70%) following local regional radiation. Those 60 or older with M or L bulk demonstrate only 25% relapse-free at 5 years, indicating a need for the investigation of other methods of management. The remaining two subgroups demonstrate an intermediate position, between the other two, with approximately 50% of the patients relapsing following treatment. The question arises from these data as to whether other treatment is likely to be more successful than local regional radiation.

TABLE I

A Comparison of the Observed and Expected Relative Death Rates by Age and Bulk[a]

	<60 Years		≥60 Years	
Bulk	O/E	No.	O/E	No.
Small	0.194	22	0.996	23
Medium or large	1.272	29	1.735	30

[a] For patients with stage IA or IIA disease and DH pathology, treated by radiation for cure. The numbers of patients in each subgroup is also given. O, Observed; E, expected.

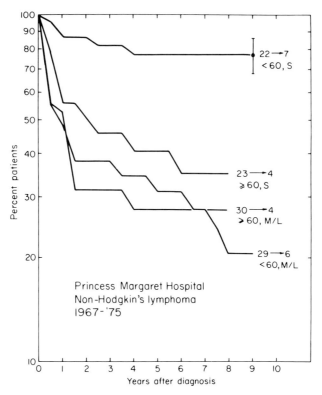

Fig. 8. The relapse-free rates for patients with stage IA or IIA DH lymphoma (group 3) treated radically with radiation, by age and bulk.

Whether radiation therapy alone is appropriate as initial treatment for patients classified as stage IA or IIA depends upon two major considerations:

1. Another modality cannot achieve the same or better outcome for less cost.
2. The overall benefit of combined therapy (radiation plus chemotherapy) is not greater than that of primary radiation therapy followed by radiation or chemotherapy for relapse.

Unfortunately, end points for measuring the cost of treatment are not available, and thus only survival can be compared. In Fig. 10 the corrected survival of all patients younger than 60, with S bulk, are shown together with that of those who had approximately 50% relapse-free rates from group 2. For the 81 (22 + 59) patients in the former grouping, the long-term survival is approximately 90% and remains essentially unchanged from 4 years after diagnosis. We argue that the management policy for these patients should be undisturbed. The 85 patients in

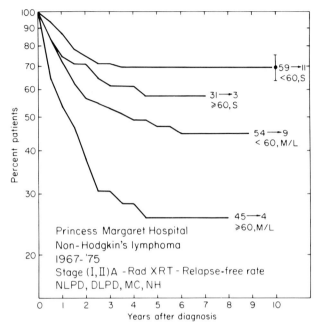

Fig. 9. The relapse-free rates for patients in group 2 by age and bulk.

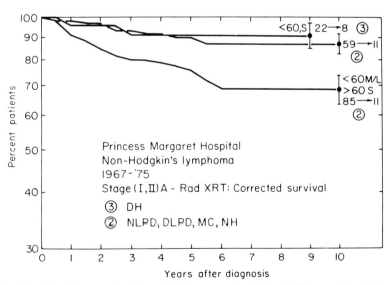

Fig. 10. The 10-year actuarial survival for group-2 patients (<60 years, S and M or L bulk) and group-3 (<60 years, S bulk) patients.

the lowermost curve are all from group 2 and are those also younger than 60 but with M or L disease, together with the remaining S bulk patients. The survival is 70% at 10 years, and there appears to be no subpopulation which dies very quickly after diagnosis and treatment. Comparing the survivals in this figure to the appropriate previous relapse-free curves indicates that approximately 40–50% of the patients who relapse are salvaged by further treatment.

The 166 patients in Fig. 10 comprise 17% of the total lymphoma population. The overall 10-year actuarial corrected survival for this group is 77%. This survival rate follows from a policy of radiation therapy alone as initial treatment, and for 61% of these patients this is all the treatment required. Tables III and IV will simplify the conclusions of this discussion after the following analysis of the remaining subgroups and of the dose–control relationships.

Figure 11 illustrates the survival curves for the remaining patients not included in Fig. 10. The only patients from group 2 are those 60 years or older with M or L bulk. The rest are all the DH patients (group 3) except those younger than 60 with S bulk. Thirty-five percent (35%) survive 8–10 years. Comparison with the relapse-free rates indicates that only 10–15% must be salvaged after treatment for relapse. The survival curves demonstrate that the fraction of the population who die soon after diagnosis and treatment lies within these sub-

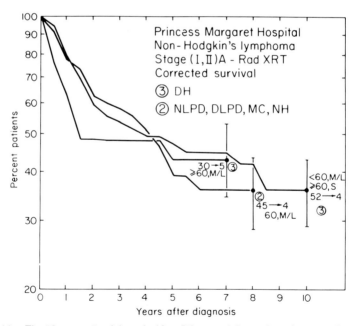

Fig. 11.   The 10-year actuarial survival for all the remaining patients in groups 2 and 3 not included in Fig. 10.

groups of patients. Clearly other approaches to management need to be studied for patients who fall into these categories. However, as the majority are 60 or older, many may not be included in prospective trials utilizing current chemotherapeutic protocols.

Radiation dose is the last factor to be discussed. Figure 12 illustrates the relationship between dose and control by involved region for patients with DH. This is similar to the method used by Fuks and Kaplan (9). The curve is for those with M or L bulk. The dose per fraction ranges between 1 and 3 Gy, with the majority at about 2 Gy. Analysis without the 1-Gy data makes no major difference to the curve. As can be seen, there is a rapid rise in control rate by involved region until the curve appears to plateau at 80–85% for doses of 40 Gy and higher. We can provide no evidence for an advantage of prescribing doses higher than 35–40 Gy. This is similar to the report by Fuks and Kaplan (9), although

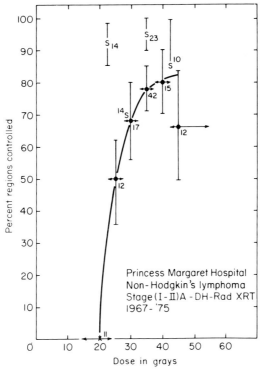

Fig. 12. The dose–regional control curve for stage IA and IIA patients with DH disease, radical radiation, and M or L bulk. Also plotted are the regional control rates for those with S disease. The number of regions at each dose level is shown. The dose range for each data point plotted is illustrated as well as 1 standard error.

they were unable to demonstrate a clear dose–control relationship for DH lymphoma. Also plotted are those with S disease, where the control rate by region involved is seen to be higher than for the M or L bulk regions at equivalent doses. The dose–control curve provides the expected local control rate for patients with stage I, M or L bulk disease. Where two regions are involved with the same bulk, the expected patient control rate is obtained by multiplying the two control rates together.

The local control rate is higher for group 2 than for group 3 (87 versus 70%). With such a high overall regional control rate in group 2 for all doses used, there are so few sites of failure at each dose level that a dose–control curve could not be established. Consequently a logrank analysis was carried out to examine the local control rate with dose, adjusted by bulk and age. The different doses used were grouped into those 34.5 Gy or less and those higher. The average dose in the former was 27.15 Gy, and the latter 37.87 Gy. The dose per fraction (f) varied between 1 and 3 Gy, the majority being about 2 Gy. No confounding of dose, bulk, and age was found, but interaction among all three was detected. For patients younger than 60, with increased bulk, no effect of dose could be demonstrated. The regional control rate, in both low- and high-dose subgroups, was 90%. However, for these 60 or older, M or L bulk was associated with a significantly higher relapse rate than with S ($p = .017$). This was not so in the high-dose subgroup where the effect of bulk disappeared (Table II). Thus, for patients 60 years or older, increasing the dose for increased bulk appears necessary to achieve a regional control rate similar to that achieved for those with S disease. These data imply that 25–30 Gy in 15–20 f is sufficient to achieve 90% local control by region except for those 60 years or older with bulky disease. When two regions are involved, the chance of control by patient falls to an estimated 81% ($0.9 \times 0.9 \times 100$). Thus, it is still appropriate to increase dosage to normal tissue tolerance when there is extensive local regional disease in order to obtain a maximum chance of control for each patient. However, even when only one region is involved, older patients require an increased dose to 35–40 Gy in 20–25 f to achieve a high local control rate if they are to be treated by radiation alone.

TABLE II

A Comparison of the Observed and Expected Regional Failure Rates

Dose (Gy)	O/E	No. of regions
≤34.50	3.4	46
>34.50	0.985	43

[a]For patients in group 2, ≥60 years, with NLPD, DLPD, MC, or NH pathology and M or L bulk, by dose and adjusted by bulk and age. O,Observed; E, expected.

TABLE III

A Summary of the Recommendations for Management of Patients with Stage IA or IIA Non-Hodgkin's Lymphoma, Small Disease[a]

Age	DLWD, DLID[b]	NLPD, MC, NH, DLPD[c]	DH[d]
<60 years	XRT	XRT	XRT
⩾60 years	XRT	XRT	XRT + ChT where possible

[a]XRT, Radiotherapy; ChT, chemotherapy.
[b]XRT, 25–30 G./15–20 f.
[c]XRT, 25–30 G./15–20 f.
[d]XRT, 25–35 G./15–20 f

IV. Conclusions

The preceding analysis of the results of radiotherapy for patients with stage IA or IIA non-Hodgkin's lymphoma seen at the PMH between 1967 and 1975 has tried to identify the factors which are important for the relapse-free survival of patients following treatment. We first examined the correlation of the extent of disease as determined by diagnostic evaluation and the relapse-free survival following local regional irradiation. Correlation was considered poor, and consequently the usefulness of clinical attributes was examined. Those with DH pathology had a higher risk of relapse, both local and distant, than other patients staged in a similar fashion. A strong interaction between bulk of disease and age was demonstrated for DH such that only one group of patients could be recog-

TABLE IV

A Summary of the Recommendations for Management of Patients with Stage IA or IIA Non-Hodgkin's Lymphoma, Medium or Large Disease[a]

Age	DLWD, DLID[b]	NLPD, MC, NH, DLPD[c]	DH[a]
<60 years	XRT	XRT	ChT + XRT
⩾60 years	XRT	XRT +ChT where possible	ChT + XRT

[a]XRT, Radiotherapy; ChT, chemotherapy.
[b]XRT, 25–30 G./15–20 f.
[c]XRT, 35–40 G./20–25 f.
[d]XRT, 35–40 G./20–25 f.

nized as having a good prognosis following radiation therapy alone as primary therapy. These were patients with S bulk, younger than 60 years of age. For patients with a NLPD, DLPD, MC, or NH pathology, the interaction of age and bulk was not so strong. Only patients 60 years or older with M or L bulk had a poor prognosis. The recommendations which follow from this analysis are summarized for the different pathologies and by bulk in Tables III and IV. They are intended for current community practice while prospective studies try to elucidate more clearly the place of radiation and chemotherapy.

References

1. H. Rappaport, *in* ''Atlas of Tumor Pathology'' Sect. 3, Fasc. 8, p. 97. Armed Forces Institute of Pathology, Washington, D.C., 1966.
2. R. S. Bush, M. Gospodarowicz, D. E. Bergsagel, and T. C. Brown, *in* ''Leukemia and Non-Hodgkin's Lymphomas. Advances in Medical Oncology, Research and Education'' (D. G. Crowther, ed), Vol. 7, p. 209. Pergamon, Oxford, 1979.
3. M. V. Peters, *Am. J. Roentgenol.,* **90,** 956 (1963).
4. M. V. Peters, R. S. Bush, T. C. Brown, and J. Reid, *Br. J. Cancer* **31,** Suppl. II, 386 (1975).
5. B. A. Chabner, R. E. Johnson, R. C. Young, G. P. Canellos, S. P. Hubbard, S. K. Johnson, and V. T. DeVita, *Cancer* **42,** 922 (1978).
6. C. S. Portlock, *Semin. Oncol.* **7,** 292 (1980).
7. R. S. Stein, J. Consar, J. M. Flexner *et al., Cancer* **44,** 2236 (1979).
8. S. Monfardini, A. Banfi, G. Bonadonna, F. Rilke, F. Milani, P. Valagussa, and A. Lattuada, *Int. J. Radiat. Oncol., Biol. Phys.* **6,** 125 (1980).
9. Z. Fuks and H. S. Kaplan, *Radiology* **108,** 675 (1973).

29

Radiation Therapy in the Treatment of Advanced Non-Hodgkin's Lymphomas

ELI GLATSTEIN

I. Introduction

During the past 15 years, developments of cancer treatment, both chemotherapeutic and radiotherapeutic, have had a major impact on the treatment of Hodgkin's disease and malignant lymphomas. The approach to patients with advanced (stage III or IV) Hodgkin's disease has been virtually revolutionized from what was formerly a palliative approach to what is now generally a curative approach.

For patients with advanced (stage III or IV) non-Hodgkin's lymphomas, the results of modern treatment are more difficult to interpret. Unequivocally, patients with advanced-stage diffuse histiocytic lymphoma have a chance for a cure with chemotherapy alone that approximates 40% (1). Yet unequivocal evidence for curability of the other advanced non-Hodgkin's lymphomas is sparse, despite modern chemotherapeutic and radiotherapeutic endeavors. To delineate properly the role of radiation therapy in the treatment of non-Hodgkin's lymphomas, the differences between Hodgkin's disease and other malignant lymphomas must be clearly defined, since past strategies of treatment have largely been extrapolations of approaches that proved effective for Hodgkin's disease. The purpose of this article is to review some of the major differences between Hodgkin's disease and malignant lymphomas of the non-Hodgkin's type and to consider some of the possible roles radiotherapy might play in adult patients with advanced non-Hodgkin's lymphomas.

II. Comparisons and Contrasts between Hodgkin's Disease and Non-Hodgkin's Lymphomas

For many years, Hodgkin's disease has been recognized as one in which patients tend to be younger, less debilitated, and more likely to have systemic symptoms than patients with other malignant lymphomas (2, 3) (Table I). The orderly progression of spread in patients with Hodgkin's disease has been known for almost two decades (4). Patients with non-Hodgkin's lymphomas are less

TABLE I

Comparison between Hodgkin's Disease and Non-Hodgkin's Lymphomas

Hodgkin's disease	Non-Hodgkin's lymphomas
Tendency to occur in younger patients	Tendency to occur in older patients
Less debilitated	More debilitated; other illnesses seen
More likely to have B symptoms (30–35%)	Less likely to have B symptoms (10–15%)
Failures more consistent with contiguous spread	Failures less consistent with contiguous spread
More likely to have local-regional presentation (60–70%)	More likely to have advanced stage at presentation (75–80%)
Greater mediastinal involvement, less marrow, mesenteric, and Waldeyer's ring involvement	Greater involvement of mesenteric nodes, Waldeyer's ring, and marrow; less mediastinal involvement
Accepted histopathological classification	At least six different histopathological classifications
Comparatively few stem cells	Presumably most cells are potentially stem cells
Immunological anergy common, dysgammaglobulinemia rare	Dysgammaglobulinemia more common, anergy common

likely to fit the concept of contiguity of spread as postulated for Hodgkin's disease. Even so, the vast majority of patients with non-Hodgkin's lymphomas at presentation who have less than stage IV disease are likely to have tumors involving contiguous sites at diagnosis (5). However, unlike patients with Hodgkin's disease, many patients who *fail* treatment are more likely to fail at noncontiguous sites than those with Hodgkin's disease. Despite this fact, a pattern of failure at relapse appears to be emerging, since patients who fail primary radiotherapy or primary chemotherapy are more likely to have their disease detected in nodes at the time of relapse, previously untreated nodes if treated with conventional irradiation (5), and previously involved sites if treated with chemotherapy (6).

Histopathologically, the classification of Hodgkin's disease has been clarified considerably, and at the present time the diagnosis and classification of this neoplasm (7) is relatively well accepted and comparatively reproducible throughout the world. In contrast, progress in the area of non-Hodgkin's lymphomas has been impeded because of the multiplicity of pathological classification systems (8) which have tended to fragment emerging information and prevent meaningful comparisons from different institutions all over the world.

In the United States, the most popular of the classification systems, the Rappaport (9), depends upon the distinction between follicular or nodular patterns of presentation compared with the diffuse replacement of nodal architecture. Actually, many nodes may have a mixture of both nodular and diffuse elements in the architectural pattern as seen under the microscope. Only relatively recently has this fully been appreciated (10), but it is easy to see how confusion can occur in a specific case concerning whether or not it should be classified as a nodular or indolent pattern versus a diffuse or aggressive pattern of lymphoma. It is not the purpose of this article to review the evidence concerning this important distinction, but merely to acknowledge that the problem of reproducible and consistent categorization exists for all histopathological classifications of non-Hodgkin's lymphomas.

Another important distinction between Hodgkin's disease and non-Hodgkin's lymphomas is the stem cell population involved. One of the confusing aspects of the histological appearance of Hodgkin's disease is the admixture of neoplastic cells with inflammatory cells. The implication of this fact is that much of the mass that we call "tumor" in Hodgkin's disease is probably inflammatory and incapable of neoplastic behavior. Thus, the true stem cell population in patients with Hodgkin's disease may be assumed to be considerably smaller than the stem cell population in patients with non-Hodgkin's lymphomas, in whom the nodal picture is usually one of extensive replacement, either nodular or diffuse, by abnormal cells lacking a major inflammatory component.

It may well be that this comparatively smaller number of neoplastic cells in Hodgkin's disease represents a major reason why modern treatments are relatively far more effective in a curative sense for Hodgkin's disease than they are for patients with non-Hodgkin's lymphomas.

Clinically, patients with non-Hodgkin's lymphomas can be expected to have advanced stage III or IV (Ann Arbor staging classification) in 70–80% of cases. This percentage is somewhat less for patients with diffuse lymphomas and somewhat higher for patients who have nodular lymphoma (2). It is one of the major paradoxes of non-Hodgkin's lymphomas that patients with nodular or comparatively indolent lymphoma tend to have more advanced stage disease at diagnosis than a population of patients with diffuse or more aggressive lymphomas. Staging laparotomies have demonstrated that patients with nodular or indolent histology who appear to have lymphoma clinically confined to the supradiaphragmatic region are likely to have occult abdominal disease at presentation, often in mesenteric nodes (2). On the other hand, staging laparotomies have failed to demonstrate that patients with diffuse or aggressive histologies have been systematically understaged by clinical techniques (2). The explanation for this apparent paradox is not clear, but perhaps reflects the limitations of light microscopy in the interpretation of pathology specimens removed at the time of laparotomy.

III. Responsiveness of Non-Hodgkin's Lymphoma to Treatment

Both radiotherapists and chemotherapists agree that any enhanced survival that can be obtained in these patients will have to come from achieving complete remission from treatment. Definitions of complete remission, i.e., total regression of all evidence of all tumor, depend upon the individual physician caring for the patient. Not only must the patient be reevaluated for the extent of disease at the completion of all treatment but, in addition, regular, careful follow-up examinations with annual bone marrow evaluations and regular surveillance films of the abdomen to monitor the retroperitoneal nodes appear to be almost as important as a careful history and physical examination for these patients.

The list of chemotherapeutic agents that have major response rates against non-Hodgkin's lymphomas is very long; however, very few of these agents have a high (>50%) probability of achieving a complete response by themselves. Even when multiple agents are combined together, the ability to *sterilize* non-Hodgkin's lymphoma appears confined to a relatively small minority of patients, although a complete response can be achieved today in the majority of patients, regardless of histology. The most frequent site of relapse after chemotherapy appears to be nodes (6) and other sites of prior involvement.

In contrast, high-dose (4000 rads or more) irradiation in the treatment of stage I, II, or III non-Hodgkin's lymphomas can not only be expected to have a high degree of complete remission but also a low rate of relapse in the treated fields (5), with the possible exception of diffuse histiocytic lymphoma (11). Many patients reported in the literature with stage I or II disease who fail high-dose radiation therapy have failed on the opposite side of the diaphragm, where radiation was not routinely employed. In the present era of intensive chemotherapy, radiation therapy applied to both sides of the diaphragm is not usually performed, although only a few studies have actually addressed the efficacy of such an approach (12). For advanced lymphoma, the limitations to radiation therapy appear to be (a) the large number and extent of sites requiring prolonged treatment, (b) the possibility of further progression in one area not actively irradiated while a different site is being treated, (c) the significant probability of occult tumor beyond the radiation portals, either other nodes or especially marrow in advanced patients, and (d) general patient status of overall performance. Yet following total lymphoid irradiation, initial relapse in treated sites is comparatively uncommon (e), the converse of the experience with chemotherapy.

IV. Primary Radiotherapy in Advanced Non-Hodgkin's Lymphomas

The results of primary radiotherapy in advanced non-Hodgkin's lymphoma classified by any of the modern classification systems are surprisingly limited. In recent years most of the published literature dealing with this form of treatment has revolved around total body irradiation (TBI). Excellent survival at 5 years has been reported along with a comparatively high complete response rate; however, long-term follow-up shows that virtually all these patients have failed their treatment (13), and thus this approach to treatment must be considered palliative. Thus, the results of TBI, usually used today for patients with an indolent or nodular histology, are comparable to what has been achieved by either single-agent or multiagent chemotherapy (14) for this group of diseases.

The results of high-dose, wide-field total lymphoid irradiation are also surprisingly limited. Wide-field approaches (15) to the abdomen appear essential in primary radiotherapeutic management of non-Hodgkin's lymphomas, because of the high propensity for mesenteric involvement, even at presentation. Thus, the techniques for primary radiotherapy in these diseases must be distinguished carefully from those employed for the treatment of Hodgkin's disease. The Stanford University group published a series of patients with stage III non-Hodgkin's lymphomas who were treated with primary, high-dose (3500 rads or more) total nodal radiotherapy alone (16). The results of treatment in patients with diffuse or aggressive histologies were considered inadequate when compared to the results of combination chemotherapy for diffuse histiocytic lymphoma. Only about 20% of the stage III patients remained free of disease at 5 years, in contrast to the approximately 40% of patients with diffuse histiocytic lymphoma, reported in other series (1), who were cured by combination chemotherapy alone. However, it should be noted that this radiotherapeutic series included *all* histologies and was not confined to diffuse histiocytic lymphoma alone. Unequivocal evidence of the curability of diffuse lymphomas other than the histiocytic type by chemotherapy alone is lacking (17, 18).

The more provocative aspect of the Stanford study was the observation that approximately 35% of nodular lymphoma patients were free of relapse at *10 years* with high-dose, wide-field radiotherapy alone. Although the numbers were modest, they compared quite favorably to the results reported with combination chemotherapy alone (16-18). More importantly, small series reported from other institutions (19, 20) appear to confirm the Stanford observations concerning the prolonged disease-free survival seen in patients with stage III nodular lymphoma who undergo wide-field, high-dose radiotherapy. It should be stressed, however, that in the natural history of patients with nodular lymphoma, 10 years is an insufficient period of time to judge reliably whether or not curative treatment has been delivered. Even so, these results in a relatively heterogeneous population of 51 patients with stage III nodular lymphoma represent a standard to which other treatments for stage III nodular lymphoma may be compared.

V. Combined Modality (Combination Chemotherapy and Radiotherapy) in the Treatment of Advanced Non-Hodgkin's Lymphomas

Given the relatively modest potentially curative results of both primary radiotherapy and primary combination chemotherapy in patients with stage III or IV advanced non-Hodgkin's lymphoma, it is surprising to see how seldom these two modalities have been combined in curative approaches for these patients. The explanation for this fact is not clear, but probably reflects initial euphoria concerning combination chemotherapy in the treatment of diffuse histiocytic lymphoma (as distinct from other histologies) and growing awareness of the potential leukemogenic consequences of combined-modality treatment in Hodgkin's disease (21). It should be noted, however, that the chemotherapy usually associated with this uncommon phenomenon includes procarbazine, a compound particularly well known for its potential leukemogenicity in animal studies (22, 23). Procarbazine is not commonly employed in the treatment of non-Hodgkin's lymphomas.

Total body irradiation has been combined with the chemotherapeutic regimen of cytoxan, vincristine, and prednisone (CVP) and compared to CVP alone in a study at the National Cancer Institute (24). The preliminary results indicated no enhanced responsiveness and no suggestion of benefit in terms of survival or freedom from relapse. The hematological toxicity was more pronounced when the two modalities were combined, as might have been predicted. This study was essentially confined to patients with nodular lymphoma.

In another study, the Stanford group combined high-dose (greater than 4000 rads) total lymphoid irradiation after two cycles of CVP chemotherapy and then followed with additional chemotherapy after the completion of irradiation for patients with stage IV nodular lymphoma (25). The complete response rate, median survival, and actuarial freedom from relapse did not differ from values for patients who were randomized to receive CVP alone or even single-agent chemotherapy. This study was considered a disappointment for combined-modality treatment. However, it should be noted that it was limited to stage IV patients, virtually all of whom had bone marrow involvement. Following the initial two cycles of chemotherapy, the bone marrow was not repeated to verify its ''control''; instead, patients automatically went to high-dose total lymphoid irradiation before CVP was reinstituted after the completion of radiotherapy. The toxicity of such treatment was moderately severe. Even so, one wonders if different results might have been achieved if patients had received enough chemotherapy to induce a *pathologically confirmed* complete remission before integrating the irradiation. The logic for such a possible study is predicated upon the fact that the rate of relapse following intensive chemotherapy for nodular lymphomas appears to be continuous (26), without plateau. Radiation therapy to nodal regions could then be investigated as ''consolidation'' after intensive chemotherapy. This approach, which has been used successfully in patients with advanced Hodgkin's disease (27), has the additional appeal of necessitating probably a lesser dose of irradiation, since patients have achieved a complete remission before initiation of the irradiation. Such an aggressive approach is in progress at the National Cancer Institute (28) for advanced-stage nodular lymphoma (Fig. 1) and is being compared to more conservative management as advocated by Portlock and Rosenberg (29).

For patients with advanced non-Hodgkin's lymphomas of unfavorable histology, the major thrust of investigation for the last decade has been predominantly with combination chemotherapy alone. Such investigation has been important in the development of several different regimens, including C-MOPP (30), BACOP (31, 32), CHOP (33), and COMLA (34), and has demonstrated unequivocally that such regimens are capable of curing a significant proportion of patients with advanced histiocytic lymphoma, approximately 40%. None of these regimens appears to have obvious superiority over the others in terms of results. Patients with large masses, bone marrow involvement, and gastrointestinal involvement appear to represent a particularly poor prognostic group (35). The use of

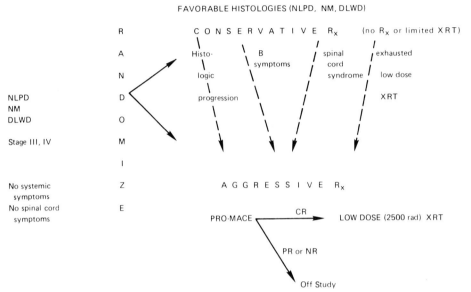

Fig. 1. National Cancer Institute. Advanced-stage (III and IV) non-Hodgkin's lymphoma with a favorable histology. NLPD, Nodular lymphocytic poorly differentiated; NM, nodular mixed; DLWD, diffuse lymphocytic well differentiated; XRT, radiotherapy; CR, complete remission; PR, partial response; NR, no response.

combined-modality treatment in these unfavorable cases has not been systematically undertaken by many investigators. The Stanford group attempted combined-modality approaches in such patients by starting with two cycles of chemotherapy before moving to high-dose total lymphoid radiation which was followed by additional chemotherapy. Such a program was compared to similar chemotherapy alone in a randomized study (12) with some suggestion of benefit, although not major. Again, the timing of the irradiation and chemotherapy and the dose of irradiation were, in retrospect, not optimal with respect to the induction of a true remission by the initial two cycles of chemotherapy. Possibly the use of a more cautiously sequenced combined-modality treatment as described above for nodular lymphomas could still prove to be useful in these patients. Another possibility is the repetitive alternation of several cycles of chemotherapy with large fields of irradiation as reported for advanced Hodgkin's disease (36).

VI. Summary

The role of radiation therapy in the management of advanced non-Hodgkin's lymphomas has not been well defined. In the past, the tendency has been to plan treatment for non-Hodgkin's lymphomas based upon the strategy that has evolved for Hodgkin's disease. Clearly, the differences between these two groups of lymphomas render the simple extrapolation of the details of sequencing of modalities and doses invalid.

The responsiveness of virtually all non-Hodgkin's lymphomas to radiation therapy is excellent; local recurrence at the sites of irradiation is relatively uncommon, with the possible exception of diffuse histiocytic lymphoma. Sites of relapse are usually seen in untreated locations, in sharp distinction to the pattern of relapse seen in patients treated with multiagent chemotherapy.

Primary radiotherapy in advanced non-Hodgkin's lymphoma has been relatively disappointing. Total body irradiation has proved to be a modest palliative maneuver, with no obvious potential for cure. On the other hand, high-dose, wide-field total lymphoid irradiation may possibly have some curative potential in patients with nodular lymphoma, although at least a 15-year follow-up is required before any such conclusion can be made. Certainly, if there is any such curative potential in primary radiotherapy alone, it would have to be restricted to patients with well-documented stage III disease who represent suitable candidates for such a form of treatment. Thus, at best, it would represent a minority of the patient population with advanced non-Hodgkin's lymphoma of the nodular type. For patients with advanced-stage diffuse lymphoma, such treatment is felt to be inappropriate, considering the accomplishments of curative chemotherapy, at least for diffuse histiocytic lymphoma.

Considering the different patterns of relapse as seen in patients with advanced lymphoma treated with radiation alone or chemotherapy alone, one is surprised to see how little investigation with combined-modality treatment has actually taken place. Certainly, the major obstacle to such investigation is determination of the optimal sequencing of chemotherapy and irradiation. Whereas definite benefits have never really been seen from combined-modality treatment as thus far carried out (almost certainly in suboptimal fashion), predictably enhanced toxicity has been seen. Yet, at the present time such studies may hold the key to a future improvement in the survival and freedom from relapse of patients with advanced non-Hodgkin's lymphomas.

References

1. D. L. Sweet and H. M. Golomb, *Semin. Oncol.* **7,** 302–309 (1980).
2. D. R. Goffinet, R. Warnke, N. R. Dunnick, R. A. Castellino, E. Glatstein, T. S. Nelson, R. F. Dorfman, S. A. Rosenberg, and H. S. Kaplan, *Cancer Treat. Rep.* **61,** 981–992 (1977).

3. C. S. Portlock and E. Glatstein, *Annu. Rev. Med.* **29,** 81–91 (1978).
4. S. A. Rosenberg and H. S. Kaplan, *Cancer Res.* **26,** 1225–1231 (1966).
5. Z. Fuks, E. Glatstein, and H. S. Kaplan, *Br. J. Cancer* **31,** 286–297 (1975).
6. P. S. Schein, B. A. Chabner, G. P. Canellos, R. C. Young, and V. T. DeVita, *Cancer* **35,** 354–357 (1975).
7. R. J. Lukes, L. F. Craver, T. C. Hall, H. Rappaport, and T. Rubin, *Cancer Res.* **26,** 1311 (1966).
8. R. F. Dorfman, *Cancer Treat. Rep.* **61,** 945–951 (1977).
9. H. Rappaport, W. J. Winter, and E. B. Hicks, *Cancer* **9,** 792–821 (1956).
10. R. A. Warnke, H. Kim, Z. Fuks, and R. F. Dorfman, *Cancer* **40,** 1229–1233 (1977).
11. Z. Fuks and H. S. Kaplan, *Radiology* **108,** 675–684 (1973).
12. E. Glatstein, S. S. Donaldson, S. A. Rosenberg, and H. S. Kaplan, *Cancer Treat. Rep.* **61,** 1199–1207 (1977).
13. S. C. Carabell, J. T. Chaffey, D. S. Rosenthal, W. C. Moloney, and S. Hellman, *Cancer* **43,** 994–1000 (1979).
14. R. C. Young, R. E. Johnson, G. P. Canellos, B. A. Chabner, H. D. Brereton, C. W. Berard, and V. T. DeVita, *Cancer Treat. Rep.* **61,** 1153–1159 (1977).
15. D. R. Goffinet, E. Glatstein, Z. Fuks, and H. S. Kaplan, *Cancer* **37,** 2797–2805 (1976).
16. E. Glatstein, Z. Fuks, D. R. Goffinet, and H. S. Kaplan, *Cancer* **37,** 2806–2812 (1976).
17. P. S. Schein, B. A. Chabner, G. P. Canellos, R. C. Young, C. W. Berard, and V. T. DeVita, *Blood* **43,** 181–189 (1974).
18. T. Anderson, R. A. Bender, R. I. Fisher, V. T. DeVita, B. A. Chabner, C. W. Berard, L. Norton, and R. C. Young, *Cancer Treat. Rep.* **61,** 1057–1066 (1977).
19. J. D. Cox, *Radiology* **126,** 767–772 (1978).
20. S. H. Levitt, C. D. Bloomfield, and C. K. K. Lee, *Radiology* **118,** 457–459 (1976).
21. C. N. Coleman, C. J. Williams, A. Flint, E. Glatstein, S. A. Rosenberg, and H. S. Kaplan, *N. Engl. J. Med.* **297,** 1249–1252 (1977).
22. M. G. Kelly, R. W. O'Gara, S. T. Yancey, and V. T. Oliverio, *Cancer Chemother. Rep.* **39,** 77–80 (1964).
23. S. M. Sieber, P. Correa, D. W. Dalgard, and R. H. Adamson, *Cancer Res.* **38,** 2125–2134 (1978).
24. H. D. Brereton, R. C. Young, D. L. Longo, L. R. Kirkland, C. W. Berard, E. S. Jaffe, V. T. DeVita, and R. E. Johnson, *Cancer* **43,** 2227–2231, (1979).
25. C. S. Portlock, S. A. Rosenberg, E. Glatstein, and H. S. Kaplan, *Blood* **47,** 747–755 (1976).
26. E. M. McKelvey and T. E. Moon, *Cancer Treat. Rep.* **61,** 1185–1190 (1977).
27. L. R. Farber, L. R. Prosnitz, E. C. Cadman, R. Lutes, J. R. Bertino, and D. B. Fischer, *Cancer* **46,** 1509–1517 (1980).
28. B. A. Chabner, *Ann. Intern. Med.* **90,** 115–117 (1979).
29. C. S. Portlock and S. A. Rosenberg, *Ann. Intern. Med.* **90,** 10–13 (1979).
30. V. T. DeVita, G. P. Canellos, B. A. Chabner, P. S. Schein, S. P. Hubbard, R. C. Young, *Lancet* **1,** 248–250 (1975).
31. P. S. Schein, V. T. DeVita, S. Hubbard, B. A. Chabner, G. P. Canellos, C. W. Berard, and R. C. Young, *Ann. Intern. Med.* **85,** 417–422 (1976).
32. A. T. Skarin, D. S. Rosenthal, W. C. Moloney, and E. Frei, *Blood* **49,** 759–770 (1977).
33. E. M. McKelvey, J. A. Gottlieb, H. E. Wilson, A. Haut, R. W. Talley, R. Stephens, M. Lane, J. F. Gamble, S. E. Jones, P. N. Grozea, J. Gutterman, C. Coltman, Jr., and T. E. Moon, *Cancer* **38,** 1484–1493 (1976).
34. E. Cadman, L. Farber, D. Berd, and J. Bertino, *Cancer Treat. Rep.* **61,** 1109–1116 (1977).
35. R. I. Fisher, V. T. DeVita, and B. L. Johnson, *Am. J. Med.* **63,** 177–182 (1977).
36. R. T. Hoppe, C. S. Portlock, E. Glatstein, S. A. Rosenberg, and H. S. Kaplan, *Cancer* **43,** 472–481 (1979).

30

The Stanford Randomized Trials of the Treatment of Hodgkin's Disease: 1967–1980

SAUL A. ROSENBERG, HENRY S. KAPLAN, RICHARD T. HOPPE, PAULA KUSHLAN, AND SANDRA HORNING

I. Introduction

The Stanford University Medical Center randomized trials of the treatment of Hodgkin's disease were initiated in 1962. At that time, primary treatment options were limited to various radiation plans for clinically staged (CS) patients of stage I, II, or III extent. These protocols were extensively revised in 1967–1968, when laparotomy staging (PS) became routine, and nitrogen mustard–vincristine–procarbazine–prednisone (MOPP) chemotherapy became available. Thereafter, patients with all stages of disease were studied. The use of MOPP as an adjuvant after irradiation was the major question tested in studies from 1968 to 1974 for patients with pathological stage (PS) I, II, and III disease, including those with limited extranodal disease, defined as the E lesion in the Ann Arbor system (1).

A pilot study on the use of irradiation as an adjuvant to MOPP for patients with PS IV disease was initiated during that period as well. In 1974, based on the preliminary results of these combined-modality studies, new protocols were initiated. These studies tested minimal radiotherapy fields followed by adjuvant MOPP for patients with PS IA and IIA disease, procarbazine–Alkeran–vinblastine (PAVe) chemotherapy as a less acutely toxic alternative to MOPP as an adjuvant for patients with PS II_E and III disease, and alternating combined-modality therapy for patients with PS IIIB and IV disease. The details and results of these randomized trials have been presented and published in previous reports (2–7).

This article will summarize and update the Stanford randomized trials for the treatment of Hodgkin's disease during the 1967–1980 period. This will provide a maximum of 12 years follow-up for the first adjuvant MOPP studies.

II. Patient Selection and Study Design

The details of patient eligibility, diagnostic studies employed, and protocol designs have been previously described (4). The major features of eligibility and the major diagnostic studies utilized were:

1. The patient was 16–65 years of age, inclusive.
2. The patient had received no prior therapy.
3. The patient's permanent residence was within 300 miles of the Stanford University Medical Center.
4. Bipedal lymphography and bone marrow biopsy were employed in all patients.
5. A staging laparotomy with a splenectomy was used increasingly in 1967 and routinely after July 1968, except for patients with PS IV disease.

The Stanford H-1 protocol, initiated in 1967 for patients with PS IA and IIA disease, compared involved-field (IF) radiotherapy with subtotal or total lymphoid irradiation (STLI or TLI). Though this was not a study of adjuvant or combined-modality therapy, the results are relevant to the general discussion.

The Stanford H-2, -3, and -4 protocol designs, initiated in 1968 for patients with PS, IB, IIB, IIIA, and IIIB with or without E lesions tested the value of six cycles of adjuvant MOP(P) (prednisone was withheld if the patient had received mediastinal irradiation) following TLI for these stages of disease.

The Stanford H-5 protocol was initiated in 1968 for patients with PS III_SA and III_SB (and II_S) disease. In this protocol, patients treated with irradiation alone received treatment to the entire liver as well as TLI.

The Stanford H-7 protocol, initiated in 1968 for patients with PS IV disease (except PS IV_H), received TLI as an adjuvant after six cycles of MOPP (H-7) or, as modified in the K-7 study, "sandwiched" after three cycles of MOPP compared to six cycles of MOPP alone.

The R-1 and K-1 protocols, initiated in 1970 for patients with PS IA and IIA disease, compared radiotherapy alone, usually STLI, to STLI followed by six cycles of adjuvant MOP(P). A small group of relatively favorable cases received only IF radiotherapy followed by six cycles of MOP(P) in the adjuvant trial. A total of 363 patients was enrolled in these studies.

In 1974, the S studies were initiated, replacing all previous studies, except for patients with PS IB and IIB disease who continued in the H-2 study. These studies have been detailed previously (6). There were eight different protocols: involved-field radiotherapy followed by adjuvant MOP(P) for PS IA and IIA disease (S-1 study); PAVe as an alternate adjuvant for MOP(P) for PS II_E and IIIA disease (S-2, S-3, and S-4 studies); alternating MOP(P) or PAVe with TLI and hepatic irradiation for PS III_SB disease (S-5 study); and various combined-modality approaches for PS IV disease (S-6, S-7, and S-8 studies) utilizing MOPP and TLI. A total of 235 patients was enrolled in these studies when they were discontinued in 1980.

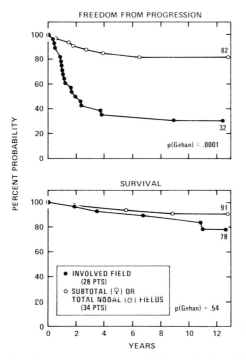

Fig. 1. Results of Stanford randomized trial for PS IA and IIA Hodgkin's disease, initiated in 1967.

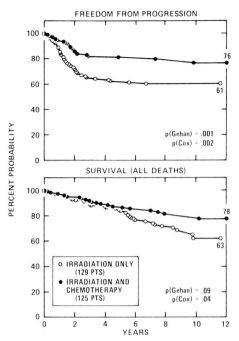

Fig. 2. Results of Stanford randomized trials of adjuvant MOP(P) chemotherapy for PS I, II, and III Hodgkin's disease, initiated in 1968 and 1970.

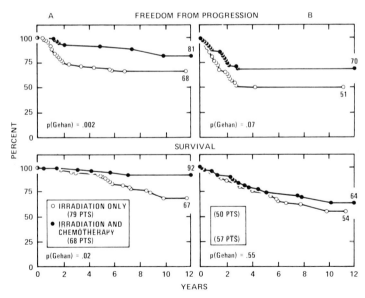

Fig. 3. Results of Stanford randomized trials of adjuvant MOP(P) chemotherapy for PS I, II, and III Hodgkin's disease, initiated in 1968 and 1970, comparing asymptomatic (A) and symptomatic (B) patients.

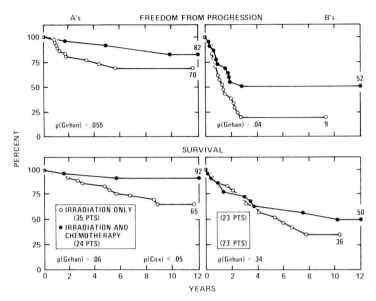

Fig. 4. Results of Stanford randomized trial for PS IIIA and IIIB Hodgkin's disease, initiated in 1968, comparing asymptomatic (A) and symptomatic (B) patients.

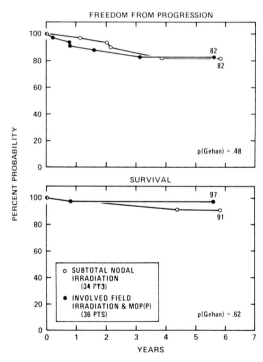

Fig. 5. Results of Stanford randomized trial for PS IA and IIA Hodgkin's disease, initiated in 1974.

517

III. Results

The major end points of these randomized trials are seen in actuarial survival and relapse-free survival (also called freedom from progression, FFP) curves.

The results of the H-1 trial (Fig. 1) are of special interest. In these relatively favorable cases, an early and highly significant advantage of STLI or TLI was evident in FFP. However, even after 12 years, a significant impact on survival is not evident, though there may be a beginning separation of the survival curves after 10 years. The importance and interpretation of these observations will be discussed.

The results of the adjuvant MOP(P) trials (H-2, -3, -4, and -5) are summarized in Fig. 2. As previously reported, when the study groups are combined, a highly significant improvement in FFP in the adjuvant MOP(P) group is evident, and a survival advantage for patients receiving MOP(P) is probable. If these results are looked at in more detail, it can be seen that the advantages of adjuvant MOP(P) are most significant for asymptomatic patients (Fig. 3), especially those with PS IIIA disease (Fig. 4). Patients with PS IIIB do poorly with TLI and hepatic irradiation alone, as compared to the combined-modality approach. It is not clear

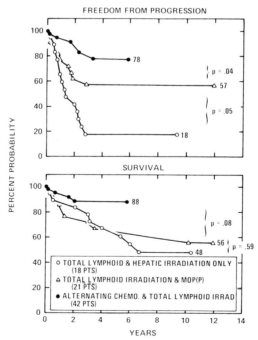

Fig. 6.   Results of Stanford randomized trials for PS IIIB Hodgkin's disease, initiated in 1968 and 1974.

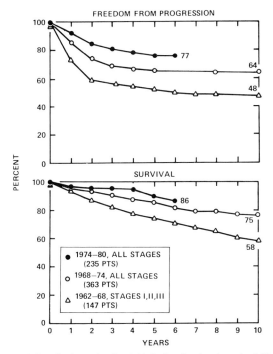

Fig. 7. Results of Stanford randomized trials for the treatment of Hodgkin's disease during three eras, 1962–1968, 1968–1974, and 1974–1980.

from these data, however, whether the combined-modality program is superior to MOPP alone for PS IIIB disease, which was not tested.

In the pilot study on 33 patients with PS IV disease (H-7, K-7) testing combined-modality therapy, there was no benefit of adjuvant radiotherapy after MOPP chemotherapy.

The results of the S-1 study demonstrate after 6 years that adjuvant MOP(P) can replace extended-field irradiation to clinically uninvolved sites without compromise of excellent disease-free and actuarial survival (Fig. 5). The PAVe adjuvant study demonstrated equivalent efficacy of PAVe and MOP(P) as adjuvants and the considerably less acute toxicity of the PAVe program (8).

The S-5 protocol of alternating chemotherapy and radiotherapy for PS IIIB disease demonstrated considerable improvement in survival and disease-free survival, as compared retrospectively to previous management programs of TLI alone or TLI followed by MOP(P) chemotherapy (Fig. 6) (9).

The combined-modality protocols of PS IV disease have too few patients enrolled to draw firm conclusions but suggest improved survival as compared to the previous H-7, K-7 series.

The overall results for all patients treated in these protocol studies have improved during the three major treatment eras (Fig. 7). The S studies enrolling patients of all stages from 1974 to 1980 have resulted in the overall probability of FFP of 77% and an actuarial survival of 86% at 6 years.

IV. Treatment Complications

The acute and late toxicity and morbidities of modern management of Hodgkin's disease are considerable and are well described in the literature. The major problems are listed in Table I. Though some of these complications are fatal, the overall survival of patients treated with these methods has continued to improve. Nonetheless, as these effects of treatment have been recognized, modifications of therapy techniques have been employed which have resulted in a marked reduction in or elimination of problems of radiation pneumonitis, radiation carditis, and bone growth abnormalities in children.

The major serious treatment complications are the long-term problems of sterility in men after combination chemotherapy and sterility in women after combined-modality therapy, which includes pelvic irradiation (10, 11), and acute myelomonocytic leukemia, especially after combined-modality therapy (12). We have also observed an increased incidence of unfavorable diffuse non-Hodgkin's lymphoma occurring many years after the combined-modality treatment programs (13).

V. Discussion

The survival of patients with Hodgkin's disease has increased dramatically during the period of these studies. This is especially true for patients with the

TABLE I

Major Complications of the Therapy of Hodgkin's Disease

Radiation pneumonitis
Radiation carditis
Radiation bone growth abnormalities in children
Hypothyroidism
Male sterility after combination chemotherapy
Female sterility after combined-modality therapy
Acute myelomonocytic leukemia
Non-Hodgkin's lymphoma, diffuse, large-cell type
Opportunistic infections
Prolonged immunosuppression
Psychosocial problems

most favorable stages of the disease, even those who have suffered one or more relapses. Patients who relapse after initial radiation programs for favorable disease have a high probability of subsequent cure (salvage) and prolonged survival as a result of MOP(P) chemotherapy. Even patients who are destined to succumb to the disease may survive for 10 or more years because of the excellent palliative programs utilized in these protocol settings.

The H-1 study is an example of the difficulty in demonstrating a survival advantage of two treatment programs, one (TLI or STLI) much superior to the other (IF) in resulting in durable initial control of the disease. Potentially curative salvage treatment programs are very effective for patients in the IF group in prolonging survival for 10 years at least after initial relapse.

This is also evident in the adjuvant MOP(P) trials. Survival advantages are not apparent or significant for the first 5 years, despite definite improvement in FFP for various stages of Hodgkin's disease as a result of combined-modality therapy. Survival advantages of 10–20% in these studies are often statistically not significant because of the limited numbers of patients studied or because adequate numbers of patients are not at risk for the full 10 years or more which may be required.

Even if a 10–20% survival advantage is eventually realized in several of these treatment groups, the long-term serious treatment complications challenge us to modify our treatment programs. We must attempt to reduce not only the acute toxicity of therapy but also the serious or fatal late complications of sterility and acute leukemia.

Undoubtedly, the alkylating agents, including procarbazine, contribute significantly to both sterility and leukemogenesis. There is abundant clinical and animal documentation of these effects. It would be desirable to have available as an adjuvant chemotherapy regimen a combination of drugs which theoretically has a much lower risk of inducing these serious problems. The adriamycin-bleomycin–vinblastine–dacarbazine (ABVD) program of Bonadonna to date has not been associated with male sterility nor secondary acute leukemia (14). Adriamycin has another potentially serious long-term problem, however, cardiotoxicity. In addition, a longer period of at least 10 years may be required to be assured of a low leukemia risk following adriamycin.

VI. Future Studies

The next series of trials of the treatment of Hodgkin's disease at Stanford, initiated in the fall of 1980, represent the fourth major change since 1962. A major feature of these studies is to test an adjuvant with less acute toxicity and less risk of inducing sterility and leukemia. Selected subgroups will be treated without exploratory laparotomy staging, because combined-modality programs appear indicated. Even more aggressive treatment programs will be compared for the most unfavorable settings of the disease. Special attention will be directed toward improved salvage programs for patients who relapse, and toward quantitating, as much as possible, treatment effects on fertility and on cardiac, pulmonary, and bone marrow function. We will also attempt to judge the psychosocial and economic impacts of these complex therapies.

Acknowledgments

This study was supported by grants CA-05838, CA-09287, and CA-21555 from the National Cancer Institute, and by a gift from the Bristol-Myers Company.

References

1. P. P. Carbone, H. S. Kaplan, K. Musshoff, *et al.*, Report of the committee on Hodgkin's disease staging classification. *Cancer Res.* **31**, 1860 (1971).
2. M. R. Moore, J. M. Bull, S. E. Jones, *et al.*, Sequential radiotherapy and chemotherapy in the treatment of Hodgkin's disease: A progress report. *Ann. Intern. Med.* **77**, 1 (1972).
3. S. A. Rosenberg, M. R. Moore, J. M. Bull, *et al.*, Combination chemotherapy and radiotherapy for Hodgkin's disease. *Cancer* (*Philadelphia*) **30**, 1505 (1972).
4. S. A. Rosenberg and H. S. Kaplan, The management of stages I, II, and III Hodgkin's disease with combined radiotherapy and chemotherapy. *Cancer* (*Philadelphia*) **35**, 55 (1975).
5. S. A. Rosenberg, H. S. Kaplan, E. Glatstein, *et al.*, The role of adjuvant MOPP in the radiation therapy of Hodgkin's disease: A progress report after eight years on the Stanford trials. *In* "Adjuvant Therapy of Cancer" Proceedings of the International Conference, Amsterdam, (S. E. Salmon and S. E. Jones, eds.), p. 505. Elsevier/North-Holland Biomedical Press, Amsterdam and New York, 1977.
6. S. A. Rosenberg, H. S. Kaplan, E. Glatstein, *et al.*, Combined modality therapy of Hodgkin's disease: A report on the Stanford trials. *Cancer* (*Philadelphia*) **42**, 991 (1978).
7. S. A. Rosenberg, H. S. Kaplan, and B. W. Brown, Jr., The role of adjuvant MOPP in the therapy of Hodgkin's disease: An analysis after ten years. *In* "Adjuvant Therapy of Cancer II" (S. E. Jones and S. E. Salmon, eds.), p. 109. Grune and Stratton, New York, 1979.
8. E. M. Wolin, S. A. Rosenberg, and H. S. Kaplan, A randomized comparison of PAVe and MOP(P) as adjuvant chemotherapy for Hodgkin's disease. *In* "Adjuvant Therapy of Cancer II" (S. E. Jones and S. E. Salmon, eds.), p. 119. Grune & Stratton, New York, 1979.
9. R. T. Hoppe, C. S. Portlock, E. Glatstein, *et al.*, Alternating chemotherapy and irradiation in the treatment of advanced Hodgkin's disease. *Cancer* (*Philadelphia*) **43**, 472 (1979).
10. R. M. Chapman, S. B. Sutcliffe, L. H. Rees, *et al.*, Cyclical combination chemotherapy and gonadal function: retrospective study in males. *Lancet* **1**, 284 (1979).
11. S. Horning, R. T. Hoppe, H. S. Kaplan, *et al.*, Female reproductive potential after treatment for Hodgkin's disease. *N. Engl. J. Med.* **304**, 1377 (1981).
12. C. N. Coleman, J. S. Burke, A. Varghese, S. A. Rosenberg, and H. S. Kaplan, this volume, Chapter 16.
13. J. G. Krikorian, J. S. Burke, S. A. Rosenberg, *et al.*, Occurrence of non-Hodgkin's lymphoma after therapy for Hodgkin's disease. *N. Engl. J. Med.* **300**, 452 (1979).
14. P. Valagussa, A. Santoro, R. Kenda, *et al.*, Second malignancies in Hodgkin's disease: Complications of certain forms of treatment. *Br. Med. J.* **280**, 216 (1980).

31

The Role of Combined Radiotherapy and Chemotherapy in the Primary Management of Hodgkin's Disease: Southwest Oncology Group Studies

CHARLES A. COLTMAN, JR., JOSEPH W. MYERS,
ELEANOR MONTAGUE, LILLIAN A. FULLER, PETRE N. GROZEA,
EDWARD J. DE PERSIO, AND DENNIS O. DIXON

I. Introduction

Properly applied radiotherapy is curative in greater than 80% of patients with stage I or II Hodgkin's disease (1). Chemotherapy consisting of mechlorethamine, vincristine, procarbazine, and prednisone (MOPP) is now curative in 55% of patients with advanced Hodgkin's disease (2). In 1971, the Southwest Oncology Group began its first combined-modality study on pathologically staged IIB, IIIA, and IIIB Hodgkin's disease (3). At that time the management of patients with stage IIB or IIIB disease with radiotherapy alone was less favorable (4). The study (CAR 1, SWOG 160) was designed to combine MOPP chemotherapy with total nodal radiotherapy in patients with laparotomy-staged IIB, IIIA, and IIIB Hodgkin's disease. The sequence of MOPP followed by radiotherapy was chosen to determine the safety and effectiveness with which total nodal radiotherapy could be delivered following MOPP chemotherapy. Further objectives were to control B symptoms promptly and to reduce bulk disease and thus minimize the size of the radiotherapy ports. This single-arm phase-1 study allowed gradual escalation of the dose of MOPP from three to six cycles as tolerance to radiotherapy was demonstrated.

A year later the Southwest Oncology Group, in February 1972, began a study of combined-modality therapy (involved-field radiotherapy plus six cycles of MOPP) in pathologically staged IA, IB, IIA, and IIB Hodgkin's disease (RAC 1, SWOG 781) (5). This study moved MOPP chemotherapy, so effective in advanced disease (2), into the management of localized Hodgkin's disease (stages I and II) and compared the standard treatment extended-field radiotherapy, to involved-field radiotherapy plus six cycles of MOPP.

The initial Southwest Oncology Group combined-modality study (CAR 1, SWOG 160) clearly demonstrated that MOPP, followed by total nodal radiotherapy, could be given to patients with stage IIB, IIIA, or IIIB disease with safety and excellent survival (3). The survival data were at least as good as those for total nodal radiotherapy followed by six cycles of MOPP (4) and clearly better than those for radiotherapy alone (6, 7).

In 1974, the Southwest Oncology Group had successfully added bleomycin, in low doses, to MOPP (MOPP 4, SWOG 774) with a complete response rate of 84%, the best group result to date (8). Based on the results of these two studies, in 1975, the group undertook a third combined-modality study (CAR 2, SWOG 7518) on Hodgkin's disease. Patients with pathologically staged IIIA or IIIB disease were randomly assigned to treatment with MOPP plus low-dose bleomycin for 10 cycles or MOPP plus low-dose bleomycin for 3 cycles followed by total nodal radiotherapy. This article will detail the current status of the first two studies and comment briefly on the preliminary results of the third.

II. Patients and Methods

A. All Studies

All three studies were conducted by the membership of the Southwest Oncology Group. All patients had histologically proven Hodgkin's disease, and tissue was submitted for review by the Pathology Panel and Repository for Lymphoma Clinical Studies. Those found not to have Hodgkin's disease on review were not eligible for the study. All patients provided a complete history and underwent a physical examination with appropriate laboratory studies. Preoperative clinical staging included isotope scans, metastatic bone survey, and a bipedal lymphograph. A full chest tomography (for those with hilar node enlargement) and a bone marrow biopsy were performed. All patients were required to undergo an exploratory laparotomy and splenectomy for complete pathological staging. Patients between the ages of 10 and 65 years (SWOG 781 and 160), free of other systemic illness and who had had no prior chemotherapy or radiotherapy, were eligible. There were no age restrictions in SWOG 7518. All patients gave their informed consent and were available for long-term follow-up.

The minimum requirements for radiotherapy included (1) supervoltage irradiation equipment with a minimum energy of 2 MeV, (2) central and off-axis tumor dose measurements, (3) beam verification films, (4) a tumor dose rate of 850–1000 rads total basic tumor dose per week, (5) a 4000- to 4500-rad total basic tumor dose, (6) additional treatment for residual disease through reduced fields at the same or a slightly higher tumor dose rate for a total of 500–2000 rads, (7) avoidance of doses above 4000 rads to the heart and spinal cord, (8) avoidance of doses over 4500 rads to the canda equina, gut, and upper mediastinum, (9) treatment of hila only if involved, (10) reduction in mediastinal fields with response of tumor, and (11) weekly complete blood counts, with radiation interrupted for granulocyte counts of $1000/\mu l$ and platelet counts of $60,000/\gamma l$.

Following the termination of all treatment, patients in all studies were followed in unmaintained remission at monthly intervals for 6 months, at two monthly intervals for 6 months, at four monthly intervals for 2 years, and yearly until relapse. No definitive secondary or tertiary therapy was prescribed at the time of relapse. In general, however, radiotherapy was used for local recurrence (marginal, geographical miss, or transdiaphragmatic extension), and MOPP chemotherapy was used for involved-field recurrences and extranodal extensions.

Freedom from relapse is defined as the time from treatment start to the time of disease progression (relapse). Freedom from relapse and overall survival curves were plotted by the method of Kaplan and Meier (9), and survival curves were compared by the Gehan modification of the generalized Wilcoxon test (10) as well as the logrank test (11). Tumor mortality refers to those patients who died of progressive Hodgkin's disease. Patients who died of causes other than Hodgkin's disease are shown as censored data on tumor mortality curves (2).

B. Stages I and II (SWOG 781)

Eligible patients with pathological stage IA, IB, IIA, or IIB Hodgkin's disease were randomly assigned to extended-field radiotherapy (mantle and paraaortic iiradiation for upper torso presentations) or to involved-field radiotherapy followed by six cycles of MOPP. Three patients with pelvic disease, other than unilateral inguinal adenopathy, received the mantle and inverted Y. Those with high neck nodes and those with unilateral inguinal adenopathy, proven by lymphography and laparotomy, were excluded from the study.

Following completion of involved-field radiotherapy and a 4-week rest period, MOPP chemotherapy, as previously described (12), was instituted for a total of six cycles. Prednisone was administered for 10 days during the first and fourth cycles at a dose of 40 mg/m^2 per day.

C. Stages IIB, IIIA, and IIIB (SWOG 160)

Eligible patients with pathological stage IIB, IIIA, or IIIB Hodgkin's disease were entered in this single-arm study. The initial treatment consisted of three cycles of MOPP (12). A minimum of 4 weeks, or until marrow recovery (maximum of 10 weeks), elapsed from the last course of MOPP to the start of radiotherapy. All patients received total nodal radiotherapy, except for those treated at the M.D. Anderson Hospital where total abdominal radiotherapy, rather than the inverted Y port, was employed (7/143 patients).

The area of major and symptomatic involvement prior to chemotherapy was the first area to be treated with radiotherapy. In the majority of patients, disease above the diaphragm was treated first with anterior and posterior extended (mantle) fields excluding normal lung. Radiation below the diaphragm started from 6 to 8 weeks following completion of the mantle port. The abdominal field covered the inguinal, femoral, and deep iliac nodes, bilaterally, together with the paraaortic nodes and the splenic pedicle. Treatment to the abdominal nodes was given in one course or, in patients with poor tolerance to radiation therapy (poor tolerance to chemotherapy, excessive weight loss, and continuing disability), in two courses. In these cases, the upper two-thirds of the abdominal nodes were treated first and, following a 4- to 8-week break, the pelvic and femoral nodes. With total abdominal radiotherapy a 3000-rad tissue dose was delivered in 4–5 weeks, and an additional 1000-rad tumor dose delivered through reduced fields to residual disease.

D. Stages IIIA and IIIB (SWOG 7518)

Eligible patients with pathological stage IIIA or IIIB Hodgkin's disease were randomly assigned to MOPP plus low-dose bleomycin for 10 cycles, as previously described (8), or to MOPP plus low-dose bleomycin for 3 cycles followed by total nodal radiotherapy. The radiotherapy consisted of an upper mantle, beginning 4 weeks (maximum 10 weeks) after the end of 3 cycles of chemotherapy, followed by an inverted Y. This study featured systematic restaging at the end of the induction phase to define the completeness of response.

III. Results

A. Stages I and II (SWOG 781)

Between February 1972 and August 1978, the 230 eligible patients with pathological stage IA, IB, IIA, or IIB disease were randomly assigned to extended-field radiotherapy (114) and involved-field radiotherapy plus six cycles of MOPP (116). Table I shows the comparability of the treatment groups with respect to sex, age, histology, stage, and mediastinal involvement. There are no statistically significant differences between the two groups. The longest follow-up is now 8 years. Figure 1 shows the freedom from relapse and survival for all 230 patients. Freedom from relapse has just reached the 75th percentile, and overall survival has not yet reached the 80th percentile. Figure 2 compares patients with stage IA or IIA disease with those with stage IB or IIB disease with respect to freedom from relapse and survival. The data show that stage IB and IIB patients have a significantly lower freedom from relapse ($p = .001$) and survival ($p < .001$) than those with stage IA or IIA disease, irrespective of treatment.

Those patients (all stages) treated by involved-field radiotherapy plus MOPP have a significantly better freedom from relapse than those treated by extended-field radiotherapy [p (logrank) $= .048$]. There is, however no survival advantage

TABLE I

Stage I and II Hodgkin's Disease (RAC 1, SWOG 781): Comparability of Treatment Groups

Characteristic	EFXRT	IF + MOPP	p Value
Sex			
Male	66	60	.88
Age			
<20	17	20	.72
20–39	78	80	.63
40–59	15	15	.59
>59	4	1	.40
Histology			
Lymphocyte predominance	6	3	—
Mixed cellularity	24	31	.59
Nodular sclerosis	81	81	.33
Stage			
IA	22	25	.53
IB	3	1	.51
IIA	69	66	.96
IIB	20	24	.82
Mediastinal involvement	62	67	.91

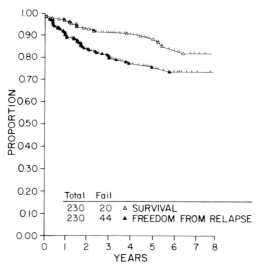

Fig. 1. Stage I and II Hodgkin's disease (RAC 1, SWOG 781). Freedom from relapse and overall survival for all 230 patients.

[p (Gehan) = .69]. This relapse-free survival advantage for the combined modality is seen among patients with stage IB or IIB disease [p (logrank) = .02] but not with stage IA or IIA disease [p (logrank) = .417] (Fig. 3). There is, however, no survival advantage in either the stage IA and IIA or IB and IIB groups.

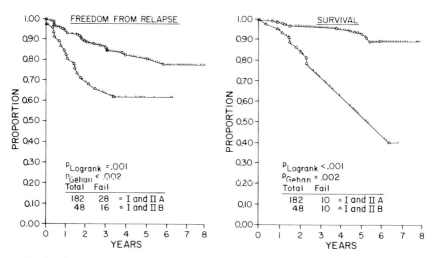

Fig. 2. Stage I and II Hodgkin's disease (RAC 1, SWOG 781). Comparison of stages IA and IIA with IB and IIB with respect to freedom from relapse and survival.

Figure 4 examines the two modalities with respect to freedom from relapse and survival among patients with mediastinal involvement. This plot takes into consideration only the presence or absence of a prominent mediastinum, not its relative size. There is a freedom-from-relapse advantage for the combined-modality compared to the extended-field radiotherapy [p (logrank) = .03], but again no survival advantage is seen [p (Gehan) = .61]. This freedom-from-relapse advantage is seen only among patients with stage IB or IIB disease [p (Gehan) = .03] and not with stage IA or IIA disease [p (Gehan) = .6]. Histology does not have an effect, as yet, on freedom from relapse or survival. Table II examines the sites of relapse in the two limbs of the study. Extranodal sites of relapse occurred almost three times as frequently among patients treated with extended-field radiotherapy (p = .014).

Table III lists the causes of death among patients on the two limbs. Ten patients have died on each limb of the protocol. A total of 10 (4.3%) died of progressive Hodgkin's disease, 4 on the extended-field radiotherapy and 6 on the involved-field radiotherapy plus MOPP limbs. Of real concern is the fact that 2 patients, on the combined-modality limb of the study, developed acute leukemia and died. The first patient was a 37-year-old male who had stage IIB Hodgkin's disease and had treatment initiated on 6/27/72. A month into involved-field radiotherapy, he developed advancing disease outside the radiotherapy field and progressed immediately to MOPP for six cycles. He remained in complete remission until 11/77, when marrow aplasia developed. Acute myelomonocytic leukemia was diagnosed in 7/78, and the patient died 12/20/78, having failed to achieve a complete remission on therapy with daunorubicin, arabinosyl cytosine,

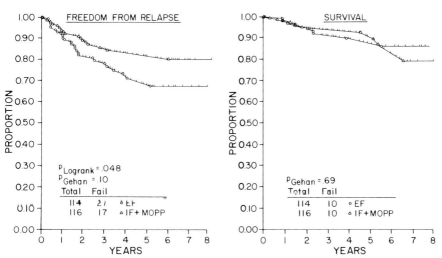

Fig. 3. Stage I and II Hodgkin's disease (RAC 1, SWOG 781). Comparison of involved-field (IF) radiotherapy plus MOPP with extended-field (EF) radiotherapy with respect to freedom from relapse and survival.

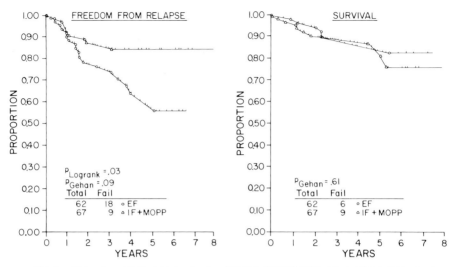

Fig. 4. Stage I and II Hodgkin's disease (RAC 1, SWOG 781). Comparison of involved-field (IF) radiotherapy plus MOPP with extended-field (EF) radiotherapy in patients with mediastinal involvement with respect to freedom from relapse and survival.

TABLE II

Stage I and II Hodgkin's Disease (RAC 1, SWOG 781): Sites of Relapse with Extended-Field Radiotherapy Compared to Involved-Field Radiotherapy plus MOPP

Site	Extended field	Involved-field + MOPP	p Value
Extranodal	17	6	.014
Lung	9[a]	4[b]	
Pleura	4	—	
Bone	1	1	
Bowel	1	—	
Epidural	1	—	
Soft Tissue	1 (chest wall)	1 (breast)	
Nodal	10	10	
Unknown	—	1	
Total	27	17	.048[c]

[a] 2/9 M+
[b] ¼P + and ¼ Brain +
[c] Logrank test.

TABLE III

Stage I and II Hodgkin's Disease (RAC 1, SWOG 781): Causes of Death among Patients Treated with Extended-Field Radiotherapy Compared to Those Treated with Involved-Field Radiotherapy plus MOPP

Cause	EFXRT (114)	IF + MOPP (116)
Progressive disease	4	6
Acute leukemia	—	2[a]
Oat cell of lung	1	—
Infection	2	1
Cardiogenic shock	1	—
Trauma	1	—
Pulmonary embolus	1	—
Unknown	—	1
	10	10

[a] $p = .50$ (Fisher exact).

and 6-thioguanine. The second patient was a 55-year-old male who had stage IIA Hodgkin's disease and began combined-modality treatment on 1/16/75. Therapy was completed 9/75, and the patient was followed in unmaintained remission until 7/6/79 when admitted with fever and chills. Bone marrow aspiration showed acute myelocytic leukemia. He was treated with one cycle of arabinosyl cytosine, for 7 days, oncovin, and prednisone. A remission was not achieved, and he died 8/20/79.

B. Stages IIB, IIIA, and IIIB (SWOG 160)

Between April 1971 and February 1975, a total of 143 eligible patients with stage IIB (20), IIIA (68), or IIIB (57) Hodgkin's disease began MOPP chemotherapy. Six patients received less than three cycles of MOPP, subsequently 72 received three cycles of MOPP, 62 received four cycles of MOPP, and finally, 6 received greater than four cycles of MOPP, followed in each group by total nodal radiotherapy. Although abdominal radiotherapy was delayed in 21 patients, and pelvic irradiation was never completed in 21 patients, there was no correlation of the delays with the number of cycles of MOPP administered.

Figure 5 shows tumor mortality (those whose death was attributable to progressive disease), compared with overall survival (death from all causes) and freedom from relapse. A total of 12 patients died without evidence of Hodgkin's disease: acute leukemia (4), pancytopenia (2), breast cancer (1), tuberculosis (1), sepsis (2), herpes zoster (1), and small-bowel obstruction (1). The current estimated 5-year survival rate is 78% with a maximum follow-up of 9 years, 2 months.

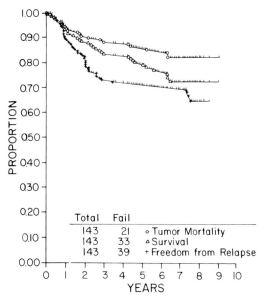

Fig. 5. Stage IIB, IIIA, and IIIB Hodgkin's disease (CAR 1, SWOG 160). Comparison of tumor mortality, overall survival, and freedom from relapse among all 143 patients.

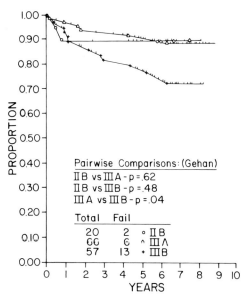

Fig. 6. Stage IIB, IIIA, and IIIB Hodgkin's disease (CAR 1, SWOG 781). Comparison of tumor mortality in stages IIB, IIIA, and IIIB.

There were no significant differences in freedom from relapse ($p > .14$) or survival ($p > .12$) with respect to stage IIB, IIIA, or IIIB. Figure 6 shows the tumor mortality by stage, and the pairwise comparisons show differences only in stage IIIA versus IIIB [p (Gehan) $= .04$]. Substages $IIIA_1$ and $IIIA_2$ show no differences in freedom from relapse or survival.

A total of seven patients who started in this protocol developed acute leukemia. Three of the leukemia patients were not included in the final evaluation because of major protocol violations. In two cases the therapist failed to irradiate the splenic pedicle, in spite of a positive spleen and/or splenic nodes. One patient had an excessive attenuation of the dose of abdominal radiotherapy. Thus 7 of 146 (4.8%) patients developed acute leukemia, 4 of 72 who had had three cycles of MOPP and 3 of 62 who had had four cycles of MOPP. There is no difference in incidence with respect to the number of cycles of MOPP ($p = .85$).

C. Stages IIA and IIB (SWOG 7518)

Between December 1974 and January 1980, a total of 113 patients were randomly assigned to MOPP plus low-dose bleomycin for 10 cycles or MOPP plus low-dose bleomycin for 3 cycles, followed by total nodal radiotherapy. Figure 7 shows the freedom-from-relapse and survival curves by treatment for the two limbs of this study. With maximum survival just beyond 4 years, there

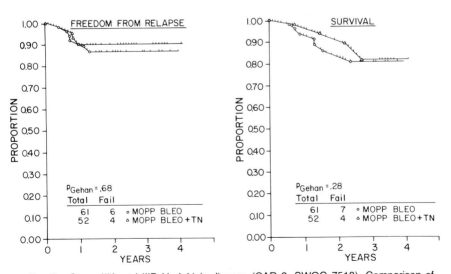

Fig. 7. Stage IIIA and IIIB Hodgkin's disease (CAR 2, SWOG 7518). Comparison of MOPP plus low-dose bleomycin (BLEO) for 10 cycles with MOPP plus low-dose bleomycin for three cycles plus total nodal (TN) radiotherapy with respect to freedom from relapse and survival.

are no differences [p (Gehan) = .68 and .28 respectively]. The overall freedom from relapse rate is 73% at 2 years, and the overall survival rate at 2 years is 81%.

IV. Discussion

The data from the stage I and II Hodgkin's disease study (RAC 1, SWOG 781) show that patients with stage I or IIA have a freedom-from-relapse and survival advantage (78 and 89%, respectively, at 8 years) over stage IB and IIB patients [p (logrank) = .001 and .001, respectively] (Fig. 2). The data for stages IA and IIA are comparable to those for radiotherapy alone at Stanford University Medical Center (1). The combined-modality treatment has a freedom-from-relapse advantage for all patients [p (logrank) = .048] (Fig. 3), but because of the effectiveness of salvage therapy there is no survival advantage [p (Gehan) = .69] in spite of the three time more frequent extranodal relapses on radiotherapy alone. This freedom-from-relapse advantage is found to pertain only to the stage IB and IIB group of patients. There are now data from three studies (2, 8, 13) which show that patients who relapse following prior radiotherapy have a significantly greater chance of achieving a complete response with combination chemotherapy than those with no prior chemotherapy.

The question of bulky mediastinal disease, as an adverse prognostic sign, was first examined by Levi *et al.* (14) in their randomized study of surgically staged IA, IIA, and IIIA Hodgkin's disease who received limited-field irradiation followed by MOPP compared with extended-field irradiation. They found a significantly higher number of marginal recurrences among those with bulky mediastinal disease (2+ to 3+). These marginal relapses occurred more frequently among those on irradiation alone ($p > .05$). The Stanford group has recently examined the prognostic importance of mediastinal involvement in pathological stage I and II disease and found that those with a mediastinal mass/thorax ratio $\geq$ 0.3 had significantly worse freedom from relapse ($p = .007$) and borderline worse survival ($p = .10$) than those treated with the combined modality. The mediastinal mass/thorax ratio could not be measured in all the patients with mediastinal involvement in the current study because of inability to obtain all initial chest X rays. There was a freedom from relapse, but no survival advantage, for those treated with combined-modality therapy, among those with prominent mediastinal masses (Fig. 4) which is seen among those with stage IB and IIB, but not stage IA and IIA disease.

The potential risk of acute leukemia developing in patients with localized Hodgkin's disease treated with combined-modality therapy has finally been realized. Two patients developed acute leukemia on the combined-modality limb while in their initial remission. The most important aspect of the study is that half of the patients received radiotherapy alone as primary therapy and are thus unlikely to be at risk for acute leukemia. In the Southwest Oncology Group review of second malignancy in Hodgkin's disease (15), no patient who received radiotherapy alone developed acute leukemia.

The phase I study of MOPP followed by total nodal radiotherapy in stage IIB, IIIA, and IIIB Hodgkin's disease (CAR 1, SWOG 160) showed that three cycles of MOPP could be safely administered prior to total nodal radiotherapy with immediate symptomatic control and reduction in the size of mediastinal masses. The relapse-free survival at 9 years of 64% is a favorable result, in spite of seven cases of acute leukemia. In the study of Kun et al. (16) six cycles of MOPP followed by total nodal radiotherapy were employed in stages IA–IIIB Hodgkin's disease. The study was terminated because of an increased incidence of local and marginal recurrences within irradiated fields and marked enhancement of normal tissue reactions, with serious morbidity in 54% of patients. Such was not the case in the present study.

Based on this study (CAR 1, SWOG 160) the Southwest Oncology Group conducted a direct comparison of chemotherapy (three cycles of MOPP plus low-dose bleomycin) plus total nodal radiotherapy with chemotherapy alone (10 cycles of MOPP plus low-dose bleomycin) (CAR 2, SWOG 7518). With preliminary data in, there are no differences in the two limbs of the study with respect to relapse-free survival or overall survival at 4 years. Preliminary data suggest that patients with nodular sclerosis histology are more likely to relapse on chemotherapy than the combined modality.

Primary radiotherapy remains the treatment of choice in pathological stage IA, IIA, IB, and IIB Hodgkin's disease. Chemotherapy alone is effective treatment for stage IIIA and IIIB disease.

References

1. R. T. Hoppe, *Semin. Oncol.* **7**, 144 (1980).
2. V. T. DeVita, R. M. Simon, S. M. Hubbard, R. C. Young, C. W. Berard, J. H. Moxley, III, E. Frei, III, PP. Carbone, and G. P. Canellos, *Ann. Intern. Med.* **92**, 587 (1980).
3. C. A. Coltman, Jr., E. Montague, and T. E. Moon, *in* "Adjuvant Therapy of Cancer" (S. E. Salmon and S. E. Jones, eds.), p. 529. Elsevier/North-Holland, Biomedical Press, Amsterdam and New York, 1977.
4. S. A. Rosenberg and H. S. Kaplan, *Cancer* **35**, 55 (1975).
5. C. A. Coltman, Jr., L. A. Fuller, R. Fisher, and E. Frei, *in* "Adjuvant Therapy of Cancer II" (S. E. Jones and S. E. Salmon, eds.), p. 129. Grune & Stratton, New York, 1979.
6. A collaborative study, *Cancer (Philadelphia)* **38**, 288 (1976).
7. R. E. Johnson and L. B. Thomas, *Radiology* **96**, 603 (1970).
8. C. A. Coltman, Jr., *Semin. Oncol.* **7**, 155 (1980).
9. E. S. Kaplan and P. Meier, *J. Am. Stat. Assoc.* **53**, 457 (1958).
10. E. A. Gehan, *Biometrika* **52**, 203 (1965).

11. R. Peta, M. C. Pike, and P. Armitage, *Br. J. Cancer* **35,** 1 (1977).
12. E. Frei, III, J. K. Luce, J. F. Gamble, C. A. Coltman, Jr., J. J. Costanzi, R. W. Talley, R. W. Monto, H. E. Wilson, J. S. Hewlett, F. C. Delaney, and E. A. Gehan, *Ann. Intern. Med.* **79,** 376 (1973).
13. S. B. Sutcliffe, P. F. M. Wrigley, and J. Peto, *Br. Med. J.* **1,** 679 (1978).
14. J. A. Levi, P. H. Wiernik, and M. J. O'Connell, *Int. J. Radiat. Oncol., Biol. Phys.* **2,** 853 (1977).
15. D. M. Toland, C. A. Coltman, Jr., and T. E. Moon, *Cancer Clin. Trials* **1,** 27 (1978).
16. L. E. Kun, V. T. DeVita, R. C. Young, and R. E. Johnson, *Int. J. Radiat. Oncol. Biol. Phys.* **1,** 619 (1976).

32

The Role of Combined Radiotherapy and Chemotherapy in the Primary Management of Non-Hodgkin's Lymphomas

G. BONADONNA, A. LATTUADA, S. MONFARDINI, E. BAJETTA, R. BUZZONI, R. CANETTA, P. VALAGUSSA, AND A. BANFI

I. Introduction

Radiotherapy (RT) has represented the conventional primary treatment for non-Hodgkin's lymphoma (NHL) with clinically localized disease (stage I or II), and with all techniques employed this approach has proved to be curative in a proportion of patients. However, even with more accurate staging procedures (bone marrow biopsy, laparoscopy, laparotomy), adequate doses through megavoltage equipment, and adoption of treatment programs including uninvolved areas, the 5-year results do not always appear satisfactory. In fact, the

TABLE I

Cumulative 5-Year Relapse-Free Survival in Stage I and II Non-Hodgkin's Lymphomas Treated with Primary Irradiation

Patient classification	CS (%)	PS (%)
Total	35–55	45–65
Stage I	50–55	65–75
Stage II	30–40	35–55
Nodular lymphoma	50–60	55–90
Diffuse lymphoma	25–45	50–65

cumulative data from the literature (1–5) show that at 5 years the total relapse-free survival (RFS) ranges from 35 to 55% in patients clinically staged (CS) and from 45 to 65% in those pathologically staged (PS) (Table I). In all published series the results vary considerably in relation to the proportion of patients having nodular or diffuse lymphoma within each staging group. The best results are usually achieved in stage I diffuse histiocytic lymphoma (DHL) staged with laparotomy. In this subgroup the large majority of patients can in fact be cured by optimal irradiation.

Because of the known reasons for irradiation failures (6, 7) and the recent progress achieved with intensive multiple-agent chemotherapy in advanced malignant lymphoma, treatment alternatives have been investigated in recent years. The first prospective controlled studies with combined RT–chemotherapy programs were initiated at the Istituto Nazionale Tumori in Milan (8–10) and at Stanford University (3) and were subsequently followed by studies by two Scandinavian research groups (11, 12). More recently, the efficacy of primary chemotherapy alone was tested in localized NHL with unfavorable histology by investigators at the M.D. Anderson Hospital (Houston, Texas) (13) and at the University of Arizona (14, 15).

This chapter will first report the updated results of the two randomized studies carried out on localized lymphomas in Milan and will also discuss the relative merits of different treatment approaches on the basis of current results.

II. Combined-Treatment Programs

Table II outlines the study design of both prospective randomized trials carried out in Milan. The first study (P 7210) was started in 1972 and utilized either RT alone or RT combined with cyclophosphamide–vincristine–prednisone (CVP) chemotherapy. The details concerning treatment methods and patient selection were reported in previous publications (8–10). Briefly, after pathological stag-

TABLE II

Milan Trials in PS I and II Non-Hodgkin's Lymphomas

Years of study	Patients evaluable	Random treatment
1972–1980 (P 7210)	96	RT → CR ⓡ $\begin{cases} \text{No further therapy, or} \\ \text{CVP} \times 6 \end{cases}$ Stratification: PS I and I_E, PS II and II_E; nodular, diffuse pattern; lymphocytic, nonlymphocytic
1976–1980 (P 7606)	82	ⓡ $\begin{cases} \text{CVP} \times 3 \to \text{RT} \to \text{CVP} \times 3, \text{ or} \\ \text{BACOP} \times 3 \to \text{RT} \to \text{BACOP} \times 3 \end{cases}$ Stratification: PS I and I_E, PS II and II_E; diffuse lymphocytic, diffuse non-lymphocytic

ⓡ Denotes randomization; CR denotes complete remission.

ing, patients were started on RT, and 4 weeks following the irradiation program complete responders were randomized to receive no further therapy or six cycles of CVP. The treatment program for most patients who failed on RT alone consisted of CVP, and further irradiation was added for patients with contiguous or marginal relapse; most patients with failure after combined therapy were started on a non-cross-resistant regimen such as adriamycin, bleomycin, and prednisone (ABP) (16). Radiotherapy was delivered with ^{60}Co teletherapy, and in 74% of patients the irradiation program included the involved areas as well as proximal clinically uninvolved lymph node-bearing region(s). The involved area(s) received 40–50 Gy and the noninvolved area(s) 35–40 Gy on a schedule of 8–10 Gy 5 days/week. The CVP treatment was administered according to the original dose schedule designed at the National Cancer Institute (NCI) (17) and shown in Table III. Pathological stage was determined in 98% of patients through bone marrow biopsy, laparoscopy (26%), and/or laparotomy (74%). Of the original 113 patients, only 96 were considered evaluable for comparative response to therapy (RT, 49; RT plus CVP, 47), since 10 patients (9%) progressed during RT. The histopathological diagnosis was formulated by utilizing the Rappaport classification. There was a preponderance of cases with diffuse histology (RT, 76%; RT plus CVP, 66%), particularly the diffuse histiocytic type. About 50% of the patients presented with extranodal involvement and Waldeyer's ring represented the single most frequent extranodal site (RT, 31%; RT plus CVP, 23%). Approximately half the patients were classified as having either PS I or II according to the Ann Arbor system.

A second randomized trial (P 7606) was started in 1976 but limited to patients with diffuse lymphoma (Table II). The purpose was twofold: (1) to compare the

TABLE III

CVP and BACOP Regimens

Treatment	Dose (mg/m^2)	Route[a]	Schedule
CVP			
Cyclophosphamide	400	po, iv	Days 1–5
Vincristine	1.2[b]	iv	Day 1
Prednisone	100	po, im	Days 1–5
Recycle on day 22			
BACOP			
Bleomycin	5	iv	Days 15 and 22
Adriamycin	25	iv	Days 1 and 8
Cyclophosphamide	650	iv	Days 1 and 8
Vincristine	1.2	iv	Days 1 and 8
Prednisone	60	po, im	Days 15–28
Recycle on day 29			

[a] po, Orally; iv, intravenously; im, intramuscularly.

[b] The dose was 1.4 mg/m^2 in the study with radiotherapy with or without CVP (six cycles).

efficacy of CVP versus that of an adriamycin-containing regimen such as the NCI combination known as BACOP (18) (Table III); (2) to limit or avoid disease progression during RT by starting treatment with chemotherapy (the so-called sandwich technique). Radiotherapy was delivered with ^{60}Co teletherapy or a 6-MeV linear accelerator on the same schedule as in the previous study (8–10).

The irradiation program included both involved areas (40–50 Gy) and proximal uninvolved (30–40 Gy) lymph node-bearing region(s). All patients were pathologically staged by combining two bone marrow biopsies with laparoscopy (two to four liver biopsies). Although both Rappaport and Kiel classifications were utilized in this study, and more recently also the new "Working Formulation," for the sake of comparison the data will be presented only in terms of the Rappaport classification.

Table IV presents the main patient characteristics of trial P 7606. From July 1976 to September 1980, a total of 104 patients were entered into the study, and 82 have completed the treatment program. All patients with lymphocytic lymphoma had the diffuse poorly differentiated subtype; in the group of nonlymphocytic lymphoma there was a preponderance of diffuse histiocytic lymphoma (total 37 of 51 or 73%). In 11 patients both nodular and diffuse patterns of growth were present within the same lymph node. Bulky disease, defined as a neoplastic lymphoid mass greater than 10 cm in the largest diameter, was observed in 10 of 82 evaluable patients (12%).

TABLE IV

Main Patient Characteristics

Characteristic	CVP group	BACOP group
Total entered	54	50
Total evaluable[a]	43	39
Median age (years)[b]	53 (16-69)	47 (18-68)
PS I	25	23
PS II	18	16
Diffuse lymphocytic lymphoma	17	14
Diffuse nonlymphocytic lymphoma	26	25
Diffuse and nodular patterns	6	5
Bulky disease (>10 cm)	5	5
Median follow-up (months)[b]	22 (2-46)	24 (4-46)

[a] Combined treatment completed as of September 30, 1980.

[b] Range is shown in parentheses.

III. Statistical Analyses

Tests of significance comparing subgroups of patients achieving and not achieving CR were done using the chi-square test with Yates' correction. Relapse-free survival distributions were calculated using the actuarial life table method starting from the end of radiation therapy for the CVP program and from the day of initial treatment for the second study up to the closing date for the present analysis (October 1, 1980). Survival distributions were always calculated starting from the day of initial treatment. The statistical significance of differences observed among various subgroups of patients was assessed by the logrank test (19). Percentages of patients free of disease or surviving are reported in the text and in the tables for two points in time (8 and 2 years, respectively), as derived from life table plots. However, p values listed represent a comparison of the complete plots.

IV. Treatment Results

A. CVP Program

During the 5 months of CVP chemotherapy extensions were documented in 5 of 47 patients (11%); during the same period of time this occurred in 17 of 49 patients (35%) treated with RT alone. Table V summarizes the comparative RFS

TABLE V

Comparative Percentages of 8-Year Relapse-Free Survival

	RFS (%)		
Patient classification	RT	RT + CVP	*p*
Total	45.9	65.3	.01
Histology			
Nodular	54.6	66.5	.57
Diffuse	44.9	64.3	.02
Lymphocytic	38.3	76.8	.04
Nonlymphocytic	50.6	57.1	.13
Stage			
I	63.6	70.6	.05
II	31.5	52.4	.05
Presentation			
Nodal	43.5	64.5	<.03
Extranodal	48.2	66.2	<.06

values. The actuarial analysis at 8 years essentially confirmed the 5-year results (9, 10). This was true also for total survival (RT, 54.8%; RT plus CVP, 77.4%; $p < .03$). The minor differences in the p value found between the 5- and the 8-year analyses are indeed attributable to the small number of patients at risk for 8 years.

Figure 1A and B graphically shows the RFS and total survival in both treatment groups. In the analysis of RFS both curves have a tendency to level off after the third year; the analysis of survival indicates that, when the primary treatment was RT alone, there was a progressive death rate up to the sixth year. This pattern of progressive mortality over time was due to nodular lymphomas and not to diffuse lymphomas whose survival curve leveled off at the third year. As already pointed out in our previous publications (9, 10), salvage therapy failed to induce a higher incidence of a second durable complete remission (CR) in patients who relapsed after RT alone (CR, 54%; median duration, 21 months) compared to RT plus CVP (CR, 50%; median duration, not reached). The similarity of survival curves after the first relapse is shown in Fig. 2. The survival of the 10 patients who had disease progression while on primary irradiation was poor, as shown in Fig. 3; this reemphasizes once more the importance of achieving prompt CR. The prognostic importance of stage is evident from the analysis of Fig. 4A and B: In spite of the improvement provided by the combined-modality approach, there remains a clear separation in the RFS and survival between stages I and II.

As already pointed out in the report on the 5-year results, treatment toxicity was moderate, and late sequelae from RT were observed in only one patient (10).

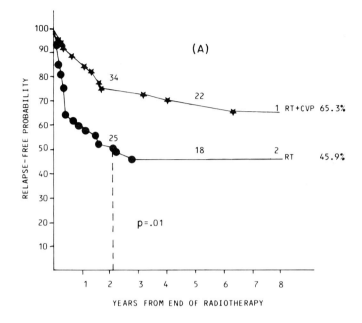

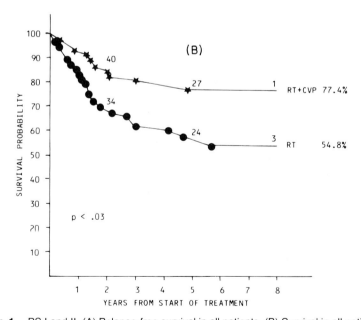

Fig. 1.   PS I and II. (A) Relapse-free survival in all patients. (B) Survival in all patients.

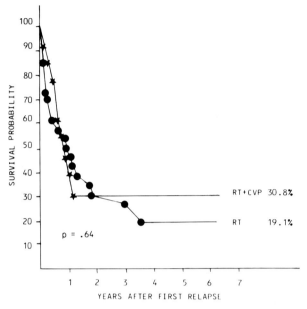

Fig. 2. PS I and II. Survival after first relapse.

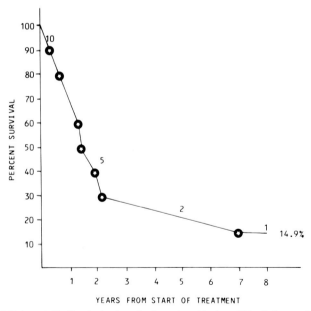

Fig. 3. PS I and II. Survival of patients not achieving CR at the end of primary radiotherapy.

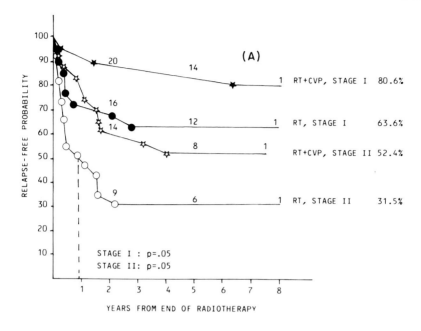

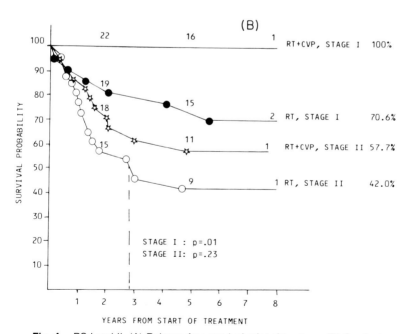

Fig. 4. PS I and II. (A) Relapse-free survival related to stage. (B) Survival.

TABLE VI

Percentages of Complete Remission Related to Subgroups

Patient classification	CVP group (%)	BACOP group (%)	p
Total	88.4	97.4	.25
Stage I	100	100	—
Stage II	72.2	93.8	.26
Lymphocytic	100	100	—
Nonlymphocytic	80.8	96.0	.21
Diffuse and nodular pattern	100	100	—
Bulky disease	100	100	—

Second neoplasms in nonirradiated areas were histologically documented in three patients given RT plus CVP. Tumors (carcinoma of the colon, urinary bladder, and hard palate) were detected after 35, 56, and 67 months, respectively, from completion of therapy.

B. CVP versus BACOP

Table VI presents the comparative percentage of CR at the end of multimodality therapy. While at the present moment no significant differences are seen among the treatment subgroups, the following observations can be made: (1) There is a constant trend in favor of BACOP compared to CVP; (2) by starting treatment with chemotherapy, disease progression while on therapy occurred in 5 of 43 patients (11.6%) given CVP and in only 1 of 39 patients (2.6%) treated with BACOP; (3) new disease manifestations always occurred at distant sites; (4) CR was always higher in PS I versus PS II, as well as in lymphocytic versus

TABLE VII

Comparative 2-Year Relapse-Free and Total Survival

Patient classification	RFS (%)			Survival (%)		
	CVP group	BACOP group	p	CVP group	BACOP group	p
Total	77.6	88.7	.38	86.0	85.6	.98
PS I	83.9	90.9	.63	94.4	90.0	.67
PS II	67.2	85.6	.42	74.9	79.6	.71
Lymphocytic	72.6	85.0	.67	100	83.0	.16
Nonlymphocytic	81.2	91.0	.44	77.8	86.9	.44

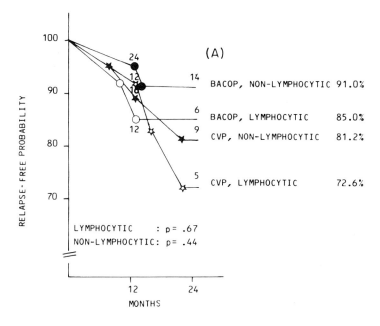

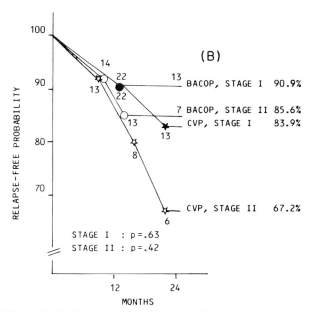

Fig. 5. PS I and II. (A) Relapse-free survival related to main histological subgroups. (B) Relapse-free survival related to stage.

nonlymphocytic lymphomas, but the difference was minimal in the BACOP group. It is interesting to note that in both series all patients with bulky disease achieved a complete response. Table VII summarizes the 2-year RFS and survival. Though at the present time none of the comparative findings is significant because of the limited number of patients at risk, the analysis of RFS always shows a trend in favor of BACOP versus CVP (Fig. 5A and B).

In both series, treatment was well tolerated and allowed the administration of a high percentage of the planned dose of all drugs. In particular, no patient developed pulmonary or cardiac toxicity or a second neoplasm.

V. Comment

Prospective randomized trials for localized lymphomas remain difficult, mainly because of the numerous histopathological subgroups and the limited proportion of patients with true PS I or II disease. This latter finding does not necessarily apply to DHL where half, if not more, of the patients with a single supradiaphragmatic adenopathy can be found to have PS I disease. Moreover, the definitive staging procedures have not yet been clearly defined, although staging laparotomy has been recently utilized only by a few research centers and abandoned in elderly patients, as well as when the treatment plan includes chemotherapy.

The few published results on the combined-modality approach probably reflect the above-mentioned difficulties and so far prevent definitive conclusions from being drawn. The results of only five prospective randomized trials have been reported in the medical literature, and in three studies including the second Milan trial (P 7606), the findings are still preliminary. For this latter reason as well as for those mentioned above, a cross-series comparison would be extremely difficult, if not totally misleading. The Stanford group has recently updated the results of a prospective randomized study (3) comparing in favorable lymphomas involved-field (IF) irradiation versus total nodal irradiation (TNI) and in unfavorable lymphomas TNI versus TNI plus CVP or cytosine arabinoside–adriamycin–thioguanine (CAT) chemotherapy. At 8 years (20) in 76 study patients less than 65 years old and staged with laparotomy, the RFS confirmed the absence of a significant difference between the two treatment groups (favorable histology: IF 77.8% versus TNI 100%, $p = .14$; unfavorable histology; TNI 66.7% versus TNI plus chemotherapy 49.5%, $p = .55$). The same applied to total survival (favorable histology: IF 56.7% versus TNI 75.8%, $p = .83$; unfavorable histology: TNI 59.2% versus TNI plus chemotherapy 45.7% $p = .55$). These findings remain difficult to compare with those observed in Milan; most probably, the limited number of patients in each subgroup could be the main reason for the somewhat contradictory results in the two trials.

Two Scandinavian groups have provided preliminary evidence that multimodality treatment can be superior to irradiation alone. Nissen (11) has utilized IF RT (40–60 Gy) with and without adjuvant chemotherapy given for a 6-week period with vincristine, prednisone, and streptonigrin followed by oral cyclophosphamide for 3 years with pulses of vincristine and prednisone. The early results showed that 11 of 28 patients (39%) relapsed in the RT group and only 1 of 29 (3.5%) did so in the RT plus chemotherapy group. With multimodality therapy the relapse rate was particularly low in PS II (1 of 11) in patients with unfavorable histology (1 of 24) and with B symptoms (0 of 6). Landberg *et al.* (12) treated 55 patients with locally extended-field RT (40 Gy) alone (29 cases) or with RT plus nine cycles of a modified CVP chemotherapy (26 cases). At 30 months, the RFS was 41% for patients without and 86% for patients with adjuvant CVP. There was no difference in the relapse rate between PS I and II patients. The diffuse lymphomas relapsed more often after RT alone (9 of 22) than after combined treatment (2 of 21), and this difference was particularly striking in DHL (RT, 5 of 10; RT plus CVP, 0 of 10). However, at 30 months, total survival was similar in both treatment groups (92 and 91%). Although not taking part in a prospective study, patients recently evaluated by Timothy *et al.* (5) had an improved RFS when different forms of chemotherapy were added to IF or extended-field RT. In fact, 12 of 13 with CS I and 6 of 8 with CS II lymphoma remained alive and disease-free at follow-up periods of 12–76 months (median, 24 months). Involved-field RT and cyclophosphamide, adriamycin, vincristine, prednisone, bleomycin (CHOP-Bleo) have also improved the 5-year survival (78%) of CS I and II patients treated at the M.D. Anderson Hospital (21, 22).

More recently, on the basis of their own brilliant results as well as those of Cabanillas *et al.* (13), Miller and Jones (14, 15) have stressed the point that initial chemotherapy with CHOP or CHOP-Bleo appears to be the treatment of choice for localized DHL, while the role of RT remains to be defined. The issue could be of considerable practical importance, but it cannot be resolved only on the basis of published results utilizing limited series of patients and without the support of a prospective randomized trial. When a staging laparotomy was performed, RT alone (IF, extended-field, and total nodal) could provide in a limited series of patients a 5-year RFS and total survival ranging from 80 to 100% in PS I DHL (20, 23). Similar results were also reported by investigators who utilized primary combination chemotherapy in clinically staged patients (15); however, their series were too small to allow for definitive conclusions in term of cure rate.

In stage II DHL, as well as in all patients with diffuse histology other than diffuse histiocytic, the results of radiotherapy alone are unsatisfactory even when patients are staged with laparotomy (20, 24). Therefore, also considering the fraction of patients with new disease manifestations before the irradiation program can be completed (10, 12, 24), the initial treatment should include combination chemotherapy. By starting chemotherapy first, the response to drug treatment can be assessed and, if the rationale of employing systemic treatment is to eradicate tumor outside the irradiated volume, it seems illogical to delay the introduction of systemic therapy. The drug regimen should include adriamycin, since this drug is very effective in diffuse lymphomas, particularly of the diffuse histiocytic type (25). The preliminary results of our second trial utilizing BACOP versus CVP provide preliminary evidence that this direction is correct. As mentioned before, whether radiation should or should not always be included in the treatment strategy utilizing initial chemotherapy should be determined, in our opinion, only from the results of a prospective randomized trial. Since one of the limitations of curative chemotherapy is represented by the presence of bulky disease, we doubt that drug treatment alone could eradicate lymphomas in a high proportion of patients with adenopathies greater than 7–10 cm in diameter or with large primary extranodal involvement. Most probably, IF radiation given after induction chemotherapy could ensure local tumor eradication in a high percentage of cases, especially with DHL.

Optimal treatment of stage I and II lymphomas with low-grade or intermediate-grade malignancy (follicular) remains at present less well defined because the usefulness of a staging laparotomy is not clear-cut and the results of adjuvant CVP appear contradictory among the published series (9–12). The treatment of choice appears to be RT, and in the Stanford experience the 8-year RFS and survival were not significantly different for patients given IF radiation and those treated with TNI. Chemotherapy could be reserved for patients with relapse, considering that moderately aggressive drug therapy resulted in a good total survival rate for this group of slow-growing lymphomas (26).

In conclusion, RT alone could still be considered the treatment of choice only in PS I DHL staged with a laparotomy. In all other situations initial chemotherapy with an adriamycin-containing regimen is recommended for improving the cure rate over that of RT alone. The actual usefulness of RT in patients started on effective chemotherapy remains to be better defined through appropriate randomized trials. At the present time, recommendations for management of follicular lymphoma remain less well defined.

References

1. G. Bonadonna, A. Lattuada, and A. Banfi, *Eur. J. Cancer* **12**, 661 (1976).
2. R. S. Bush, M. Gospodarowicz, J. Sturgeon, *et al., Cancer Treat. Rep.* **61**, 1129 (1977).
3. E. Glatstein, S. S. Donaldson, S. A. Rosenberg, *et al., Cancer Treat. Rep.* **61**, 1199 (1977).
4. S. Hellman, J. T. Chaffey, D. S. Rosenthal, *et al., Cancer* **39**, 843 (1977).
5. A. R. Timothy, T. A. Lister, D. Katz, and A. E. Jones, *Eur. J. Cancer* **16**, 799 (1980).
6. Z. Fuks, E. Glatstein, and H. S. Kaplan, *Br. J. Cancer* **31**, Suppl. II, 286 (1975).
7. Z. Fuks and H. S. Kaplan, *Radiology* **108**, 675 (1973).

8. A. Lattuada, G. Bonadonna, F. Milani, *et al., in* "Adjuvant Therapy of Cancer" (S. E. Salmon and S. E. Jones, eds.), p. 537. Elsevier/North-Holland Biomedical Press, Amsterdam, 1977.

9. G. Bonadonna, A. Lattuada, S. Monfardini, *et al., in* "Adjuvant Therapy of Cancer II" (S. E. Salmon and S. E. Jones, eds.), p. 145. Grune & Stratton, New York, 1979.

10. S. Monfardini, A. Banfi, G. Bonadonna, *et al., Int. J. Radiat. Oncol., Biol. Phys.* **6,** 125 (1980).

11. N. I. Nissen, *Antibiot. Chemother. (Basel)* **24,** 73 (1978).

12. T. G. Landberg, L. G. Håkansson, T. R. Möller, *et al., Cancer* **44,** 831 (1979).

13. F. Cabanillas, G. P. Bodey, and E. J. Freireich, *Proc. Am. Assoc. Cancer Res.* **20,** 19 (1979).

14. T. P. Miller and S. E. Jones, *Lancet* **1,** 358 (1979).

15. T. P. Miller and S. E. Jones, *Cancer Chemother. Pharmacol.* **4,** 67 (1980).

16. S. Monfardini, G. Tancini, M. De Lena, *et al., Med. Pediatr. Oncol.* **3,** 67 (1977).

17. C. M. Bagley, V. T. DeVita, C. W. Berard, and G. P. Canellos, *Ann. Intern. Med.* **76,** 227 (1972).

18. P. S. Schein, V. T. DeVita, S. Hubbard, *et al., Ann. Intern. Med.* **85,** 417 (1976).

19. R. Peto, M. C. Pike, P. Armitage, *et al., Br. J. Cancer* **35,** 1 (1977).

20. S. A. Rosenberg, personal communication.

21. L. M. Toonkel, L. M. Fuller, J. F. Gamble, *et al., Cancer* **45,** 249 (1980).

22. L. I. Heifetz, L. M. Fuller, R. W. Rodgers, *et al., Cancer* **45,** 2778 (1980).

23. J. D. Bitran, H. M. Golomb, J. E. Ultmann, *et al., Cancer* **42,** 88 (1978).

24. P. Kushlan, C. N. Coleman, E. J. Glatstein, *et al., Proc. Am. Soc. Clin. Oncol.* **19,** 337 (1978).

25. V. T. DeVita, R. I. Fisher, and R. C. Young, *in* "Recent Advances in Cancer Treatment" (H. J. Tagnon and M. J. Staquet, eds.), p. 39. Raven, New York, 1977.

26. R. Hoppe, P. Kushlan, H. Kaplan, *et al., Blood* (in press).

33

In Vivo Effects of Murine Hybridoma Monoclonal Antibody on Human T-Cell Neoplasms

RICHARD A. MILLER AND RONALD LEVY

I. Introduction

Numerous reports have demonstrated the antitumor effects of passive antibody administration. In animals, antisera reactive with tumor cells have lead to unequivocal inhibition of tumor growth *in vivo* (1-7). Similar studies in humans have provided evidence for definite, albeit short-lived, antitumor effects of heterologous antisera (7-12). In one study, treatment of a patient with Sézary syndrome with antithymocyte globulin resulted in a 75% reduction in lymphadenopathy and complete resolution of skin erythema (13). Despite these results, serotherapy has not been developed in the treatment of human cancer. The major reasons for this have been the difficulty in preparing xenogeneic antisera with specificity for tumors and the fear of administering large amounts of foreign protein to patients.

The hybridoma technique developed by Köhler and Milstein provides a method for the production of virtually unlimited amounts of pure monoclonal antibodies (14). With this technique, it is possible to produce antibodies of a defined class, avidity, and specificity. Bernstein *et al.* (15) have shown the utility of monoclonal antibodies in the treatment of a mouse lymphoma. They demonstrated that monoclonal antibodies directed against a normal T-cell differentiation antigen (Thy 1.1) could inhibit the growth of a transplantable mouse lymphoma which expressed high levels of this antigen. In some instances, these antibodies were capable of curing mice with tumor transplant doses 100-fold greater than the LD_{100}.

We have developed a murine monoclonal antibody, L17F12, which reacts with a normal human T-cell differentiation antigen (16). We find increased amounts of this antigen on the malignant cells of patients with cutaneous T-cell lymphomas and some T-cell leukemias. A protocol for the treatment of T-cell neoplasms with this antibody has been established, and in this article we describe our experience using monoclonal antibody in the treatment of two patients. The clinical effects, immunological analysis, and problems encountered during this therapy are discussed.

Case Reports

Patient BC was a 64-year-old female with a 12-year history of mycosis fungoides treated with electron-beam, orthovoltage radiotherapy and alkylating agents. Since 1978 she has had progressive lymphadenopathy and cutaneous tumor growth. She was admitted to Stanford University Hospital for a trial of antibody therapy, in March 1980, with rapidly growing, ulcerating skin tumors and circulating Sézary cells in her blood.

Patient CE was a 67-year-old male with a 9-month history of adult T-cell leukemia and skin rash. After failing to respond to several chemotherapeutic agents, he was admitted to Stanford University Hospital with a rising white blood

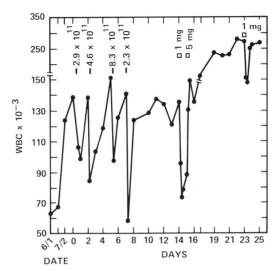

Fig. 1. Clinical course of Patient CE. Changes in the WBC are indicated over the period of time in which leukophereses and antibody therapy were performed. Each leukopheresis was performed over a 4- to 6-hour period with the number of cells removed indicated on the graph. Three separate doses of antibody were given as indicated.

cell count (WBC) and a falling platelet count and hematocrit. During the 2-week period preceding hospitalization, his WBC rose from 60,000/mm³ to 135,000/mm³ with 93% abnormal lymphocytes. Ninety-five percent of his mononuclear cells formed E rosettes with sheep erythrocytes. On physical examination, he was found to have lymphadenopathy, hepatosplenomegaly, and a diffuse violaceous skin rash involving the face, neck, arms, and trunk. Laboratory studies included a platelet count of 66,000/mm³, elevated serum lactate dehydrogenase, and alkaline phosphatase, and a normal serum creatinine. Leukopheresis was performed to reduce his tumor burden using a Haemonetics Model 30 cell separator. Each pheresis removed between 2.3×10^{11} and 8.3×10^{11} cells, dropping his WBC as shown in Fig. 1. Within 36 hours of each pheresis, his WBC returned to pretreatment levels. After four leukophereses with a total removal of 1.8×10^{12} cells over an 8-day period, his WBC had not been reduced and there was no evidence of a clinical response. Therefore leukopheresis therapy was abandoned.

II. Materials and Methods

A. Antibody Purification

Hybridoma L17F12 has been previously described (16). It secretes a mouse IgG2a antibody which is specific for mature human T cells. L17F12 hybridoma cells were grown in the peritoneal cavity of BALB/C mice. Ascites was collected aseptically, and the immunoglobulin fraction was prepared by $(NH_4)_2 SO_4$ precipitation and dialyzed against saline. This resulted in an antibody preparation that was greater than 90% pure as determined by sodium dodecyl sulfate (SDS) polyacrylamide gel electrophoresis (16). After ultracentrifugation to remove microaggregates, the preparation was passed through a 0.45-μm Swinnex filter (Nagle Company, Rochester, New York). Cultures for aerobic and anaerobic bacteria, fungus, mycobacteria, and mycoplasma were negative. Endotoxin was absent as determined by the *Limulus* amebocyte lysate assay (Amsco Medical Products, Erie, Pennsylvania).

B. Serum and Tumor Cell Preparation

Serum samples were prepared from peripheral blood and stored at $-20°C$. In Patient CE, tumor cells were obtained by Ficoll–Hypaque separation of heparinized blood (17); greater than 90% of the mononuclear cells had abnormal morphology. These cells were stored in liquid nitrogen in RPMI-1640 medium with 100 μg/ml penicillin, 100 units/ml streptomycin, 15% heat-inactivated fetal calf serum (FCS, Flow Laboratories, McLean, Virginia), and 10% dimethyl sulfoxide. At the time of testing, cells were rapidly thawed at 37°C, diluted with medium, and separated over a cushion of Ficoll–Hypaque to remove dead cells. Leukemic cells prepared in this manner were greater than 95% viable as determined by trypan blue dye exclusion. Large numbers of pretreatment cells were obtained by leukopheresis into containers with hydroxyethyl starch. After allowing the red blood cells to sediment, the buffy coat cells were cryopreserved as described above.

C. Complement-Mediated Cytotoxicity

Fifty microliters of L17F12 hybridoma culture fluid supernatant were added to plastic tubes (Falcon, No. 2058, Oxnard, California) containing 2×10^6 leukemia cells from Patient CE and incubated on ice for 20 minutes. After washing twice with Dulbecco's phosphate-buffered saline (DPBS) containing 5% FCS, 50 μl of a 1:2 dilution of complement (either rabbit serum prescreened to be nontoxic to human lymphocytes or fresh CE serum) was added to the cell pellet and incubated at 37°C for 60 minutes. The cells were then washed twice and resuspended in 0.1 ml of DPBS, and fluorescein diacetate (1 mg/ml acetone) was added to a final concentration of 10 μg/ml. After 5 minutes at 4°C, the cells were washed and the percent viability was determined by enumerating fluorescent cells (live) with a fluorescence-activated cell sorter (18) (FACS III, Becton Dickinson Electronics Laboratory, Mt. View, California).

D. Immunofluorescence Staining

Cells (2×10^6) were placed in plastic tubes and incubated with $50\mu l$ of hybridoma culture fluid supernatant at 4°C for 20 minutes. They were washed twice and incubated for another 20 minutes with 50 μl of biotinylated (affinity-purified) goat anti-mouse immunoglobulin ($50 \mu g/ml$) which had been absorbed to remove reactivity with human serum. The cells were washed twice and then reacted with 50 μl fluorescein–avidin (19) ($50 \mu g/ml$, Vector Laboratories, Burlingame, California). After the cells were washed, they were fixed in 1% formaldehyde in phosphate-buffered saline (PBS) and analyzed for fluorescent staining with the FACS. In some experiments, purified L17F12 antibody rather than hybridoma culture supernatant was used for the first stage of immunofluorescence staining. In addition to staining with L17F12, anti-human immunoglobulin light-chain antisera and monoclonal anti-Ia antibody (20) were tested. Immunofluorescence staining of frozen tissue sections has been described (21).

E. Assay for Free L17F12 Antibody in Serum

Measurements of circulating free antibody were made using a cell-binding radioimmunoassay (22). The CE cells were fixed with 0.125% glutaraldehyde and used in all subsequent cell-binding assays. Cells (2×10^5) were added to wells of round-bottom polyvinyl chloride microtiter plates (Cooke Laboratory Products, Alexandria, Virginia) and incubated overnight at 4°C with 20 μl of CE serum samples or purified L17F12 antibody. After washing, 25 μl of ^{125}I-labeled goat anti-mouse immunoglobulin ($1-2 \times 10^5$ cpm) was added and incubated for at least 4 hours. After the plates were washed, wells were cut out using a hot-wire device and transferred to tubes for gamma counting.

F. Assay for Free Antigen in Serum

With the use of a cell lysate prepared from CE cells, a competition cell-binding radioimmunoassay was used to measure free circulating L17F12 antigen. CE cells in DPBS containing 4×10^8 cells/ml were mixed 1:1 with detergent consisting of 1.0% Nonident P-40 (B.D.H. Chemicals, Ltd., Poole, England), 0.2% Brij 36 (Atlas Powder Company, Buena Vista, Mexico), and 3×10^{-3} M phenylmethylsulfonyl fluoride (Sigma Chemical Company, St. Louis, Missouri) in DPBS. After incubation for 1–2 hours at 4°C, nuclei and cell debris were removed by centrifugation at 10,000 g. The resulting supernatant was used as a standard source of L17F12 antigen and represented the lysate of 2×10^8 cells/ml. The antigen preparation or CE serum was mixed with an equal volume of a dilution of L17F12 hybridoma culture fluid, which barely saturated 2×10^5 target cells. After incubation for 16–24 hours at 4°C, 2×10^5 CE cells were added and incubated for an additional 18 hours at 4°C. The amount of L17F12 antibody binding to CE cells was determined as described above using ^{125}I-labeled goat anti-mouse immunoglobulin. A titration curve using the CE cell lysate preparation showed maximum blocking of L17F12 antibody binding to CE cells at a lysate dilution of 1:16 (1.25×10^7 cells/ml lysate). Quantitation of circulating free antigen was made by comparing the blocking with a 1:4 dilution of CE serum samples to the maximum blocking seen with the standard antigen.

G. Assay for Human Anti-mouse Antibody

An immunoprecipitation method was used to detect a human anti-mouse antibody response by Patient CE. Purified L17F12 antibody was labeled with ^{125}I by the chloramine-T method (23). Then 5 μl (1.5×10^6 cpm for 0.5 minute) was added to 50 μl of CE serum samples and incubated overnight at 4°C. Then 50 μl of goat anti-human immunoglobulin, absorbed on a column of L17F12 coupled to Sepharose, was then added and incubated for 16–24 hours at 4°C. The resulting precipitate was washed three times with PBS and counted in a gamma counter. Pretreatment CE serum served as a control.

In order to quantitate the antibody response, various concentrations of purified goat anti-mouse immunoglobulin (absorbed with human serum coupled to Sepharose) were added to pretreatment CE serum samples containing ^{125}I-labeled L17F12. Immunoprecipitates were formed as above by adding 50 μl of rabbit anti-goat immunoglobulin (absorbed against human serum and L17F12). With this method, an exponential standard curve, relating the amount of anti-mouse antibody to ^{125}I-labeled L17F12 in the precipitates, was obtained. From this curve, one could estimate the amount of human anti-L17F12 antibody present.

H. Antigenic Modulation

Antigenic modulation was studied *in vitro* by culturing 2×10^6 cells in 1 ml of medium in plastic tubes with various concentrations of L17F12 antibody. Control cells were incubated with medium alone or an indifferent antibody. After various times in culture, immunofluorescence staining was performed as described above.

I. ^{111}In Oxine-Labeled Lymphocytes

Peripheral blood mononuclear cells were obtained from Patient CE as described above and labeled with 300 μCi of ^{111}In oxine (Diagnostic Isotopes, Belleville, New Jersey). The methods of labeling, infusion into the patient, scanning, and radiopharmacokinetic analysis have been reported (24). Measurements of radioactivity of whole-blood samples taken at various times before and after antibody treatment were made. Since fluctuations in WBC would affect radioactivity in the blood, measurements of radioactivity were normalized to a WBC of 100,000 cells/mm³. *In vitro* viability studies on labeled and unlabeled cells showed no differences up to 1 week in culture.

J. Method of Administration

In Patient BC, antibody was diluted with normal saline and given by intramuscular injection or by slow intravenous injection. In Patient CE, antibody was diluted into 250 ml of normal saline containing 5% human albumin (Plasbumin, Cutter Laboratories, Berkeley, California). This was delivered by continuous intravenous infusion over 6 hours, using a volumetric infusion pump (IMed Corporation, San Diego, California).

III. Results

A. Characterization of Tumor Cells

With immunofluorescence staining, cells and frozen tissue sections obtained from a cutaneous tumor of Patient BC stained brightly with L17F12 antibody. When stained for surface immunoglobulin and Ia antigen, CE cells were negative, but were strongly positive for the L17F12 antigen. *In vitro* CE cells did not spontaneously proliferate nor did they proliferate in response to phytohemagglutinin or to L17F12 antibody (data not shown).

B. *In Vivo* Therapy

One milligram of antibody, diluted in 1 ml of normal saline, was given by intramuscular injection into the gluteal region of Patient BC. No local or systemic toxicity was noted, and no clinical effect was observed. One day later, a similar 1-mg dose was given intravenously. Forty-five minutes later the patient experienced chills and fever lasting 3 hours, but no hypotension. One hour after the administration of antibody, the peripheral blood Sézary cell count dropped from 1100 to 70 cells/mm³ but then returned to pretreatment levels (Fig. 2). There was no effect on other white blood cells or platelets. No further antibody therapy was undertaken.

Prior to the administration of antibody, CE serum was analyzed for circulating free antigen which was not found (see below). We considered the absence of circulating free antigen to be a necessary condition before embarking upon *in vivo* therapy. After an observation period of 6 days with a stable WBC, the patient was given 1 mg of antibody. Therapy with antibody produced no fever,

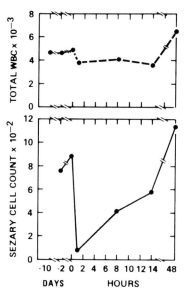

Fig. 2. Effect of antibody on WBC and Sézary cell count in Patient BC. One milligram of antibody produced a rapid fall in Sézary cell count without affecting other white blood cells.

chills, bronchospasm, hypotension, or other symptoms, Within 3 hours of the start of antibody administration the WBC had fallen from 135,000 to 95,000/mm³ and reached a nadir of 73,800/mm³ at 6 hours. However, the WBC returned to 88,700/mm³ by the next day, a response similar to that seen after leukapheresis. A 5-mg dose of antibody was then given, but this time the WBC did not fall and continued to rise to pretreatment levels. Again, the patient experienced no symptoms as a result of antibody therapy.

Following treatment, Patient CE developed transient and reversible renal dysfunction as measured by a gradual decrease in creatinine clearance from 100 ml/minute to a minimum of 54 ml/minute at 24 hours. Forty-eight hours after treatment, creatinine clearance had returned to 80 ml/minute and remained at pretreatment levels thereafter. Transient and reversible hepatic dysfunction was also observed as the SGOT rose from 49 to 219 and the alkaline phosphatase from 172 to 450 (mU/ml). Within 48–72 hours, liver function tests returned to pretreatment levels.

C. Assay for L17F12 Antibody in Serum and on Leukemia Cells of Patient CE

Using a cell-binding radioimmunoassay capable of detecting 10–20 ng/ml, we were unable to find any free L17F12 antibody in serum samples obtained before,

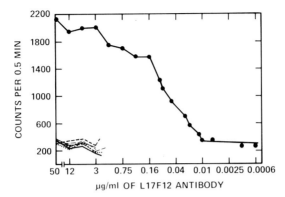

Fig. 3.   Assay for free L17F12 antibody in the serum of Patient CE. A titration curve using purified L17F12 antibody in a cell-binding radioimmunoassay is shown (solid circles). Six serum samples obtained before, during, and after the first course of antibody (both 1- and 5-mg doses) were tested and showed no free antibody.

during, and after treatment (Fig. 3). Our inability to detect free antibody was not surprising considering the dose and the patient's large number of circulating cells. It was likely that 1 mg of antibody (approximately 4×10^{15} molecules) was completely absorbed by the approximately 7×10^{11} circulating cells. Thus about 5×10^3 antibody molecules were available for each circulating leukemic cell, but it is doubtful that they could have been distributed evenly among all cells. We were also unable to detect murine antibody on circulating CE cells by immuno-fluorescence staining with a goat anti-mouse immunoglobulin reagent (data not shown). The number of antibody molecules on each cell could have been below the limit of detectability. Moreover, it is likely that antibody-coated leukemic cells were removed immediately from the circulation.

D. Detection of Free Antigen Released during Treatment with Antibody

No free L17F12 antigen was detectable in the serum of Patient CE prior to therapy. With antibody treatment, however, free antigen became detectable with maximum amounts found 24 hours after the beginning of treatment (Fig. 4). The 5-mg dose of antibody was inadvertently given at a time when large amounts of circulating free antigen were present. Conceivably, this was responsible for the lack of effect seen with this dose, since the administered antibody would have been blocked from binding to cells. Of note was the decrease in renal function seen during the time when free antigen was present, presumably a result of immune complex deposition in the kidney. The mechanism for release of free antigen into the circulation was unclear but was likely a consequence of cell destruction.

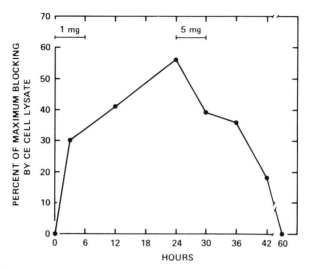

Fig. 4. Release of free antigen into the serum during treatment with monoclonal antibody. A cell lysate prepared from CE cells was used as a standard source of antigen in a competition cell-binding radioimmunoassay. Quantitation of circulating free antigen was made by comparison of blocking with CE serum samples to the maximum blocking seen with the standard antigen. Results are expressed as percentage of blocking seen with the standard antigen. Before treatment, no free antigen was detected. Following 1 mg of antibody, free antigen became readily detectable but was cleared from the serum by 60 hours.

E. Antigenic Modulation

At various times during and after antibody therapy, CE leukemic cells were sampled and stained by indirect immunofluorescence with L17F12 antibody. As shown in Fig. 5, the intensity of fluorescence progressively decreased at 1, 6, and 12 hours after treatment with the 5-mg dose. There was no change seen during, or 1 hour after, the 1-mg dose. CE cells were found to have reexpressed fully the L17F12 antigen by 72 hours following the 5-mg dose (data not shown).

Antibody-induced loss of antigen *in vivo* was studied further *in vitro*. Using a range of purified antibody concentrations that could have been achieved *in vivo*, we found that antigenic modulation was both time- and dose-dependent. As seen in Fig. 6, greater modulation was seen with either increasing antibody concentration or time of incubation. This correlated with our *in vivo* findings of progressively greater antigenic modulation following the 5-mg dose. This provided an additional explanation for the lack of effect seen with the larger dose of antibody. As more surface antigen was lost, leukemic cells became less sensitive to the effects of antibody. We considered it possible that during modulation surface antigen was shed into the serum providing the source of free L17F12 antigen. However, at the time maximum free antigen was found, no antigenic

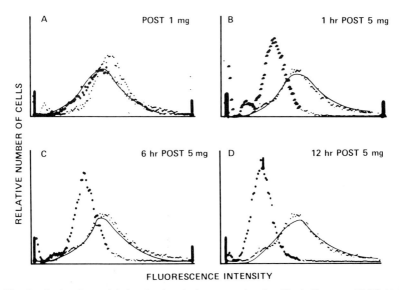

Fig. 5. Antigenic modulation *in vivo* during monoclonal antibody therapy. FACS histograms of L17F12 immunofluorescence-stained CE cells taken immediately after 1 mg (A) and, at various times, after 5 mg of antibody (B-D). Solid black line indicates staining of pretreatment samples. CE cells showed progressively lesser amounts of antigen over a period of 12 hours following the 5-mg dose.

modulation was observed on circulating cells (24 hours after the 1-mg dose). This does not exclude the possibility that cells sequestered in extravascular compartments could have modulated and shed antigen.

F. [111]In Oxine-Labeled Lymphocyte Scan

In order to follow the fate of tumor cells during antibody therapy, we injected ^{111}In-labeled CE leukemic cells into the patient 2 days prior to therapy. Radioactivity in peripheral blood samples was measured serially before and after antibody therapy. Before treatment, the radioactivity in the blood and the WBC remained constant (Fig. 7). With antibody treatment there was a fall in the WBC, but the radioactivity in the blood, normalized for the WBC, was constant. This indicated that both labeled and unlabeled cells were removed from the circulation equally in response to the antibody. However, as the WBC rebounded, there was a fall in normalized counts per minute, indicating that the proportion of labeled cells decreased. Thus the increase in the WBC represented the appearance of a new population of leukemic cells and not just a return of previously sequestered cells. Whole-body scans performed before and after antibody administration revealed intense uptake in the liver and spleen.

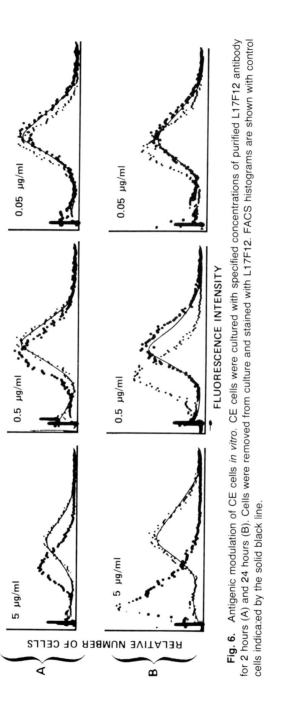

Fig. 6. Antigenic modulation of CE cells *in vitro*. CE cells were cultured with specified concentrations of purified L17F12 antibody for 2 hours (A) and 24 hours (B). Cells were removed from culture and stained with L17F12. FACS histograms are shown with control cells indicated by the solid black line.

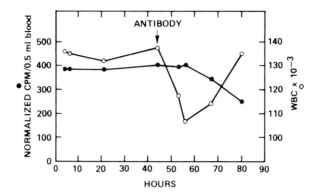

Fig. 7. With the use of ^{111}In oxine-labeled lymphocytes, the fate of tumor cells during treatment with monoclonal antibody was studied. Radioactivity measured in whole-blood samples was normalized to a WBC of 100,000/mm[3]. With the fall in WBC induced by antibody, no change in normalized whole-blood radioactivity was seen. As the WBC returned, there was a drop in the normalized radioactivity, which indicated that a new population of cells had returned to the circulation.

G. Mechanism of Cell Elimination by L17F12 Antibody

In vitro CE cells were killed by L17F12 antibody and rabbit complement but not when autologous serum was used as the complement source (Table I). This made it unlikely that the drop in the WBC seen *in vivo* was a result of complement-mediated cytotoxicity. Moreover, serum C3 and C4 complement levels (measured by radial immunodiffusion) did not fall during antibody treatment. The mechanism of cell elimination was unclear, but cell-mediated immune reactions must have been involved.

TABLE I

Complement-Mediated Cytotoxicity of CE Cells[a]

Serum complement source	Percent viability (%)
CE	95
Rabbit	4
Control	>99

[a] CE and rabbit sera were used at 1:2 dilution. Control cells were treated with L17F12 antibody and then medium. Cells treated with rabbit serum alone had a viability of 96%. The percentage of fluorescent cells was determined by FACS analysis of 10,000 cells.

TABLE II

Anti-Mouse Antibody Response of Day 5 Serum IgM and IgG Fractions

Immunoprecipitation of[a]	Mean cpm ± SD in immunoprecipitates[b]
Pretreatment serum	6,438 ± 914
Unfractionated serum	22,617 ± 2719
IgM fraction	17,506 ± 1003
IgG fraction	7,400 ± 1120

[a] Immunoprecipitation performed as described in Section II using ^{125}I-labeled L17F12 antibody. Immunoglobulin fractions tested at 10 mg/ml concentrations.

[b] Duplicate samples.

H. CE Anti-Mouse Antibody Response

Serum samples were analyzed for the appearance of antibodies directed against the L17F12 antibody for as long as 3 weeks after the last antibody treatment. Anti-mouse antibodies became detectable 5 days after the first dose of L17F12 antibody but were undetectable thereafter. In order to quantitate this response, a standard curve using known amounts of goat anti-mouse antibody was produced. From this curve, we estimated that the patient made an anti-mouse antibody response of approximately 0.5 μg/ml (in contrast to approximately 0.5 mg/ml in a typical hyperimmune antiserum). We examined the nature of this anti-mouse antibody response further by fractionating CE day-5 serum into IgG or IgM using size-exclusion chromatography on Sephadex G-200. As shown in Table II, the anti-mouse antibody activity was limited to the IgM fraction.

I. Second Trial of Antibody Treatment

Following the second dose of antibody, Patient CE was treated with high-dose methotrexate and L-asparaginase chemotherapy. He failed to respond to these treatments, as his WBC rose to 275,000/mm^3. Another 1-mg dose of antibody was given 7 days after the first trial. Again, no symptoms were noted, and this time no change in renal or hepatic function occurred. Once again, the WBC dropped dramatically to 148,000/mm^3 and then rebounded to pretreatment levels (Fig. 1). No free antigen was detected during this treatment course. Immediately after treatment, CE cells once again showed evidence of antigenic modulation.

IV. Discussion

In this study, we reported on the *in vivo* effects of murine hybridoma monoclonal antibody in two patients with T-cell neoplasms. Both patients were ideal candidates for this trial, because their neoplastic cells expressed large amounts of the L17F12 antigen although this antigen was not found circulating in their serum. Another report on therapy using a hybridoma monoclonal antibody has appeared (25). In that study, high doses of antibody (75–1500 mg) were required before an effect on the WBC was seen because large quantities of circulating antigen interfered with the ability of antibody to reach the target cells. In the current study, 1 mg was sufficient to cause dramatic reductions in circulating tumor cells. As in the study by Nadler *et al.,* we could not detect free antibody in the serum (25). Undoubtedly, most of the antibody was bound to target cells. We were also unable to detect murine antibody on leukemia cells sampled during therapy. Either these amounts were below the limits of detection or antibody-coated cells were removed immediately from the peripheral blood.

During the first course of treatment, free L17F12 antigen was found in the serum of Patient CE. This presumably was the result of tumor cell destruction and antigen release. A decrease in creatinine clearance was seen coincident with the detection of antigen. A second dose of antibody, given at that time, caused a further reduction in renal function. This decrease in renal function, also seen by Nadler et al, is probably the result of immune complexes filtered by the kidney (25). Immune complex deposition also could have been responsible for the transient hepatic dysfunction. With the second trial of antibody therapy no free antigen was found, and no renal or hepatic dysfunction was noted.

During exposure to L17F12 antibody *in vivo,* CE leukemia cells were found to undergo antigenic modulation. This was not seen during or after the first 1-mg dose but occurred during the 5-mg dose. In *in vitro* studies, antigenic modulation was found to be time- and dose-dependent. Similar results have been described by Old *et al.* (26, 27) in mice with TL antigen-positive leukemia and by Ritz *et al.* (28) using an antibody against human acute lymphoblastic leukemia (ALL). After antigenic modulation, cells were no longer destroyed by anti-TL antibody in mice treated for TL-positive leukemia (27). As in the TL system of mice, antigenic modulation in our patient was a reversible phenotypic change and did not represent immunoselection. This mechanism of antigenic modulation is under further study in our laboratory and has been found to occur for the L17F12 antigen on all normal and neoplastic T cells tested *in vitro.* Many other, but not all, T-cell antigens also modulate rapidly.

In Patient CE, ^{111}In oxine-labeled leukemia cells provided a means of evaluating the mechanism of elimination of cells from the circulation. Radioactivity in peripheral blood samples was normalized to minimize changes due to fluctuations in the WBC. That labeling did not affect cell viability or function was tested *in vitro* and by findings *in vivo* of identical changes in the WBC and radioactivity. After antibody therapy, the normalized radioactivity remained constant, while the WBC fell. The return of a new population of white blood cells was proven by the fall in normalized radioactivity as the WBC rose. The mechanism of tumor cell eradication was not clear, but complement appeared to have no role. Perhaps antibody-coated leukemia cells were removed in the liver by cell-mediated mechanisms. This could have been responsible for the transient elevation of liver enzyme.

The administration of murine antibody to humans would be expected to produce a host immune response. To minimize this, we chose to give low-dose ultracentrifuged antibody by the intravenous route, since this has been shown to be tolerogenic in animals (29, 30). In Patient CE we were able to find a small, temporary antibody response to the murine L17F12 antibody of 0.5μg/ml of serum. This response was seen 5 days after the first dose of antibody and was shown to be IgM. The absence of a later humoral response and failure to make IgG might be related to a failure to switch from IgM to IgG production. This could have occurred because regulatory T cells were affected by antibody treatment or because of the immunosuppressive effects of the chemotherapy the patient received. At any rate, this transient anti-mouse immune response was weak and did not affect a second trial of antibody which successfully lowered the WBC.

It is useful to compare the clinical response of antibody therapy to the leukaphoresis performed on Patient CE. The rapid return of WBC seen after antibody therapy was similar to that seen after leukopheresis (Fig. 1). Based on changes in the WBC, antibody eliminated about 5×10^{11} cells, making it as effective as a single leukopheresis. A similar conclusion has been made by Hamblin *et al.* (31) in a study using highly purified sheep anti-idiotype antibody in the treatment of a patient with CLL. After four leukophereses of 1.8×10^{12} cells, no change in tumor burden was appreciated by clinical evaluation. It is likely that the number of cells eradicated by two courses of antibody therapy represented only a small percentage of the patient's total tumor burden. Obviously, a greater clinical impact could be achieved in patients with small tumor burdens or with repeated courses of antibody.

Heterologous antithymocyte globulin (ATG) has been used in the treatment of cutaneous T-cell lymphomas (13, 32, 33). Several patients responded to doses of 200–1000 mg, but serious toxicity, related to the large amounts of foreign protein, was noted (13, 32). Hybridoma monoclonal antibody may alleviate this problem, since it can be prepared in a highly purified form (our preparation was greater than 90% pure versus the approximately 1–5% purity of ATG) which does not contain other irrelevant or dangerous cross-reactive antibodies. Although our first patient experienced fever and chills after a 1-mg dose given intravenously, this was not seen in our second patient who was given the antibody by slow intravenous infusion.

We conclude from the results of this study that specific immunotherapy with murine hybridoma monoclonal antibody can be safely performed. In order for this treatment modality to be successful, there are problems which must be solved. These problems include: (1) the presence or release of circulating free antigen, (2) antigenic modulation, and (3) a host anti-mouse immune response. We do not feel that these problems are insurmountable. Plasmapheresis could be used to lower the amounts of free antigen, and proper doses and schedules could minimize the effects of antigen release. Antigenic modulation could be circumvented by proper scheduling and could be monitored *in vitro*. Not all antibodies cause antigenic modulation, so other antibodies could be developed. A host anti-mouse humoral response was not a problem in our study. It may be that this problem is clinically insignificant. Alternatively, recently described human–human hybridomas could be used to develop human antitumor antibodies (32). Such antibodies, however, will not alleviate the problems of free antigen and antigenic modulation. Other approaches might be to combine antibodies of different specificities or to combine chemotherapy and/or radiotherapy with antibody therapy.

Based on these concepts, we have begun treatment of a patient with advanced, refractory cutaneous T-cell lymphoma. Administration of eight courses of the L17F12 antibody over a 4-week period has produced a dramatic clinical response with marked reduction in lymphadenopathy and regression of cutaneous tumors and plaques. The problems of antigen release and antigenic modulation have occurred but have been obviated by proper doses and schedules. To date, this patient has not demonstrated a clinically significant anti-mouse immune response and has tolerated each treatment without any side effects.

V. Summary

A murine monoclonal antibody directed against a normal T-cell differentiation antigen was given to two patients with T-cell neoplasms. Immunofluorescence staining showed increased amounts of this antigen in each patient's tumor cells. The first case, a patient with mycosis fungoides, had a dramatic but temporary fall in circulating Sézary cells. In a patient with T-cell leukemia, two courses of *in vivo* therapy were given using a 1-mg dose. Each produced a prompt and dramatic fall in the WBC with a return to pretreatment levels over the ensuing 24 hours—a pattern similar to that seen with leukopheresis. After the first dose of antibody, circulating free antigen became detectable in the serum, and a transient decline in creatinine clearance was noted. A 5-mg dose of antibody given at that time was ineffective, presumably because it was blocked by free antigen. Antigenic modulation by leukemia cells was found transiently following each course of antibody. A weak and clinically insignificant host anti-mouse antibody response was found 5 days after the first treatment. This patient tolerated antibody therapy without difficulty. Monoclonal antibodies offer promise as an immunotherapeutic approach to cancer, but the problems encountered here must be addressed.

References

1. G. Möller, *Nature* (*London*) **204**, 846 (1965).
2. J. J. Collins, F. Sanfilippo, L. Tsong-Chow, R. Ishizaki, and R. S. Metzgar, *Int. J. Cancer* **21**, 51 (1978).
3. W. P. Drake, P. C. Ungaro, and M. R. Mardiney, *JNCI, J. Natl. Cancer Inst.* **50**, 909 (1973).
4. C. Hu and T. J. Linna, *Ann. N.Y. Acad. Sci.* **277**, 634 (1976).
5. L. J. Old, E. Stockert, E. A. Boyse, and G. Geering, *Proc. Soc. Exp. Biol. Med.* **124**, 63 (1967).
6. G. R. Pearson, L. W. Redmon, and L. R. Bass, *Cancer Res.* **33**, 171 (1973).
7. P. W. Wright and I. D. Bernstein, *Prog. Exp. Tumor Res.* **25**, 140 (1980).
8. G. A. Currie, *Int. J. Cancer* **26**, 141 (1972).
9. A. Fefer, *Cancer Res.* **36**, 182 (1971).
10. R. B. Herberman, G. N. Rogentine, and M. E. Oren, *Clin. Res.* **17**, 328 (1969).
11. S. A. Rosenberg and W. D. Terry, *Adv. Cancer Res.* **25**, 323 (1977).
12. P. W. Wright, K. E. Hellström, I Hellström, and I. D. Bernstein, *Med. Clin. North Am.* **60**, 607 (1976).
13. R. I. Fisher, T. T. Kubota, G. L. Mandell, S. Broder, and R. C. Young, *Ann. Intern. Med.* **88**, 799 (1978).
14. G. Köhler and C. Milstein, *Nature* (*London*) **256**, 495 (1975).
15. I. D. Bernstein, M. R. Tam, and R. C. Nowinski, *Science* **207**, 68 (1980).
16. E. G. Engleman, R. Warnke, R. I. Fox, and R. Levy, *Proc. Natl. Acad. Sci. U.S.A.* **78**, 1791 (1981).
17. A. Boyum, *Scand. J. Clin. Lab. Invest.* **21**(97), 77 (1968).
18. M. F. Loken and L. A. Herzenberg, *Ann. N.Y. Acad. Sci.* **83**, 43 (1975).
19. R. Heitzman and F. M. Richards, *Proc. Natl. Acad. Sci. U.S.A.* **71**, 3537 (1975).
20. R. Warnke, R. A. Miller, T. Grogan, M. Pederson, J. Dilley, and R. Levy, *N. Engl. J. Med.* **303**, 293 (1980).
21. R. Warnke, M. Pederson, C. Williams, and R. Levy, *Am. J. Clin. Pathol.* **70**, 867 (1978).
22. R. Levy and J. Dilley, *J. Immunol.* **119**, 387 (1977).
23. F. C. Greenwood, W. M. Hunter, and J. S. Glover, *Biochem. J.* **89**, 114 (1963).
24. R. A. Miller, C. N. Coleman, H. D. Fawcett, R. T. Hoppe, and I. R. McDougall, *N. Engl. J. Med.* **303**, 89 (1980).
25. L. M. Nadler, P. Stashenko, R. Hardy, W. D. Kaplan, L. N. Button, *et al.*, *Cancer Res.* **40**, 3147 (1980).
26. L. J. Old, E. Stockert, E. A. Boyse, and J. H. Kim, *J. Exp. Med.* **127**, 523 (1968).
27. E. A. Boyse, E. Stockert, and L. J. Old, *Proc. Natl. Acad. Sci. U.S.A.* **58**, 954 (1967).
28. J. Ritz, J. M. Pesando, J. Notis-McConarty, and S. F. Schlossman, *J. Immunol.* **125**, 1506 (1980).
29. D. W. Dresser and G. Gowland, *Nature* (*London*) **203**, 733 (1964).
30. D. W. Dresser, *Immunology* **5**, 345 (1962).
31. J. T. Hamblin, A. K. Abdul-Ahad, J. Gordon, F. K. Stevenson, and G. T. Stevenson, *Br. J. Cancer* **42**, 495 (1980).
32. L. Olsson and H. S. Kaplan, *Proc. Natl. Acad. Sci. U.S.A.* **77**, 5429 (1980).

34

A Survey of Pediatric Hodgkin's Disease at Stanford University: Results of Therapy and Quality of Survival

SARAH S. DONALDSON AND HENRY S. KAPLAN

I. Historical Perspective

Several series have appeared in the literature during the past few years describing the results of therapy of Hodgkin's disease in children. The major series containing the largest numbers of children are summarized in Table I. Because staging and treatment policies have changed over recent years, the majority of these retrospective series are heterogeneous with respect to therapy; thus, they must be analyzed carefully.

The early studies of the 1960s dealt with clinically staged patients, including those studied with lymphangiography and bone marrow biopsy; most of these patients received radiotherapy and often palliative single-drug chemotherapy (1–4). The Memorial Hospital (New York) experience with 86 children included

MALIGNANT LYMPHOMAS

TABLE I

Results of Therapy in Large Retrospective Series of Hodgkin's Disease in Children

Investigator	No. of patients	Stages[a]	Years	Survival/relapse-free survival (%)	
				5 Years	10 Years
Tan et al. (1),	86	CS I–IV	1960–1969	62/?	50/?
New York	45	PS I–IV	1970–1974	82/?	
Donaldson et al. (2), Stanford	79	Mixed, CS, PS I–IV	1962–1972	89/66	70/41
	41	PS I–IV	1968–1972	93/82	
Smith and Rivera (3), Memphis	57	Mixed CS, PS I–IV	1967–1972	86/79	—
Smith et al. (4), London	59	Mixed CS, PS I–IV	1941–1975	85/?	—
Botnick et al. (6), Boston	52	PS I–III	1969–1975	98/90	—
Olweny et al. (8), Kampala	48	CS I–IV	1967–1977	67	—
Jenkin and Berry (5), Toronto	52	PS I–IV	1969–1977	92/57	89/54
	41	CS I–IV	1973–1977	89/85	

[a] CS, Clinical stage; PS, pathological stage.

49 (57%) who had undergone lymphangiography (1). Treatment in this series was extended-field radiotherapy for 51 children, with 6 receiving total nodal irradiation and 27 receiving limited-field irradiation only. Chemotherapy was reserved for those with disseminated disease. Surgical staging was employed for the 45 patients diagnosed during the years 1970–1974.

In the Stanford University Medical Center series of 79 children, all were clinically staged with lymphangiography and bone marrow biopsy, and 41 of 79 (52%) were surgically staged with splenectomy (2). Most of these children participated in randomized studies testing varying treatment regimens involving primary radiotherapy; multiagent chemotherapy has been used since 1968 as an adjuvant to irradiation in those with advanced disease.

During this era the St. Jude's Children's Research Hospital (Memphis, Tennessee) group relied largely on clinical staging, with protocol patients receiving high-dose radiotherapy to varying volumes depending on stage as well as chemotherapy which consisted of vincristine and cytoxan (3).

The Royal Marsden Hospital (London) group incorporated a variety of staging and therapeutic policies including radiotherapy and limited used of multiagent chemotherapy (4). In all these series, despite the variations in staging evaluation and treatment, 5-year survival rates ranged between 62 and 93%, and 5-year relapse-free survival rates between 57 and 79%.

At the Princess Margaret Hospital in Toronto a 92% 5-year survival rate and a 57% relapse-free survival rate were achieved in pathologically staged patients treated with extended fields and high-dose radiotherapy (5). Similarly, the Stanford group (2) observed 93% survival and 82% relapse-free survival rates at 5 years when pathological staging was employed. Thus, when pathological staging was uniformally used in children, 5-year survival rates increased to 92–93% and 5-year relapse-free survival rates to 57–82%.

The most favorable results from this era were reported by Botnick and colleagues at the Joint Center for Radiation Therapy (Boston) in a series of 52 children with pathological stage I–III disease (6). Those with stage I or IIA disease received extended-field radiotherapy alone; those with stage IIIA disease received total nodal radiotherapy, and those with systemic symptoms received total nodal radiotherapy plus nitrogen mustard, vincristine, procarbazine, and prednisone (MOPP). After a median follow-up interval of 3 years, 90% of these children were continuously free of disease, and 98% were alive without evidence of disease. These data further support the use of surgical staging and extended-field radiotherapy for early-stage disease, and combined-modality treatment for advanced disease. Thus, although treatment policies vary from institution to institution, centers with large numbers of children continue to show improved survival and freedom from relapse among pathologically staged patients using high-dose, large-volume radiotherapy for regionally localized disease and combined-modality treatment for advanced disease.

Whereas 2- and 5-year survival data are plentiful, 10-year survival data have been sparse and are only now beginning to emerge with continued follow-up of children treated during the late 1960s and 1970s. Tan et al. (1) showed that, for children clinically staged and treated initially primarily with extended-field radiotherapy, a 50% survival could be expected, with flattening of the survival curve after 9 years following diagnosis. In their series of 41 consecutive protocol patients and 11 nonprotocol patients, Jenkin and Berry (5) have reported 10-year relapse-free survival and survival rates of 54 and 89%, respectively. Patients who relapsed were generally then treated with MOPP and additional radiation. They demonstrated that salvage therapy was effective in maintaining a median duration of second remission of only 3 years; more than half of the children who experienced a first relapse had subsequent multiple relapses (5).

The Stanford experience supports these observations. Figure 1 shows our data on 171 consecutive children systematically staged, treated, and followed by a single team of physicians between 1962 and 1980. The actuarial 5-, 10-, and 15-year survival rates were 90, 80, and 70%, respectively, with corresponding freedom-from-relapse rates of 75, 66, and 66%, respectively. Although most

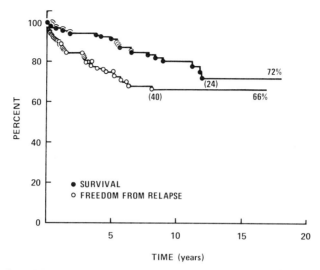

Fig. 1. Actuarial analysis of survival and freedom from relapse among 171 consecutive children, 15 years of age or less, seen, treated, and followed at Stanford between 1962 and 1980.

relapses occur within the first 3 years after diagnosis, late relapses can occur, with the latest in the Stanford pediatric series being observed 8 years following initial treatment. In general, late relapses occurred in patients who were not surgically staged initially and to whom no subdiaphragmatic radiation had been given. Thus these 15- to 18-year follow-up data in a large, consecutive series of children demonstrate the reality of long-term cure.

During the decade 1967–1977, at the Uganda Cancer Institute in Kampala, children with Hodgkin's disease were treated with MOPP chemotherapy (7) alone because radiation therapy facilities were nonexistent (8). These children were not subjected to surgical staging. Data from this group revealed that 42 of 48 (88%) achieved complete remission, with 31 of 42 (74%) remaining in first remission in excess of 5 years. The 5-year survival rate for the entire group was 67%, with 75% of stage I and II patients and 60% of stage III and IV children surviving. Although this patient population differs from the United States, Canadian, and British children in terms of genetic and environmental factors as well as histological subtype, the data support the conclusion that chemotherapy clearly is effective in pediatric Hodgkin's disease. The experience of the Southwest Oncology Group (SWOG) with 233 patients of all ages with advanced Hodgkin's disease treated with MOPP alone for six cycles reinforces the Uganda data; in this series, survival as a function of age was best for younger patients as compared to those in their middle or later adult years (9). Of 56 patients less than 20 years of age in the SWOG study, only 11 failed MOPP therapy, yielding an actuarial 7- to 8-year survival in the range of 65%, as compared to 55, 32, and 25% for those 20–40, 40–60, or greater than 60 years of age, respectively.

In light of the emerging effectiveness of chemotherapy and the increased use of combined-modality therapy, the group at Princess Margaret Hospital (Toronto) introduced a policy of involved-field radiation alone for clinical stage I patients and extended-field radiation and six cycles of MOPP chemotherapy for those with clinical stage II through IV disease (5, 10). Extended-field treatment included mantle and paraaortic fields with doses in the range of 3500 rads, which was gradually reduced to 2000–2500 rads. Since all patients received systemic chemotherapy, pathological staging was not employed. In this series of 41 children, the 5-year survival rate of 89% was comparable to their previous experience, but the relapse-free survival rate improved to 85% at 5 years. Only 1 of 32 children with clinical stage I–IVA disease relapsed in a nonirradiated lymph node. However, 4 of 9 clinical stage IVB children relapsed, making the relapse-free survival in the range of 50% for this unfavorable group.

II. Disease Characteristics

Although it was once thought that children with Hodgkin's disease fared less well than adults (11–14), and that the disease in childhood displayed characteristics that differed significantly from the disease seen in the adult population (15), the large series reviewed in Table I indicates that the natural history and response to treatment in children do *not* differ from those in adults. With respect to disease presentation, the areas of initial involvement and extension of disease are similar to those seen in adults. Figure 2 shows the documented frequency of involvement of various lymph node and extralymphatic sites at the time of presentation among 129 surgically staged children with Hodgkin's disease at Stanford. Supradiaphragmatic disease was common, with nearly 80% of children having disease on one or both sides of the neck at diagnosis. Extranodal extension to the pericardium, pleura, and pulmonary parenchyma was observed in the presence of massive mediastinal and/or hilar disease. No children in this series had epitrochlear, brachial, or popliteal adenopathy at presentation.

However, clinical staging including physical examination, chest radiographs and whole lung tomograms, a lymphangiogram, and a bone marrow biopsy is accurate in only approximately 70% of these patients, as shown in Fig. 3. Of the 129 patients, 90 were accurately staged clinically, 25% were upstaged, and an additional 5% were downstaged on the basis of surgical findings. Occult splenic disease was detected in 42 of these 129 children (33%) which would not have been apparent by clinical staging. Three of these children additionally had liver disease proven at a staging laparotomy.

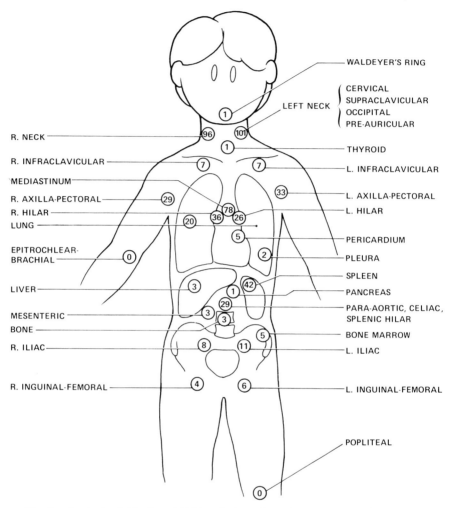

Fig. 2. Anatomic distribution of 490 lymphatic and extralymphatic sites of documented involvement in 129 surgically staged children with Hodgkin's disease.

Special attention does need to be given to children, however, in terms of the potential complications of treatment and their late effects. In this area, children represent both a challenge and a dilemma in treatment planning. As it is clear that 9 of 10 children carefully staged and treated will be long-term survivors, we must look to the quality of survival and carefully analyze the effects of our therapies which now yield such gratifying results.

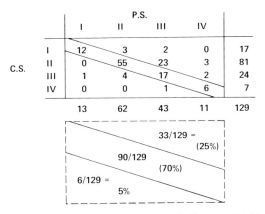

Fig. 3. Accuracy of clinical staging among 129 surgically staged children with Hodgkin's disease.

III. Effects of Treatment

In a patient population undergoing active growth and development, one must give special consideration to tissue development and organ function when planning treatment programs. Perhaps of greatest concern in children is the impairment of bone growth and development known to accompany high-dose, large-volume irradiation (16, 17). This is particularly marked when high doses (greater than 3500 rads) are administered to the total axial skeleton. Such treatment results in a disproportionate alteration in sitting height (crown-to-rump measurement) as compared to standing height. This abnormality is particularly marked in children less than 6 years of age and those in adolescence (11–13 years) at the time of treatment, during which time bone growth is particularly active. Growth impairment more than 2 standard deviations below the mean can be expected in these age groups when high doses of radiation are delivered to the axial skeleton. Abnormal development is particularly marked following typical mantle-field irradiation, which may result in a small thorax, short clavicles, narrow shoulders, and atrophy of the soft tissues of the neck. However, if radiation doses are reduced to less than 2500 rads to the axial skeletal, these bone growth defects are greatly diminished, standing heights being at or within 1 standard deviation of the mean and sitting heights being in the range of 1–2 standard deviations from the mean for all patients (16, 17).

Abnormalities in cardiac or pulmonary function which accompany high-dose, large-volume radiation may be particularly serious and severe. It is not obvious that children are more prone to injury in these tissues than adults, although they do have a projected long-term survival during which additional late effects could occur. The risks of pulmonary and cardiac injury noted and reported a decade ago (18–22) have been greatly minimized by refinements in the techniques of radiotherapy (23). With respect to the pediatric population, these techniques have emphasized megavoltage radiation, multiple shrinking fields, thin organ blocks, beam-shaping devices, and aids to immobilization (24). These methods help to accomplish effective shielding of lungs, heart, kidneys, and other vital organs and tissues, thus effectively minimizing late effects of radiation on organ growth and function.

Endocrine effects of aggressive treatment are largely related to thyroid and gonadal dysfunction. Among 119 children at Stanford studied with thyroid function tests, 77 (65%) were found to be chemically abnormal with elevated thyroid-stimulating hormone (TSH) or depressed thyroxine (T4) levels (25). This abnormality is directly related to both the dose of radiotherapy administered and the length of time of follow-up. The likelihood of thyroid injury among children receiving thyroid doses greater than 2600 rads was greater than among children who received less than 2600 rads. The natural history of this chronic radiation-induced thyroid dysfunction is not known. However, in the Stanford series there were 27 of 73 children (37%) with elevated TSH levels in whom spontaneous recovery occurred. Two of 119 children developed thyroid nodules, both shown to be benign thyroid adenomas at thyroidectomy. Although the risk of thyroid malignancy in this group of children is too small yet to be determined (26), we recommend thyroid replacement therapy for children who are chemically (elevated TSH with normal or depressed T4) or clinically hypothyroid, since the long-term carcinogenic risk of unopposed stimulation of the thyroid gland in childhood is unknown.

Gonadal injury following therapy is an increasing problem which must be addressed before therapeutic decisions are made. The technique of ovarian transposition (oophoropexy) with appropriate gonadal shielding has allowed the preservation of ovarian function in young women with Hodgkin's disease (27). Figure 4 shows the menstrual status of a series of girls, 13 years of age or greater at the time of analysis, and the impact of chemotherapy when added to radiation therapy. When oophoropexy was undertaken, followed by gonadal shielding to the pelvis, 100% of girls treated with radiation alone in the Stanford series maintained normal menses. When chemotherapy was added to this regimen, 21 of 27 (78%) maintained normal menses. The greatest insult occurred in those who had pelvic irradiation plus six cycles of MOPP, of whom only 6 of 11 (54%) maintained normal menses. Thus, the impact of aggressive therapy on ovarian function in children appears to be less than that in adults (28, 29). Of interest is that 8 of these young women later became pregnant. Three pregnancies were terminated with therapeutic abortions; the remaining five resulted in normal, healthy, full-term babies.

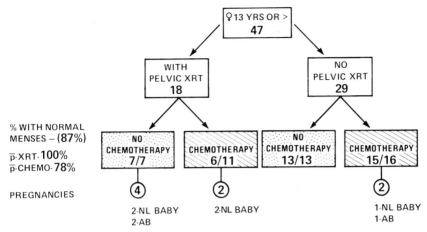

Fig. 4. Fertility as measured by menstrual status in 47 girls, 13 years of age or greater. XRT, Radiotherapy; AB, abortion; NL, normal.

The available data on male fertility are more limited and require longer follow-up. Incidental irradiation to the testis from an inverted-Y field can cause oligospermia or azospermia; however, this effect is often transient and full recovery may occur (30). With testicular shielding the gonadal dose can be kept to less than 100 rads during total nodal irradiation and complete recovery of spermatogenesis expected within 2 years after treatment (31). With subtotal nodal irradiation, where the pelvic lymph nodes are not treated, testicular doses are between 10–30 rads, with good recovery of testicular function within 9–18 months. However, testicular injury following MOPP chemotherapy appears to be more severe, with less likelihood of recovery from azospermia. Ugandan adolescent boys with Hodgkin's disease were studied for hormonal abnormalities following full courses of MOPP chemotherapy. Nine of 13 pubertal boys (10–16 years of age at the time of treatment) developed moderate to severe gynecomastia, complete germinal aplasia, a 10-fold increase in serum follicle-stimulating hormone (FSH) levels, a 3-fold increase in mean luteinizing hormone (LH) levels, and decreased serum testosterone levels (32). In contrast, the prepubertal boys showed no change in serum gonadotrophin levels and did not develop gynecomastia. In North America gynecomastia appears to be less common following MOPP therapy. However, it is clear that germ cell depletion and Leydig cell dysfunction are expected and unavoidable consequences of a full course of MOPP chemotherapy. The data available from large groups of adult males reveal that the probability of recovery of spermatogenic function and fertility is low. Insufficient numbers of boys prepubertal at the time of treatment have been followed long enough to indicate whether the late effects for this subgroup will be distinctly different from those for adolescent or adult males.

Among the Stanford pediatric population, gonadal function data are available on only eight boys (Fig. 5). Of four who received pelvic lymph node irradiation, one had a subsequent testicular biopsy at the time of an incidental hydrocele repair which showed absence of spermatogenesis. Three other boys who had pelvic radiation later fathered normal children. Of four postpubertal boys who received six courses of MOPP chemotherapy in whom semen analyses were performed, all showed absolute azospermia at follow-up periods of 4, 5, 7, and 9 years following chemotherapy.

Serious bacterial infections appear in approximately 10–12% of children with Hodgkin's disease (33, 34). In the Stanford series of 181 children, there were 27 episodes of infection in 22 patients, 15 of which represented bacteremia and/or meningitis (33). The likelihood of developing serious bacterial infection was related to the intensity of the treatment administered, regardless of whether or not the patient had undergone a previous splenectomy. The risk of serious bacterial infection after irradiation was 1.4% in splenectomized and 2.8% in nonsplenectomized children. All children with *Streptococcus pneumoniae* or *Hemophilus influenzae* bacteremia and/or meningitis had previously undergone a splenectomy. The incidence of serious bacterial infection has decreased almost to zero since we instituted the routine administration of prophylactic penicillin. A prospective investigation of the efficacy of pneumococcal vaccine undertaken at Stanford in children with Hodgkin's disease demonstrated significant differences in antibody response among children immunized prior to splenectomy and treatment as compared to those immunized after splenectomy, radiation, and chemotherapy (35). The duration of response was variable, and the response to any one antigen did not necessarily correlate with the response to other antigens.

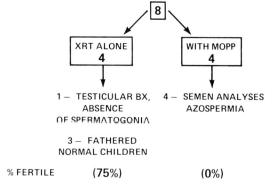

Fig. 5. Fertility in 8 boys as measured by semen analyses, testicular biopsy (BX), or ability to father a child. XRT, Radiotherapy.

Thus, one cannot rely on the presently available pneumococcal vaccine as the sole means of protection against pneumococcal infections in asplenic children with Hodgkin's disease.

Viral infections, particularly those with *Herpes zoster varicella* (HZV) virus, were more frequent in children treated with aggressive chemotherapy and radiation therapy as compared to those treated with radiation therapy alone, regardless of whether or not a splenectomy had been performed (36). The Stanford review of 181 children revealed an incidence of HZV of 56% among those receiving chemotherapy and radiation therapy as compared to 23.8% among those who received extended-field radiotherapy alone and 11.1% in those receiving local-field radiation alone. Twenty-seven percent of the children developed disseminated infection. However, development of HZV infection was not related to subsequent relapse or death due to Hodgkin's disease.

Of greatest concern in the selection of treatment regimens for children with a high probability of long-term survival is the risk of developing a second malignant tumor following successful treatment of the first. The secondary neoplasms which have been reported have largely been secondary hematological malignancies. The initial Stanford review by Coleman *et al.* (37) of 680 previously untreated patients demonstrated 8 cases of leukemia occuring among the 330 patients treated with both radiation and chemotherapy. The actuarial risk of developing leukemia in this group was 2.9% at 5 years and 3.9% at 7 years. There were no cases of leukemia among patients treated with radiation alone, nor in the small group treated with MOPP chemotherapy alone. However, we subsequently saw cases of leukemia following MOPP chemotherapy alone. A later analysis of a large, overlapping series of Stanford patients revealed 7 cases of non-Hodgkin's lymphoma among patients who had received both radiotherapy and chemotherapy (38).

An analysis of our pediatric population of 171 children revealed that 4 children (2.3%) developed second malignant tumors (Table II). These included 1 case of

TABLE II

Second Malignant Tumors

Treatment	Number	Percentage
All treatments	4/171	2.3
Radiation alone	0/59	0
MOPP alone	0/1	0
Combined-modality therapy	4/111	3.6
Low-dose XRT and MOPP	0/46	0
High-dose XRT and MOPP	4/65	6
High-dose XRT and MOPP, planned	1/29	3
High-dose XRT and MOPP, for relapse	3/36	8

acute monocytic leukemia, 1 case of non-Hodgkin's lymphoma (undifferentiated lymphoma), and 2 sarcomas, 1 chondrosarcoma and 1 an unclassifiable sarcoma. There were no second malignant tumors among the 57 patients treated with radiation alone, and only 1 child was treated with chemotherapy alone. Thus, all four malignant tumors arose in the 111 children who had received combined-modality treatment. No cases of second malignant tumors were seen in the subset who had received low-dose radiation and MOPP.[1] All four second tumors were in patients who had received high-dose total lymphoid irradiation with MOPP. The unclassifiable sarcoma arose within the abdominal irradiation field after a 5-year disease-free interval in a child with pathological stage IIB mixed cellularity Hodgkin's disease who had been treated with total lymphoid irradiation and adjuvant MOPP. This tumor was nonresponsive to further chemotherapy. The three other cases of a second malignant tumor arose in children initially treated with radiation who then relapsed and received chemotherapy for salvage, giving an incidence of 3/36 (8%) among this subset of children. The one case of leukemia developed within 4 years after initial diagnosis, the lymphoma after 10 years, and the chondrosarcoma after 9 years in a boy with multiple enchondrosis (Ollier's disease).

IV. Current Approach

The present challenge in the treatment of children with Hodgkin's disease is to delineate a program which will ensure continuation of our present excellent survival and disease-free survival figures while minimizing the risks of acute and chronic complications. Ten years ago, it appeared that the most significant untoward late effect of treatment was the profound impairment of bone growth that could be anticipated in youngsters given high-dose total lymphoid irradiation. At that time a pilot program was devised at Stanford (23) to ascertain whether multiple cycles of MOPP combination chemotherapy could replace part of the radiation dose in pathologically staged children. During the past 10 years 46 pathologically staged children have been treated with low-dose radiotherapy and MOPP. Radiation volumes were determined by the pathological stage. Involved-field radiation was given to those with pathological stage I or IIA disease, subtotal nodal radiation to those with stage $I_E A$ or $II_E A$ disease (localized extranodal extension), and total nodal radiation to those with systemic symptoms or with stage III disease. Patients with stage IIIB or IV disease received radiation to known sites and MOPP in an alternating "ping-pong" sequence with two cycles of drug followed by one region of radiation, another two cycles of drug, etc., until the total plan was completed (39). Radiation doses were determined on the basis of the child's bone age, using doses of 1500 rads for those with a bone age

[1]See Note Added in Proof on p. 588.

of less than 6 years, 2000 rads for those 6–10 years, and 2500 rads for those 11–14 years of age. When necessary, massive lymphadenopathy not overlying the axial skeleton was locally supplemented to 3000–3500 rads. All patients received six cycles of MOPP chemotherapy.

Actuarial analyses of survival and freedom from relapse are shown in Fig. 6. The stages of the patients are shown in the inset. Survival and relapse-free survival at 10 years were 96% and 93%, respectively. There were only three relapses. Two of these occurred in children having extensive stage IV disease at diagnosis, including bone marrow involvement, who failed to respond to MOPP chemotherapy, were never disease-free, and died within 6 months of diagnosis. The third relapse occurred in a girl with stage $III_{EE}B$ disease involving the lung and pericardium. She had a recurrence at 18 months in an irradiated neck node and has apparently been salvaged with further radiation.

Although the maximal follow-up in this group is 10 years, the median follow-up is only 3 years; thus, longer evaluation will be necessary to ascertain the ultimate disease status and late complications of treatment. However, it appears that low-dose irradiation and six cycles of MOPP are highly effective for control of most lymph node sites. Figure 7 shows the status of control of 151 involved lymph node regions in these 46 children. Sites were scored as involved on the basis of palpable disease considered positive on physical examination and of radiographic extent of disease as determined by chest X-ray, whole-lung tomograms, and lymphangiogram; each lymph node region was scored individually as in the Ann Arbor staging system (40). There has been only one relapse among 151 irradiated nodal sites, for a local relapse rate of 0.6%. This failure occurred

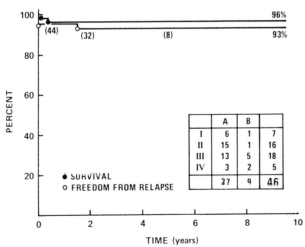

Fig. 6. Actuarial analysis of survival and freedom from relapse among 46 children treated with low-dose radiation with MOPP.

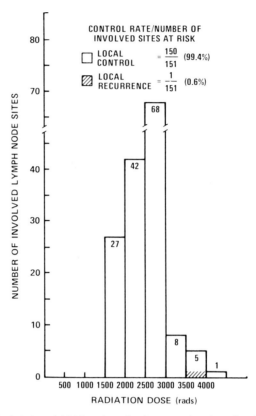

Fig. 7. Control status of 151 lymph node sites as a function of radiation dose and six cycles of MOPP among 46 children.

in a massively enlarged cluster of lymph nodes treated to 3500 rads plus six cycles of MOPP.

To date this treatment plan has been well tolerated. There have been no complications from surgical staging and no serious bacterial infections in children who have received prophylactic antibiotics. The acute morbidity of treatment has largely been related to nausea and vomiting, peripheral neuropathy, hair loss, and bone marrow suppression from chemotherapy. These have all been reversible and have not been considered severe. Early thyroid dysfunction following thyroid doses of less than 2500 rads has appeared in only 4 of 24 (17%) children tested. The follow-up interval is too short to ascertain the impact of gonadal function in prepubertal patients.

The ultimate assessment of growth preservation will require many patients and long-term follow-up. However, Fig. 8 shows 9-year follow-up height and weight measurements for a child who at age 4 was found to have pathological stage III$_S$B Hodgkin's disease and was treated with low dose (2000 rads) total lymphoid irradiation followed by six cycles of MOPP chemotherapy. The child's weight and standing height, after being slightly subnormal for a few years, are now within less than 1 standard deviation from the mean. The sitting height was unchanged for approximately 3 years but is now increasing parallel to the mean. This youngster remains relapse-free 10 years following treatment, with height and weight within the range of normal. Thus, the combination of low-dose

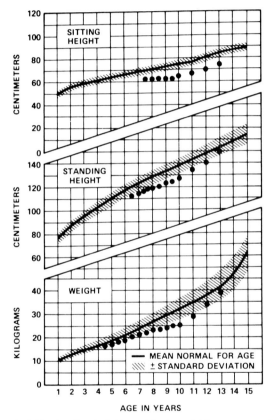

Fig. 8. Sitting height, standing height, and body weight measurements of a boy with pathological stage III$_S$B Hodgkin's disease treated with low-dose (2000 rads) total lymphoid irradiation followed by six cycles of MOPP chemotherapy. The solid lines and shaded areas are the mean plus or minus the standard deviation for age. The patient's body weight and standing height, after being slightly subnormal for a few years, are again within less than 1 standard deviation from the mean; the sitting height remained static for about 3 years but is now increasing parallel to the normal curve. The boy, treated at age 4, remains free of disease at age 14. [Reprinted by permission from H. S. Kaplan (23).]

irradiation and chemotherapy has been effective in achieving apparent cure without the known bone growth sequelae of high-dose radiation. Developmental impairment of these children has been minimal or absent. To date we have seen no second malignant tumors in this group, but the mean follow-up period is still too short to feel secure, since the median interval from the diagnosis of Hodgkin's disease to the diagnosis of leukemia in an earlier study was 41 months (37).

V. Future Considerations

Despite the impressive evolving body of data underscoring the successes achieved in Hodgkin's disease, there is still room for further improvement. Several major questions need to be addressed in future investigations of the optimal management of children with Hodgkin's disease.

1. Are there subsets of patients in whom staging laparotomy can appropriately be omitted? Staging laparotomy can only be defended if the information discovered will aid in treatment planning. There are some subsets of patients in whom the detection of subdiaphragmatic disease is very uncommon. Experience in adults has demonstrated that the likelihood of discovering subdiaphragmatic disease is in the range of 2% among those few patients who have lymphocyte predominance Hodgkin's disease confined to the upper right neck (near the angle of the mandible) and a negative chest X-ray and lymphangiogram (23). Another group with a small likelihood of subdiaphragmatic disease includes the rare patients with nodular sclerosing Hodgkin's disease confined to the mediastinum, with no cervical-supraclavicular adenopathy, after very careful neck examination, and a negative lymphangiogram. There have been only 2 of 171 children in the Stanford series with clinical stage IA lymphocyte predominance disease confined to the upper right neck and only 1 of 171 children with nodular sclerosing Hodgkin's disease confined to the mediastinum.

Patients who clearly have stage IV disease with multiple pulmonary or osseous disease benefit from combined-modality therapy. Patients with massive intrathoracic disease and/or massive splenic disease are also best handled with combined-modality therapy rather than radiation alone. In such a setting surgical staging may not change a treatment program and thus may not be essential in the evaluation.

As mentioned, Jenkin and Berry of the Princess Margaret Hospital reported an excellent 89% survival and a 85% freedom from relapse among 41 children with stage I–IV disease who were clinically staged without laparotomy. These children were treated with extended-field irradiation to doses of 2000–3500 rads, supplemented with six cycles of MOPP for those with clinical stage II–IV disease

(5). The policy at Stanford has been to limit the volume of radiation as well as the dose *even further* in children known to have early disease on the basis of surgical staging. Thus, a child with pathological stage IIA disease at Stanford receives a minimantle or a mantle field depending on the sites of involvement and six cycles of MOPP, whereas at the Princess Margaret Hospital such a patient is given a treatment program including extended-field radiation (a mantle, paraaortic and splenic field) plus six cycles of MOPP. Since the Stanford survival and relapse-free survival rates (Fig. 6) compare favorably with those of the Toronto series, and since there have been no deaths due to sepsis in splenectomized children treated with prophylactic penicillin, there appears to be no strong argument for abandoning staging laparotomy as part of our overall management policy.

2. Can we better tailor our therapy to the stage and extent of disease? Here the answer lies again in one's philosophy of treatment. Whereas subsets of patients have been shown to require combined-modality treatment for maximal local control, i.e., those with massive intrathoracic disease or massive splenic disease (41), other patients do not require combined-modality treatment. The Stanford S1 study randomized patients with pathological stage IA or IIA disease between subtotal lymphoid irradiation and involved-field radiation plus MOPP and failed to show a significant difference in efficacy of these treatment arms (23). Patients with stage IB or IIB disease (the Stanford H2 study) randomized between total lymphoid irradiation alone versus total lymphoid radiation plus MOPP also failed to show an advantage from chemotherapy (23). Thus, radiation alone is sufficient for these groups, and chemotherapy can safely be omitted. However, adequate irradiation requires high-dose, large-volume treatment. The use of low-dose irradiation plus MOPP offers at least equal assurance of local control without the penalty of bone growth impairment in children.

3. How can we improve our cure rates for those with stage IV marrow-positive disease? Overall experience shows that MOPP chemotherapy alone is not adequate for patients with Hodgkin's disease involving the bone marrow (42). It may be that alternating MOPP with other combination chemotherapy regimens such as adriamycin, bleomycin, vinblastine, and dacarbazine (ABVD) (43) or using different timing schedules may improve upon this subset which carries a poor prognosis.

4. Are there other combinations of chemotherapeutic agents which have a decreased risk of inducing sterility? Prospective randomized trials with a long-term careful follow-up will be necessary to search for drug combinations as effective as MOPP but with fewer sequelae on gonadal tissue. Since the pediatric population represents a small percentage of the general population with Hodgkin's disease, it is probable that we must look to the adult experience for these answers.

5. Can we minimize the possibility of second malignant tumor induction? A longer follow-up interval will be required to validate our preliminary impression

that the Stanford policy of surgical staging, low-dose, limited-field irradiation, and MOPP chemotherapy has been successful in decreasing or eliminating the risk of the induction of second malignant tumors.

6. How can we quantitate acute and late treatment morbidity? A major unsolved problem with respect to pediatric Hodgkin's disease is to define the risk/benefit ratio of our treatments as they apply to this population with projected long-term survival. It is not possible to equate or compare accurately the consequences of a 2–3 month period of irradiation to those of a 6-month program of chemotherapy or a 9-month program of combined-modality treatment. It is difficult to choose between the bone growth impairment resulting from high-dose radiation and the sterility induced by MOPP chemotherapy. Inability to continue school or work, a change in body image, or the emotional impact of having a malignant disease are other aspects of childhood Hodgkin's disease which require consideration when deciding upon treatment programs. The successful treatment programs of yesterday and today have raised new questions for tomorrow regarding the quality of survival and the price of success.

Note Added in Proof

Since the submission of this paper, one child treated with low-dose radiation and MOPP has developed acute myelogenous leukemia, and a second has a bone marrow suggestive of pre-leukemia, demonstrating that children are also at risk for induction of second malignant tumors after treatment with combined modality therapy.

References

1. C. Tan, G. J. D'Angio, P. R. Exelby, P. H. Lieberman, R. C. Watson, W. C. Cham, and M. L. Murphy, The changing management of childhood Hodgkin's disease. *Cancer* **35**, 808–816 (1975).
2. S. S. Donaldson, E. Glatstein, S. A. Rosenberg, and H. S. Kaplan, Pediatric Hodgkin's disease. I. Results of therapy. *Cancer* **37**, 2436–2447 (1976).
3. K. L. Smith, and G. Rivera, Comparison of the clinical course of Hodgkin's disease in children and adolescents. *Med. Pediatr. Oncol.* **2**, 361–370 (1976).
4. I. E. Smith, M. J. Peckham, T. J. McElwain, J. C. Gazet, and D. C. Austin, Hodgkin's disease in children. *Br. J. Cancer* **36**, 120–129 (1977).
5. R. D. T. Jenkin and M. P. Berry, Hodgkin's disease in children. *Semin. Oncol.* **7**, 202–211 (1980).
6. L. E. Botnick, R. Goodman, N. Jaffe, R. Filler, and J. R. Cassady, Stages I–III Hodgkin's disease in children. Results of staging and treatment. *Cancer* **39**, 599–603 (1977).
7. V. T. DeVita, A. Serpick, and P. P. Carbone, Combination chemotherapy in the treatment of advanced Hodgkin's disease. *Ann. Intern. Med.* **73**, 881–895 (1970).
8. C. L. Olweny, E. Katongole-Mbidde, C. Kiire, S. K. Lwanga, I. Magrath, and J. L. Ziegler, Childhood Hodgkin's disease in Uganda. A ten year experience. *Cancer* **42**, 787–792 (1978).

9. C. A. Coltman, Chemotherapy of advanced Hodgkin's disease. *Semin. Oncol.* **7**, 155–173 (1980).

10. D. Jenkin, M. Freedman, P. McClure, V. Peters, F. Saunders, and M. Sonley, Hodgkin's Disease in children: Treatment with low dose radiation and MOPP without staging laparotomy. A preliminary report. *Cancer* **44**, 80–86 (1979).

11. K. Ziegler, "Die Hodgkinsche Krankheit." Fisher, Jena, 1911.

12. C. A. Smith, Hodgkin's disease in childhood; clinical study with resumé of literature to date. *J. Pediatr.* **4**, 12–38 (1934).

13. H. Charache, Hodgkin's disease in children. *N.Y. State J. Med.* **46**, 507–509 (1946).

14. K. H. Vogelgesang and A. Többen, Ein Beitrag zur Prognose und Therapie der Lymphogranulomatose. *Strahlentherapie* **101**, 77–87 (1956).

15. R. C. Young, V. T. DeVita, and R. E. Johnson, Hodgkin's disease in childhood. *Blood* **42**, 163–174 (1973).

16. J. C. Probert and B. R. Parker, The effects of radiation therapy on bone growth. *Radiology* **114**, 155–162 (1975).

17. J. C. Probert, B. R. Parker, and H. S. Kaplan, Growth retardation in children after megavoltage irradiation of the spine. *Cancer* **32**, 634–639 (1973).

18. R. J. Carmel and H. S. Kaplan, Mantle irradiation in Hodgkin's disease. An analysis of technique, tumor eradication, and complications. *Cancer* **37**, 2813–2825 (1976).

19. H. S. Kaplan and J. R. Stewart, Complications of intensive megavoltage radiotherapy for Hodgkin's disease. *Natl. Cancer Inst. Monogr.* **36**, 439–444 (1973).

20. K. E. Cohn, J. R. Stewart, L. F. Fajardo, and E. W. Hancock, Heart disease following radiation. *Medicine (Baltimore)* **46**, 281–298 (1967).

21. J. R. Stewart, K. E. Cohn, L. F. Fajardo, E. W. Hancock, and H. S. Kaplan, Radiation-induced heart disease; a study of twenty-five patients. *Radiology* **89**, 302–310 (1967).

22. L. F. Fajardo, J. R. Stewart, and K. E. Cohn, Morphology of radiation-induced heart disease. *Arch. Pathol.* **86**, 512–519 (1968).

23. H. S. Kaplan "Hodgkin's Disease," 2nd ed. Harvard Univ. Press, Cambridge, Massachusetts, 1980.

24. S. S. Donaldson, E. Glatstein, and H. S. Kaplan, Radiotherapy of childhood lymphoma. *In* "Trends in Childhood Cancer" (M. M. Donaldson and H. G. Seydel, eds.), pp. 38–66. Wiley, New York, 1976.

25. L. S. Constine, S. S. Donaldson, I. R. McDougall, and H. S. Kaplan, Thyroid dysfunction after radiotherapy in children with Hodgkin's disease. *Int. J. Radiat. Oncol. Biol. Phys.* **6**, 1357 (abstr.) (1980).

26. I. R. McDougall, C. N. Coleman, J. S. Burke, W. Saunders, and H. S. Kaplan, Thyroid carcinoma after high-dose external radiotherapy for Hodgkin's disease. Report of three cases. *Cancer* **45**, 2056–2060 (1980).

27. G. R. Ray, H. W. Trueblood, L. P. Enright, H. S. Kaplan, and T. S. Nelson, Oophoropexy: A means of preserving ovarian function following pelvic megavoltage radiotherapy for Hodgkin's disease. *Radiology* **96**, 175–180 (1970).

28. L. G. Sobrinho, R. A. Levine, and R. C. DeConti, Amenorrhea in patients with Hodgkin's disease treated with antineoplastic agents. *Am. J. Obstet. Gynecol.* **109**, 135–139 (1971).

29. M. C. Morgenfeld, V. Goldberg, H. Parisier, S. C. Bugnard, and G. E. Bur, Ovarian lesions due to cytostatic agents during the treatment of Hodgkin's disease. *Surg., Gynecol. Obstet.* **134**, 826–828 (1972).

30. B. Speiser, P. Rubin, and G. Casarett, Aspermia following lower truncal irradiation in Hodgkin's disease. *Cancer* **32**, 692–698 (1973).

31. T. L. Thar, and R. R. Million, Complications of radiation treatment of Hodgkin's disease. *Semin. Oncol.* **7**, 174–183 (1980).

32. R. T. Sherins, C. L. M. Olweny, and J. C. Ziegler, Gynecomastia and gonadal dysfunction in adolescent boys treated with combination chemotherapy for Hodgkin's disease. *N Engl. J. Med.* **299,** 12–16 (1978).

33. S. S. Donaldson, E. Glatstein, and K. L. Vosti, Bacterial infections in pediatric Hodgkin's disease: Relationship to radiotherapy, chemotherapy, and splenectomy. *Cancer* **41,** 1949–1958 (1978).

34. R. R. Chilcote, R. L. Baehner, D. Hammond, and Children's Cancer Study Group, Septicemia and meningitis in children splenectomized for Hodgkin's disease. *N Engl. J. Med.* **295,** 798–800 (1976).

35. S. S. Donaldson, K. L. Vosti, F. R. Berberich, R. S. Cox, H. S. Kaplan, and G. Schiffman, Response to pneumococcal vaccine among children with Hodgkin's disease. *Rev. Infect. Dis.* **3,** 5133–5143 (1981).

36. F. Reboul, S. S. Donaldson, and H. S. Kaplan, *Herpes zoster* and *varicella* infections in children with Hodgkin's disease: An analysis of contributing factors. *Cancer* **41,** 95–99 (1978).

37. C. N. Coleman, C. J. Williams, A. Flint, E. J. Glatstein, S. A. Rosenberg, and H. S. Kaplan, Hematologic neoplasia in patients treated for Hodgkin's disease. *N. Engl. J. Med.* **297,** 1249–1252 (1977).

38. J. G. Krikorian, J. S. Burke, S. A. Rosenberg, and H. S. Kaplan, The occurrence of non-Hodgkin's lymphoma following therapy for Hodgkin's disease. *N. Engl. J. Med.* **300,** 452–458 (1979).

39. R. T. Hoppe, C. S. Portlock, E. Glatstein, S. A. Rosenberg, and H. S. Kaplan, Alternating chemotherapy and irradiation in the treatment of advanced Hodgkin's disease. *Cancer* **43,** 472–481 (1979).

40. H. S. Kaplan and S. A. Rosenberg, The treatment of Hodgkin's disease. *Med. Clin. North Am.* **50,** 1591–1610 (1966).

41. R. T. Hoppe, S. A. Rosenberg, H. S. Kaplan, and R. S. Cox, Prognostic factors in pathological stage IIIA Hodgkin's disease. *Cancer* **46,** 1240–1246 (1980).

42. C. S. Portlock, S. A. Rosenberg, E. Glatstein, R. Levy, and H. S. Kaplan, Failure of initial therapy for stages I, II and III Hodgkin's disease: Salvage management. *Proc. Am. Soc. Clin. Oncol.* **18,** 342 (abstr.) (1977).

43. A. Santoro, G. Bonadonna, V. Bonfante, and P. Valagussa, Non-cross-resistant regimens (MOPP and ABVD) versus MOPP alone in stage IV Hodgkin's disease (HD). *Proc. Am. Soc. Clin. Oncol.* **21,** 470 (abstr.) (1980).

35

Pediatric Non-Hodgkin's Lymphomas: The Children's Cancer Study Group Experience—An Interim Report

R. D. T. JENKIN, J. R. ANDERSON, R. CHILCOTE, P. COCCIA,
P. EXELBY, J. KERSEY, J. KUSHNER, A. MEADOWS, S. SIEGEL,
J. WILSON, S. LEIKIN, AND D. HAMMOND

I. Introduction

During the early 1970s it became clear that the classic 10–15% cure rate for children with non-Hodgkin's lymphoma, obtained with radiation treatment with or without resection, was progressively improving with the addition of systemic treatment.

In general, modified childhood leukemia regimens together with radiation treatment were utilized. The earliest and most important demonstration of a major improvement was by Wollner, who in 39 children demonstrated a 73% disease-free rate with 56+ to 88+ months' follow-up. She utilized a 10-drug leukemia program intensified with cyclophosphamide and radiation treatment to sites of bulk disease (1). Wollner obtained equally good results when the disease was predominantly intraabdominal (2).

Another approach stemmed from the treatment experience with childhood African lymphoma (Burkitt's lymphoma). In North American patients Ziegler (3) demonstrated the effectiveness of cyclophosphamide–methotrexate–vincristine regimens with or without prednisone and emphasized the excellent results, more than 80% survival, obtained when the total body burden of tumor cells was low, that is, in localized disease, compared with cases involving a large body burden, about 40% survival, and questioned the need for treatment prolonged beyond 6 months.

Djerassi demonstrated that high doses of methotrexate alone gave very high initial complete response rates (4).

More recently, Weinstein and his colleagues in Boston obtained an 82% 2-year survival rate with the combination of adriamycin with vincristine, prednisone, L-asparaginase, and 6-mercaptopurine. Burkitt's-type lymphoma did less well and is now not treated with this regimen (5, 6).

Murphy utilized a cyclophosphamide-intensified leukemic regimen for localized disease and a cyclophosphamide- and adriamycin-intensified regimen for more advanced disease and obtained a 90% disease-free survival rate at 2 years for patients in stages I and II and 39% for stages III and IV. In advanced disease she was not able to demonstrate any benefit from the addition of radiation treatment but obtained suggestive evidence that elective central nervous system (CNS) treatment was necessary (7).

In 1975 it appeared to the investigators of the Children's Cancer Study Group (CCSG) that the most important research objective was to determine optimal systemic treatment. In practice it was necessary to confirm Wollner's observations with the LSA_2-L_2 regimen. A new treatment regimen was designed having origins in the work of Ziegler and Djerassi and utilizing cyclophosphamide, methotrexate in maximal dosage without citrovorum rescue, vincristine, and prednisone (COMP). Initially the toxicity and effectiveness of the new treatment regimen was studied by the CCSG and was shown in a pilot study to be effective without unreasonable toxicity (8). Subsequently CCSG investigators compared the LSA_2-L_2 regimen to COMP in a prospective randomized trial. In view of the heterogeneity of the childhood non-Hodgkin's lymphomas it was elected to concentrate on a single two-arm study and to determine some of the biological features of this spectrum of malignancies. Radiation treatment and central nervous system (CNS) prophylaxis were therefore standardized in this study in the fashion described by Wollner for the LSA_2–L_2 regimen.

This article will describe the interim results of this study.

II. Children's Cancer Study Group Trial (CCG-551)

The investigators of the CCSG opened a prospective randomized treatment trial for children with non-Hodgkin's lymphoma in April 1977. All children were eligible for this trial provided only that they were newly diagnosed, previously untreated patients less than 17 years old with less than 25% lymphoma cells in the bone marrow.

Trial patients were randomized after stratification for extent of disease (localized and nonlocalized); principal anatomical site of disease (mediastinum, abdomen, nodal, and other); institutional histological diagnosis (Rappaport); bone marrow status (M1 or M2); CNS disease at diagnosis (present or absent); and age (above and below age 13). Randomization was to one of two treatment arms: regimen I (cyclophosphamide, vincristine, methotrexate, and prednisone) and regimen II (the 10-drug LSA_2–L_2 regimen of Wollner) (Table I). The LSA_2–L_2 regimen was modified by dose reduction for cytosine arabinoside and 6-thioguanine in intensification, to 100 and 50 mg/m^2, respectively. Later the duration of treatment for these two drugs was reduced from 4 weeks to 2 weeks because of hematological toxicity.

Both treatment regimens included similar elective CNS treatment with maintained intrathecal methotrexate and the same radiation treatment, that is, radiation to all sites of known disease for localized presentations and to sites of bulk disease, defined as masses greater than 3.0 cm in diameter, in nonlocalized presentations. Thus CNS prophylaxis and radiation treatment were not planned study variables.

Between April 1977 and September 1979, inclusive, 329 children were entered in the study and formed the basis of this interim report, an analysis in September 1980.

III. Results

A. Overall

The 2- and 3-year survival rates, respectively, were 65 and 62%, and the relapse-free survival rates were 59 and 57% (Fig. 1).

Very few new events were seen after 24 months. It is anticipated that the

TABLE I

Regimen I (COMP) and Regimen II (LSA$_2$–L$_2$): Drug Dosage and Schedule[a]

Induction	Consolidation	Maintenance
Regimen I (COMP)		
CPM: 1.2 gm/m², iv, day 1	—	CPM: 1.0 gm/m², iv, day 1, repeat every 28 days
VCR: 2.0 mg/m² (max. 2.0 mg), iv, weekly on days 3, 10, 17, and 24		VCR: 1.5 mg/m², iv (max. dose 2.0 mg), day 1, and 15. Repeat every 28 days
MTX: 6.25 mg/m², it, day 5 and on days 31 and 34 during PDN withdrawal		MTX: 6.25 mg/m², it, day 29, repeat every 28 days
MTX: 300 mg/m², iv, on day 12 (60% of dose as iv push and 40% as 4-hr infusion)		MTX: 300 mg/m², iv, day 15, (60% of dose iv push, 40% as 4-hr infusion): repeat every 28 days
PDN: 60 mg/m² (max. 60 mg), po, daily, in 4 divided doses, days 3–30, decremental doses to 0 days 31–37.		PDN: 60 mg/m² (max. dose 60 mg), po, daily × 5. First cycle start day 29, repeat every 28 days
XRT		

Regimen II (LSA₂-L₂)

CPM: 1.2 gm/m², iv, day 1

VCR: 2.0 mg/m² (max. dose 2.0 mg), iv, weekly on days 3, 10, 17, and 24

MTX: 6.25 mg/m², IT, day 5, repeat on days 31 and 34 during PDN withdrawal

PDN: 60 mg/m² max. dose 60 mg), po, daily in 4 divided doses, days 3–30, decremental doses to 0 days 31–37

DNM: 60 mg/m², iv, days 12 and 13

ARA-C: 100 mg/m², iv, daily × 5 (Mon.–Fri.) for 4 weeks[b]

6-TG: 50 mg/m², po, 8–12 hr after each ARA-C injection

L-Asp: 6000 IU/m²/day × 14, im, on completion of ARA-C + 6-TG

MTX: 6.25 mg/m², it, twice, 3 days apart, beginning 2–3 days after last L-Asp injection

BCNU: 60 mg/m², iv, single dose 2–3 days following completion of it MTX

Cycle:
(1) TG-CPM—TG, 300 mg/m², po, daily × 4 days, followed by CPM, 600 mg/m², iv, single dose, day 5

(2) HU-DNM—HU, 2.4 g/m², po, daily × 4 days, followed by DNM, 45 mg/m², iv, day 5

(3) MTX-BCNU—MTX, 10 mg/m², po, daily × 4 days, followed by BCNU, 60 mg/m², iv, day 5

(4) ARA-C-VCR—ARA-C, 150 mg/m², iv, daily × 4 days, followed by VCR 2.0 mg/m², (max. dose 2.0 mg), iv, day 5

(5) MTX: 6.25 mg/m², it, 2 doses 3 days apart

[a] Duration of treatment was 18 months. CPM, Cyclophosphamide; VCR, vincristine; MTX, methotrexate; PDN, prednisone; ARA-C, cytosine arabinoside; 6-TG, 6-thioguanine; L-Asp, L-asparaginase; BCNU, 1,3-bis (2-chloroethyl)-1-nitrosourea; HU, hydroxyurea; DNM, daunomycin; iv, intravenously, it, intrathecally; po, orally; im, intramuscularly.

[b] See text.

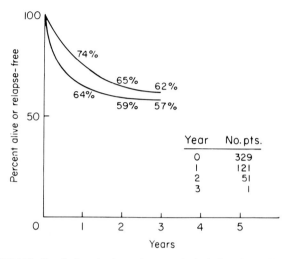

Fig. 1. CCG-551. Survival and relapse-free survival of all patients. The number of patients alive at each year is indicated.

2-year relapse-free rates in this study will approximate the final cure rates. All subsequent data reported will relate to relapse-free survival rates.

B. Localized versus Nonlocalized Disease

One hundred and one patients had localized disease (101/329, 31%) at diagnosis. The anatomical sites and extent of disease included in this subset were the

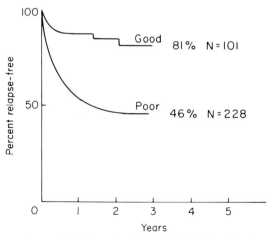

Fig. 2. Relapse-free survival for patients with localized (good) and nonlocalized (poor) disease at diagnosis.

gastrointestinal tract with or without involved mesenteric nodes, Waldeyer's ring with or without involved cervical nodes, lymph node presentations confined to a single region or two adjacent regions, and any of the rare extralymphatic sites provided that the disease was limited to a single site with or without involved regional nodes. Mediastinal mass presentations were specifically excluded and classified as nonlocalized.

The 3-year relapse-free survival rate was 81%. Only two events occurred after 18 months (Fig. 2).

Conversely, 228 patients (69%) had nonlocalized disease. The 3-year relapse-free survival rate was 46% (Fig. 2).

C. Sex, Site, Histology, and Surface Markers

This study confirmed the male preponderance of childhood non-Hodgkin's lymphoma, 252 boys (77%) compared with 77 girls (23%). Three-year relapse-free survival rates were girls 60% and boys 55%. Univariant analysis by site, histology, and the presence or absence of T- or B-cell surface characteristics has not yet produced meaningful data.

D. Bone Marrow Involvement

The presence of bone marrow involvement was an adverse prognostic factor. Forty-four patients (13%) with a positive bone marrow at diagnosis had a 21% 3-year relapse-free survival rate compared with 62% for 285 patients (87%) with an M1 marrow at diagnosis (Fig. 3).

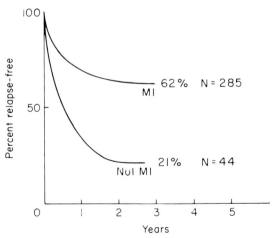

Fig. 3. Relapse-free survival by the presence (Not M1) or absence (M1) of bone marrow involvement at diagnosis.

TABLE II

The Correlation between Institutional and Review Histological Diagnosis[a]

Institution histology	Review histology					
				Undifferentiated		
	Unclassified	Lymphoblastic	Histiocytic	BKT	Pleomorphic	Total
Unclassified	2	4	1	0	1	8
Lymphoblastic	4	70	8	15	26	123
Histiocytic	0	2	22	3	11	38
Undifferentiated						
BKT	0	5	0	25	29	59
Pleomorphic	0	1	2	2	2	7
Total	6	82	33	45	69	235

[a] BKT, Burkitt's type.

E. Histological Diagnosis

The review histological diagnosis did not correlate well with the institutional diagnosis (Table II). Thus a diagnosis of lymphoblastic disease was made in 82/235 (35%) patients on review compared with 123/235 (52%) patients at the institutions.

While these differences may be mainly semantic, they are important in view of the relevance of histological classification to treatment in this study. Blind review of our material has confirmed internal consistency in making the distinction between lymphoblastic and nonlymphoblastic disease and in making a diagnosis of undifferentiated or histiocytic disease. Only in attempting the subdivision of undifferentiated lymphomas into pleomorphic or Burkitt type was there difficulty. It is not known at this time whether there is merit in seeking this subdivision.

Review histology and principal site of disease were related in this study: Mediastinal presentations ($N = 53$) 81% lymphoblastic; gastrointestinal tract and abdominal presentations ($N = 74$) 82% undifferentiated and 91% nonlymphoblastic.

F. Regimen I versus Regimen II: Overall

There was no difference in 3-year relapse-free survival rates by regimen: regimen I 56% and regimen II 59% (Fig. 4).

G. Regimen I versus Regimen II: Localized Disease

Both regimens were effective. The 3-year relapse-free survival rates were regimen I 83% and regimen II 80%.

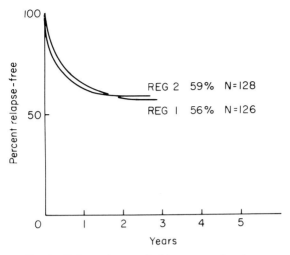

Fig. 4. Relapse-free survival by treatment regimen.

H. Regimen I versus Regimen II: Nonlocalized Disease by Histology

For patients with lymphoblastic disease, a significant difference was found in 3-year relapse-free survival rates: regimen II ($N = 32$) 76% and regimen I ($N = 27$) 27% (Fig. 5). Conversely, for all patients with nonlymphoblastic disease regimen I was superior: regimen I ($N = 42$) 56% and regimen II ($N = 35$) 29% (Fig. 6).

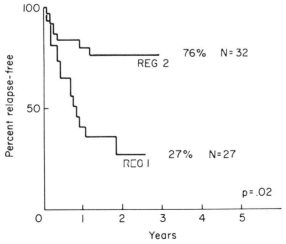

Fig. 5. Relapse-free survival for patients with nonlocalized lymphoblastic disease by treatment regimen.

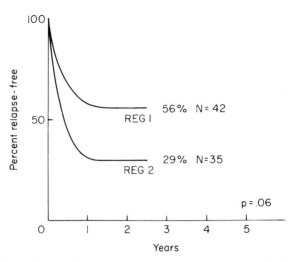

Fig. 6. Relapse-free survival for patients with nonlocalized nonlymphoblastic disease by treatment regimen.

While the size of the subsets becomes very small, the same trend favoring superior relapse-free survival rates for regimen I were seen for each of the histological subdivisions: undifferentiated pleomorphic, regimen I (N = 18) 59% and regimen II (N = 14) 30%; undifferentiated Burkitt's type, regimen I (N = 11) 61% and regimen II (N = 10) 23%; and histiocytic lymphoma, regimen I (N = 11) 54% and regimen II (N = 9) 26%.

IV. Summary

To date this study has confirmed that a modified LSA_2-L_2 treatment (regimen II) will produce improved results in children with non-Hodgkin's lymphoma and has demonstrated that similar overall results may be obtained with a four-drug program, regimen I (COMP). The important observation is that each of the regimens was, for nonlocalized disease, histology-specific, with regimen I (COMP) superior for nonlymphoblastic disease and regimen II (LSA_2-L_2) superior for lymphoblastic disease.

These regimens produced equally good results in patients with localized disease. Nonlymphoblastic disease is the common form (82%) in localized disease. It was of interest that for patients with localized nonlymphoblastic disease only 1 of 29 relapsed when treated with regimen I compared with 5 of 24 treated with regimen II, a result consistent with those obtained for patients with nonlocalized disease.

At this point the duration of treatment in this study, 18 months, appears at least adequate, in that relapse after 2 years is uncommon. This duration may be excessive. To examine this point the current CCSG study for patients with localized disease utilizes regimen I and is comparing durations of 6 and 18 months.

The positive definition of the malignant diseases encompassed by the negative term "non-Hodgkin's lymphoma" remains an important scientific objective. This study will provide data in support of this objective, since a treatment-specific disease response may be an important parameter in the final multivariate analysis of this study which hopefully will have as an outcome better disease definitions.

The important practical outcome of this study is that a further quantum jump in survival rates may be anticipated when optimal treatment programs specific for major subsets of patients within non-Hodgkin's lymphomas are utilized.

References

1. N. Wollner, P. R. Exelby, and P. H. Lieberman, Non-Hodgkin's lymphoma in children. *Cancer* **44**, 1990–1999 (1979).
2. N. Wollner, A. E. Wachtel, P. R. Exelby, and D. Centore, Improved prognosis in children with intra-abdominal non-Hodgkin's lymphoma following LSA_2-L_2 protocol chemotherapy. *Cancer* **45**, 3034–3039 (1980).
3. J. L. Ziegler, Treatment results of fifty-four American patients with Burkitt's lymphoma are similar to the African experience. *N. Engl. J. Med.* **297**, 75–80 (1977).
4. I. Djerassi and J. S. Kim, Methotrexate and citrovorum factor rescue in the management of childhood lymphosarcoma and reticulum cell sarcoma. (Non-Hodgkin's lymphomas). *Cancer* **38**, 1043–1051 (1976).
5. H. Weinstein, Z. Vance, N. Jaffe, D. Buell, J. Cassady, and D. Nathan, Improved prognosis for patients with mediastinal lymphoblastic lymphomas. *Blood* **53**, 687–694 (1979).
6. H. J. Weinstein and M. P. Link, Non-Hodgkin's lymphoma in childhood. *Clin. Haematol.* **8** (3), 699–716 (1979).
7. S. B. Murphy and H. O. Hustu, A randomized trial of combined modality therapy of childhood non-Hodgkin's lymphoma. *Cancer* **45**, 630–637 (1980).
8. A. T. Meadows, R. D. T. Jenkin, J. R. Anderson, R. Chilcote, P. Coccia, P. Exelby, J. Kushner, S. Leikin, S. Siegel, J. S. Wilson, and D. Hammond, A new therapy schedule for pediatric non-Hodgkin's lymphoma: Toxicity and preliminary research. *Med. Pediatr. Oncol.* **8** (1), 15–24 (1980).

36

LSA$_2$-L$_2$ in Childhood Non-Hodgkin's Lymphoma

NORMA WOLLNER

I. Introduction

This article will concern itself with a review of the present status of the use of the LSA$_2$-L$_2$ treatment protocol and the reasons for this approach as far as radiation therapy and surgery are concerned.

II. Historical Background

A. Age and Sex Incidence

Non-Hodgkin's lymphoma is a disease that affects mostly males (male/female ratio 2:1) (1, 2). In both sexes the age incidence is almost uniform from age 4 on

MALIGNANT LYMPHOMAS

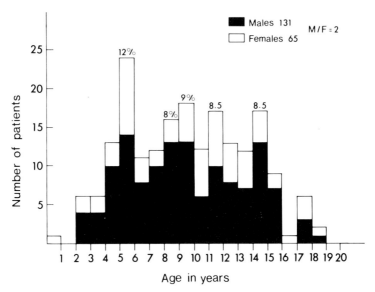

Fig. 1. Non-Hodgkin's lymphoma in children, 1964–1979.

to adulthood (Fig. 1). Seldom is the disease seen below the age of 1 year, and in this particular age group the lymphoma is quite aggressive and disseminated at diagnosis; the same is true of leukemia.

In non-Hodgkin's lymphoma the age incidence is an even distribution, with perhaps a peak at age 5. Whereas in leukemia the age incidence is bimodal, in Hodgkin's disease the incidence is higher at age 10 onward.

B. Clinical Staging

Non-Hodgkin's lymphoma is a disease quite different from Hodgkin's disease; that is, there is early dissemination to the bone marrow and to the central nervous system, a prevalence of extranodal disease, and a rapid and a fatal clinical course when untreated (and occasionally when treated). Therefore, to use the Ann Arbor staging is in some cases inadequate and difficult.

In 1971 (3) we devised a staging system later simplified (1974) (4) and now revised to conform to all possible initial primary sites (Table I).

In 196 patients reviewed (Table II) only 19% had early-stage disease of which only 8% had localized disease or stage I.

The majority of the patients (159/196) had extensive disease. Sixty-four of these patients had marrow involvement, an incidence of 32% of marrow replacement at the time of diagnosis (5–8). Five or 3% had initial central or peripheral nervous system involvement at diagnosis.

TABLE I

**Memorial Sloan-Kettering Cancer Center (1980):
Staging Non-Hodgkin's Lymphoma**

Stage	Criteria
I	Disease localized to one site or intraabdominal tumor completely resected
II	One site involved with regional node extension or two nodal sites involved on same side of diaphragm or intraabdominal lesion tumor completely resected
III	Tumor present on both sides of diaphragm or primary mediastinal involvement or inoperable intraabdominal disease
IV	Central nervous system involvement at diagnosis, primary epidural involvement, or bone marrow involvement at diagnosis
	A. Less or equal to 25% blasts at one or all marrow sites examined
	B. More than 25% blasts at all marrow sites examined

A further refinement of stage IVB (that is, patients with more than 25% blasts in the bone marrow), which is considered leukemia by most but lymphoma with marrow metastases by us, is:

1. Bulky disease in one area if nodal (3 cm or larger), with minimal or absent nodal involvement elsewhere. Bone marrow replacement (total or partial), with or without peripheral circulating blasts at the time of diagnosis.

2. If primary mediastinal disease, 50% or greater volume of the thoracic cavity involved by tumor, with or without pleural effusion. Bone marrow involvement (partial or total), with or without circulating blasts.

3. Unquestionable non-Hodgkin's lymphoma at the primary site, such as primary nasopharyngeal, mandible, gastrointestinal tract, liver, ovarian, breast,

TABLE II

**Non-Hodgkin's Lymphoma in Children
(1964–1979): Stages**

Stage	No. of patients	Percentage
I	15	
		19
II	22	
III	90	46
IV	5	
IVA	31	35[a]
IVB	33	

[a] Of the 196 patients, only 17% could be considered by some as high-risk leukemia.

thyroid, or skeletal disease. Initial bone marrow involvement (partial or total), with or without peripheral blood involvement.

4. Multiple primary sites usually extranodal, with rapid onset and extensive enough in the areas involved to suggest a sarcomatous process with marrow involvement (partial or total with or without hepatosplenomegaly).

It should be understood that a staging system that is so complicated is used only for uniformity of scientific work and comparison of results. Eventually non-Hodgkin's lymphoma will be staged as follows: I—localized (the present I and II); II—disseminated (the present III); and, III—disseminated disease with initial marrow and central nervous system involvement.

When this is achieved and is easily applicable by all, we will know that this disease is finally understood.

C. Primary Sites

A primary site is defined as that with the largest volume at diagnosis. At times, the symptoms and signs noticed by patients or parents are in adjacent areas, such as primary nasopharyngeal involvement causing stuffy nose and noisy breathing, but unless it causes deformity of facial features or bleeding, it will be noticeable as such only when neck nodes become apparent. Also, such is the case of some primary mediastinal disease brought to the attention of the physician because of low cervical or supraclavicular nodes.

If multiple primary sites are involved at the time of diagnosis, then the largest tumor is considered the primary site. In some instances there is disseminated disease with equal aggressiveness of the tumor in most areas, making determination of the primary site difficult. If pathologists can consider some tumors unclassifiable, then clinicians may consider a primary site unknown. These are nevertheless, rare events.

In Table III, the intraabdominal site is the most common primary site. Within the abdominal cavity organs such as the spleen, liver, kidneys, ovaries, and paraaortic nodes can be the initial site of disease. The most common intraabdominal site nevertheless is the gastrointestinal tract. Within the gastrointestinal tract (9, 10), the ileocecal region is more often involved. It is not unusual that, even with a distinct primary lesion in the ileocecal region, other distant areas in the ileum, jejunum, and duodenum may be involved as well, giving rise to multiple primary intestinal lesions.

Also, in some patients, usually young ones (where abdominal distention may not be considered unusual), the extent of disease in the abdomen is so diffuse that a primary site cannot be identified. Therefore we prefer to consider all these different primary sites primary intraabdominal. Mediastinal and peripheral nodal sites are equally represented. Mediastinal disease usually is very extensive within the thoracic cavity, involving all mediastinal structures and the pericardium with

TABLE III

Non-Hodgkin's Lymphoma in Children
(1964–1979): Primary Sites

Primary site	No. of patients	Percentage
Intraabdominal	63	32
Mediastinal	43	22
Peripheral nodal	44	22
Nasopharyngeal	13	7
Skeletal	19	10
Subcutaneous	8	4
Breast	1	0.5
Thyroid	1	0.5
Epidural	3	1.5
Testicular	1	0.5
Total	196	100

extension to the pleural surfaces. Some patients also have extensive disease outside the thoracic cavity on diagnosis. Peripheral nodal disease, nevertheless, is usually diagnosed earlier, because it is visible to parents and physicians earlier. It is believed that delay in diagnosis is responsible for dissemination to the bone marrow and the central nervous system. This is not necessarily true, as shown in our data:

1. In primary intraabdominal (occult) disease the incidence of initial marrow involvement (10/63) is 16%. The incidence of central nervous system involvement at diagnosis is 7%.

2. In primary mediastinal (occult) disease initial bone marrow involvement (17/43) is 39%, while central nervous system metastasis is 0%.

3. In primary peripheral nodal (visible) disease the initial incidence of bone marrow involvement is 50% (22/44) and central nervous system involvement is 0%. The reasons for this are not known.

Other uncommon primary sites are nasopharyngeal, skeletal, subcutaneous, and epidural. Rarer primary sites are the thyroid in a 5-year-old boy, the testicles at age 5, and the breast at age 4. The patient with primary testicular involvement had no other evidence of disease at the time of diagnosis at age 5. The patient with primary breast disease had it in one breast at age 4.

Histology

Based on a modified Rappaport histological classification, the most common histological type was diffuse lymphocytic and lymphoblastic, poorly differentiated (Table IV). Only one patient had nodular disease.

TABLE IV

Sequence of Clinical Events in Non-Hodgkin's Lymphoma in Children (1964–1970)

Local recurrence	80%
Median time	2 months
Bone marrow involvement	70%
Median time	3 months
Central nervous system involvement	45%
Median time	4 months

All these cases will eventually be reclassified in a new 1980 histological working classification.

D. Review of LSA$_2$-L$_2$ Protocol Changes

1. 1971–December 1973

In 1964, major advances were being made in leukemia, providing patients with a better quality of survival. This was not so for non-Hodgkin's lymphoma which was still poorly understood as a disease entity separate from Hodgkin's lymphoma. The uncertainty of distinguishing those with early marrow involvement from leukemia selected out patients with earlier disease, and the staging and treatment offered was similar to that of Hodgkin's disease. The results were dismal, and the quality of survival was appalling. The advent of cyclophosphamide, and its use in Burkitt's lymphoma in Africa, did little to improve the results in American children when the drug was used alone.

The analysis of 61 patients from 1964 to 1970 diagnosed, staged, and treated at Memorial Sloan-Kettering Cancer Center with what we still consider adequate clinical and radiological staging is analyzed in Fig. 2. The lower curve shows disease-free actuarial survival of the 61 patients to be 11%, with 7 patients alive at 10 years without evidence of recurrence. Five of these 7 had stage I disease—3 primary peripheral nodal, 2 intraabdominal, 1 tonsillar and 1 primary in the mandible. The other two were stage III and IV, respectively, and were treated with cyclophosphamide and concomitant radiation therapy. The stage III case involved diffuse undifferentiated primary ovarian disease, and the stage IV diffuse undifferentiated primary tonsillar involvement.

The sequence of events in these 61 patients can be seen in Table V. In this group of patients initial bone marrow involvement (stages IVA and IVB) was seen in 12/61 cases or 20%. Initial central nervous system involvement was seen in 1/61 or 1%. Bone marrow involvement *de novo*, as far as treatment failure is concerned, appeared in 52% and recurred in all but one patient (18%).

Bone marrow seldom was a site of the first event. In 85% of the cases it followed local recurrence. Therefore the foremost problem was the lack of con-

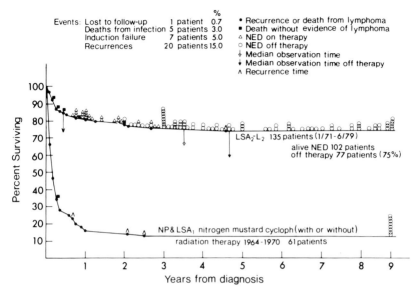

Events: Lost to follow-up 1 patient 0.7
Deaths from infection 5 patients 3.0
Induction failure 7 patients 5.0
Recurrences 20 patients 15.0

• Recurrence or death from lymphoma
■ Death without evidence of lymphoma
△ NED on therapy
○ NED off therapy
↓ Median observation time
↓ Median observation time off therapy
∧ Recurrence time

LSA$_2$-L$_2$ 135 patients (1/71-6/79)
alive NED 102 patients
off therapy 77 patients (75%)

NP & LSA$_1$ nitrogen mustard cycloph (with or without)
radiation therapy 1964-1970 61 patients

Fig. 2. Non-Hodgkin's lymphoma in children. Effect of treatment on survival.

trol of primary disease (80% of the patients) within a short period of time (2 months), inevitably followed by bone marrow or central nervous system metastases alone or in combination. The incidence of central nervous system involvement *de novo* was 44%. Therefore the incidence of bone marrow and central nervous system metastases was almost equal (52 and 44%), both occurring 1–1.5 months after local recurrence. Fifty percent of the patients were dead within the first 3 months, and 88% within the first year (12). It follows therefore that, if success in controlling this disease was the goal, several points were to be considered:

1. Effective and rapid local and systemic control of disease.

2. Protection of bone marrow from involvement or disappearance of evidence of initial involvement by the end of the first month.

3. Protection from initial central nervous system involvement and/or development of central nervous system involvement during the treatment.

If this could be accomplished within 1 month and maintained, perhaps the results and quality of survival could be improved. In 1970, the L$_2$ protocol for leukemia was devised (13–15), and it was particularly interesting to us because it used the most effective known agents in combination and in sequence, with a rapid change in drugs and pulse maintenance by different drugs at the maximal tolerated dosage. This treatment was ideal for marrow protection and/or marrow remission, but it was not enough for initial bulky disease. Our previous experi-

TABLE V

LSA$_2$–L$_2$ Treatment

Year	Induction[a]	Consolidation[b]	Maintenance	Radiation	Surgery
1971–1973	Cyclophosphamide; rest 3 days Prednisone for 4 weeks Vincristine four times weekly Daunomycin twice IT methotrexate three times	Cytosine arabinoside, 15 doses Thioguanine, 15 doses L-Asparaginase, 12 doses BCNU IV once IT methotrexate twice	Thioguanine Cyclophosphamide Hydroxyurea Daunomycin Methotrexate BCNU Cytosine arabinoside Vincristine IT methotrexate	To abdomen for inoperable cases All nasopharyngeal Bulky primary site (only the largest in multiple areas involved) No radiation to mediastinum Dosage intended; 3500–4500 rads Timing induction consolidation, and maintenance	Diagnostic only
1974	Same, but no interval between cyclophosphamide and prednisone	Same	Same	No radiation therapy to abdomen 2000 rads to all involved areas during induction and early consolidation (if multiple areas are to be irradiated)	Diagnostic Markers For extensive intra-abdominal involvement at the time of third vincristine treatment in induction to evaluate degree of response and need for further radiation

[a] 1971–1973, followed by 4–7 days rest; 1974, followed by 2 days rest.
[b] 1971–1973, followed by 7 days rest; 1974, followed by 2 days rest.

ence with cyclophosphamide suggested that this drug provided a quick and appreciable reduction in bulky disease, but alone it led to local recurrence before the next dosage of chemotherapy could be given. It also led to early tumor resistance if given at constant intervals in the same dosage. It was known that radiation therapy was an effective modality of treatment, even though not curative. Based on this information and these ideas in 1971 we proposed the LSA$_2$-L$_2$ which consisted of cyclophosphamide–L$_2$ and in some cases radiation therapy (12).

a. Chemotherapy. (January 1971–December 1973). Table V is self-explanatory. The reason for the 3-day delay between cyclophosphamide and the induction was to determine the rapidity and completeness of the response to cyclophosphamide and its implications for survival. We have found that, in non-Hodgkin's lymphoma, the rapidity and completeness of response has no prognostic significance. This is not difficult to understand if one recognizes that, even though non-Hodgkin's lymphoma responds well to most agents, it also becomes rapidly resistant to them, and it can regrow as fast as it can be destroyed. The intervals between induction and consolidation were maintained as in the L$_2$. The dosages of drugs such as daunomycin, *N, N*-bis(2-chloroethyl)-*N*-nitrosourea (BCNU), and oral methotrexate were also maintained, and it soon became obvious that in stage IV disease treatment for 3 years required a total dosage of daunomycin of more than 500 mg/m^2, which would be undesirable, especially if permanent and irreversible cardiac damage was to be avoided. As far as oral methotrexate and BCNU are concerned, the oral toxicity of the former and the bone marrow toxicity of the latter delayed the administration of further chemotherapy.

b. Radiation Therapy. The role of radiation therapy in advanced non-Hodgkin's lymphoma was unclear (16, 17). For those with stage IV disease, radiation was given only to a bulky area where compression to vital organs could be a potential problem. There was no intent of cure, since it would be impossible to deliver 4500 rads (the dosage then accepted to be curative) to multiple sites. Prior to 1971, since there were no survivors with stage IV non-Hodgkin's lymphoma, radiation therapy was hence given as a palliative local measure but not for curative purposes. In primary intraabdominal tumors, where disease was inoperable and extensive (most of them with ascites and potentially perforating tumors) the fear of complete obstruction of the urinary tract, as well as bowel perforation, led us to deliver radiation therapy within the induction phase. The results as published were poor; neither radiation or chemotherapy could be given as planned in the first 2 weeks because of severe and nonmeasurable clinical toxicity (18).

Mediastinal primary sites did not receive 4500 rads, since we felt that both chemotherapy and radiation therapy would produce severe bone marrow depression and delay chemotherapy. All other sites were irradiated with 4500 rads. The local morbidity for primary nasopharyngeal disease with this dosage of radiation therapy was unacceptable and became apparent 5 years after treatment. This was evidenced by lack of growth of facial bones, lack of body growth, lack of sexual maturation, cataracts, and malposition of permanent teeth with severance of their roots and microphthalmia.

c. Surgery.   From 1971 to 1973 the role of surgery was diagnostic, and it was used for emergency interventions such as bowel perforation or obstruction. Complete surgical excision was only possible for localized primary intraabdominal lesions.

2. *From 1974 to the Present*

From 1974 to the present (ongoing protocol) the following modifications were made:

a. Chemotherapy.   This remained unchanged except for a 24-hour interval between cyclophosphamide and vincristine instead of 3 days. Chemotherapy was administrated in conjunction with antibiotics and white cell, platelet, and blood transfusions in stages III and IV throughout severe pancytopenia. When renal shutdown ensued within 24 hours after cyclophosphamide, the remainder of the chemotherapy was given without much delay (2–3 days) together with vascular or peritoneal dialysis. There was no rest period between induction and consolidation, and consolidation and maintenance, except for 48 hours after intrathecal therapy. The L-asparaginase dosage was reduced to 200 units/kg or 6000 units/m^2 intramuscularly in 1975 because of difficulties with allergic reactions with the intravenous route. In maintenance, all drugs and dosages have remained the same except:

1. Daunomycin was decreased to 15 mg/m^2 or 0.5 mg/kg. A total dose was not to exceed 500 mg/m^2 for all cases, except for mediastinal disease where total dosage was reduced to 350 mg/m^2 because of cardiac irradiation.
2. Methotrexate by oral route was reduced to 5 mg/day for 4 nights instead of 10 mg/m^2.
3. BCNU was decreased to 30 mg/m^2 or 1 mg/kg only in maintenance.

The duration of the treatment continues to be 2 years for stages I, II, III, and 3 years for stage IV.

b. Radiation Therapy.   All primary sites received 2000 rads in 2 weeks at the start of induction. When multiple areas were involved, all the patients received radiation in a noncontinuous fashion or in a continuous field when a mantle was used.

Because of the poor results for extensive intraabdominal involvement with combined radiation and chemotherapy treatment, we decided to administer only chemotherapy in a very aggressive manner, in spite of renal shutdown and bowel perforation, since supportive therapy is easily available at a cancer center. During induction and between the third and fourth vincristine treatments, when the bone marrow has recovered, evaluation and degree of completeness of response to chemotherapy is done through a second-look operation. When residual tumor is present, radiation therapy is given to a total of 2000 rads to the tumor area outlined by surgical clips. If there is no residual tumor, no radiation therapy is needed, sparing the patient delayed toxicity to the bowel from unnecessary radiation.

c. Surgery.   Surgery has become more sophisticated, being used for adequate initial biopsies or repeat biopies for markers and other studies, such as electron microscopy and cell cultures. A repeat biopsy should be done only if the patient can withstand it, or if there will be no more than a 24-hour delay in the onset of chemotherapy. If the marrow is involved, cell marker studies on the bone marrow, blood, cerebrospinal fluid, and biopsy tissue should be correlated.

In extensive intraabdominal lesions we have already discussed the role of second-look surgery. In 19 patients reexploration was possible (50%). Only two patients had residual tumor, not palpable clinically. We know that a negative cranial transaxial tomogram (CTT), gallium scan, upper gastrointestinal and barium enema or sonogram is helpful, but still not 100% conclusive, if small nodes remain positive. A positive study may not be significant either, since we have found residual large masses which contain no active tumor but phagocytes and necrotic tissue. We have encountered so far no morbidity with second-look operations. We feel that the mortality of undiscovered inadequately treated disease, if no second-look operation is performed, is not ideal therapy. The results of the LSA$_2$-L$_2$ in cases of primary intraabdominal involvement, even when extensive, is excellent, but there still remains a small percentage of patients in which failure is the result. A better understanding of the meaning of the presence of residual disease at second-look operations warrants continuing this approach.

Recently we have heard of "debulking" at the time of diagnosis. Only a nonsurgeon can speak of debulking an extensive primary intraabdominal tumor. It cannot be done, and the barrier between the peritoneal cavity and the skin and subcutaneous tissue is often broken when an attempt to remove large tumors is made. If chemotherapy is successful, why not do what has been done in the past, that is, remove a potentially disastrous lesion such as an obstructive, near-perforation, bowel lesion, or biopsy suspicious areas?

If an ovarian site is being dealt with, then an oophorectomy is indicated, but only on the affected side.

III. Results of the LSA$_2$-L$_2$

One hundred thirty five patients were entered from January 1971 to August 1979. All were previously untreated. The ages ranged from 8 months to 18 years, and the male/female ratio was 1.75:1 (Table VI). Primary sites are shown in Table VII, histology is shown in Table VIII, and stages in Table IX.

The upper curve in Fig. 2 shows the disease-free survival of 135 patients to be 75% with a median observation time for the entire group of $3\frac{1}{2}$ years; 102 patients are alive without recurrent lymphoma from 12+ months to 112+ months. Seventy-seven patients are off therapy (75%) with a median observation time of almost 5 years.

The one patient reported as lost to follow-up in the upper curve at the time of this report was found to be alive with no evidence of disease 5 years after diagnosis. Five patients died from infection: one patient died with disseminated chicken pox (unknown exposure during induction); one patient with ataxia telangiectasia died of a fulminating pulmonary infection 8 months after diagnosis, without any evidence of lymphoma; one patient died from adenovirus pneumonitis 3 months after onset of therapy; one patient died of pentamidine shock for treatment of *Pneumocystis carinii* at a time when we were not giving Bactrim prophylaxis; and the last patient died of a disseminated measles infection 24 months after diagnosis during the last cycle of chemotherapy.

Seven patients failed to achieve a remission at the end of 1 month, an induction failure of 5%; 15% (20 patients) experienced recurrence with a median time for recurrence of 3 months; thus the failure rate was 20%. Some of these failures, we believe, could have been avoided. Failure to deliver adequate treatment was due to the fact that no radiation therapy was given during induction (1974) when there was still resistance to the irradiation of all areas if cyclophosphamide caused a marked reduction in the size of the tumor. Nevertheless, 10% of the patients still constitute a puzzle and, even though histologically or biologically similar to other patients, their disease escapes aggressive management. In these patients, refinements of immunological parameters, cell biology, and other studies may

TABLE VI

LSA$_2$-L$_2$ Treatment at Memorial Sloan-Kettering Cancer Center (1971–1979)

Patients entered	135 (all previously untreated)
Age range	8 months–18 years
Median age	9 years
Males	86
Females	49
Male/female ratio	1.75/1
Median age, males	9
Median age, females	10

TABLE VII

LSA$_2$-L$_2$ Treatment at Memorial Sloan-Kettering Cancer Center (1971–1979): Primary Sites

Site	No. of patients
Intraabdominal	42
Mediastinal	31
Peripheral nodal	31
Nasopharyngeal	10
Skeletal	10
Subcutaneous	7
Epidural	2
Breast	1
Testicular	1
Total	135

eventually provide us with a clue. In spite of all this, I still believe that some patients, no matter how they are classified by cell markers, histology, primary site, or stage, simply will not be curable by this protocol. If one could tell beforehand which patients will fail, a different approach could be entertained. The difficulty is that, if no complete response is evidenced within a month, then we believe it is too late to treat the disease by a different protocol. There is no way we can tell before that time who will not do well. We have looked at prognostic factors such as age (Fig. 3) and sex (Fig. 4) and found no differences in survival, contrary to what has been published (19).

TABLE VIII

LSA$_2$-L$_2$ Treatment at Memorial Sloan-Kettering Cancer Center (1971–1979): Histology

Type	No. of patients
Diffuse lymphoblastic	34
Convoluted (17)	
Nonconvoluted (17)	
Diffuse lymphocytic, poorly differentiated	37
Diffuse histiocytic	24
Diffuse undifferentiated	23
Non-Hodgkin's lymphoma	13
Diffuse plasmacytic	2
Diffuse mixed	1
Nodular mixed	1
Total	135

TABLE IX

**LSA$_2$-L$_2$ Treatment at Memorial Sloan-Kettering Cancer Center (1971–1979):
Stage at Diagnosis**

Stage	No. of patients	Percentage
I	3	21 or 16
II	18	
III	58	43
IVA	22	
		56 or 41
IVB	32	
IV	2	

[a] Early stages or good prognosis, 16%; poor prognosis, 84%.

A. Primary Sites

Among the primary sites with larger numbers of patients there is no difference
in disease-free survival (Fig. 5). For rarer primary sites such as subcutaneous and
skeletal, we feel that the number of patients is too small to draw any conclusions.
For primary skeletal disease we have accidentally learned that perhaps no radiation therapy is as effective as, if not better than, radiation therapy plus
chemotherapy. This was observed in a baby 8 months old with multiple bone

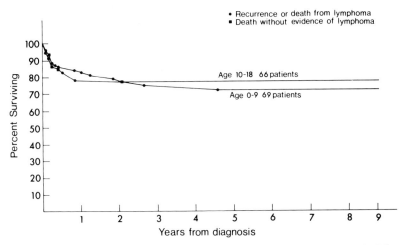

Fig. 3. Non-Hodgkin's lymphoma in children, 1971–1979. Disease-free survival, by age
groups, after LSA$_2$-L$_2$ treatment.

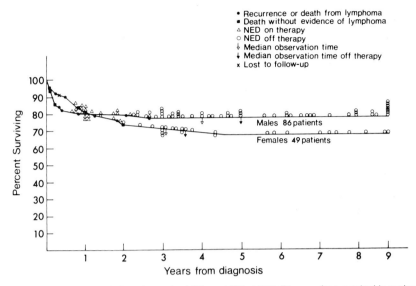

Fig. 4. Non-Hodgkin's lymphoma in children, 1971–1979. Disease-free survival in males and females after LSA$_2$-L$_2$ treatment.

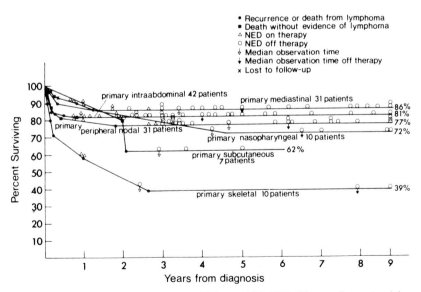

Fig. 5. Non-Hodgkin's lymphoma in children, 1971–1979. Disease-free actuarial survival, by primary sites, after LSA$_2$-L$_2$ treatment.

lesions and massive replacement of the bone marrow in whom radiation therapy was not possible and to whom chemotherapy alone was given. At the beginning of maintenance, a follow-up skeletal survey showed that all the bone lesions that were present before had healed. The same happened to a 4-year-old girl with three bones affected, all in the epiphyseal lines, in whom chemotherapy alone caused resolution of the lytic lesions and the formation of scar tissue. These patients are still being treated, and more patients and a longer follow-up are needed for definite conclusions.

B. Stages

In 21 patients with stage I or II disease there were two noteworthy events (Fig. 6). One patient died of disseminated intravascular coagulation and chicken pox in the second month, and the other, who had primary nasopharyngeal stage II disease, had testicular involvement at 3 months. In the latter patient, the possibility of initial testicular involvement was very high and therefore his staging should have been stage III. When cyclophosphamide is given, if there is testicular involvement, there is an immediate response with a decrease in the size of the testes usually lasting for 2–3 months. So far, we have not found testicular relapse, early or late during chemotherapy, unless the testes were involved initially and radiation therapy was not given. We believe also that initial testicular involvement, as well as initial central nervous disease, has to be treated early in

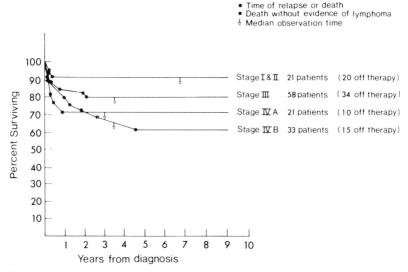

Fig. 6. Non-Hodgkin's lymphoma in children, 1971–1979. Disease-free survival, by stages, after LSA₂-L₂ treatment.

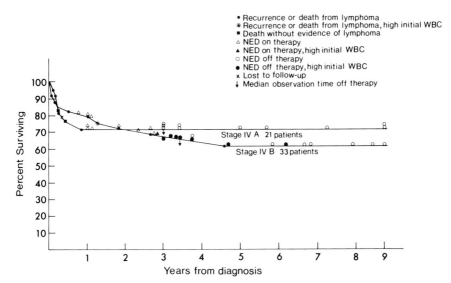

Fig. 7. Non-Hodgkin's lymphoma in children, 1971–1979. Disease-free survival after LSA$_2$-L$_2$ treatment of patients with initial marrow involvement.

the course of therapy with a combination of radiation and more intensive central nervous system prophylaxis in the form of intrathecal methotrexate for successful control.

The remaining stages show no major differences in disease-free survival. Figure 7 shows more clearly the similarity between the disease-free survival of these two groups, that is, stages IVA and IVB. Also, on the stage IVB curve one can see that eight or nine patients with initial white counts of more than 50,000 and multiple bulky sites of disease (solid circles) have survived free of recurrence.

IV. Summary and Conclusions

The LSA$_2$-L$_2$ still continues to be the therapy of choice for non-Hodgkin's lymphoma in children. Even though the number of patients with different histological types does not approach that of large studies, one must consider that there is a common denominator among all these different histological subtypes, namely, the investigator and the institution. The demands made at our institution in regard to quality control in the treatment of all patients are rigorous and uniform, and even so there are some protocol violations which one cannot avoid. If this is true at an institution that has lived through and utilized the LSA$_2$-L$_2$, I wonder what the situation is at institutions that have no such controls. One may ask:

1. Are patients with stages I and II being overtreated by the LSA$_2$-L$_2$, since today 80–90% survive free of disease with this and other protocols (20, 21)? When we reviewed the results of radiation therapy alone, surgical excision alone, and minimal chemotherapy, such as induction with nitrogen mustard or cyclophosphamide followed or not followed by minimal maintenance therapy with 6 MP and methotrexate for a few months, we found that in 16 patients so treated the disease-free survival was 40%. For such early disease, this is a poor survival, and we therefore would rather overtreat 40% in order to save 90%. There is no way in which we can obtain 100% survival. Today, even with the best available knowledge and techniques, radiological and clinical staging is still perhaps not adequate. Or maybe a patient's personal individual response, or lack of it, is responsible for unexpected failures. In parameningeal disease, stages I and II, protection of the central nervous system is mandatory. In primary gastrointestinal disease, perhaps if surgical staging is done by a surgeon knowledgeable of the natural history of this disease, we could accept no central nervous system protection and less intensive, or the same, chemotherapy, except for a shorter period of time (22).

2. Is radiation therapy a necessary tool in the treatment of non-Hodgkin's lymphoma? We believe in a multimodal approach. In our hands 2000 rads with the LSA$_2$-L$_2$ produces no prohibitive toxicity, no fatalities, and no severe immunological deficits. Even Weinstein (23), who in his original publication advocated no radiation therapy for primary mediastinal disease, has since had some recurrences with a fatal outcome (24). He and his group advocate radiation therapy if no complete response is obtained within a month. I feel that, by that time, all is lost and the patient's disease is irretrievable. In Murphy's (22) report stating that the addition of radiation therapy to chemotherapy contributed nothing to the eventual outcome of the disease, one must read carefully between the lines and conclude that, first, chemotherapy was stopped for the administration of radiation therapy and, second, the radiation therapy dosage was far in excess of what we give at our institution. In a forthcoming publication, we will show that for primary mediastinal disease that receives radiation therapy, recurrence at this site is unusual as a first event, and that it usually happens as a result of recurrence or de novo disease elsewhere. That is not the problem. We feel that it is desirable not only to control bulky local disease but also to prevent de novo disease elsewhere leading to certain death. It will be impossible to ascertain the validity of such statements with the number of patients studied so far, whether at our institution or in cooperative study groups. The proof will only come with a very large randomized study, which in my opinion should be carried out at a large cancer center where quality control can be ascertained.

3. What is the prognostic significance of histology (25)? Statements have been made that only diffuse lymphoblastic convoluted or nonconvoluted disease responds well to the LSA₂-L₂ and, since most mediastinal tumors are supposedly diffuse lymphoblastic, the results are good. The disease-free survival in 31 patients with primary mediastinal disease treated with the LSA₂-L₂ is 86%. However, in these 31 patients, 14 had diffuse lymphoblastic, convoluted, or nonconvoluted histology, and 17 had other histological types such as diffuse lymphocytic poorly differentiated, diffuse histiocytic, and diffuse undifferentiated. The survival for the diffuse lymphoblastic group is 80% as opposed to 90% for other types of histology. Therefore, histology does not have prognostic significance in primary mediastinal disease where most results have been successful as opposed to those for other histological types. For instance, in primary peripheral nodal disease, for a total of 31 patients (Fig. 8) the disease-free survival is 76% with a median follow-up of 4¼ years, with 18 of the 23 survivors off therapy. The median observation time for the patients off therapy is almost 6 years. In Fig. 9 the disease-free survival for primary peripheral nodal disease in relation to histology suggests that all histological subtypes except diffuse histiocytic have a good prognosis. Since the histiocytic group is so controversial, this is not surprising.

4. Primary intraabdominal (26, 27): Figure 10 shows that in 42 patients treated with the LSA₂-L₂ disease-free survival is 80%. The median observation time for the entire group is 40+ months, and for those off therapy 48+ months. In Fig. 11

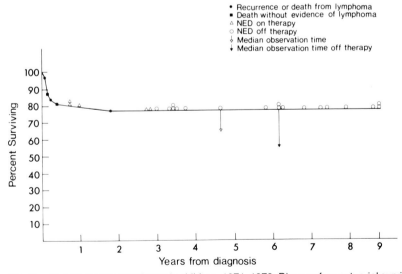

Fig. 8. Non-Hodgkin's lymphoma in children, 1971–1979. Disease-free actuarial survival after LSA₂-L₂ treatment of 31 patients with primary peripheral nodal involvement.

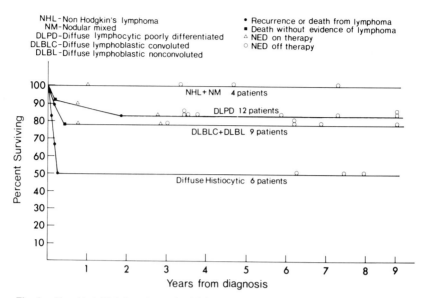

Fig. 9. Non-Hodgkin's lymphoma in children, 1971–1979. Disease-free actuarial survival after LSA$_2$-L$_2$ treatment of patients with primary peripheral nodal involvement.

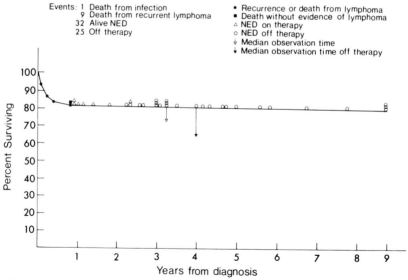

Fig. 10. Non-Hodgkin's lymphoma in children, 1971–1979. Disease-free actuarial survival after LSA$_2$-L$_2$ treatment of 42 patients with intraabdominal involvement.

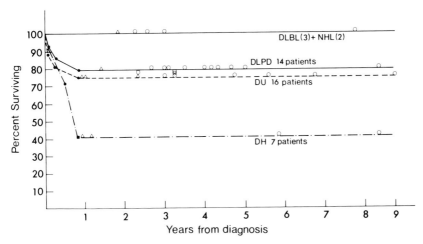

Fig. 11. Intraabdominal non-Hodgkin's lymphoma in children, 1971–1979. Disease-free survival after LSA₂-L₂ treatment in relation to histology.

one can see that it is not the diffuse undifferentiated group or the American Burkitt's intraabdominal lymphoma group that does not respond to the LSA₂-L₂ but a diffuse histiocytic group with a survival of only 40%. Why? In this small group there was one patient to whom radiation therapy was given concomitantly with the induction of the LSA₂-L₂ (that is, a patient treated in the early phase of the LSA₂-L₂) and another patient in whom the primary splenic site was not disclosed initially but only discovered when relapse occurred. Unfortunately, this could not be helped, since up to that time no primary splenic involvement had ever been seen in children. For this patient, the approach should have been a splenectomy done at the time of initial marrow remission, that is, within a month, thus avoiding the recurrence within 4 months at the primary site. Figure 12 shows that staging or, perhaps more accurately, the amount of initial bulky disease has a prognostic significance since stage IV patients have done poorly. Whether this is true or not is still difficult to say since the number of patients with intraabdominal disease with initial marrow and central nervous system involvement is small.

5. What are the reasons for second-look operations and how can they be justified? We have explained the reasons for second-look operations. We feel that patients, nevertheless, have to be carefully screened and that only those with massive residual bulky disease at the time of diagnosis should be reexplored at the end of induction. We can easily say this now, while in the early phases of the

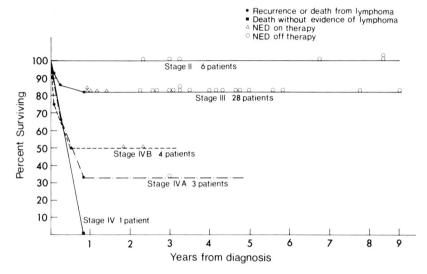

Fig. 12. Non-Hodgkin's lymphoma in children, 1971–1979. Disease-free actuarial survival after LSA$_2$-L$_2$ treatment of 42 patients with intraabdominal primary involvement in relation to stage.

LSA$_2$-L$_2$ without irradiation the quality and degree of response were still unknown, and thus some patients were reexplored when today they would not be. Since most cases of Burkitt's lymphoma were considered by others to be nonresponsive to the LSA$_2$-L$_2$, we felt that they should have had a second look when the criterion of initial bulky residual disease was met in order to prove that response to the LSA$_2$-L$_2$ was complete and therefore feasible. There is still a lot of work to be done; histology has to be looked upon with critical eyes. We are still in the process of reviewing all cases and reclassifying them in presently known histological classifications and also the 1980 working classification. With this, once more, we will look upon the role of histology as a prognostic factor.

The role and significance of cell markers is still incipient. The role of radiation therapy will probably remain an open question. When? How much?

One question, nevertheless, is easy to answer, at least for us, with the LSA$_2$-L$_2$. The most important prognostic factors are (1) the quantity of initial bulky disease, and (2) treatment.

In order to acieve maximum cell kill, the LSA$_2$-L$_2$ in combination with moderate dosage radiation therapy (2000 rads in 2 weeks) has produced good results and, so far, little morbidity.

As we have said many times, the LSA$_2$-L$_2$ with or without radiation therapy produces severe toxicity, mainly in patients with extensive disease and in those with inoperable intraabdominal disease, and they should be treated only at a cancer center where available ancillary supportive therapy is easily and immediately accessible.

References

1. M. L. Brecher, L. F. Sinks, R. R. M. Thomas, and A. I. Freeman, Non-Hodgkin's lymphoma in children. *Cancer (Philadelphia)* **41**, 1997-2001 (1978).

2. M. P. Sullivan and J. J. Butler; Non-Hodgkin's lymphoma of childhood. *In* "Clinical Pediatric Oncology" (W. W. Sutow, T. J. Vietti, and D. J. Fernback, eds.), 2nd ed., pp. 444-466. Mosby, St. Louis, Missouri, 1977.

3. N. Wollner, J. H. Burchenal, P. H. Lieberman, P. Exelby, G. D'Angio, and M. L. Murphy, Non-Hodgkin's lymphoma in children, *Med. Pediatr. Oncol.* **1**, 235-263 (1975).

4. N. Wollner, J. H. Burchenal, P. H. Lieberman, P. Exelby, G. D'Angio, and M. L. Murphy, Non-Hodgkin's lymphoma in children. A comparative study of two modalities of therapy. *Cancer (Philadelphia)* **37**, 123-134 (1976).

5. N. Wollner, Central nervous system and bone marrow involvement in childhood non-Hodgkin's lymphoma. *In* "Leukemia and Lymphoma in the Nervous System" (C. Pochedly, ed.), pp. 152-175. Thomas, Springfield, Illinois, 1977.

6. M. L. Brecher, L. F. Sinks, R. R. M. Thomas, and A. I. Freeman, Non-Hodgkin's lymphoma in children. *Cancer (Philadelphia)* **41**, 1997-2001 (1978).

7. A. Watanabe, M. P. Sullivan, W. W. Suton, and J. R. Wilbur, Undifferentiated lymphoma, non-Burkitt's type, and bone marrow involvement in children. *Am. J. Dis. Child.* **125**, 57-61 (1973).

8. J. J. Hutter, B. E. Favor, M. Nelson, and C. P. Holton, Non-Hodgkin's lymphoma in children; correlation of CNS disease with initial presentation. *Cancer (Philadelphia)* **36**, 2132-2137 (1975).

9. J. L. Ziegler, Similar treatment results in Americans and Africans with Burkitt's lymphoma. *N.Engl. J. Med.* **297**, 75-80 (1977).

10. C. L. Berry and J. W. Keeling, Gastrointestinal lymphoma in childhood. *J. Clin. Pathol.* **23**, 459-463 (1970).

11. N. Wollner, P. R. Exelby, and P. H. Lieberman, Non-Hodgkin's lymphoma in children. A progress report on the original patients treated with the LSA$_2$-L$_2$ protocol. *Cancer (Philadelphia)* **44**, 1990-1999 (1979).

12. N. Wollner, P. R. Exelby, P. H. Lieberman, G. D'Angio, and M. L. Murphy, Non-Hodgkin's lymphoma in children: A comparative study of two modalities of therapy. *Cancer (Philadelphia)* **37**, 123-134 (1976).

13. B. C. Clarkson and J. Fried, Changing concepts of treatment in acute leukemia. *Med. Clin. North Am.* **55**, 561-600 (1971).

14. B. C. Clarkson, Cell-cycle kinetics - Clinical applications. *In* "Antineoplastic and Immunosuppressive Agents," *Handb. Exp. Pharmakol.* [N.S.] **38**, 1974.

15. M. Haghbin, C. Tan, B. Clarkson, V. Miké, J. H. Burchenal, and M. L. Murphy, Intensive chemotherapy in children with acute lymphoblastic leukemia (L-2 protocol). *Cancer (Philadelphia)* **33**, 1491-1498 (1974).

16. R. D. T. Jenkin, Radiation in the treatment of non-Hodgkin's lymphoma in children. *Semin. Oncol.* **4**, 311-315 (1977).

17. S. C. Carabell, J. R. Cassady, H. J. Weinstein, and N. Jaffe, The role of radiation therapy in the treatment of pediatric non-Hodgkin's lymphoma. *Cancer (Philadelphia)* **42**, 2193-2205 (1978).

18. N. Wollner, A. Wachtel, P. Exelby, and D. Centore, Improved prognosis in children with intra-abdominal non-Hodgkin's lymphoma following LSA$_2$-L$_2$ protocol chemotherapy. *Cancer (Philadelphia)* **45,** 3034–3037 (1980).

19. J. L. Ziegler, Treatment results of 54 American patients with Burkitt's lymphoma are similar to the African experience. *N. Engl. J. Med.* **297,** 75–80 (1977).

20. R. J. A. Aur, H. O. Hustu, J. V. Simone, C. B. Pratt, and D. Pinkel, Therapy of localized and regional lymphosarcoma of childhood. *Cancer (Philadelphia)* **27,** 1328–1331 (1971).

21. M. L. Brecher, L. F. Sinks, R. R. M. Thomas, and A. I. Freeman, Non-Hodgkin's lymphoma in children. *Cancer (Philadelphia)* **41,** 1997–2001 (1978).

22. S. B. Murphy and O. H. Hustu, A randomized trial of combined modality of therapy of childhood non-Hodgkin's lymphoma. *Cancer (Philadelphia)* **45,** 630–637 (1980).

23. H. J. Weinstein, Z. B. Vance, N. Jaffe, D. Buell, J. R. Cassady, and D. G. Nathan, Improved prognosis for patients with mediastinal lymphoblastic lymphoma. *Blood* **53,** 687–694 (1979).

24. H. J. Weinstein, L. M. Cassady, R. Nadler, R. Levey, and F. S. Coral, Prolonged remissions in patients with mediastinal lymphoblastic lymphoma. *Proc. Am. Assoc. Cancer Res. Am. Soc. Clin. Oncol.* **21,** 433 (abstr.) (1980).

25. S. B. Murphy, G. Frizzera, and A. E. Evans, A study of childhood lymphoma. *Cancer (Philadelphia)* **36,** 2121–2131 (1975).

26. R. S. Bush, and C. L. Ash, Primary lymphoma of the gastrointestinal tract. *Radiology* **92,** 1349–1354 (1969).

27. R. D. T. Jenkin, M. J. Sonley, C. A. Stephens, J. M. M. Darte, and M. V. Peters, Primary gastrointestinal tract lymphoma in childhood. *Radiology* **92,** 763–767 (1969).

37

Evaluation and Prevention of Anthracycline Cardiotoxicity

MICHAEL R. BRISTOW

The cardiotoxic properties of anthracyclines are well known. Although anthracyclines may produce acute and subacute cardiac effects (1, 2), it is the chronic dose and time-related cardiomyopathic effects (3) that are the most common and most troublesome. The purposes of this article are first to outline the pathophysiology of anthracycline cardiomyopathy and then to comment briefly on pathogenesis and prevention.

I. Pathophysiology

A. Anthracycline-Mediated Myocardial Morphological Damage

The cardiac morphological effects of anthracyclines have been well described (4–7). The characteristic myocardial lesion is myofibrillar dropout, often of single cells surrounded by other cells that appear entirely normal. The cellular damage is best identified by electron microscopy, although in advanced stages the characteristic vacuolated cell is readily identified by light microscopy. This histological abnormality may also be observed in cardiomyopathies of other types, but in these instances it is not the predominant cellular effect.

The characteristic histological picture of anthracycline cardiomyopathy is readily identified in endomyocardial biopsy material obtained from the apical portion of the right ventricular septum (5–7). The material so obtained can be quantified for the degree of the anthracycline effect (7), which makes possible a prospective study of the dose–effect and structure–function relationships of anthracycline cardiomyopathy in humans. An analysis of these relationships in individual patients forms the basis for precise assessment of the risk status for developing heart failure with the addition of further drug, as will be discussed below.

We quantify right ventricular endomyocardial biopsy material on a 0–3 basis: 0, normal; 1, a minimal effect; 2, a moderate degree of damage; and 3, severe morphological changes. Grade-2 changes have now been further subdivided by M. Billingham to include early (grade-2A) and late (grade-2B) degrees of moderate abnormality. In our experience quantification of the morphological effects is the single most predictive, most reliable information available in anthracycline cardiomyopathy and is the key element in our dose limitation technique and experimental studies.

B. Dose–Effect and Structure–Function Relationships

The first important observation on anthracycline cardiomyopathy was made by Lefrak and associates at the M. D. Anderson Hospital (3). In a review of the incidence of heart failure in the first group of patients treated with adriamycin in the United States these workers noted that anthracycline-associated heart failure was dose-related, and that the incidence increased dramatically at doses greater than 550 mg/m^2. The dose-related nature of anthracycline cardiomyopathy is the single most consistent finding in this disorder and is observed whether one is measuring the incidence of heart failure, degree of morphological damage, or frequency and severity of functional abnormalities.

The relationship betwen heart failure incidence and adriamycin dose observed by Lefrak and his associates was that of a parabolic function, i.e., a relationship having a threshold or unchanging portion at lower values of x (dose) but which increases exponentially at higher values of x. A parabolic relationship is a commonly observed mathematical form for data derived from biological systems, usually because it is the lower portion of a dose–response curve which has been prevented from reaching a maximum and defining a rectangular hyperbola. The practical implication of the shape of the dose–heart failure incidence relationship in adriamycin cardiomyopathy is that a point will be reached that is at a threshold for observing y (heart failure). In uncomplicated cases this point is at 550 mg/m^2 (3, 8).

Figure 1 illustrates that the parabolic nature of the cardiac function–adriamycin dose relationship is also observed in a plot of the incidence of catheterization abnormalities versus adriamycin dose. Figure 1 is a polynomial regression plot for the probability of abnormal catheterization at rest versus cumulative adriamycin dose. Note that patients who have received previous mediastinal radiation have their cardiac function–dose relationships shifted to the left, indicating a greater drgree of catheterization abnormality per adriamycin dose. Previous mediastinal radiation also reduces the coefficient of variation of the data and yields a higher correlation coefficient for a smaller n. Figure 2 is an attempt to quantify catheterization data in a manner similar to endomyocardial biopsy and ranks catheterization abnormalities on a 0–3 basis in patients who have had hemodynamics determined both at rest and with exercise. The scale is set to correspond to biopsy: 1, a minor abnormality that would not be associated with symptoms; 2, a moderate abnormality that would be associated with symptoms in

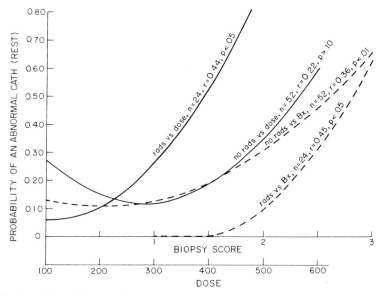

Fig. 1. Polynomial regression analyses of rest catherterization data versus biopsy (BX) score and adriamycin (doxorubicin) dose in 74 patients. "Rads" refers to patients with previous mediastinal irradiation.

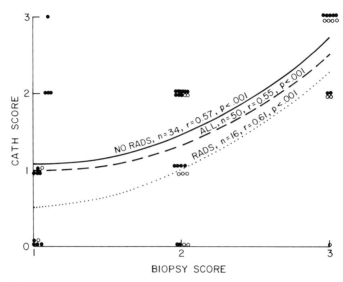

Fig. 2. Catheterization data quantified on a 0–3 basis (0, normal; 1, mild abnormality; 2, moderate abnormality; 3, severe abnormality) and plotted versus biopsy score. Lines give polynomial regression analyses, "rads" = previous mediastinal irradiation.

some patients; 3, the equivalent of heart failure. The structure–function relationship depicted by Fig. 2 is similar to that in Fig. 1, a nonlinear relationship.

Anthracycline-related myocardial damage is also dose-related, as demonstrated in Fig. 3. In contrast to the parabolically shaped cardiac function–dose relationship, there is a near-linear relationship between biopsy "score" and adriamycin dose. Note that, despite the highly significant r value by polynomial regression analysis, the scattergram reveals a good deal of individual variation. This is not due to sampling error of the biopsy, as patients studied serially show the expected progression with dose and there is a good correlation between biopsy score and catheterization abnormalities. The scatter in the biopsy-versus-dose data plotted in Fig. 3 is due to individual variability in sensitivity to the cardiomyopathic effects of anthracyclines.

Figure 3 demonstrates the morphological basis for setting the empiric limit for adriamycin at 550 mg/m². This drug dose produces an average biopsy score of +2, or a moderate amount of damage. As will be shown subsequently, this degree of damage is at the threshold for developing significant performance abnormalities. Above a dose of 550 mg/m² a biopsy score of +3 is approached, which is the morphological equivalent of heart failure.

Also note that at 550 mg/m² there are many individuals who have a minimal degree (+1) of morphological damage, most of whom (in the absence of other types of heart disease) could safely receive more adriamycin. In Fig. 1 there are a few $+3$ biopsy scores at doses ≤ 550 mg/m^2; all these patients developed heart failure.

Figure 1 also plots catheterization data against biopsy score. Note that a parabolic relationship is again obtained and that the regression line is now statistically significant. The improvement in the analysis as compared to dose is due to the more direct measurement of the structure–function relationship. That is, the heart failure–dose and abnormal cardiac function–dose relationships are actually a reflection of the performance–morphological abnormality relationship. When the data are analyzed for degree of morphological damage, this relationship is examined directly, which eliminates the variability introduced by plotting against dose.

The nonlinear nature of the cardiac function–dose relationship places limitations on the use of cardiac monitoring by measuring parameters. The parabolic nature of this relationship means that functional measurements will not change until some critical degree of damage is reached, after which deterioration in cardiac function will proceed quite rapidly. In other words, measurements made prior to this critical degree of damage, at a point where the structure–function curve is flat, cannot predict when the sudden change in performance will occur. Because the dose at which this critical degree of damage is reached is quite variable, measurements of cardiac function will need to be performed quite often if this sudden deterioration in function is going to be detected in time to prevent heart failure.

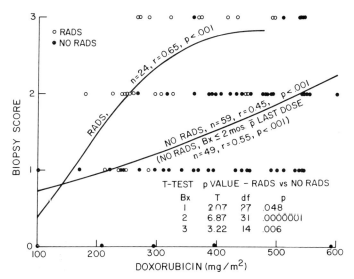

Fig. 3. Scattergram and polynomial regression analyses of biopsy–adriamycin dose data. "Rads" refers to patients who had received mediastinal irradiation.

C. Radiation and Other Risk Factors

Figure 3 demonstrates the effect of previous mediastinal radiation on anthracycline-associated morphological damage. Patients with previous mediastinal radiation have higher biopsy scores per amount of adriamycin received, which leads to a left shift in the regression line describing the data. The regression line is also steeper than that for the nonradiation relationship, indicating that a potentiation of morphological damage occurs during the entire course of adriamycin treatment. As noted in Fig. 1, mediastinal radiation has a similar effect on cardiac function.

In our experience, the potentiating effect of radiation occurs whether radiation is given before or after adriamycin and may occur even when radiation has been administered years previously. The effects are dose-related, so when feasible, radiation therapists should strive to lower the dose delivered to the left ventricle.

At our institution, the mantle technique of mediastinal radiation delivers approximately 3000 rads to the right ventricle and 1500 rads to the left ventricle. This leads to a slightly greater potentiation of morphological as compared to catheterization abnormalities, because the endomyocardial biopsy is taken from the right ventricle and the majority of catheterization abnormalities derive from parameters of left-ventricle dysfunction. This point is emphasized in Fig. 1, which shows that the catheterization–biopsy relationship is right-shifted in patients with previous mediastinal radiation (less catheterization abnormality per degree of biopsy change).

Because of the effects of mediastinal radiation on anthracycline cardiotoxicity, we use cardiac monitoring in all these patients (see below). If radionuclide ejection fractions and/or endomyocardial biopsies are not available, patients with previous mediastinal radiation should be empirically dose-limited to 350 mg/m^2.

Other risk factors for anthracycline-associated heart failure appear to lower the dose or degree of morphological damage at which heart failure develops rather than potentiate the cell damage. These include advanced age and underlying heart disease associated with subclinical myopathy, which can involve patients with a history of coronary, valvular, or myocardial heart disease and patients with a long-standing history of hypertension (9).

II. Pathogenesis

A. Etiology

Several hypotheses on the pathogenesis of anthracycline cardiomyopathy have been proposed; some of them are listed in Table I. At the cellular level, the most compelling of these is free-radical formation as proposed by Meyers and associates at the National Cancer Institute. Meyer's group has demonstrated that high doses of adriamycin can cause toxic lipid peroxidation products to be

TABLE I

Proposed Hypotheses for Anthracycline Cardiotoxicity

Inhibition of macromolecular synthesis (11)
Calcium overload (12)
Inhibition of mitochondrial enzyme function (13, 14)
Production of free radicals (10, 15)
Release of toxic vasoactive substances (16, 17)

formed, and that this formation, the associated mortality, and some of the cardiac morphological damage may be prevented by free-radical scavengers (10). The strength of this hypothesis is that it provides a cellular mechanism for the induction of damage. The weakness is that free-radical scavengers have not been shown to prevent cardiomyopathy in chronic models given conventional doses of adriamycin.

Our group has proposed an etiological hypothesis of anthracycline cardiotoxicity that appears to be operative in conventional animal models given pharmacological doses of adriamycin (4). This hypothesis, which involves the release of active substances and subsequent production of myocardial injury is attractive in that it involves a mechanism separate from any postulated antitumor effect. This mechanism therefore allows prevention of anthracycline cardiotoxicity with preservation of the antitumor response. It should be emphasized that this hypothesis does not include a cellular basis for toxic damage, but merely states that the damage is caused by the release of a vasoactive substance rather than by the anthracycline molecule itself. Thus it is not incompatible with other mechanisms proposed in Table I.

The hypothesis of vasoactive substance-induced cardiac damage originated with an investigation into the acute cardiovascular effects of adriamycin (17). We felt that it was unlikely that the acute, subacute, and chronic cardiovascular effects of anthracyclines were totally unrelated and that careful study of the acute effects might reveal a potential mechanism of chronic cardiotoxicity. What we found was that all the acute cardiovascular effects in dogs were due to the release of histamine, catecholamines, and prostaglandins and that adriamycin alone had no effect on cardiovascular function (17). We then demonstrated that the release of histamine and catecholamines also occurred in NZW rabbits under the conditions in which anthracycline cardiomyopathy is created, and that blockade of the effects of histamine and catecholamines provided near total protection against cardiomyopathy (16).

Several potential methods of preventing anthracycline cardiomyopathy derive from this hypothesis. These include:

1. Blockade of histamine and catecholamine receptors, as originally done in animals, possibly coupled with inhibition of prostaglandin synthesis.

2. Alteration in pharmacokinetics—lower doses or slow infusions of adriamycin release lower amounts of vasoactive substances per adriamycin dose or plasma concentration times time (17).

3. Development of an analogue devoid of release properties.

4. Inhibition of the release of vasoactive substances. Adriamycin releases cardiac histamine in animals (16) and humans (F. R. MacKintosh and M. Bristow, unpublished observations), and this release can be prevented by cromolyn sodium (W. S. Sageman and M. Bristow, unpublished observations). Studies are under way testing this as a protective strategy in rabbits.

B. Prevention of Anthracycline Cardiotoxicity

This discussion will be confined to methods shown to prevent anthracycline-associated cardiac damage in conventional animal models or in humans.

1. Prevention by Cardiac Monitoring

Cardiac monitoring can prevent anthracycline cardiotoxicity in a population of patients by selecting patients who can safely receive more drug. If done properly, with monitoring, as much or more anthracycline can be administered as by empiric dose limitation (8). Figure 4 shows how this occurs. The morphological

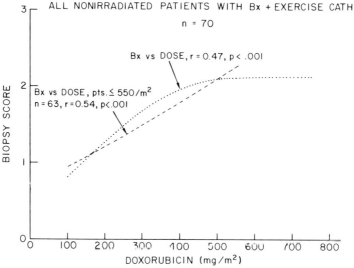

Fig. 4. "Prevention" of adriamycin (doxorubicin)-induced cardiac damage by cardiac monitoring. Dotted line is polynomial regression analysis of biopsy (Bx) score versus adriamycin dose data and includes seven patients taken to doses >550 mg/m^2 because of favorable biopsy data. Note that the regression line plateaus at a biopsy score of 2, reflecting the exclusion of patients with severe damage.

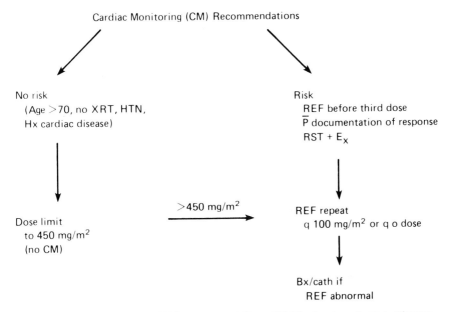

Fig. 5.   Cardiac monitoring (CM) recommendations. "Risk" refers to patients > 70 years old with previous mediastinal radiation, underlying heart disease, and a history of hypertension. REF refers to the radionuclide ejection fraction, measured at rest and during exercise.

damage–dose relationship "plateaus" in patients given doses of adriamycin > 500 mg/m², because these patients had relatively little cardiac damage when cleared for further drug administration. Administration of adriamycin in excess of 500 mg/m² then results in a degree of cardiac damage similar to that in other patients at lower doses, so the progression of damage in the general population is halted at 500 mg/m².

The cardiac monitoring protocol currently in use at Stanford is given in Fig. 5. We monitor only risk factor patients and rely on radionuclide ejection fractions performed at rest and exercise as a noninvasive screen (9). Nonrisk factor patients cross over to the risk factor group at >450 mg/m², and all abnormal ejction fractions are followed by biopsy or catheterization if there is a compelling reason to administer more drug.

2. Alteration of Pharmacokinetics

Evidence is mounting that avoidance of peak blood levels of anthracycline associated with standard dose infusion techniques may be cardiomyopathy "sparing." Patients given low-dose weekly (as opposed to the standard dose of 3–4 weeks) (18) or given 48 to 96-hour infusions (19) appear to have less cardiomyopathy. Whether this is due to prevention of the release of vasoactive substances or to avoidance of another pathogenic mechanism is unknown, but slow infusion at the same dose appears to yield equal or greater adriamycin (AUCs) (R. Benjamin, personal communication). This argues against avoidance of a direct concentration-related mechanism of cardiotoxicity and for an indirect mechanism not related to the anthracycline AUC. Such a mechanism could be a direct cardiotoxic property characterized by a higher threshold of expression than that of the antitumor properties, with consequent sparing of cardiomyopathy by avoidance of peak blood levels that result from rapid infusion. A second possibility is that slow infusion reduces the release of vasoactive substances, as occurs in animals (17). The release mechanism thus becomes desensitized to the effect of adriamycin, and less release of histamine and other vasoactive hormones results in less cardiac damage.

3. Blockade of Effects of Vasoactive Substance

As detailed earlier, blockade of the cardiovascular effects of vasoactive substances can prevent anthracycline cardiomyopathy in rabbits. The use of this approach clinically awaits completion of a study on the nature and duration of anthracycline-associated vasoactive substance release in humans, and a demonstration of which receptor subtypes are crucial to the development of cardiac damage. Preliminary data in humans indicate that (1) adriamycin releases histamine and catecholamines in a manner similar to that in animals, (2) adriamycin releases cardiac histamine, (3) histamine release is completed within 4 hours, but catecholamine release may last longer, and (4) the release of histamine and catecholamines can cause hemodynamic effects.

Recent studies on NZW rabbits indicate that blockade of α-adrenergic and H_1 and H_2 histaminic receptors is crucial to prevention of cardiomyopathy, but that β-blockade is not. This raises the possibility that coronary circulation effects of vasoactive substances are more important than myocardial effects in the pathogenesis of anthracycline cardiomyopathy.

III. Conclusions

Although cardiotoxicity is potentially a serious problem when administering anthracyclines, knowledge of the pathophysiology and associated risk factors should allow aggressive use of these important agents in the treatment of neoplastic diseases. Moreover, it is highly likely that in the near future prevention strategies will be developed that will reduce or completely eliminate this problem.

References

1. M. R. Bristow, P. D. Thompson, R. P. Martin, J. W. Mason, M. E. Billingham, and D. C. Harrison, Early anthracycline cardiotoxicity. *Am. J. Med.* **65**, 823–832 (1978).

2. M. R. Bristow, M. E. Billingham, J. W. Mason, and J. R. Daniels, Clinical spectrum of anthracycline antibiotic cardiotoxicity. *Cancer Treat. Rep.* **62**, 873-879 (1978).

3. E. A. Lefrak, A. Pitha, S. Rosenheim, and J. Gottlieb, A clinicopathologic analysis of adriamycin cardiotoxicity. *Cancer (Philadelphia)* **32**, 302-314 (1973).

4. R. S. Jaenke, An anthracycline antibiotic-induced cardiomyopathy in rabbits. *Lab. Invest.* **30**, 292-304 (1974).

5. M. E. Billingham, M. R. Bristow, E. Glatstein, J. W. Mason, M. A. Masek, and J. R. Daniels, Adriamycin cardiotoxicity: endomyocardial biopsy evidence of enhancement by irradiation. *Am. J. Surg. Pathol.* **1**, 17-23 (1977).

6. M. R. Bristow, J. W. Mason, M. E. Billingham, and J. R. Daniels, Doxorubicin cardiomyopathy: evaluation by phonocardiography, endomyocardial biopsy, and cardiac catheterization. *Ann. Intern. Med.* **88**, 168-179 (1978).

7. M. E. Billingham, J. W. Mason, M. R. Bristow, and J. R. Daniels, Anthracycline cardiomyopathy monitored by morphologic changes. *Cancer Treat. Rep.* **62**, 865-872 (1978).

8. M. R. Bristow, Pathophysiological basis for cardiac monitoring in patients receiving anthracyclines. *In* "Anthracyclines: Current Status and New Developments" (S. T. Crooke and S. D. Reich, eds.), Academic Press, New York, 1980.

9. M. Bristow, Rational system for cardiac monitoring in patients receiving anthracyclines. *ASCO Abstr., 16th Annu. Meet., Am. Soc. Clin. Oncol.* p. 356 (1980).

10. C. E. Myers, W. P. McGuire, R. H. Liss, I. Ifrim, K. Grotzinger, and R. C. Young, Adriamycin: The role of lipid peroxidation in cardiac toxicity and tumor response. *Science* **197**, 165-167 (1977).

11. S. H. Rosenoff, E. Brooks, F. Bostick, and R. C. Young, Alterations in DNA synthesis in cardiac tissue induced by Adriamycin in vivo—relationship to fatal toxicity. *Biochem. Pharmacol.* **24**, 1898-1901 (1975).

12. H. M. Olson, D. M. Young, D. J. Prieur, A. F. LeRoy, and R. L. Reagan, Electrolyte and morphologic alterations of myocardium in Adriamycin-treated rabbits. *Am. J. Pathol.* **77**, 439-450 (1974).

13. M. E. Ferrero, E. Ferrero, G. Gaja, and A. Bernelli-Zazzera, Adriamycin: Energy metabolism and mitochondrial oxidations in the heart of treated rabbits. *Biochem. Pharmacol.* **25**, 125-130 (1976).

14. Y. Iwamoto, I. L. Hansen, T. H. Porter, and K. Folkers, Inhibition of coenzyme Q_{10}-enzymes, succinoxidase and NADH-oxidase, by Adriamycin and other quinones having antitumor activity. *Biochem. Biophys. Res. Commun.* **58**, 633-638 (1974).

15. N. R. Bachur, S. L. Gordon, and M. V. Gee, Anthracycline antibiotic augmentation of microsomal electron transport and free radical formation. *Mol. Pharmacol.* **13**, 901-910 (1977).

16. M. R. Bristow, W. A. Minobe, M. E. Billingham, J. B. Marmor, G. A. Johnson, B. M. Ishimoto, W. S. Sageman, and J. R. Daniels, Anthracycline-associated cardiac and renal damage in rabbits: evidence for mediation by vasoactive substances. *Lab. Invest.* (in press).

17. M. R. Bristow, W. S. Sageman, R. H. Scott, M. E. Billingham, R. E. Bowden, R. S. Kernoff, G. H. Snidow, and J. R. Daniels, Acute and chronic cardiovascular effects of doxorubicin in the dog: the cardiovascular pharmacology of drug-induced histamine release. *J. Cardiovasc. Pharmacol.* **2**, 487-515 (1980).

18. A. J. Weiss and R. W. Manthel, Experience with the use of adriamycin in combination with other anticancer agents using a weekly schedule, with particular reference to lack of cardiac toxicity. *Cancer (Philadelphia)* **40**, 2046-2052 (1977).

19. C. S. Benjamin, M. S. Ewer, B. MacKay, M. K. Ali, S. S. Legha, and M. Valdivieso, An endomyocardial biopsy study of anthracycline-induced cardiomyopathy—detection, reversibility and potential amelioration. *ASCO Abstr. 15th Annu. Meet. Am. Soc. Clin. Oncol., 1979* p. 372 (1979).

38

Early and Late Effects of Lymphoma Treatment in the Expectation of Cure

ARVIN S. GLICKSMAN AND THOMAS F. PAJAK

I. Introduction

Over the last decade, there has been widespread acceptance of intensive treatment for Hodgkin's disease and non-Hodgkin's lymphoma, since it is associated with an increasing number of patients surviving their illness. Fifteen years ago, a standard textbook on medicine characterized Hodgkin's disease as a uniformly fatal illness with only a rare survivor under unusual circumstances (1). Now, we

MALIGNANT LYMPHOMAS

Copyright © 1982 by Academic Press,Inc.
All rights of reproduction in any form reserved.
ISBN 0-12-597120-6

can expect at least half of all patients with Hodgkin's disease to be cured of this illness, regardless of stage, after treatment with intensive radiotherapy and chemotherapy (2). Similarly, in many forms of non-Hodgkin's lymphoma 35–40% of patients can be expected to survive their illness (3). Morbidities associated with intensive treatement are more readily accepted, since there is an anticipated favorable outcome. For the most part, the acute reactions are annoying and transient, needing relatively simple measures, some supportive care, and much patience. Long-term survivors, however, in growing numbers can be expected to manifest some of the resultant morbidity associated with the achievement of cure. Just about every organ has some late sequelae of radiation, chemotherapy, or both. In many instances, these sequelae are extremely grave and life-threatening in themselves.

II. The Integument

Uniformly, epilation can be expected to occur in an area of irradiation which receives 3500–4000 rads. This is transitory, and regrowth of hair can be expected in approximately 3 months. Not infrequently, the new growth of hair is somewhat different in texture and color, and it may take as long as 6 months or a year for the new hair to become indistinguishable from normal hair growth. Epilation is also frequently associated with many chemotherapeutic agents regularly used in the treatment of lymphoma. Cytoxan, adriamycin, and vincristine will result in epilation, with return of the hair 3–6 months after cessation of drug administration.

Since the introduction of megavoltage radiation, skin problems from radiotherapy are distinctly infrequent. Only occasionally are transient erythemas likely to occur. Moist desquamation is rarely seen and is limited to intertriginous zones. However, the addition of chemotherapy may induce an enhanced radiation effect and in some instances a recall of radiation erythema. Adriamycin can do this. We have recently observed it with a newer *Vinca* alkaloid, vindesine. Telangiectasia and fibrosis are rarely seen after megavoltage radiation, although they can occur, particularly with cobalt-60 irradiation.

III. The Respiratory System

Standard mantle therapy of 3500–4000 rads using a 4-MeV linear accelerator will deliver approximately 500 rads to the whole lung, derived almost entirely from scatter and to a lesser degree from a small amount of radiation transmitted through the blocks. Depending upon the size of the mediastinal disease and the generousness with which the hilar adenopathy is encompassed, symptomatic radiation effects on the lung can be expected to occur in no more than 5% of patients (4). However, if careful respiratory function studies are performed, as many as 50% of patients will show transient changes in total lung capacity, compliance, and gas diffusion (5–8). These changes can be detected as early as 8 weeks after the completion of radiotherapy and usually disappear within 2 years (9, 10). For patients whose symptoms are moderately severe, steroids may be helpful, but withdrawal of steroids must be done cautiously, since exacerbation of symptomatic pneumonitis may occur if they are abruptly discontinued.

When patients with pulmonary nodes are treated with whole-lung radiation in doses up to 2500 rads in 4 weeks (no inhomogeneity corrections having been applied), the risk of radiation-induced lung disease increases with the dose, so that as many as one-quarter of the patients may develop signs, but less than 10% may be sufficiently symptomatic to require supportive measures. When whole-lung irradiation is performed, the use of a transmission block so that the dose is delivered at a rate of less than 100 rads/day will diminish the frequency with which radiation pneumonitis is seen but will not irradicate it (11).

Some chemotherapeutic agents have been implicated in developing respiratory system changes. The most important agent in this regard is bleomycin, the effects of which appear to be dose-dependent (12). Severe life-threatening pneumonitis is associated with doses of over 200 units/m^2. In patients who are to receive both radiation and a bleomycin-containing drug combination, the possibility exists that there will be increased pulmonary damage. Other chemotherapeutic agents such as cytoxan, N,N-bis(2-chloroethyl)-N-nitrosourea (BCNU), and actinomycin D can enhance radiation toxicity to the lung and recall prior exposure (13). Therapy consisting of mechlorethamine, vincristine, procarbazine, and dacarbazine (MOPP) has been reported on occasion to induce pulmonary toxicity itself and also when associated with radiation. This may be due to the abrupt withdrawal of the steroid component of this combination rather than the vincristine or procarbazine toxicity to the lung, directly.

IV. Cardiovascular Effects

For most patients, the treatment of Hodgkin's disease requires that the heart and great vessels be included in the field of maximal irradiation (3500–4000 rads in most settings). Between 6 months and a year after mantle therapy with such irradiation doses, 10–15% of patients may develop a pericardial rub. This is a dose-related reaction. When the radiation is diminished to below 300 rads, the incidence falls considerably (14, 15). Shielding part of the heart by the introduction of a subcarinal block has all but eradicated the development of radiation pericarditis.

Acute pericarditis can develop during the course of radiation or as late as 4 or 5 years later. The disease is usually self-limited. For patients who develop pericardial effusion and constrictive pericarditis, a pleural-pericardial window or pericardial stripping may be life-saving (16–18).

In some cases, however, the process continues on to chronic pericardial disease (19). In point of fact, this may be appreciably more frequent than previously appreciated. In a recent report from the Princess Margaret Hospital, 12 patients with a negative cardiac history and normal physical examinations, echocardiographic abnormalities including pericardial thickening and reduction in right ventricular wall motion were detected in 10 of 12 patients who had been treated 10–16 years previously with radiotherapy with mantle therapy for Hodgkin's disease (20).

Case reports of premature myocardial infarction in patients who received radiation therapy to the chest have been appearing regularly over the last 15 years (21–23). While diffuse interstitial myocardial fibrosis has been seen frequently in patients who have received doses in excess of 3500 rads to the heart, vascular changes are less frequently observed (24). Intimal proliferation is a response to irradiation. Whether these cells are more sensitive to even modest changes in cholesterol levels and therefore more apt to induce atheromatous changes is the basis of investigative studies currently in progress (25, 26).

Radiation can induce vascular changes in large vessels as well as in small arteries (27). Vascular changes in the aorta have been reported in patients who have received total nodal irradiation. So-called pulseless disease, the aortic arch syndrome (28), and carotid artery disease have been reported after radiation for Hodgkin's disease and non-Hodgkin's lymphoma (29). On occasion, successful surgical reconstructions have been possible when the syndrome was clinically suspected and investigated with arteriography. Vascular grafts may be more difficult because of perivascular fibrosis but have been successfully reported in many instances.

Chemotherapeutic agents also produce cardiomyopathies. In a unique case, MOPP therapy induced a myocardial infarction-like syndrome on three separate occasions in the same patient (30). In view of the large number of patients who received MOPP therapy before and after this case report, this must have been an extremely rare event. Much more frequent and important is the myocardial injury associated with anthracyclines, adriamycin, and daunomycin (31). The particular injury produced by adriamycin is clearly dose-related and as far as is currently known is not reversible. Both adriamycin and radiation produce injuries to the heart which are additive rather than synergistic. Where it is anticipated that the patient will require both adriamycin and radiation, dose accommodations of each are necessary to allow for adequate therapeutic effect without fatal cardiomyopathy.

V. Hepatopathologies

At one time, the liver was considered to be a relatively radio-resistant organ. Ingold and associates (32) described the histopathology of radiation hepatitis which occurs in patients in whom the entire liver has received doses of over 3000 rads. Characteristically central vein thrombosis occurs with swelling of the liver cells. Marked alkaline phosphatase elevation occurs as the liver becomes enlarged and tender and may be associated with ascites and jaundice. The liver scan will show nonfunctioning parenchyma. When central axial nodes are irradiated, only a section of the liver is in the field. Little will be noted clinically, although the liver scan and some enzymes may be abnormal (33). For the most part, this is transient, although it can last as long as 2 years. In instances where lymphoma involved the liver and radiation was used, doses below 2500 rads were tolerable, as in the experience of the Cancer and Leukemia Group B (CALGB) and of Memorial Sloan-Kettering Cancer Center in New York. Earlier experience from Stanford University Medical Center clearly indicated that doses over 3000 rads, or 2000 rads plus radioactive gold, could produce late hepatic fibrosis.

In another experience of the CALGB vincristine concurrent with doses of radiation below 2000 rads was associated with severe and life-threatening toxicity in 16 of 35 patients at risk (34). Cassady and co-workers at Children's Hospital in Boston also found an increase in hepatic toxicity in children with Wilms tumor of the right side when vincristine was given as part of their treatment regimen (35). Fatal radiation hepatitis has been reported in a patient following therapy with adriamycin, bleomycin, vincristine, and dacarbazine (ABVD) and 2400 rads to the liver. Another case of hepatitis associated with adriamycin has been reported with doses of radiation under 2500 rads (36). One may expect that other agents may sensitize the liver to radiation in this era of combined-modality therapy and result unexpectedly in severe hepatic injury.

VI. Genitourinary Problems

The serious nature of the late complications of irradiation of the kidneys at moderate doses is so well known to radiotherapists that radiation nephritis is now an extremely rare event (37). Kaplan reports that there was not one case in 1,200 patients treated for Hodgkin's disease at Stanford (38) For the most part, axial node irradiation can be delivered limiting the dose of radiation to the kidneys to scatter. In patients who have not had a splenectomy, most of the left kidney may receive the full brunt of the irradiation dose, as was probably the case in the patient described by Danforth in 1975 who was found, 7 years subsequent to radiotherapy for stage IIIA Hodgkin's disease, to have total destruction of the left kidney (39). In patients with abdominal presentation of non-Hodgkin's lymphoma, the dose to the kidney is generally restricted to less than 1750 rads when abdominal bath irradiation is given. Even in combination with the usual chemotherapeutic agents used for this disease, there has not been a reported incidence of radiation nephritis where the dose to the renal parenchyma was under 2000 rads (40).

Hemorrhagic cystitis from long-term cytoxan therapy has been well documented over the last decade (41, 42). In one report examining the records of over 19,000 cancer patients, Fairchild et al. found a ninefold increase in bladder cancer in patients who received cyclophosphamide (43). To put this into proper perspective, however, case 3 in the report of Wall and Claussen in 1975 is useful (44). This involved a 27-year-old man with stage IVB Hodgkin's disease who received 147 gm of cyclophosphamide over 3 years, which had to be discontinued because of hemorrhagic cystitis. Over the next $10\frac{1}{2}$ years, he received 23 gm of chlorambucil. Upon the reappearance of hematuria, a well-differentiated epidermoid carcinoma of the bladder was discovered. He was subjected to a total cystectomy which revealed extensive in situ carcinoma. While one is concerned over the need to perform a total cystectomy in a 40-year-old patient, the prospect of this for 13 years after the appearance of stage IVB Hodgkin's disease is an achievement not likely a generation ago. It is interesting to note that hemorrhagic cystitis has been reported following a year of MOPP therapy, but this must be a very rare event (45).

Since many patients successfully treated for Hodgkin's disease are young and in the child-bearing period, a good deal of attention must be given to attempts to preserve reproductive integrity. When radiotherapy is used, the problem is somewhat different for males and females and is age- and dose-dependent (46). In males, fractionated doses of radiation appear to be more destructive than single doses in terms of sperm production (47). Periaortic irradiation will result in between 20 and 40 rads on the testis from scatter. When pelvic irradiation is added, the dose will increase to as much as 300–400 rads unless special protective devices are used. In most studies, (Table I) fractionated doses of under 100 rads will produce temporary aspermia in 100% of patients, but recovery will begin approximately 1 year later. With doses of 100–200 rads, temporary aspermia will persist for as long as 2 years. After doses of between 200 and 300 rads, 3 years may be required for recovery, and over 5 years for doses in excess of this, if occurs at all (48, 49). Serum follicle-stimulating hormone (FSH) levels will be elevated until the damaged seminiferous epithelium has been repaired and returns to normal function.

In females, fractionated doses of radiation will produce temporary or permanent sterility, depending upon the dose and age of the patient (Table II). Generally speaking, lower doses are more likely to produce permanent amenorrhea in older women. A dose of 150 rads over a 4-week period appears to have no

TABLE I

Sperm Counts after Testicular Irradiation

Dose (rads)	Effect	Duration
10–25	Oligospermia	6 Months (100% recovery)
25–50	Aspermia	1 Year (100% recovery)
50–100	Aspermia	18 Months to 2 years; persistent aspermia or oligospermia at 4 years
100–150	Aspermia	18 Months to 4 years; aspermia or oligospermia may be present beyond 4 years
200–300	Aspermia	Permanent in many cases; no recovery seen at 4 years, but could occur as late as 10 years

permanent deleterious effects in young women but can produce sterilization in women over the age of 35. A dose of 250–500 rads is likely to sterilize women over 35 permanently, but only about half of women under 35. The remainder will have transient amenorrhea. Doses of 1000–3000 rads are likely to produce permanent sterility in all women so exposed.

Preservation of ovarian function can be achieved by surgical procedures which

TABLE II

Ovarian Function after Irradiation

Dose (rads)	Age	Effect	Duration
50	All	None	Normal pregnancies reported
50–100	All	Normal menses, amenorrhea	Temporary; most patients have return of normal menses
100–200	Under 35	Normal menses	—
	Over 35	Amenorrhea	May be temporary, but there may be permanent sterilization in at least half the patients
200–500	Under 35	Amenorrhea	Temporary in some; permanent in about half; normal menses return in about half
500–700	Under 35	Amenorrhea	Permanent in most patients; 25% may have return of menses after 2–3 years
	Over 35	Amenorrhea	Permanent
1250–1500	Over 35	Amenorrhea	Permanent

place the ovaries at sites that are likely to receive only scatter irradiation (50). The midline oophoropexy has been most widely used for this purpose, although movement of the ovaries laterally to the iliac fossa has been used in some institutions with successful preservation of ovarian function. With midline oophoropexy and shielding during irradiation, approximately two-thirds of women maintain normal ovarian function and subsequent pregnancies are possible. To date, the offspring appear to be normal as well (51).

It is now clearly appreciated that chemotherapeutic effects on the gonads can be expected to be long-term and, in many instances, produce complete destruction of reproductive potential (52, 53). In the male, chlorambucil and cyclophosphamide (54, 55) have resulted in sterility, and testicular atrophy occurred in a carefully studied group of men treated with combination chemotherapy, MOPP, and CVP. Sherins and DeVita showed that azospermia persisted for approximately 2 years after intensive chemotherapy, but that return to normal function could be anticipated (56). Serum levels of testosterone and luteinizing hormone (LH) were generally normal, but FSH elevation was observed during the period of azospermia (57). In prepubescent boys treated with cyclophosphamide, no abnormalities of LH, FSH, or testosterone were found 8 months to 7 years after treatment (58). Similarly, MOPP therapy in six prepubescent boys tested showed no change in serum gonadotropins, while 9 of 13 pubescent boys had moderate to severe gynecomastia, germinal aplasia, elevation in FSH and LH, and reduced testosterone levels 2 years after combined chemotherapy (59).

In young females, primary ovarian failure has been reported after single-drug or combined chemotherapy (60). Elevated FSH and LH levels were found in amenorrheic females previously treated for Hodgkin's disease. Although the disappearance of oocytes can be anticipated, some patients may develop only irregularity of their menses, and pregnancies have been reported. Single agents, such as cyclophosphamide, have produced the same effects with approximately 75% of patients becoming amenorrheic, with elevated FSH levels, but this can be transitory, and successful pregnancies can occur.

Teratogenic effects of low-dose radiation have not been clearly identified. However, where chemotherapy and radiation were used, Holmes and Holmes found a significant increase in fetal abnormalities in cases where either the father or the mother had received chemotherapy and radiation treatment (61), although there has been some question concerning the statistical methods in this report (62). In men who wish to procreate, it is advisable to suggest the use of a sperm bank prior to the onset of any treatment. This will preclude both the problem of azospermia or oligospermia and the teratogenic effects of the treatments applied.

VII. Endocrine Problems

Clinically significant thyroid dysfunction has been associated with the treatment of lymphoma (63). Between 15 and 20% of young patients treated for

Hodgkin's disease may develop hypothyroidism (64). However, at least 50% of patients who have had radiation and lymphangiography have elevated thyroid-stimulating hormone (TSH) and another 20% may have an altered response to thyrotropin-releasing hormone (TRH) (65). This is of major concern, because of the carcinogenic potential of prolonged TSH elevation (66). These patients require careful observation and exogenous thyroid replacement, even though they appear euthyroid clinically. Incidental cases of thyroid cancer have started to appear, although the overall incidence is not yet apparent (67). We observed one case of hyperthyroidism in a young girl after treatment for stage IIA nodular sclerosing Hodgkin's disease who, 2 years later, developed thyroid carcinoma (68).

Another aspect of injury to the thyroid is Glatstein's observation that approximately 50% of patients who developed radiation pericarditis also had evidence of irradiation-induced hypothyroidism, which may implicate the abnormality in endocrine dysfunction as a cocausal factor in development of the pericarditis (63).

Pituitary function is temporarily altered during combined chemotherapy which includes steroids, as manifested by loss of diurnal cortisol variations, suggesting significant hypothalamic-pituitary suppression. However, patients do not develop hypoadrenalism with abrupt withdrawal of steroids on MOPP therapy. A Cushing's syndrome appearance and osteoporosis can occur. MOPP therapy has been found to depress TSH and TSH response to TRH (69). This does not decrease the elevated TSH in patients treated by both radiotherapy and chemotherapy. However, no case of thyroid cancer in a patient treated with both radiation and MOPP has yet been reported (70).

VIII. Central Nervous System Problems

Neurological sequelae of radiation, both acute and late, can occur. In the acute phase, Lhermitte's syndrome can occur with mantle therapy. This is characterized by an electric shock on bending the head, which can be extremely frightening to the patient. In a classic paper, Arthur Jones called attention to this phenomenon and, at the same time, pointed out that it is transitory and does not proceed to any serious, permanent sequelae (71). Lhermitte's syndrome has been reported to occur as frequently as 10–15%.

On the other hand, the late complications of radiation involving the central nervous system (CNS) are much more devastating, irreversible, and untreatable. These late complications, particularly transverse myelitis, have been reported with a frequency of as high as 3% and as low as 0.5% (72, 73). Occasionally, single-extremity paresis has been reported. For the most part, technological considerations are responsible for these differences. Careful attention to the physical and technical application of adjacent fields can reduce the possibility of an overdose to the spinal cord (74). The 3-and-2 technique developed by Nisce and D'Angio at Memorial Sloan-Kettering further diminishes the prospect of either a cold-spot gap or an overlap hot spot in the area of the spinal cord (75). Other technical considerations include the use of a posterior cervical block in the mantle technique, which diminishes the dose to the cervical spinal cord, and treating each field every day (76).

Intrathecal methotrexate, which is most frequently used in the management of acute lymphocytic leukemia, but is also a part of the treatment of some childhood lymphomas, has been reported to produce paraplegia (77). This has been associated with abnormal cerebrospinal fluid dynamics and may also have been part of the problem of the diluent, since preservative-free methotrexate in approximately 1000 children treated in CALGB protocols has not resulted in a single case to date (78). Another common neurotoxic effect of methotrexate is leukoencephalopathy, which may be more of a problem in children with leukemia than in those treated for lymphoma.

Vincristine neurotoxicity has been well documented (79). For the most part it is transient, but long-term weakness has been noted in some cases. Essentially 100% of patients develop decreased reflexes to some degree. Paresthesias will occur in well over half of patients; motor weakness will afflict one-third of patients, and constipation is also likely to occur with doses of 1 mg/m^2. The severity of the neurotoxicity is dose-related, and it is generally believed to be reversible, although long-term follow-up has not indicated a 100% return to function in 100% of patients.

IX. Psychosocial Problems

Many patients treated for Hodgkin's disease are adolescents and young adults. For them a life-threatening illness is an implausible event, for it is very difficult for them to accept their own mortality. This is an unusual form of denial and serves well as a coping mechanism. Rarely does it interfere with treatment.

One of the more difficult problems for youngsters is alopecia. We recently had a 16-year-old girl who found an old Greek fishing cap which she wore continuously for 6 months. She wore it to school; she wore it at mealtime, and I am sure she wore it to bed at night. With this cap on her head, she felt she could carry on her everyday activities and meet her peers. Another young man of 24 with stage II diffuse histiocytic lymphoma was told by his medical oncologist that he would require chemotherapy and that he would lose his hair and become sterile. He categorically refused all treatment. It took 2 weeks of intensive work by our team of psychologists and social workers to bring him back into a therapeutic program. Other than these isolated problems, for the most part, these young people accept intensive treatment regimens faithfully. Almost apologetically, they admit to tiredness, loss of appetite, nausea, and vomiting. Frequently, they resist changes in their lifestyle, supportive measures, or antinausea medication.

This cooperative attitude, requiring trust and confidence in treatment programs which have been described as causing transient disabilities but likely to be curative, may be shaken when the patient develops a recurrence. Although salvage therapy for Hodgkin's disease has achieved excellent results, for a young patient the necessity for restarting treatment can be shattering. Now the oncologist is looked upon with some distrust and hostility. In a national study on Hodgkin's disease where involved-field versus extended-field treatment was studied, as many as one-third of the patients developed a recurrence with involved-field therapy (73). However, most of these patients could be treated with another local field of radiotherapy. For such patients, survival appears to be uneffected by local recurrence and local treatment. In the Stanford experience, stage I and IIA Hodgkin's disease patients received chemotherapy after radiotherapy only after a recurrence, with excellent survival (80). However, we are uncertain of the psychological impact of the need for a second go-round with therapy and how we can factor this into the quality of the survival of the patients. To answer these questions, we have undertaken a psychosocial study of CALGB patients in the current stage I and II Hodgkin's protocol.

The late psychological impact in children up to the age of 15 has been studied 10 years after treatment for cancer (81). It appears that, except for the physical disabilities associated with cure of the neoplasm, most of the survivors have made excellent adjustments and are living essentially normal lives. However, a closer examination and study of another group of 114 survivors of childhood malignancies, a high rate of adjustment problems was noted (82). In the latter study, there was a high degree of anxiety and depression. In a study recently completed in our department using the Taylor Scale of Manifest Anxiety and the Center for Epidemiology Depression Scale (CES-D) we found no more anxiety and depression in the patients, their relatives who brought them in for treatment, or the staff who treated them (Table III). In fact, the anxiety and depression levels were comparable to those which would be found in a random sample of people interviewed at a shopping mall (83). The least anxious or depressed group are the patients with Hodgkin's disease. For the most part, they have already heard that their illness can be effectively treated, albeit with intensive, prolonged therapy. They receive tremendous support from their primary caregivers, usually parents, and from the staff at the hospital. Peer acceptance is not strained and, if

TABLE III

Psychosocial Problems in Cancer Treatment

	Anxiety (%)	Depression (%)
Patients	5	24
Visitors	3	22
Staff	1	6

anything, can be characterized as almost casual. Finally, our adolescent and young adult group sessions with a staff psychologist have given us insights enabling us to head off potential problems rather than allowing them to build up (84).

X. Skeletal Problems

Soon after the discovery of X rays, the impairment they can produce in growing bone was appreciated (85). Among the effects seen in young children receiving axial node irradiation and pelvic irradiation are diminished height, particularly sitting height, in practically all growing children, and scoliosis and kyphosis occasionally (86, 87). With the doses of radiation used in the management of lymphomas, osteonecrosis is not a problem. Dental problems, however, secondary to radiation effects on the mandible and maxilla will occur, with malformation of the erupting permanent teeth in young patients. Xerostomia, secondary to impaired saliva formation, and changes in the consistency of saliva can contribute to severe dental decay if appropriate prophylactic and persistent oral hygiene measures are not instituted early after radiotherapy (88).

Late adverse effects on bone of combination chemotherapy used routinely in the management of lymphomas have been reported. Avascular necrosis of the femoral head has been seen approximately 1 and 2 years after both MOPP and COPP (89, 90). It has been postulated that the steroid may be the responsible agent. Although only about 10 cases have been reported, a larger number of unrecorded instances probably exists at major centers treating large numbers of patients with intermittent high-dose steroids for malignant lymphomas. Infrequent as it may be, it may be severe enough to require correction by surgical intervention (91, 92).

XI. Hematological Problems

As much as 75% of adult marrow may be included in total nodal irradiation techniques, less in children because of marrow activity in long bones. When orthovoltage techniques were used, Sykes and her colleagues showed that it was unlikely that regeneration of marrow would occur with doses above 3000 rads (93, 94). In patients studied as long as 13 years after 4000-rad treatment, no regeneration of the sternal marrow could be discerned. More recently, experimental systems have indicated that mouse marrow will regenerate after 3000-rad treatment in 9–12 months (95) and that some regeneration will be seen using iron-59 uptake studies, even after therapy with 4000–5000 rads (96). Cionini noted normal marrow activity between 6 and 9 months after mantle and inverted-Y therapy using cobalt-60 irradiation with doses of 3500–400 rads (97). However, this is not to be considered to indicate that the marrow will function as if it had not been previously irradiated. It is appreciably more difficult to deliver MOPP therapy after total nodal irradiation (98, 99). Most patients will not tolerate full-dose chemotherapy, and significant prolonged leukopenia and thrombocytopenia may preclude the continuation of drug therapy beyond the second or third cycle at any dose whatsoever. With a combination of drugs including nitrosourea, it was found in the CALGB that there was unacceptable toxicity from the sequence of chemotherapy and radiotherapy, although the alternate sequence was toxic but manageable when the interval was long enough (100). On the other hand, there is extensive experience that salvage therapy with chemotherapy after radiotherapy can be accomplished in a large number of cases with an impressive second chance for long-term survival and possibly a cure, except in patients with bone marrow recurrence (101).

XII. Immunological Problems

Patients with widespread cancer have been found to be immunosuppressed, apparently by virtue of the presence of the malignant tumor burden (102–104).

In patients with lymphoma, immunosuppression has been found even in patients with very localized disease, and of course the very treatment of this disease is immunosuppressive in itself. Impairment of the immune system in patients with lymphoma is manifested by diminution of T cells found in most patients with Hodgkin's disease (105). An elevated B-cell population has been found in most patients with lymphoma. Further suppression of T-cell activity after radiotherapy can be quite prolonged (106).

Part of the modern management of Hodgkin's disease includes careful staging and, for many patients, a splenectomy is part of the procedure. Postsplenectomy septicemia and meningitis can occur in as many as 10% of children (107, 108). Although, in a careful study from Stanford, there was no difference in the probability of bacterial infection with or without splenectomy, overwhelming infection occurred only in patients who had had a splenectomy, and approximately 1% mortality was associated with this problem (109, 110).

The most frequent bacterial infections appear to be those sensitive to penicillin, and prophylactic penicillin has been advised. The use of polyvalent pneumococcal vaccine has been widespread, although its efficacy in preventing serious illness is yet to be established (111, 112).

By far the most frequent viral disease is herpes zoster–varicella infection which in one series occurred in 17% of Hodgkin's patients and 9% of non-Hodgkin's patients who had their spleens in place and was significantly higher in splenectomized patients (113). Foregoing splenectomy but subjecting the organ to therapeutic doses of radiation can induce splenic atrophy and the same risk of overwhelming sepsis (114). In most patients who develop zoster it occurs within the first 2 years of treatment. Those in whom zoster occurs many years later are frequently found to have a recurrence of their lymphoma shortly thereafter. Whether passive immunization with a transfer factor can be protective in this setting, as has now been reported in childhood leukemia, will need to be carefully investigated (115). It would be a welcome addition to our therapeutic armament if indeed this were the case.

XIII. Second Malignant Neoplasms

Over the years it has been well recognized that patients with one primary neoplasm have a high susceptibility to a second neoplasm (116). In studies on patients with Hodgkin's disease and lymphoma treated before the era of intensive chemotherapy and/or radiation, there was a two- to threefold increase in second malignant neoplasms represented almost entirely by skin cancer (117). In a recent report from Memorial Sloan-Kettering, Brody and Shottenfeld compared the periods 1950–1954, 1960–1964, and 1968–1972 (118). They found a marked increase in second malignant neoplasms in the more recent studies, particularly in leukemia. Arseneau and his colleagues at the National Cancer Institute were the first to implicate the intensive radiotherapy and intensive chemotherapy being used to cure patients as a significant hazard in leukemogenesis (119). Subsequent studies from many other centers have substantiated these observations (120–122). Acute nonlymphocytic leukemia occurs within the first 5 years after treatment (123–126). Furthermore, of some concern is a second undifferentiated lymphomatous neoplasm occurring after a 5-year interval, which has been reported by the Stanford group and others (127).

An analysis of the recent experience of the CALGB in studies on advanced Hodgkin's disease performed between 1966 and 1974 (128) has been performed to gain insight into the risk attributable to each component of curative treatment, induction chemotherapy, radiotherapy, and maintenance chemotherapy.* Protocol 6604 randomly assigned stage III patients to either total nodal radiation, involved-field radiation, and/or chemotherapy. The chemotherapy consisted of 4 weeks of vinblastine followed by one course of nitrogen mustard. Protocols 6712, 6951, and 7251 were for patients with stage IIIB and IV Hodgkin's disease. All but two induction programs contained an alkalating agent, a vinca alkaloid, and procarbazine. Approximately 25–30% of the patients in each of these studies received MOPP as their induction program. The 1969 study em-

*We are grateful to Drs. R. Cooper, L. Stutzman, N. Nissen, B. Hoogstraten and A. Gottlieb, and Mr. O. Glidewell whose studies in the CALGB were included in these analyses.

ployed maintenance therapy with vinblastine or chlorambucil. The 1972 study utilized as maintenance therapy either vinblastine alone or vinblastine with the induction regimen repeated every 8 weeks. Fifteen hundred and fifty-four patients were entered; 130 were disqualified, and 97 were excluded for previous protocol entry reasons, leaving a total of 1324 evaluable cases.

Eight hundred and one patients achieved complete remission in these four studies. Complete remission was defined as normalization of all initially documented disease parameters. Systematic restaging was not required.

In this discussion, only patients whose complete remission terminated in a second malignancy will be considered. The mean follow-up time for complete remission was 44 months. To date, there have been 10 patients with acute myeloid leukemias occurring while the patients were in continuous complete remission. The median time from the entrance into the study to the diagnosis of acute myelogenous leukemia (AML) was 55 months, with a range of 10–80 months. Three other patients developed AML after relapse of the Hodgkin's disease. The relative risk ratio for these 10 patients was 162.9 which is highly significant. The life table estimate was 5.6%. At the same time, 15 other second malignancies were recorded (Table IV). The relative risk ratio was 2.0 and has now achieved a level of statistical significance. Since the relative risk analysis may underestimate the expected second malignancy if the data are diluted by patients with a short follow-up time, an analysis by the number of years under study was done (Table 5). This failed to reveal any bias introduced by potential latency in the data.

There were three components of the treatment these patients received, induction chemotherapy, radiotherapy, and maintenance chemotherapy. Each of these

TABLE IV

CALGB Hodgkin's Disease Studies: Second Malignancies Other Than Acute Myelogenous Leukemia

Malignancy	No. of cases
Chronic myelocytic leukemia	1
Chronic lymphocytic leukemia	1
Colon	2
Melanoma	1
Adenocarcinoma of the lung	1
Thyroid	1
Cervix	1
Vulva	1
Bladder	1
Squamous cell, skin	3
Osteogenic sarcoma	1
Basal cell (hand)	1

TABLE V

CALGB Hodgkin's Disease Studies: Occurrence of Second Malignancies While in Continuous Complete Remission

Type	Number observed	Number expected	Relative risk ratio	Significance level	Lifetable estimate (%)
AML	10	0.061	162.9	.001	5.6 ± 2.6
Non-AML	15	7.5	2.0	.010	9.6 ± 2.9
Combined	25	7.6	3.3	.01	14.7 ± 3.6

has been examined as a hazard factor in the development of genous leukemia (AML). For the 801 patients in complete remission, 10 of whom developed AML, a comparison of no radiotherapy versus any radiotherapy had a p value of .49 (not significant). MOPP and MVPP induction therapy versus the nitrosourea induction regimens used had a p value of .006 (highly significant). No maintenance versus chlorambucil maintenance had a p value of .015 (clearly significant), and chlorambucil maintenance versus non-chlorambucil maintenance had a p value of .0078 (highly significant). Prolonged chlorambucil maintenance appears to be chiefly responsible for inducing a high number of cases of AML during complete remission. Five of the 10 cases of AML developed in patients in complete remission who had received no prior radiotherapy. Thus prolonged chemotherapy in itself is associated with the development of AML. In chlorambucil-maintained patients, the inclusion of nitrogen mustard in the induction regimen or prior radiotherapy is associated with an appreciably increased relative risk ratio of developing AML during complete remission (Table VI).

Clearly, the development of a second malignant neoplasm represents one of the most disturbing of all the late consequences of successful treatment of lymphoma. The increase in skin cancer, which is very successfully treated, is not

TABLE VI

CALGB Hodgkin's Disease Studies: Occurrence of Acute Myelogenous Leukemia during Complete Remission in 801 Patients after Various Components of Treatment

Treatment	Probability [a]
No radiotherapy versus any radiotherapy	.49
MOPP AND MVPP induction versus nitrosourea induction	.006
No maintenance versus CLB maintenance	.015
CLB maintenance versus VLB, etc., maintenance	.0078

[a] Mantel–Haenzel analysis.

very worrisome. However, there is cause for concern about the increasing incidence of leukemia and non-Hodgkin's lymphoma which are extremely difficult to treat and carry a very high mortality rate. In the most recent studies, approximately 5% of patients successfully treated for lymphoma appear to develop this problem (129). If, in an attempt to prevent the development of a second malignant neoplasm, less intensive treatment is delivered, resulting in a 5-10% diminution in survival, we have accomplished nothing (130).

The use of alternative treatment programs must be carefully evaluated. Whether one can use less radiation either in a diminished volume or a diminished dose alone or in combination with chemotherapy needs to be carefully assessed before changes in policy are introduced. The use of maintenance chemotherapy in Hodgkin's disease has been shown to add nothing to survival and has been abandoned. Alternatives to MOPP induction chemotherapeutic combinations may diminish the prospect of a second neoplasm. The nitrosourea combinations used in the CALGB were clearly associated with less leukemogenesis without the risk of diminished efficacy in Hodgkin's disease. Early data from Milan with ABVD points in the same direction, although these data rest heavily on patients treated less than 3 years ago (131).

It is only as a consequence of the success of so many investigators over the last 20 years that so many patients have survived intensive treatment, only a small number of whom have some troublesome problems. Many of these problems have been solved by careful attention to the details of treatment, to alternate treatment programs, or to diminution of treatment dose or combinations. We need to be aware of the implications of treatment programs as manifested by late effects but cannot sacrifice patients to lesser treatments just to avoid untoward consequences. Only with carefully designed studies, particularly prospective randomized clinical trials, can we undertake to explore the questions: Is less better? Are there better treatment combinations? This is the challenge of the next decade.

References

1. C. V. Moore, Hodgkin's Disease. *In* "Textbook of Medicine" (R. Cecil and R. Loeb, eds.), 11th ed., Saunders, Philadelphia, Pennsylvania, 1963.
2. H. S. Kaplan, "Hodgkin's Disease," 2nd ed. Harvard Univ. Press, Cambridge, Massachusetts, 1980.
3. R. A. Sueuli and J. E. Ultmann, Non Hodgkin's lymphomas: historical perspective and future prospects. *Semin. Oncol.* **7,** 223-233 (1980).
4. W. M. Wara, T. L. Phillips, L. W. Margolis, and V. Smith, Radiation pneumonitis: a new approach to the derivation of time–dose factors. *Cancer,* (*Philadelphia*) **32,** 547-552 (1973).
5. C.P.C., *N. Engl. J. Med. NEJM,* **283,** 191-201 (1970).
6. J. J. Lokich, H. Bass, F. Eberly, D. Rosenthal, and W. C. Moloney, The pulmonary effect of mantle irradiation in patients with Hodgkin's disease. *Radiology* **108,** 398-402 (1973).

7. R. F. Evans, R. H. Sagerman, T. L. Ringrose, J. H. Auchincloss, and J. Bowman, Pulmonary function following mantle field irradiation for Hodgkin's disease. *Radiology* **111**, 729-731 (1974).

8. H. Host and J. R. Vale, Lung function after mantle-field irradiation in Hodgkin's disease. *Cancer (Philadelphia)* **32**, 329-332 (1973).

9. H. I. Libshitz, A. B. Brosof, and M. E. Southard, Radiographic appearance of the chest following extended field radiation therapy for Hodgkin's disease. *Cancer (Philadelphia)* **32**, 207-215 (1973).

10. C. Lassvik, B. Rosengren, and B. Wranne, Pulmonary gas exchange following irradiation of cervical, mediastinal, hilar and axillary nodes. *Acta Radiol.: Ther., Phys., Biol.* **16**, 27-31 (1977).

11. H. S. Kaplan, "Hodgkin's Disease," 2nd ed., p. 422. Harvard Univ. Press, Cambridge, Massachusetts, 1980.

12. J. F. Holland and E. Frei, "Cancer Medicine," p. 823. Lea & Febiger, Philadelphia, 1973.

13. R. B. Weiss and F. M. Muggia, Cytotoxic drug-induced pulmonary disease (Update 1980). *Am. J. Med.* **38**, 259-266 (1980).

14. R. Stewart, K. E. Cohn, L. F. Fajardo, E. W. Hancock, and H. S. Kaplan, Radiation-induced heart disease. *Radiology* **89**, 302-310 (1967).

15. K. E. Cohn, J. R. Stewart, L. F. Fajardo, and E. W. Hancock, Heart disease following radiation. *Medicine (Baltimore)* **46**, 281-297 (1967).

16. D. S. Masland, C. T. Rotz, and T. H. Harris, Postradiation pericarditis with chronic pericardial effusion. *Ann. Intern. Med.* **69**, 97-102 (1968).

17. R. H. Pierce, M. D. Haferman, and A. R. Kagan, Changes in the transverse cardiac diameter following mediastinal irradiation for Hodgkin's disease. *Radiology* **93**, 619-624 (1969).

18. M. K. Ali, K. G. Khalil, *et al.*, Radiation-related myocardial injury: Management of two cases. *Cancer (Philadelphia)* **38**, 1941-1946 (1976).

19. W. Markiewicz, E. Gladstein, *et al.* Echocardiographic detection of pericardial effusion and pericardial thickening in malignant lymphoma. *Radiology* **123**, 161-164 (1977).

20. D. J. Perrault , B. W. Gilbert, M. D. Levy, J. Herman, and A. G. Adelman, Long-term effects of upper mantle radiation on the heart in patients with lymphoma. *Proc. Am. Assoc. Cancer Res. Am. Soc. Clin. Oncol.* ASCO **21**, 349, Abstr. C-297 (1980).

21. R. T. W. Prentice, Myocardial infarction following radiation. *Lancet* **2**, 388 (1965).

22. M. R. Dollinger, M. A. Lavine, and L. V. Foye, Myocardial infarction due to postirradiation fibrosis of the coronary arteries. *JAMA, J. Am. Med. Assoc.* **195**, 316-319 (1966).

23. D. L. Rodgers, Precocious myocardial infarction after radiation treatment for Hodgkin's disease. *Chest* **70**, 675-677 (1976).

24. L. F. Fajardo, J. R. Stewart, and K. E. Cohn, Morphology of radiation-induced heart disease. *Arch. Pathol.* **86**, 512-519 (1968).

25. R. A. Reynolds, G. L. Gold, and W. C. Roberts, Coronary heart disease after mediastinal irradiation for Hodgkin's disease. *Am. J. Med.* **60**, 39-45 (1976).

26. A. Steinfield and A. Most; personal communication.

27. G. Nylander, F. Pettersson, and J. Swedenborh, localized arterial occlusion in patients treated with pelvic-field radiation for cancer. *Cancer (Philadelphia)* **41**, 2158-2161 (1978).

28. W. J. Heidenberg, A. Lupovitch, and N. Tarr, Pulseless disease complicating Hodgkin's disease. *JAMA, J. Am. Med. Assoc.* **195**, 488-491 (1966).

29. G. D. Silverberg, R. H. Britt, and D. R. Goffinet, Radiation-induced carotid artery disease. *Cancer (Philadelphia)* **41**, 130-137 (1978).

30. P. Weinstein, E. Greenwald, and J. Grossman, Unusual cardiac reaction to chemotherapy following mediastinal irradiation in a patient with Hodgkin's disease. *Am. J. Med.* **60**, 152-156 (1976).

31. G. Bonnadonna and S. Manfardini, Cardiac toxicity of daunomycin. *Lancet* **1**, 837 (1969).

32. J. A. Ingold, G. B. Reed, H. S. Palan, and M. A. Bagshaen, Radiation hepatitis. *Am. J. Roentgenol., Radium Ther. Nucl. Med.* **93**, 200-208 (1965).

33. M. Tefft, A. Mitus, L. Das, G. F. Vawter, and R. M. Filler, Irradiation of the liver in children: Review of experience in the acute and chronic phases, and in the intact normal, and partially resected. *Am. J. Roentgenol., Radium Ther. Nucl. Med.* **108**, 365-383 (1970).

34. A. S. Glicksman and H. W. Grunwald, Vincristine enhanced hepatic radiation toxicity. *Proc. Am. Assoc. Cancer Res. Am. Soc. Clin. Oncol.* ASCO **20**, 318, Abstr. C-114 (1979).

35. A. W. Malcolm, N. Jaffee, J. Folkman, and J. R. Cassady, Bilateral Wilms' tumor. *Int. J. Radiat. Oncol., Biol. Phys.* **6**, 167-174 (1980).

36. L. E. Kun and B. M. Camitta, Hepatopathology following irradiation and adriamycin. *Cancer (Philadelphia)* **42**, 81-84 (1978).

37. C.P.C., *N.Engl. J. Med.* **278**, 1343-1349 (1972).

38. H. S. Kaplan, "Hodgkin's Disease," 2nd ed., p. 434. Harvard Univ. Press, Cambridge, Massachusetts, 1980.

39. D. N. Danforth and N. Javadpour, Total unilateral renal destruction caused by irradiation for Hodgkin's disease. *Urology* **5**, 790-293 (1975).

40. D. N. Churchill, K. Hong, and M. H. Gault, Radiation nephritis following combined abdominal radiation and chemotherapy (bleomycin-vincristine). *Cancer (Philadelphia)* **41**, 2126-2164 (1978).

41. P. H. L. Worth, Cyclophosphamide and the bladder. *Br. Med. J.* **3**, 182 (1971).

42. G. A. Dale and R. B. Smith, Transitional cell carcinoma of the bladder associated with cyclophosphamide. *Urology* **112**, 603-604 (1974).

43. W. V. Fairchild, C. R. Spence, H. D. Solomon, and M. Gangai, The incidence of bladder cancer after cyclophosphamide therapy. *J. Urol.* **122**, 163-164 (1979).

44. R. L. Wall and K. P. Clauden, Carcinoma of the urinary bladder in patients receiving cyclophosphamide *N.Engl. J. Med.* **293**, 271-273 (1975).

45. J. E. Royal and R. A. Seeler, Hemorrhagic cystitis with MOPP therapy. *Cancer (Philadelphia)* **41**, 1261-1264 (1978).

46. P. Ash, The influence of radiation on ferility in man. *Brt. J. Radiol.* **53**, 271-278 (1980).

47. C. C. Kushbaugh and G. W. Cassarett, The effects of gonadal irradiation in clinical radiation therapy: a review. *Cancer (Philadelphia)* **37**, 1111-1120 (1976).

48. B. Speiser, P. Rubin, and G. W. Cassarett, Aspermia following lower truncal irradiation in Hodgkin's disease. *Cancer (Philadelphia)* **32**, 692-698 (1973).

49. E. W. Hahn, S. Feingold, and L. Nisce, Aspermia and recovery of spermatogenesis in cancer patients following incidental gonadal irradiation during treatment: a progress report. *Radiology* **119**, 223-225 (1976).

50. T. D. Winstanly, M. J. Peckham, D. E. Austin, M. A. F. Murray, and H. S. Jacobs, Reproductive and endocrine function in patients with Hodgkin's Disease: Effects of oophoropexy and irradiation. *Br. J. Cancer* **33**, 226-231 (1976).

51. O. LeFloch, S. S. Donaldson, and H. S. Kaplan, Pregnancy following oophoropexy and total nodal irradiation in women with Hodgkin's disease. *Cancer (Philadelphia)* 2263-2268 (1976).

52. P. Richyer, J. C. Calamera, M. C. Morgenfeld, A. Kierszenbaum, J. Lavieri, and R. Mancini, Effect of chlorambucil on spermatogenesis in the human with malignant lymphoma. *Cancer (Philadelphia)* **26**, 1026-1030 (1970).

53. L. Sorbinho, P. Levine, and R. Deconti, Amenorrhea in patients with Hodgkin's disease treated with antineoplastic agents. *Am. J. Obstet. Gynecol.* **109**, 135-139 (1971).

54. K. F. Fairley, J. U. Barrie, and W. Johnson, sterility and testicular atrophy related to cyclophosphamide therapy. *Lancet* **1**, 568-569 (1972).

55. P. H. Feng, Cyclophosphamide and infertility. *Lancet* **1**, 840-841 (1972).

56. R. J. Sherins and V. T. DeVita, Effect of drug treatment for lymphoma on male reproductive capacity. *Ann. Intern. Med.* **79**, 216–220 (1973).

57. G. Asbjornsen, K. Molne, P. Klepp, and A. Aakvaag, Testicular function after combination chemotherapy for Hodgkin's disease. *Scand. J. Haematol.* **16**, 66–69 (1976).

58. R. J. Sherins, C. L. Olweny, and J. L. Seigler, Gynecomastia and gonadal dysfunction in adolescent boys treated with combination chemotherapy for Hodgkin's disease. *N.Engl. J. Med.* **229**, 12–16 (1979).

59. R. T. Kirkland, A. M. Bongiovanni, D. Cornfeld, J. B. McCormick, J. S. Parks, and A. Tenore, Gonadotropin responses to luteinizing-releasing factor in boys treated with cyclophosphamide for nephrotic syndrome. *J. Pediatr.* **89**, 941–944 (1976).

60. G. L. Warne, K. F. Fairley, J. B. Hobbs, and F. I. R. Martin, Cyclophosphamide induced ovarian failure. *N. Engl. J. Med.* **289**, 1159–1162 (1973).

61. G. E. Holmes and F. F. Holmes, Pregnancy outcome of patients treated for Hodgkin's disease. *Cancer (Philadelphia)* **41**, 1317–1322 (1978).

62. R. Simon, Statistical methods for evaluating pregnancy outcomes in patients with Hodgkin's disease. *Cancer (Philadelphia)* **45**, 2890–2892 (1980).

63. E. Glatstein, S. McHardy-Young, N. Brast, J. R. Eltringham, and J. P. Kriss, Alterations in serum thyrotropin (TSH) and thyroid function following radiotherapy in patients with malignant lymphoma. *J. Clin. Endocrinol. Metab.* **32**, 833–841 (1971).

64. Z. Fuks, E. Glatstein, G. W. Marsa, M. S. Bagshaw, and H. S. Kaplan, Long-term effects of external radiation on the pituitary and thyroid glands. *Cancer (Philadelphia)* **37**, 1152–1161 (1976).

65. D. Nelson, K. V. Reddy, R. E. O'Mara, and P. Rubin, Thyroid abnormalities following neck irradiation for Hodgkin's disease. *Cancer (Philadelphia)* **42**, 2553–2562 (1978).

66. S. M. Shalet, J. D. Rosenstock, C. G. Beardwell, D. Pearson, and P. H. Jones, Thyroid dysfunction following external irradiation to the neck for Hodgkin's disease in childhood. *Clin. Radiol.* **28**, 511–515 (1977).

67. Z. Weshler, D. Krasnpkuki, Y. Peshin, and S. Biran, Thyroid carcinoma induced by irradiation for Hodgkin's disease. *Acta Radiol.: Oncol., Radiat. Phys., Biol.* **17**, 383–386 (1978).

68. J. J. Nickson and A. S. Glicksman; unpublished case.

69. A. Naysmith, B. W. Hancock, D. R. Cullen, J. Richmond, and C. E. Wilde, Pituitary function in patients receiving intermittent cytotoxic and corticosteroid therapy for malignant lymphoma. *Lancet* **1**, 715–717 (1976).

70. S. C. Schimpff, P. H. Wiernick, J. Wiswell, and P. Salvatore, Radiation-related thyroid dysfunction in Hodgkin's disease. *Proc. Am. Assoc. Cancer Res. Am. Soc. Clin. Oncol.* **19**, 376, Abstr. C-279 (1978).

71. A. Jones, Transient radiation myelopathy with reference to Lhermitte's sign of electrical paresthesia. *Br. J. Radiol.* **37**, 727–744 (1964).

72. H. S. Kaplan and J. R. Stewart, Complications of intensive megavoltage radiotherapy for Hodgkin's disease. *Natl. Cancer Inst. Monogr.* **36**, 439–444 (1973).

73. A collaborative study, Survival and complications of radiotherapy following involved and extended field therapy of Hodgkin's disease, stages I and II. *Cancer (Philadelphia)* **38**, 288–305 (1976).

74. R. D. Marks, S. K. Agarwal, and W. C. Constable, Increased rate of complications as a result of treating only one prescribed field daily. *Radiology* **107**, 615–619 (1973).

75. H. Rosillo-Poussin, L. Z. Niesce, and B. J. Leem, Complications of total nodal irradiation of Hodgkin's disease, stage III and IV. *Cancer (Philadelphia)* **42**, 437–441 (1978).

76. S. Hopfan, A. Reid, L. Simpson, and P. J. Ager, Clinical complications arising from overlapping of adjacent radiation fields—physical and technical consideration. *Int. J. Radiat. Oncol., Biol. Phys.* **2**, 801–808 (1977).

77. R. G. Gagliano and J. J. Constanzi, Paraplegia following intrathecal methotrexate. *Cancer* **37**, 1663–1668 (1976).
78. E. S. Henderson, Acute lymphoblastic leukemia *in* "Cancer Medicine" (J. M. Holland and E. Frei, eds.), pp. 1173–1199. Lea & Febiger, Philadelphia, Pennsylvania, 1973.
79. H. D. Weiss, M. D. Walker, and P. H. Wiernik, Neurotoxicity of commonly used antineoplastic agents. *N.Engl. J. Med.* **291**, 127–133 (1974).
80. H. S. Kaplan, "Hodgkin's Disease," 2nd ed., p. 522. Harvard Univ. Press, Cambridge, Massachusetts, 1980.
81. H. A. Holmes and F. F. Holmes, After ten years, what are the handicaps and lifestyles of children treated for cancer. *Clin. Pediatr.* **14**, 819–823 (1975).
82. J. E. O'Malley, G. Koocher, D. Foster, and L. Slavin, Psychiatric sequelae of surviving childhood cancer. *Am. J. Orthopsychiatry* **49**, 608–616 (1979).
83. J. Goodwin, A. S. Glicksman, and D. Slaby, Arts perceptions in a health care facility, in press.
84. R. M. Tull and S. LaFarge, Use of videotape with adolescent oncology patients. Behavioral Medical Society, 1980.
85. G. Perthes, Ueber den Einfluss der Roentgen Strahleb auf Epitheliale Gerwebe, insbedondere auf da carcinoma. *Arch. Klin. Chir.* **71**, 955–1000 (1903).
86. H. W. C. Ward, Disordered vertebral growth following irradiation. *Br. J. Radiol.* **38**, 459–646 (1965).
87. J. C. Probert and B. R. Parker, The effects of radiation therapy on bone growth. *Radiology* **114**, 115–162 (1975).
88. S. Dreisen, T. E. Daly, J. B. Drave, *et al.*, Oral complications of cancer radiotherapy. *Postgrad. Med.* **61**, 85–92 (1977).
89. D. C. Ihde and D. T. DeVita, Osteonecrosis of the femoral head in patients with lymphoma treated with intermittent combination chemotherapy. *Cancer (Philadelphia)* **36**, 1585–1588 (1975).
90. D. L. Sweet, D. G. Roth, R. K. Desser, J. B. Miller, and J. E. Ultman, Avascular necrosis of the femoral head with combination therapy. *Ann. Intern. Med.* **85**, 67–68 (1976).
91. A. R. Timothy, A. K. Tucker, J. S. Malpas, P. F. Wright, and S. B. J. Sutcliff, Osteonecrosis after intensive chemotherapy for Hodgkin's disease. *Lancet* **1**, 154 (1978).
92. N. M. Albala, A. Steinfeld, and M. T. Khilnani, Osteonecrosis in patients with Hodgkin's disease following combined chemotherapy. *Pediatr. Med. Oncol.* (in press).
93. M. P. Sykes, F. Chu, H. Savel, G. Bonnadonna, and H. Mathis, The effects of varying dosages of irradiation upon sternal-marrow regeneration. *Radiology* **83**, 1084–1087 (1964).
94. M. P. Sykes, F. Chu, T. S. Gee, and S. McKenzie, Follow-up on the long term effects of therapeutic irradiation on bone marrow. *Radiology* **113**, 179–180 (1974).
95. D. F. Nelson, J. T. Chaffet, and S. Hellman, Late effects of X-irradiation on the ability of mouse bone marrow to support hematopoiesis. *Int. J. Radiat. Oncol., Biol. Phys.* **2**, 39–45 (1977).
96. P. Rubin, N. A. Elbadawi, R. A. E. Thomson, and R. A. Cooper, Bone marrow regeneration from cortex following segmental fractionated irradiation. *Int. J. Radiat. Oncol., Biol. Phys.* **2**, 27–38 (1977).
97. L. Cionini, Bone marrow damage following total nodal radiation in Hodgkin's disease patients. *Br. J. Radiol.* **46**, 67–68 (1973).
98. J. M. Vogel, H. R. Kimball, H. T. Foley, S. M. Wolff, and S. Perry, Effect of extensive radiotherapy on the marrow frabulocyte reserves of patients with Hodgkin's disease. *Cancer (Philadelphia)* **21**, 708–804 (1968).
99. E. G. Bell, J. G. Mcafee, and W. C. Constable, Local radiation damage to bone and marrow demonstrated by radioisotopic imaging. *Radiology* **92**, 1083–1088 (1969).

100. A. J. Gottlieb, C. D. Broonfield, A. S. Glicksman, N. Nissen, and T. F. Pajak, "Nitrosoureas in the Therapy of the Lymphomas - A Summary of the Cancer and Leukemia Group B Experience," Nitrosourea Symposium. Academic Press, New York (in press).

101. H. S. Kaplan, "Hodgkin's Disease," 2nd ed., pp. 529-535. Harvard Univ. Press, Cambridge, Massachusetts, 1980.

102. W. Meyer and B. Leventhal, in "Late Effects of Cancer Therapy Complications of Cancer" (M. D. Abeloff, ed.), pp. 397-416. Johns Hopkins Univ. Press, Baltimore, Maryland. 1979.

103. B. G. Leventhal, J. Mirro, and G. S. Yarbro, Immune reactivity to tumor antigens in leukemia and lymphoma. Semin. Hematol. 15, 157-179 (1978).

104. J. J. Twomey and L. Rice, Impact of Hodgkin's disease upon the immune system. Semin. Oncol. 7, 114-125 (1980).

105. R. Steele and T. Han, Effects of radiochemotherapy and splenectomy on cellular immunity in long-term survivors of Hodgkin's disease and Non-Hodgkin's lymphoma. Cancer (Philadelphia) 42, 133-139 (1978).

106. Z. Fuks, S. Strober, A. M. Bobrove, T. Sasuzuki, A. McMichael, and H. S. Kaplan, Long term effects of radiation on T and B lymphocytes in peripheral blood of patients with Hodgkin's disease. J. Clin. Invest. 58, 803-814 (1976).

107. R. M. Sutherland, J. A. McCredie, and W. R. Inch, Effect of splenectomy and radiotherapy on lymphocytes in Hodgkin's disease. Clin. Oncol. 1, 274-284 (1975).

108. R. Feld and G. P. Bodey, Infections in patients with malignant lymphoma treated with combination chemotherapy. Cancer (Philadelphia) 39, 1018-1025 (1977).

109. S. S. Donaldson, E. Glatstein, and K. L. Vosti, Bacterial infections in pediatric Hodgkin's disease. Cancer (Philadelphia) 41, 1949-1958 (1978).

110. D. M. Allen, L. Stutsman, L. E. Blumenson, M. L. Brecher, P. R. M. Thomas, J. E. Allen, T. C. Jewett, and A. I. Freeman, The incidence of post-splenectomy sepsis and Herpes zoster in children and adolescents with Hodgkin's disease. Med. Pediatr. Oncol. 7, 285-297 (1979).

111. G. R. Siber, S. G. Weitzman, A. C. Aisenberg, H. J. Weinstein, and G. Schiffman, Impaired antibody response to pneumococcal vaccine after treatment for Hodgkin's disease. N. Engl. J. Med. 299, 442-448 (1978).

112. C. V. Broome, R. R. Facklam, and D. W. Fraser, Pneumococcal disease after pneumococcal vaccination. N.Engl. J. Med. 303, 549-552 (1980).

113. S. Monfardini, E. Bajetta, C. Arnold, R. Kenda, and G. Bonadonna, Herpes zoster-varicella infection in malignant lymphomas—influence of splenectomy and intensive treatment. Eur. J. Cancer 11, 51-57 (1975).

114. M. O. Dailey, C. N. Coleman, and H. S. Kaplan, Radiation-induced splenic atrophy in patients with Hodgkin's disease and non-Hodgkin's lymphomas. N. Engl. J. Med. 302, 215-217 (1980).

115. R. W. Steele, M. G. Myers, and M. M. Vincent, Transfer factor for the prevention of varicella-zoster infection in childhood leukemia. N. Engl. J. Med. 303, 355-359 (1980).

116. S. Warren and T. Ehrenriech, Multiple primary malignant tumors and susceptability to cancer. Cancer Res. 4, 554-560 (1944).

117. J. Berg, The incidence of multiple primary cancers in the development of further cancer in patients with lymphoma, leukemia and myeloma. JNCI, J. Natl. Cancer Inst. 38, 741-752 (1967).

118. R. S. Brody and D. Schottenfeld, Multiple primary cancers in Hodgkin's disease. Semin. Oncol. 7, 187-201 (1980).

119. J. C. Arseneau, R. W. Sponzo, D. L. Levin, L. E. Schnipper, H. Bonner, R. C. Young, G. P. Cancellos, R. E. Johnson, and V. T. DeVita, Non-lymphomatous malignant tumors complicating Hodgkin's disease. N. Engl. J. Med. 287, 1119-1122 (1972).

120. C. P. Burns, R. L. Stjernholm, and R. W. Kellermeyer, Hodgkin's disease terminating in acute lymphosarcoma cell leukemia. Cancer (Philadelphia) 27, 806-811 (1971).

121. C.P.C., *N. Engl. J. Med.* **290**, 1012–1017 (1974).

123. G. B. Hutchinson, Late neoplastic changes following medical irradiation. *Cancer (Philadelphia)* **37**, 1102–1107 (1976).

124. E. C. Cadman, R. L. Capizzi, and J. R. Bertino, Acute non-lymphocytic leukemia (a delayed complication of Hodgkin's disease therapy: analysis of 109 cases). *Cancer (Philadelphia)* **40**, 1280–1296 (1977).

125. C. N. Coleman, C. J. Williams, A. Flint, E. J. Glatstein, S. A. Rosenberg, and H. S. Kaplan, Hematologic neoplasia in patients treated for Hodgkin's disease. *N. Engl. J. Med.* **297**, 1249–1252 (1977).

126. S. B. Kapadia, J. R. Krause, L. D. Ellis, S. F. Pain, and N. Wald, Induced acute non-lymphocytic leukemia following long term chemotherapy: a study of 20 cases. *Cancer (Philadelphia)* **45**, 1315–1321 (1980).

127. J. G. Krikorian, J. S. Burke, S. A. Rosenberg, and H. S. Kaplan, Occurrence of non-Hodgkin's lymphomas after therapy for Hodgkin's disease. *N. Engl. J. Med.* **300**, 452–458 (1979).

128. T. Pajak, N. I. Nissen, L. Stutzman, B. Hoogstraten, M. R. Cooper, L. P. Glowienka, O. Glidewell, and A. Glicksman, Acute myeloid leukemia (AML) occurring during complete remission (CR) in Hodgkin's disease. *Proc. Am. Assoc. Cancer Res. Am. Soc. Clin. Oncol.* **20**, 394, Abstr. C-425 (1979).

129. D. M. Toland, C. A. Coltman, and T. E. Moon, Second malignancies complicating Hodgkin's disease: the southwest oncology group experience. *Cancer Clin. Trials* **1**, 27–33 (1978).

130. G. J. D'Angio, H. W. Clatworthy, A. E. Evans, W. A. Newton, and M. Tefft, Is the risk of morbidity and rare motality worth the cure?. *Cancer (Philadelphia)* **41**, 377–380 (1978).

131. P. Valagussa, A. Santoro, R. Kenda, F. F. Bellant, F. Franchi, A. Banfi, F. Rilke, and G. Bonadonna, Second malignancies in Hodgkin's disease: a complication of certain forms of treatment. *Br. Med. J.* **280**, 216–219 (1980).

39

Late Complications of Treatment of Children With Leukemia and Lymphoma

JOSEPH V. SIMONE

I. Introduction

It is precisely because of the success of treatment of children with leukemia and lymphoma that we now have concerns for the late effects of therapy. Before 1970, so few patients survived these diseases that there was virtually no literature on the late effects of therapy. As a result of studies begun in the early 1960s, a progressive improvement in the duration of relapse-free survival has occurred, so that now one might expect approximately 50% of children with acute lymphoblastic leukemia (ALL) to survive for more than 5 years even after cessation of therapy (1). Even better results are now attained in the treatment of some children with Hodgkin's disease (2) and non-Hodgkin's lymphomas (3).

In many of the centers at which these children are treated, there has been a vigilant approach to the possibility that late side effects will emerge. This is accomplished by systematic follow-up, even long after active therapy has been discontinued, and by active studies searching for possible side effects that might not be apparent in routine medical examinations. In some cases, however, even the most careful examinations will not uncover latent side effects, because they require a period of time to emerge.

For purposes of this article, a late effect is defined as any undesirable effect of therapy that leaves a patient with a condition that threatens life or results in noticeable functional impairment even after all treatment has been discontinued. A late effect may begin to emerge during treatment, which raises the issue of whether the treatment, the disease, or the constitution of the patient is responsible. For example, if a second malignancy appears within 1 year after diagnosis of the first, it would be difficult to blame the second malignancy on therapy alone.

D'Angio has written an excellent review of the late complications observed in long-term survivors of leukemia and lymphoma (4).

II. Late Effects—Factors

A variety of factors influence the likelihood and impact of therapeutic late effects. Some of these factors are common to both children and adults: dose of radiation or chemotherapy, genetic predisposition, specific combinations of therapy employed, and frequency of short-term complications. However, the age and developmental stage of the patient are major factors in pediatric oncology, since cytostatic agents can have an even greater effect on organ development and growth in the child. Equally important is the interference of the disease and its treatment with the normal progression of children through the developmental stages within the family, school, and society. This has not been studied well and deserves significantly more effort.

III. Handicaps in the Study of Late Effects

The study of late effects is compromised of a variety of factors: (1) These studies require systematic long-term follow-up; this means not losing patients to follow-up, which requires a very diligent and persistent staff with good patient rapport. (2) The long latency period between therapeutic intervention and secondary effects weakens causal attribution, making direct relationships most difficult and unconvincing. (3) Since there may be many causes of a particular complication, e.g., second malignancies, it may be impossible to separate the factors from one another, no matter how well the patients are followed. (4) The numerical denominator of the population of patients from which the complication group is drawn may be poorly defined, and so a hazard rate may be very difficult to deduce. There is an irony in these handicaps. There is no risk of late effects in the child who dies of cancer in a short time. Treatment must be effective enough to promote long-term survival, and only with this success comes the risk of secondary failure involving serious late effects.

IV. Types of Late Effects

Late effects include: (1) second malignancy, (2) impaired growth, (3) gonadal dysfunction, (4) central nervous system (CNS) disorders, (5) psychosocial disorders, (6) other organ dysfunctions, and (7) chronic infection or its sequelae. Brief mention will be made of each except for second malignancy and CNS disorders which will be discussed in more detail.

V. Second Malignancy

The risk of a second cancer is obvious, since potentially carcinogenic chemotherapy and radiation are employed to treat the primary malignancy. It is also possible that patients develop a first cancer because of genetic susceptibility and may therefore be more likely to develop a second malignancy. This may be so even if one excludes the obvious and marked susceptibility in patients with genetic disorders such as bilateral retinoblastoma who subsequently develop osteosarcoma.

In this article, I have reviewed all patients who have had more than one malignancy on record at St. Jude Children's Research Hospital (Memphis, Tennessee). These data are shown in Table I. From February 1962 to September 1980 a total of 3579 children with cancer were admitted to St. Jude. Of these, 1722 had leukemia [1301 with acute lymphoblastic leukemia (ALL)], 209 had non-Hodgkin's lymphoma, 241 had Hodgkin's disease, and 1407 had other malignant tumors. As shown in the table, 18 patients are recorded as having two malignancies. One patient with retinoblastoma developed ALL, one with neuroblastoma developed acute myelogenous leukemia (AML), and one with a thymoma developed non-Hodgkin's lymphoma. This latter case is open to question, although the slides have been reviewed repeatedly and it appears that the patient had two almost simultaneous malignancies.

Of 1301 children with ALL admitted to St. Jude between 1962 and 1980, 9 subsequently developed a second malignancy. Although the follow-up time is relatively brief, the calculated hazard rate at 11 years shows a probability of

666   JOSEPH V. SIMONE

TABLE I

Children with Leukemia or Lymphoma and Another Malignant Neoplasm[a]

Patient no.	First malignancy	Age (yr–months)	Second malignancy	Age (yr–months)
0248	Retinoblastoma	2–11	ALL	8–2
0286	ALL	4–2	Hepatocellular carcinoma	19–1
0638	Hodgkin's	15–5	Osteosarcoma (clavicle)	25–2
0902	Hodgkin's	19–1	AML	26–2
1009	ALL	10–8	Cervical carcinoma (*in situ*)	21
1075	ALL	3–10	Juvenile CML	7–4
1370	ALL	2–7	Non-Hodgkin's lymphoma (brain)	4–5
1635	Hodgkin's	18	AML	34
2370	Hodgkin's	12–8	Basal cell carcinoma (neck)	22
2963	Hodgkin's	20	AML	25
3219	ALL	8–3	AML	8–10
3658	Neuroblastoma	4–0	AML	9–5
3843	ALL	6–11	Hodgkin's	8–0
3846	ALL	4–0	Non-Hodgkin's lymphoma (brain)	8–9
4720	Thymoma	11–6	Non-Hodgkin's lymphoma	11–9
5496	Hodgkin's	9–9	Papillary thyroid carcinoma	19
5719	ALL	7–2	Paraganglioma	81
5794	ALL	3–3	Hodgkin's	5–5

[a] From February 1962 through September 1980, a total of 3579 children with cancer were admitted to St. Jude Children's Research Hospital: 1722 with leukemia (1301 with ALL), 209 with non-Hodgkin's lymphoma, 241 with Hodgkin's disease, and 1407 with other malignant tumors.

developing a second malignancy of 0.03. However, one must examine these cases individually, because it appears that some could not possibly be treatment-related. Two patients developed Hodgkin's disease 1 and 2 years following a diagnosis of ALL while receiving treatment for ALL. Although it is certainly possible, it is unlikely that a second malignancy occurring less than 2 years after the beginning of chemotherapy was a direct result of treatment unless there was some highly unlikely predisposition. One patient developed juvenile chronic myelogenous leukemia (CML), diagnosed 3 years after the initial diagnosis of ALL, but with symptoms in retrospect that began to appear within 18 months of the diagnosis of ALL. Since this patient was seen a number of years ago, chromosome studies were not performed, and one suspects that he might have had a stem cell disorder with both manifestations resulting from the same disease process. Two patients developed what was diagnosed at the time as a reticulum cell sarcoma of the brain 2 and 5 years following the diagnosis of ALL and cranial irradiation. Once again, although it is possible that these were treatment-related, it seems especially unlikely in the patient who was only 2 years from the diagnosis of ALL. The patient who developed carcinoma of the liver had chronic active hepatitis for 15 years. Although not a direct effect of treatment, it is clearly treatment-related. The number of patients with second malignancies is relatively small (and we are grateful for that), so that direct attribution to specific therapeutic measures is hazardous. Undoubtedly, more cases will occur as we continue to follow these long-term survivors, but it does not appear that we are seeing a major, preventable problem at this time. The hazard of 3% at 11 years indicates a retrospective estimate of the likelihood of two malignancies occurring in a patient, not necessarily the hazard of treatment causing a second malignancy.

Among the 241 children with Hodgkin's disease, we have observed 6 cases of second tumors. The hazard rate at 10 years is calculated to be 0.05. In contrast to the patients with ALL, it appears that all cases of second malignancy in our patients with Hodgkin's disease could be treatment-related. First, the latent period of 5–16 years with a median of 9 years seems to be appropriate. Second, the types of second malignancies also fit: three cases of AML 5, 7, and 16 years after the diagnosis of Hodgkin's disease; and three solid tumors, all at the port of radiation, including osteosarcoma of the clavicle, basal cell carcinoma at the back of the neck, and a papillary thyroid carcinoma. Just last week another second malignancy in a patient with Hodgkin's disease was diagnosed at St. Jude, and it is not included in these data. This patient has an osteosarcoma of the scapula, also at the port of prior radiation. The follow-up period in these patients is relatively short, but it appears that the cumulative risk of secondary malignancy will be similar to what has been observed in adult patients.

VI. Impaired Growth

Since children are by definition growing and developing, any cytotoxic treatment may impair the normal growth and/or development of organs or tissues. This may be reflected in disturbances of linear growth due to chronic undernutrition and the effects of chemotherapy (5), or to radiation of the growing vertebral spine (6). In some cases, catch-up growth is observed after cessation of chemotherapy (7). Segmental irradiation of the vertebral spine can also lead to unequal growth of various segments, leading to relative shortness of trunk segments or the uneven growth of one side, resulting in scoliosis. Cranial radiation may also lead to some deficit in growth hormone responsiveness, especially when the fractions are relatively large (7).

Growth must be followed closely using appropriate growth grids, because in some cases short stature may be improved using growth hormone.

VII. Gonadal Dysfunction

Gonadal function may be impaired by the direct effect of irradiation or by the effect of chemotherapeutic agents, particularly aklylating agents. The sensitivity of the gonads to these consequences depends to some degree on the age of the patient and degree of development of gonadal function. Adolescent boys given nitrogen mustard–vincristine–procarbazine–prednisone (MOPP) therapy for Hodgkin's disease have had hormonal dysfunction as well as germinal aplasia (9). Although multiple-agent chemotherapy may not affect the fertility of girls as much (10), there have been no large-scale systematic studies on fertility in survivors of childhood cancer. It will be difficult, because of the great diversity of treatment regimens employed and the large numbers of patients required to obtain meaningful correlations.

VIII. Central Nervous System Disorders

Neuropsychological disorders have been a major concern of pediatric on-cologists ever since patients with cranial radiation have survived their disease. While some early studies showed minimal subjective disorders (11, 12), later studies with more sophisticated methods have turned up a number of potential problems in some patients. This topic was reviewed in detail in a recent publica-tion on the CNS complications of malignant disease (13). Autopsy studies have shown that necrotizing leukoencephalopathy and other pathological changes may be found in children with leukemia who have received cranial irradiation and chemotherapy (14, 15). Clinical neurological complications were reported in patients who received cranial irradiation or repeated intravenous and intrathecal doses of methotrexate (16, 17). The most direct evidence for a pathogenesis for leukoencephalopathy, however, was observed in a study performed at St. Jude Hospital (18). In this study, 228 patients with ALL were to receive identical remission induction therapy followed by cranial irradiation (2400 rads) with five doses of intrathecal methotrexate. They were subsequently randomized to receive one of four drug regimens during remisson: methotrexate weekly by vein in maximum tolerated doses, methotrexate plus mercaptopurine, methotrexate, mercaptopurine, and cyclophosphamide, or all three of these agents plus cytosine arabinoside. In each group, chemotherapy was to be increased to maximum tolerated dosage. Consequently, patients receiving methotrexate alone could tol-erate much more of the drug than patients receiving other agents with overlap-ping toxicity. In this study, leukoencephalopathy occurred during initial com-plete remission only in the group given methotrexate alone. The only apparent difference was the dose of methotrexate these patients received, 40–80 mg/m^2 per week by vein compared to 10–30 mg/m^2 per week in the other groups. Our interpretation of these data is that cranial irradiation is a permissive agent rather than a sole cause of leukoencephalopathy. In this study, relatively high doses of methotrexate intravenously and weekly were the ultimate cause of demyeliniza-tion. This is supported by the study of McIntosh et al. (16) which demonstrated a correlation between cumulative dose of systemic methotrexate and neuropsychological disorders.

Abnormalities in computerized tomographic brain scans have been observed in patients given cranial irradiation for ALL (19). The significance of some of these observations is unknown, since modest dilatation of ventricles has been observed with scans in patients taking steroids and even in normal children.

Of greater concern, however, is the intellectual development of children treated for childhood leukemia. Although a large-scale prospective study has not been done, there is evidence from retrospective studies that a certain proportion of children suffer difficulties in school performance and in neuropsychological function using a variety of test instruments. Eiser and Lansdown demonstrated that children who had received cranial irradiation under 5 years of age subsequently had some impairment in neuropsychological tests. Those who were over 5 years of age at the time of irradiation appeared to function normally in these tests (20). A retrospective study by Goff *et al.* (21) at St. Jude Hospital demonstrate that 21 long-term survivors of ALL who had been off therapy for at least 3 years did not function as well as new patients in a variety of test instruments. As shown in Table II, the long-term survivor group had an average score significantly lower than that of new patients in the Wexler IQ tests and wide-range achievement tests. In examination of motor speed and tactile motor problem solving, the long-term survivors functioned at about the same level as new patients (Table III). However, another group of 22 patients who required additional CNS irradiation and/or intrathecal chemotherapy because of one or more CNS relapses functioned significantly less well in these tests when compared to either new patients or long-term survivors who had not had a CNS recurrence. In these studies, as well as in those of Eiser and Lansdown, patients who were younger at the time of irradiation were more likely to have difficulty in

TABLE II

Results of Neuropsychological Tests in Children with Acute Lymphocytic Leukemia[a]

Test	New patients	Long-term survivors
Wechsler full-scale IQ	103 ± 15	86 ± 17
Wechsler verbal IQ	101 ± 14	86 ± 16
Wechsler performance IQ	105 ± 16	90 ± 17
Arithmetic	10 ± 3	7 ± 3
Wide-range achievement		
Reading	50 ± 14	41 ± 13
Spelling	47 ± 14	41 ± 10
Arithmetic	45 ± 8	39 ± 9

[a] Data are for 90 new patients and 21 long-term survivors. Values are means standard deviation. All differences are significant at the 0.05 level by Student's *t* test.

TABLE III

Motor Speed and Tactile-Motor Problem-Solving Abilities in Children with Acute Lymphocytic Leukemia[a]

Test	New patients	Long-term survivors	Added CNS therapy[b]
Finger oscillation dominance	47 ± 14	49 ± 16	36 ± 16
Nondominant	47 ± 17	48 ± 17	32 ± 16
Tactual performance dominance	37 ± 19	36 ± 17	29 ± 18
Nondominant	40 ± 20	37 ± 17	28 ± 18
Both hands	45 ± 18	40 ± 16	30 ± 20
Total	39 ± 21	34 ± 15	24 ± 18

[a] Data are for 61 new patients, 21 long-term survivors, and 22 patients given added CNS therapy. Values are means ± 1 standard deviation.

[b] Values for this group are significantly lower than for either of the other groups in each category ($p < .05$ by Student's t-test).

the function tests. These results have been of sufficient concern to investigators that a variety of alternative means of preventive CNS therapy are under study. These include lower doses of irradiation, intrathecal methotrexate alone throughout the course of treatment, infusions of intravenous methotrexate, and combinations of these approaches. It is too early to determine whether neuropsychological side effects will be observed with these alternative approaches. Means of predicting the possibility of neuropsychological complications are important for obvious reasons. A recent publication indicates that patients who develop a somnolence syndrome, a transient disorder occurring approximately 6–8 weeks after cranial irradiation and previously thought to be of no consequence, may have a greater likelihood of developing complications (22). A large prospective study is now under way at St. Jude to study the effects of high-dose methotrexate infusion without irradiation compared to 1800 and 2400 rads of cranial irradiation.

IX. Psychological Disorders

Having a child with cancer under the threat of death has an obvious major impact on the child and family. The disease puts enormous stress on the family unit and often leads to separation or divorce. Although this is a common observation among pediatric oncologists, systematic preventive measures have been sporadic and of uncertain effectiveness.

X. Other Organ Dysfunctions

Pediatric oncologists have major concerns about the late sequelae of chemotherapy and radiation therapy on the function of organs such as the heart, lungs, and liver. Although limited doses of anthracyclines are used to avoid acute heart failure, the ultimate effect of these "safe" doses on the growing and developing heart is unknown. Will these children be more susceptible to myocardial or vascular disorders later in life should they survive?

XI. Chronic Infection or Sequelae

Although this is not as great a concern as some of the other factors, we have recently lost two patients from chronic active hepatitis and a third who had chronic hepatitis for 15 years after the diagnosis of leukemia and eventually died of a hepatocellular carcinoma. These and other infections are of major concern, and continuous efforts must be made in an attempt to obviate these problems. Another concern is the risk of overwhelming sepsis in patients who have had a splenectomy for Hodgkin's disease. Once again, although this is not an overwhelming problem, it is real and does occur. It is not clear that a patient is ever safe from this possibility, regardless of how long the time from splenectomy.

XII. Reducing Late Effects

The manner of reducing late effects is fairly obvious in principle and difficult in practice. They include eliminating unnecessary agents, reducing dosage when possible, shortening the duration of therapy, identifying risk factors in the patient before treatment, ensuring systematic follow-up, not only for information but for the possibility of remedial intervention, (e.g., patients who have school problems may be helped if the problems are identified early), and finally, maintaining and improving the cure rate by further refinements in therapy.

It would be wrong if this article left a pessimistic impression. As stated earlier, there is a risk of late effects only in children who survive cancer. Thus, they and we are victims of success when problems do occur. Nonetheless, significant refinements which reduce the intensity and duration of therapy have already been made. These changes must be made cautiously and usually require long periods of study, especially in ALL and Hodgkin's disease. Vigorous clinical research continues at centers and in cooperative groups to improve the efficacy and safety of treatment.

Acknowledgments

Dr. Stephen George provided the statistical analysis of the data reported here. This work was supported by Cancer Center core grant CA 21765, Leukemia Program Project grant CA 20180, CA 24079, and ALSAC.

References

1. J. V. Simone, The treatment of acute lymphoblastic leukemia. *Br. J. Haematol.* **45**, 1–4 (1980).
2. S. S. Donaldson, E. Glatstein, S. A. Rosenberg, and H. S. Kaplan, Pediatric Hodgkin's disease. II. Results of therapy. *Cancer* **37**, 2436–2447 (1976).
3. N. Wollner, P. R. Exelby, and P. H. Lieberman, Non-Hodgkins lymphoma in children: A progress report on the original patients treated with the LSA₂L₂ protocol. *Cancer* **44**, 1990–1999 (1979).
4. G. J. D'Angio, Complications of treatment encountered in lymphoma-leukemia long-term survivors. *Cancer* **42**, 1015–1025 (1978).
5. R. J. A. Aur, J. V. Simone, H. O. Hustu, T. Walters, L. Borella, C. Pratt, and D. Pinkel, Central nervous system therapy and combination chemotherapy of childhoood lymphocytic leukemia. *Blood* **37**, 272–281 (1971).
6. J. C. Probert, B. R. Parker, and H. S. Kaplan, Growth retardation in children after megavoltage irradiation of the spine. *Cancer* **32**, 634–639 (1973).
7. C. R. Sunderman, and H. A. Pearson, Growth effects of long-term antileukemic therapy. *J. Pediatr.* **75**, 1058–1062 (1969).
8. S. M. Shalet, C. Beardwell, J. Twomey, P. Morris-Jones, and D. Pearson, Endocrine function following the treatment of acute leukemia in childhood. *J. Pediatr.* **90**, 920–923 (1977).
9. J. L. Ziegler, R. J. Sherrins, and C. L. M. Olweny, Gynecomastia and gonadal dysfunction in adolescent boys treated with MOPP. *Proc. Am. Soc. Clin. Oncol.* **18**, 286 (1977).
10. E. S. Siris, B. G. Leventhal, and J. L. Vaitukaitis, Effects of childhood leukemia and chemotherapy on puberty and reproductive function in girls. *N. Engl. J. Med.* **294**, 1143–1146 (1976).
11. S. S. Soni, G. W. Marten, S. E. Pitner, D. Duenas, and M. Powazek, Effects of central nervous system irradiation on neuropsychologic functioning of children with acute lymphocytic leukemia. *N. Engl. J. Med.* **293**, 113–118 (1975).
12. M. Verzosa, R. J. A. Aur, J. V. Simone, H. O. Hustu, and D. Pinkel, Five years after central nervous system irradiation of children with leukemia. *Int. J. Radiat. Biol., Oncol. Phys.* **1**, 209–215 (1976).
13. Monograph of the International Symposium on the CNS Complications of Malignant Diseases, Southampton, England, J. M. A. Whitehouse and H. E. M. Kay, eds., "Central Nervous System Complications of Malignant Disease." Macmillan, New York, 1979.
14. R. A. Price and P. A. Jamieson, The central nervous system in childhood leukoencephalopathy. *Cancer* **35**, 306–318 (1975).
15. R. A. Price and D. A. Birdwell, The central nervous system in childhood leukemia. III. Mineralizing microangiopathy and dystrophic calcification. *Cancer* **42**, 717–728 (1978).
16. S. McIntosh, S. Rothman, N. Rosenfield, D. Fisher, K. Ritchey, and H. Pearson, Systemic methotrexate and chronic neurotoxicity in childhood leukemia—A preliminary report. *Proc. Am. Assoc. Cancer Res.* **19**, 362 (1978).
17. A. T. Meadows and A. E. Evans, Effects of chemotherapy on the central nervous system: A study of parenteral methotrexate in long-term survivors of leukemia and lymphoma in childhood. *Cancer* **37**, 1079–1085 (1976).
18. R. J. A. Aur, J. V. Simone, M. S. Verzosa, H. O. Hustu, L. F. Barker, D. P. Pinkel, G. Rivera, G. V. Dahl, A. Wood, S. Stagner, and D. Mason, Childhood acute lymphocytic leukemia. Study VIII. *Cancer* **42**, 2123–2134 (1978).
19. N. Peylan-Ramu, D. G. Poplack, P. A. Pizzo, B. T. Adornato, and G. CiChiro, Abnormal CT scans of the brain in asymptomatic children with acute lymphocytic leukemia after prophylactic treatment of the central nervous system with radiation and intrathecal chemotherapy. *N. Engl. J. Med.* **298**, 815–818 (1978).

20. C. Eiser and R. Lansdown, Retrospective study of intellectual development in children treated for acute lymphoblastic leukemia. *Arch. Dis. Child.* **52,** 525–529 (1977).

21. J. R. Goff, H. R. Anderson, Jr., M. Powazek, and G. W. Marten, Distractability and memory deficits in long-term survivors of acute lymphoblastic leukemia. *J. Behav. Dev. Pediatr.* (in press). Currently available in 1979 Annual Report, St. Jude Children's Research Hospital, Memphis, Tennessee.

22. L. T. Ch'ien, R. J. A. Aur, S. Stagner, K. Cavallo, A. Wood, J. Goff, S. Pitner, H. O. Hustu, M. J. Seifert, and J. V. Simone, Long-term neurological implications of somnolence syndrome in children with acute lymphocytic leukemia. *Ann. Neurol.* **8,** 273–277 (1980).

Index